D1370075

PEDIATRIC BOARD CERTIFICATION REVIEW

AN EXCELLENT GUIDE

AN ESSENTIAL TOOL FOR BOARD CERTIFICATION

THIRD EDITION

by

D. KANJILAL, M. D.

AN EASY-TO-USE ELECTRONIC EDITION FOR IBM/COMPATIBLE COMPUTERS
IS ALSO AVAILABLE

RIVERCROSS PUBLISHING, INC.
NEW YORK
for
DURGA PUBLISHER INC.

Third Edition - 1996

ISBN: 0-944957-61-7
Library of Congress Catalog Card Number: 95-51199

Available at Barnes & Noble Bookstores and through other book and library dealers. To contact Barnes & Noble in New York call (212) 807-0099 or FAX (212) 633-2522; in Pennsylvania call (215) 707-3157.

This book and the software are available at special discount for bulk purchases by libraries, hospitals or other educational institutions. Please contact Durga Publisher, Inc., 84-21 37th Avenue, Suite 152, Jackson Heights, NY 11372.

```
            Library of Congress Cataloging-in-Publication Data

      Kanjilal, D., 1954-
           Pediatric board certification review / by D. Kanjilal. -- 3rd ed.
            p.    cm.
           "An easy-to-use electronic edition for IBM/compatible computers is
      also available."
           Includes index.
           ISBN 0-944957-61-7 (cloth : alk. Paper)
           1. Pediatrics--Examinations, questions, etc.   I.  Title.
           [DNLM:  1.  Pediatrics--examination questions.   WS  18.2 K16p  1996]
      RJ48.2.K364   1996
      618.92'00076--dc20
      DNLM/DLC
      for Library of Congress                                   95-51199
                                                                  CIP
```

Dedication

Devoted to Srimod Durga Prasanna Paramhansa Dev and Lokenath Baba

Dedicated to my parents Bimalendu and Asha Kanjilal, to my wife Debjani, to my children Nivedita, Anirban, to my brothers Debabrata, Subrata, Asoke, to my sister Shibani

Dedicated to all the readers.

INTRODUCTION

You have in your hands the third edition of Pediatric Board Certification Review. Readers of earlier editions have called and written to say that this Review has helped them not only pass, but score high in the Pediatric Board examination. Their success has con- firmed the relevance of the Review's material to the exam. Their insights have inspired suggestions to improve future editions. The present volume is in many ways my response to those suggestions.

Besides information from journals published since the second edition, almost 350 diagrams (including those of x-rays, sonograms, CT scans, various syndromes, and skin lesions), 62 graphs, 81 tables, 11 EKG's, and answers to almost 4,000 questions distinguish this edition. As traditional topics must, of course, figure in any review of this type, there has been no neglect of audiometry, tympanometry, growth curves, BAER, flow volume curves, hematologic peripheral blood smears, glucose filtrative curves, L:S ratio curves, postnatal development of organs, fetal hemoglobin curves, renograms, radionuclide renography, urodynamic studies, and cardiac shunts for congenital heart diseases. I am confident that in no other single volume can one find so much information of this type. (If you need more in-depth discussion of a topic, however, by all means consult your textbooks! This book complements them. It does not replace them.)

Every important area of pediatrics has been treated, sometimes separately by system, sometimes intersystemically. Several important points are repeated and highlighted throughout the text. Diverse materials from all of them are found in a new "Miscellaneous" section. Since the Board exam does not follow any predictable order, let alone the order of a preparation guide, you should get a sense of what that's like *before* you walk into the examination room. This new section will provide that experience. If you do not find any important topic in any chapter, then please look into the "Miscellaneous" section.

Since every day brings new discoveries in the world of pediatric medicine, books like this one quickly become outdated. I cannot print a new edition every month, but I can make an electronic edition available for the computer-literate every six months or so. All items in the software version of the book, including color and black-and-white diagrams, have been indexed for fast and accurate searches from a keyboard.

My fellow physicians should note that this book presupposes a baseline knowledge of pediatrics.

I extend my sincere thanks to Anthony Flood for his editorial help; to L. Janacek for the clear diagrams; and to Preeti Agarwal and Atul Kumar for their excellent desktop publishing expertise.

Good luck to those who apply themselves diligently to this book!

D. Kanjilal, M.D.

TABLE OF CONTENTS

TABLE OF CONTENTS

DESCRIPTION	PAGE

TABLE OF CONTENTS

TABLE OF CONTENTS

DESCRIPTION   **PAGE**

TABLE OF CONTENTS

TABLE OF CONTENTS

TABLE OF CONTENTS

DESCRIPTION   **PAGE**

TABLE OF CONTENTS

DESCRIPTION   **PAGE**

TABLE OF CONTENTS

TABLE OF CONTENTS

TABLE OF CONTENTS

DESCRIPTION   **PAGE**

TABLE OF CONTENTS

TABLE OF CONTENTS

DESCRIPTION   **PAGE**

TABLE OF CONTENTS

DESCRIPTION   **PAGE**

TABLE OF CONTENTS

DESCRIPTION   **PAGE**

TABLE OF CONTENTS

DESCRIPTION   **PAGE**

TABLE OF CONTENTS

TABLE OF CONTENTS

TABLE OF CONTENTS

DESCRIPTION   **PAGE**

TABLE OF CONTENTS

DESCRIPTION   **PAGE**

TABLE OF CONTENTS

DESCRIPTION   **PAGE**

TABLE OF CONTENTS

TABLE OF CONTENTS

DESCRIPTION   **PAGE**

TABLE OF CONTENTS

DESCRIPTION   **PAGE**

TABLE OF CONTENTS

DESCRIPTION   **PAGE**

TABLE OF CONTENTS

DESCRIPTION   **PAGE**

TABLE OF CONTENTS

TABLE OF CONTENTS

TABLE OF CONTENTS

DESCRIPTION   **PAGE**

TABLE OF CONTENTS

DESCRIPTION   **PAGE**

TABLE OF CONTENTS

DESCRIPTION   **PAGE**

TABLE OF CONTENTS

DESCRIPTION   **PAGE**

TABLE OF CONTENTS

DESCRIPTION   **PAGE**

TABLE OF CONTENTS

DESCRIPTION | **PAGE**

TABLE OF CONTENTS

DESCRIPTION   **PAGE**

TABLE OF CONTENTS

TABLE OF CONTENTS

DESCRIPTION   **PAGE**

TABLE OF CONTENTS

TABLE OF CONTENTS

DESCRIPTION   **PAGE**

TABLE OF CONTENTS

DESCRIPTION   **PAGE**

TABLE OF CONTENTS

TABLE OF CONTENTS

TABLE OF CONTENTS

DESCRIPTION   **PAGE**

TABLE OF CONTENTS

DESCRIPTION   **PAGE**

TABLE OF CONTENTS

TABLE OF CONTENTS

DESCRIPTION   **PAGE**

TABLE OF CONTENTS

TABLE OF CONTENTS

DESCRIPTION   **PAGE**

TABLE OF CONTENTS

DESCRIPTION   **PAGE**

TABLE OF CONTENTS

DESCRIPTION **PAGE**

TABLE OF CONTENTS

TABLE OF CONTENTS

TABLE OF CONTENTS

DESCRIPTION   **PAGE**

TIPS FOR THE EXAMINATION

1. First answer which comes in your mind is probably the right answer.

2. Any definitive statement is usually the wrong answer (e.g., diarrhea in newborn is always noninfectious; cardiac disease must be present in Down syndrome).

3. When there is a choice between either observation or refer to a subspecialist (e.g., orthopedic or surgeon), then observation is probably the right answer.

4. Any eye unjury should be referred to ophthalmologist, any acute surgical condition should be refereed to surgeon.

5. All the masses or swelling need not to be examined by a surgeon (e.g., small midline mass under the tongue, diagnosis is usually the ectopic thyroid, thyroid scan is necessary; a 2 year old child who appears as female has bilateral inguinal mass, diagnosis is testicular feminization syndrome, here sonogram and chromosome studies should be done).

6. When there is a choice between either observation (i.e., do not do anything) or do something, then observation is the right answer (e.g. 2 years old with lumber lordosis and protuberant abdomen, diagnosis is normal condition. There is no need to refer to orthopedic).

7. Always try to remember what is normal in different clinical conditions in any particular age group.

8. You must know the following in every disease condition:

    a. Most common cause.
    b. Most common organism in an infection.
    c. Most common clinical presentation.
    d. Preferred investigation of choice.
    e. Preferred treatment of choice.
    f. Prophylactic treatment.
    g. Most common prognostic sequela.
    h. Most common pathological findings in tumors.
    i. Isolation precautions in communicable diseases.
    j. Prevention in H. influenzas, Meningococcus, Pneumococcus, T.B., chicken pox, AIDS, and hepatitis.

9. The following are not very important:

    a. Epidemiology
    b. Incidence (except Down syndrome, Klinefelter syndrome, Turner syndrome, pyloric

stenosis when either of the two parents are affected, insulin dependent diabetic parents, overall incidence of congenital malformation).

c.   Dosage of antibiotics and other medicines.

10.   In the examination there are several questions, each of which has long descriptions followed by four or five questions: First find out that all the questions given has any relation with the description, if there is no relation then don't read the lengthy description, just answer the questions. But if there is a relation, then underline the abnormal findings (e.g., important history like exposure to any drugs or to any disease or any pertinent family history etc., important physical findings like trismus, fever, referred pain to the knee, hematuria etc., pertinent abnormal laboratory values like low MCV, high WBC count, low platelet count, abnormal electrolytes, abnormal radiological findings, abnormal urinalysis etc.,) and try to make a diagnosis. Once you know the diagnosis, then you will be able to answer those questions. Remember, questions given are very tricky but every disease has its own characteristics (e.g., trismus for peritonsillar abscess, very low MCV in thalassemia, and midline scalp defect in trisomy 13).

11.   In some questions you might see that out of the five choices in the answer, one answer you have never heard of and other choices did not match with the description. The answer you never heard of is probably the right answer.

12.   Very few questions are repeated from the first half to the second half of the test or from the first day to the second day. If you don't know certain answers, please refer to standard textbooks of Pediatrics.

13.   Have a good night sleep before the examination.

CARDIOVASCULAR

1. A **newborn** shows signs of **cyanosis, dyspnea at birth,** examination reveals **pansystolic murmur (characteristic)** audible along the (L) sternal border, **single** 2nd heart sound, (L) ventricular heave.

    CHEST X-RAY: Pulmonary **undercirculation, square shaped** heart.
    EKG: Characteristic (L) axis deviation, (L) ventricular hypertrophy; almost **absent** (R) ventricular force.
    MOST LIKELY DIAGNOSIS: Tricuspid atresia.

    Remember (L) axis deviation is **absolute feature of tricuspid atresia.** It can also be seen in **Endocardial cushion defect** and **Pompe disease.** In Endocardial cushion defect, (R) ventricular **force is present.** Pompe disease is **not** present at birth, **few months later** develop **severe** cardiomegaly and failure; other feature is **hypoglycemia.** Tricuspid atresia in **older child** presents with above features and **polycythemia, clubbing.**

    TREATMENT:
    a. **MEDICAL: Immediately give PGE$_1$** (prostaglandin) to keep the **duct** open, so blood flows from aorta to pulmonary artery, **oxygen** for hypoxia, Sodium bicarbonate for metabolic acidosis.
    b. **SURGICAL:** No definitive surgery.
        1ST STAGE: Balloon septostomy if gradient between (R) atrium and (L) atrium to increase pulmonary blood flow, or Anastomosis of aorta and pulmonary artery, or modified Blalock-Taussig shunt.
        2ND STAGE: Fontan operation (anastomosis of pulmonary artery and (R) atrium around 1 year of age.)

    Most common complication of PGE$_1$: Apnea. Use of PGE$_1$ more than 4 to 5 days consecutively can cause **hypertrophic pyloric stenosis.**

2. **Most common associated cardiac** lesion in transposition of great **vessels:** VSD (Ventricular Septal Defect).

3. **Blood circulation** in heart in **Tricuspid Atresia:** (R) atrium to (L) atrium to (L) ventricle to aorta or through VSD into pulmonary artery.

4. **Most common** cause of **death** with congenital cyanotic heart disease **under 1 year of age: Transposition of great vessels.**

5. A newborn shows signs of **cyanosis** but the **lower** extremities **less** cyanotic than upper extremities.

    MOST LIKELY DIAGNOSIS: Transposition of great vessels. Blood flow from (L) ventricle (oxygenated) to pulmonary artery through PDA (Patent Ductus Arteriosus) to lower extremities.

6. When **Transposition** of great vessels presents along **with VSD.**

    MOST LIKELY COMPLICATION: Early cardiac failure. In this case **sign of cardiac failure** (like dyspnea, rales) **more prominent** than cyanosis.

7. **Blood circulation** in heart in Transposition of great vessels: (R) atrium to (R) ventricle to aorta to **systemic circulation,** (L) atrium to (L) ventricle to **pulmonary** artery to lungs. These are **two different** circulations, mixing of blood **is only possible** when there is VSD, ASD (Atrial Septal Defect), or foramen ovale.

8. **Associated cardiac** anomalies with **single ventricle: Transposition of arteries, pulmonary stenosis,** single atrium, atrial septal defect, endocardial cushion defect.

9. **Transposition** of great vessels with VSD: **Right and left heart failure** is **major clinical** presentation than cyanosis, which is the major finding without VSD. Examination reveals **hyperdynamic** precordium and **pansystolic** murmur of VSD in (L) lower sternal border.

    CHEST X-RAY: Increased pulmonary vascularly and **cardiomegaly.**
    EKG: (R) ventricular hypertrophy.
    Remember equal (R) and (L) ventricular pressure, pulmonary **hypertension.**
    DIAGNOSIS CONFIRMED BY: Echocardiogram.

    TREATMENT:
    a. **First** pulmonary artery **banding** to reduce pulmonary circulation **with or without** atrial septectomy followed by **Mustard procedure** at the earliest opportunity.
    b. **Alternative surgery** is total correction which means arterial switch and VSD closure.

10. **Transposition** of great vessels and **PDA: First week** of life: Some benefit because of some blood flow from pulmonary artery (oxygenated) to aorta (deoxygenated).

    After one week: PDA has no benefit, but rather **enhances** clinical **deterioration,** because **most** of the blood goes from aorta to pulmonary artery to cause pulmonary overflow of blood.

11. Name a type of transposition of great vessels which may **mimic** tetralogy of Fallot: Transposition with **pulmonic stenosis.**

12. Most common **associated** cardiac anomaly in truncus arteriosus: VSD.

13. A **new born** with **cyanosis** within **1st week** of life, cyanosis **progressively gets worse,** also dyspnea. Examination reveals **lower** extremities **less** cyanotic than upper extremities, **hyperactive** precordium, either **no** murmur or PDA murmur of grade 3/6, 2nd heart sound **single** or split.

    CXR: Egg shaped heart, increased pulmonary flow, **narrow** mediastinum.

EKG: Mild (R) ventricular hypertrophy.

ABG: PaO$_2$ 15 to 30 mm of Hg (very hypoxic), O$_2$ saturation 30 to 70%

IN 100% OXYGEN: PaO$_2$ only increases slightly.

MOST LIKELY DIAGNOSIS: Transposition of great vessels.

TREATMENT:

a. **Initially PGE$_1$ immediately** in cyanotic child.

b. **SURGICAL PROCEDURE OF CHOICE: Arterial switch operation as soon as possible.**

c. **METABOLICALLY STABLE CHILD: Balloon atrial septostomy** (Rashkind) through cardiac cath. It is **initial procedure of choice.**

d. **MUSTARD OPERATION (BAFFLE PROCEDURE):** Atrial baffle connecting systemic venous blood flow through mitral valve into (L) ventricle and pulmonary venous blood flow through tricuspid valve into (R) ventricle. This surgical procedure is usually done from the 6th to the12th month. **Obstruction is** a possible **complication** of this procedure.

14. What is the defect in **Ebstein anomaly: Atrialization of ventricle: downward displacement of tricuspid valve inside** the (R) ventricle, so (R) atrium is **huge** and (R) ventricle is **small** or **rudimentary.** Pulmonary **hypertension** is one of the presentations.

15. **Most common** complication of **Ebstein** anomaly: **Arrhythmias** (example **most common** is **ectopic beat;** supraventricular tachycardia, atrial flutter and fibrillation).
WPW (Wolff-Parkinson-White) syndrome (9% cases).
RBBB (Right bundle brunch block) in older child.

16. Truncus arteriosus and pulmonary **pressure:**

a. **NORMAL PULMONARY PRESSURE: Huge blood flows** into pulmonary circulation from both ventricles results in **dyspnea, rales, congestive failure.**

b. **INCREASED PULMONARY PRESSURE: Decreased** pulmonary flow, results in **cyanosis.**

17. What is **pseudotruncus:** Pulmonary **atresia with VSD,** where blood flows from aorta **through PDA** into the main or (R) and (L) pulmonary artery.

18. Single ventricle, **defect** and **blood flow:** Blood from (R) and (L) atrium goes through either **single** or two atrioventricular valve into the single ventricular chamber from which aorta and pulmonary artery arise.

19. Hypoplastic (L) heart syndrome associated with: **Hypoglycemia;** metabolic acidosis due to hypoxia.

20. Truncus arteriosus, **defect** and **blood flow:** Single trunk of blood vessel arises from ventricle and supplying every organ (systemic, pulmonary and coronary artery) of the body.

21. A newborn shows signs of **massive** cardiomegaly (occupying the whole chest), **cyanosis** due to (R) to (L) shunt through foramen ovale, **arrythmia (most common is extra systole**

or ectopic beat). Examination reveals **systolic murmur** with or without thrill heard over the **whole anterior (L) chest wall** and **sounds like pericardial friction rub** due to tricuspid insufficiency or gallop with diastolic murmur at (L) lower sternal border.

MOST LIKELY DIAGNOSIS: Ebstein anomaly.
Older children may shows signs of **fatigue only** in mild cases along with arrythmia. **Some newborns spontaneously improve** around 1 month of age when pulmonary **pressure drops to normal.**

DIAGNOSIS:
CHEST X-RAY: Huge cardiomegaly, **reduce** pulmonary flow.
EKG: (R) atrial hypertrophy (tall P wave), arrythmia, RBBB (Right bundle branch block).
CARDIAC CATHETERIZATION: Causes arrythmia. Try to avoid it.
DIAGNOSIS CONFIRMED BY: Echocardiogram.

TREATMENT:
a. **NEWBORN: Oxygen** for hypoxia, **sodium bicarbonate** for metabolic acidosis, **PGE$_1$** to improve pulmonary circulation through ductus arteriosus. If pulmonary **hypertension,** give **tolazoline.**
b. **BIGGER CHILD OR NOT RESPONSIVE TO MEDICAL TREATMENT:** Prosthetic valve or tricuspid valvuloplasty.

22. **Most common syndrome** associated with pulmonary **arteriovenous fistula:** Rendu-Osler-Weber syndrome (hereditary hemorrhagic telangiectasia) found in 50% of cases.

23. Few months old child present with **congestive heart failure (dyspnea, rales),** dyspnea, no (or mild) cyanosis, recurrent respiratory infections. Examination reveals hyperactive precordium, **wide pulse pressure,** systolic ejection murmur with thrill in (L) sternal border due to VSD, single loud 2nd heart sound with or without split, rarely mid-diastolic apical rumbling murmur due to tricuspid insufficiency.

MOST LIKELY DIAGNOSIS: Truncus arteriosus.

DIAGNOSIS:
CHEST X-RAY: Moderate cardiomegaly, huge pulmonary flow.
EKG: Most common (R) ventricular hypertrophy, rarely biventricular.
HYPEROXIA TEST: No improvement.
DIAGNOSIS CONFIRMED BY: Echocardiogram.

TREATMENT:
a. First 12 months of age, medical management with digoxin and lasix.
b. AROUND 1 YEAR OF AGE, SURGICAL MANAGEMENT: Total correction (disconnect pulmonary artery from trunk then connect to (R) ventricle by ventriculostomy by dacron or aortic homograft).

24. An **infant** shows signs of progressively worsening **severe cyanosis,** dyspnea, fatigue, clubbing. Examination reveals polycythemia, **systolic ejection** murmur with **single 2nd** heart sound with or without click due to pulmonic stenosis, (L) parasternal **heave** with

thrill.

MOST LIKELY DIAGNOSIS: Single ventricle with **pulmonic stenosis.** (Board exam usually does not test knowledge of this).

25. **Most common** type of **ectopia cordis:** Sternum is split and heart is projected outside the chest.

26. An infant shows signs of **very mild** cyanosis with **congestive** cardiac failure (dyspnea, rales), **poor** growth, **recurrent** respiratory **infections.** All of the above due to **pulmonary overcirculation.** Examination reveals (L) parasternal **heave, less** prominent systolic ejection murmur, **loud 2nd** heart sound with split, **3rd heart** sound followed by middiastolic murmur.

    MOST LIKELY DIAGNOSIS: Single ventricle.
    CHEST X-RAY: Moderate cardiomegaly, increase pulmonary flow.
    EKG: Biventricular hypertrophy, **'Q' wave** present in **most cases.**
    DIAGNOSIS CONFIRMED BY: Echocardiogram.

    TREATMENT:
    a. **First pulmonary artery banding** to reduce pulmonary blood flow.
    b. THEN **DEFINITIVE** REPAIR: Convert single ventricle into systemic ventricle and **fontan operation** which is anastomosis of (R) atrium and pulmonary artery.

27. Eisenmenger syndrome, **defect** and **blood flow: Pulmonary hypertension** with **reversed** shunting (pulmonary artery to aorta through PDA, right atrium to left atrium if septal defect, right ventricle to left ventricle is septal defect) or **bidirectional** shunting. Usually present in **2nd or 3rd decade** of life with cyanosis, dyspnea initially then develop chest pain, syncope and hemoptysis.

    TREATMENT: Only medical management. Surgery is **contraindicated** because closure of PDA, ASD, VSD will **cause (R) heart failure** due to pulmonary hypertension.

28. **Most common congenital** cardiac defect: VSD.

29. A newborn appears in **1st week** of life with **dyspnea,** poor feeding. Examination reveals **grayish blue color of the skin, weak peripheral pulses or absent pulses,** (R) ventricular **heave, and or** short middiastolic murmur.

    MOST LIKELY DIAGNOSIS: Hypoplastic left heart syndrome.
    CHEST X-RAY: Moderate to severe **cardiomegaly, increase** pulmonary vascularity.
    EKG: (R) ventricular hypertrophy, **small (L) ventricular pattern,** bilateral hypertrophy.
    HYPEROXIA TEST: No improvement.
    DIAGNOSIS CONFIRMED BY: Echocardiogram.

    TREATMENT:
    a. MEDICAL: PGE_1 to keep the **duct open,** so blood flows from pulmonary artery to aorta.

b. SURGICAL: **Procedure of choice** is **Norwood operation.**
    i. **NORWOOD STAGE I:** Anastomosis of narrow ascending aorta with pulmonary artery at **birth.**
        NORWOOD STAGE II: Fontan procedure (anastomosis of right atrium with pulmonary artery) done 6-24 months of age.
    ii. HEART **TRANSPLANT.**
    iii. **If** mitral atresia or stenosis present: Balloon atrial septostomy.

PROGNOSIS: Very poor, **high mortality.**

30. **Hypoplastic left** heart syndrome, **defect** and **blood flow:** It includes **hypoplastic (L) ventricle,** hypoplastic **ascending** aorta, mitral atresia or **stenosis.**

    Most of blood flows from (L) atrium to (R) atrium, then to (R) ventricle, to pulmonary artery, to PDA, to aorta.

31. Pulmonary arteriovenous **fistula** and **features: Cyanosis, dyspnea, bleeding** (epistaxis, hematemesis, melena), **CNS symptoms** (diplopia, convulsion, motor weakness) due to thrombosis, emboli, abscess. Examination reveals **continuous murmur over the fistula region.**

    CHEST X-RAY: Opacity over fistula area.
    EKG: Normal.
    DIAGNOSIS CONFIRMED BY: Pulmonary **arteriography.**
    TREATMENT: Excision of fistula.

32. **Most common prognosis** of VSD: Usually (50%) **closed spontaneously by 1 year of age** (other complication infective endocarditis less than 1%, pulmonary hypertension and stenosis, respiratory infection). VSD is a **benign** lesion.

33. **Newborn with VSD: Asymptomatic, no** murmur present because in the first 3 days of life, pulmonary pressure is usually higher than is systemic pressure, so (L) to (R) shunt does **not** occur in 1st 3 days of life. When pulmonary pressure **drops below** systemic pressure then (L) to (R) shunt begin.

34. **L-Transposition** of great arteries **means:** Ventricular version (**right ventricle on left side and vice versa)** and pulmonary artery arise from (R) side of heart (left ventricle), aorta arise from (L) side of heart (right ventricle).

    (**Most** of the transposition is **D-transposition:** Both ventricles are **placed normally).**

35. An infant who is **asymptomatic** receives normal physical checkup, examination reveals loud **harsh pansystolic** murmur in (L) **lower sternal** border and thrill.

    MOST LIKELY DIAGNOSIS: VSD.

    4 to 6 weeks old child with **duskyness while** crying or during infection, **large VSD with increased pulmonary flow** due to (L) to (R) shunt, shows signs and **symptoms** of **poor**

feeding, dyspnea, poor growth, sweating and recurrent respiratory **infections. No** cyanosis present. It is **acyanotic** heart disease. **Unlike** Tetralogy, which may present as **cyanotic** heart disease.

CHEST X-RAY: Normal or increased heart size and pulmonary flow.
EKG: Normal or **biventricular** hypertrophy, broad notch `P' wave indicates (L) atrial enlargement.
DIAGNOSIS CONFIRMED BY : Echocardiogram.

TREATMENT:
a.   **ASYMPTOMATIC: No** treatment necessary, because in 50% of cases it spontaneously closes by 1 year of age.
b.   **CARDIAC FAILURE:** Give Digoxin and lasix. If no improvement within 2 or 3 days then **Surgical closure** of VSD. It should be done **before 2 years** of age when pulmonary **hypertension** develops.
c.   **PULMONARY HYPERTENSION: First pulmonary artery banding** to **reduce** pulmonary overflow, then surgical repair of VSD.

(VSD **is commonly** given in Board examination).

36.   Cause of **death** in A-V canal due to: Congestive cardiac failure.

37.   **Asymptomatic ASD** (atrial septal defect) management: **Asymptomatic ASD:** Need **open heart** surgery to close the atrial septal defect. It should be done **before** the patient **enter the school. Pulmonary hypertension** is the **most** important **complication of ASD,** it develop in **childhood.**

38.   A **child** present with history of **tiring easily after walking upstairs or running.**

Examination **reveals systolic ejection** murmur with or without thrill, which is best heard in **(L) upper sternal border, widely split** 2nd heart sound in **all phases** of respiration. It is due to **increased flow through pulmonary artery,** normal peripheral pulses.

MOST LIKELY DIAGNOSIS: Atrial septal defect (ostium secundum defect).
CHEST X-RAY: Mild cardiomegaly, **increased** pulmonary flow.
EKG: (R) ventricular hypertrophy, (R) atrial enlargement.
DIAGNOSIS CONFIRMED BY: Echocardiogram.

TREATMENT: Surgical repair of ASD by open heart surgery **before** child begins school. After that, pulmonary **hypertension usually develops.**

39.   **Functional closure** of PDA occurs: Soon after birth.

40.   Most common **cardiac** lesion in Rubella: PDA.

41.   **Most common cardiac** anomaly in **preterm:** PDA.

42.   **Most common** cardiac anomaly in **Down** syndrome: **Endocardial cushion defect**

(common atrioventricular canal and ostium primum defect).

Common atrioventricular canal: defect in **interatrial** and **interventricular** septum with **single atrioventricular** valve.

Ostium primum: Defect in lower portion of atrial septum, cleft in the anterior leaflet of mitral valve.

Clinical presentation of ostium primum defect same as ostium secundum defect of ASD. In both the defect is (L) to (R) shunt, **acyanotic,** but rather pulmonary hypertension. Common A-V canal presents with congestive cardiac failure (dyspnea, rales), recurrent respiratory infections. Examination reveals large heart, harsh systolic murmur with thrill due to VSD, split 2nd heart and pulmonary systolic ejection murmur due to increased pulmonary flow.

EKG IN A-V CANAL: Characteristic (L) axis deviation.
DIAGNOSIS CONFIRMED BY: Echocardiogram.
TREATMENT: Total surgical correction.

43.   PDA in **fullterm** and **premature** infant

In fullterm: Defect in muscular and endothelial layer, so it cannot close spontaneously.
In premature: **Normal** ductal structure, **usually** closes **spontaneously within first 4 weeks** of life.

44.   **Most frequent** complication of PDA in later part of childhood: Infective endocarditis.

45.   **Most common** cardiac anomaly in **fullterm:** VSD.

46.   A child shows signs of **growth** failure, recurrent pulmonary **infection, gets tired** from participating in outdoor sports.   or

A child may be completely **asymptomatic.** Examination reveals **harsh** systolic murmur or **grating** or **swishing** type present in (L) **upper sternal border around 2nd intercostal space,** may be with **thrill, bounding** peripheral pulse; **machinery** murmur found in **older** children.

MOST LIKELY DIAGNOSIS: PDA
CHEST X-RAY: Increased pulmonary flow, heart size **normal or increased.**
EKG: Normal or (L) ventricular hypertrophy.
DIAGNOSIS CONFIRMED by **Echocardiogram.**

TREATMENT:
a.   **PREMATURE:** 1st **Fluid restriction and diuretics.** If these fail, give **indomethacin;** if this fails, then **surgical ligation.**
b.   **FULLTERM:** First **indomethacin,** if this fails, then **ligation.**
c.   **ALL CHILDREN: Surgical ligation.**

47.   Name **one congenital** heart disease where the child is **well-developed and healthy:**

Pulmonic stenosis.
(Most cardiac diseases are associated with **poor** growth and development.)

48. A **premature** with RDS (Respiratory Distress Syndrome) on mechanical ventilator, suddenly **requires higher oxygen** on mechanical ventilator. Examination reveals equal **bounding** peripheral pulse.
MOST LIKELY DIAGNOSIS: PDA.
CHEST X-RAY: Worsening of RDS.

49. What improvement seen after surgical ligation of PDA? Child **gains weight;** has less respiratory infection.

50. Operative **complication** of surgical PDA ligation: Phrenic nerve paralysis.

51. What happened to **asymptomatic** PDA in **premature:** Spontaneously closed **within first 4** weeks of life.

52. **Side** effects of **indomethacin:** Oliguria, increased serum urea nitrogen and creatinine, low platelet and platelet dysfunction, but it does not cause clinically significant bleeding.

53. **Pulmonary stenosis (PS)** associated with the disease: **Noonan syndrome,** Neurofibromatosis.

54. **Most common** type of **pulmonic stenosis: Valvular stenosis.**

55. **Most common complication** of pulmonic stenosis: Congestive cardiac failure.

56. An **infant** shows signs of **cyanosis, dyspnea,** and right ventricular failure, but the infant is **well-developed** and **well-nourished;** examination reveals **systolic ejection murmur** heard best **during expiration, split 2nd heart sound.**

    MOST LIKELY DIAGNOSIS: Pulmonic stenosis.
    CHEST X-RAY: Diminished pulmonary circulation, cardiomegaly.
    EKG: (R) ventricular hypertrophy.
    DIAGNOSIS CONFIRMED BY: Echocardiogram.

    TREATMENT:
    a. **Mild and asymptomatic** patient can lead **normal** life, **no** surgery necessary.
    b. **Moderate to severe with symptomatic** patient:

    TREATMENT OF CHOICE: Balloon pulmonary valvotomy.

57. Peripheral pulmonic stenosis commonly found in: Congenital **Rubella.**

58. **Coarctation** of the aorta **most commonly** found in: Turner syndrome (45X0).

59. **Most common site of coarctation: Just below** the origin of (L) subclavian artery found in **98% cases (post ductal** type).

60. Most **serious** complication of **coarctation** of aorta: **Congestive cardiac failure** due to hypertension. Intracranial hemorrhage may also occur.

61. **Classic sign** of coarctation of aorta: **Reduced** pulse and blood pressure more in **lower** extremities than upper extremities.
    (Normally lower extremities B.P. is **10-20 of Hg higher** than upper extremities).

62. A child in **2nd decade** of life shows signs and symptoms of severe **headache, nose bleed, cold feet.** Examination reveals **more diminished pulse and blood pressure** in **lower** extremities than upper extremities, **systolic ejection murmur** heard in **interscapular** region in the back.

    MOST LIKELY DIAGNOSIS: Coarctation of the aorta.

    Usually present in **2nd decade** of life. Cold feet **due to poor circulation.** Throbbing headache and epistaxis due to **hypertension** in the **upper part** of the body. **Newborn** present with congestive cardiac failure.

    CHEST X-RAY: Notching of the inferior border of ribs due to enlarged collateral blood vessels.
    EKG: Normal or (L) **ventricular hypertrophy,** rarely (L) bundle branch block.

    TREATMENT:
    a. **UNCOMPLICATED** PATIENT: Medical treatment.
    b. **COMPLICATED** PATIENT: **Surgical excision** of **coarctation** segment and **primary** anastomosis is the **procedure of choice.** If **not** feasible, then use patch in the obstructed area. Optimal age for surgery **between 3 to 6 years** because less operative complication.

63. **Most commonly** associated **cardiac** anomaly in coarctation of aorta: Aortic **valve** abnormalities **(mostly bicuspid).**

64. **Chest x-ray** showing 'snow man sign' is characteristics of: **Dilated** (L) and (R) superior vena cava and **dilated** (L) innominate vein.

65. **Scimitar syndrome: Chest x-ray finding** of **crescentic** shadow of vascular density along the (R) heart border due to anomalous **pulmonary veins** draining into the **inferior vena cava.**

66. **Most common site** of pulmonary venous drainage in **TAPVR** (total anomalous pulmonary venous return):
    (L) superior vena cava **(43%** cases).
    (Right superior vena cava only 12%).

67. **Most dangerous** type of TAPVR (total anomalous pulmonary venous return):

    Obstructive type: Diminished venous return to heart, so **reduced** pulmonary circulation.
    Non obstructive type: **Increased** pulmonary circulation.

68. Name a **congenital** cardiac lesion where (R) side of the heart **oxygen content and oxygen saturation is higher** than (L) side of the heart: TAPVR (Total Anomalous Pulmonary Venous Return). (In **normal** person and in **all others** congenital cardiac anomalies **oxygen** is **lower** in (R) heart than (L) heart).

69. **Complication** of **aortic valvotomy** in neonate in congenital aortic stenosis: Residual **obstruction** and aortic **incompetence.**

70. A **child** with history of sudden death was brought to the emergency room. This child is **a known cardiac** patient and waiting for the **surgery** to be done next month.

    MOST LIKELY CARDIAC DEFECT IS: Congenital aortic stenosis.

71. **Three** types of **clinical** presentation of TAPVR.

    a. **SEVERE OBSTRUCTIVE** TYPE: Obstruction to pulmonary venous return, **infradiaphragmatic** type (pulmonary veins drain **below** the diaphragm), present with **severe cyanosis** and **tachypnea. No** murmur present, it is present in **neonatal period. Diminished** pulmonary circulation, small heart.
    b. **MILD TO MODERATE** OBSTRUCTIVE TYPE: Usually **early in life** shows signs of **congestive** cardiac failure, pulmonary hypertension, **systolic murmur** along (L) sternal border and gallop, **mild** cyanosis. **Mildly** diminish pulmonary **circulation, normal** heart size.
    c. NON-OBSTRUCTIVE TYPE: Usually does not manifest **until late childhood, no** pulmonary hypertension, no cyanosis, **Pulmonary overcirculation, enlarged heart,** (R) ventricular hypertrophy.

72. **Management of TAPVR :**

    a. IF **GRADIENT** BETWEEN (R) ATRIUM AND (L) ATRIUM: Balloon septostomy, so blood goes from (R) atrium **to (L) atrium.**
    b. IF CARDIAC **FAILURE (CONGESTIVE):** Digoxin and Lasix.
    c. IF THE INFANT IS **GETTING WORSE:** Surgery immediately, anastomosis of pulmonary veins to (L) atrium.

73. **Most common** type of **congenital** aortic stenosis: **Valvular** stenosis. (Other type is subvalvular).

74. A child with **normal** growth and development, **asymptomatic,** came for routine physical. Examination reveals **systolic ejection murmur with thrill** present in aortic area **radiate towards** neck (R) side and down the (L) sternal border towards apex.

    MOST LIKELY DIAGNOSIS: Congenital aortic stenosis.

    Most of the **congenital** aortic stenosis are **asymptomatic, except** in **critical** aortic stenosis which present in **early infant age** with **(L) ventricular failure** (dyspnea, rales, tachypnea). **Sudden death** occurs in **aortic stenosis.**

CHEST X-RAY: Cardiomegaly, prominent ascending aorta, calcification of valve in children.
EKG: Normal or (L) ventricular hypertrophy.
DIAGNOSIS CONFIRMED BY: Echocardiogram.
TREATMENT: Aortic valvotomy is **procedure of choice.**

75. **Most common** cardiac anomaly with **William syndrome: Supravalvular aortic stenosis** with **hypercalcemia.** (Characteristic facial features are: hypertelorism, prominent upper lip, flat bridge of the nose, short and upturned nose.)

76. **Most common** cause of **mitral valve prolapse: Congenital**
(Other **causes** are **rheumatic or viral).**

77. **Most common** cause of **primary pulmonary** hypertension: **Unknown.**

78. An **adolescent female** with history of **backache** for few weeks; examination reveals **scoliosis, late systolic murmur** at the **apex with click; murmur** was **prolonged when patient stood.**

     MOST LIKELY DIAGNOSIS: Mitral valve prolapse.

     It is **more common** in **female** with **scoliosis** (probably because **both** the structures develop from **mesoderm,** here vertebrae and mitral valve).

     CHEST X-RAY: Normal.
     EKG: Diphasic T wave in lead II, III, AVF, V6 is **characteristics,** may be normal.
     DIAGNOSIS CONFIRMED BY: **Echocardiogram** shows **posterior movement** of posterior mitral valve leaflet in mid **or** late systole or prolapse of both mitral valve leaflet throughout systole.

     TREATMENT: No specific treatment, but **prophylactic antibiotics** to prevent endocarditis as in the case of any other congenital cardiac lesion (organic).

79. What other **organ** defect **is associated with scoliosis in a female adolescent? Cardiac, mitral valve prolapse.** (When female present **with mitral valve prolapse,** then **also look for scoliosis.)**

80. **Most common cardiac anomaly** in Marfan syndrome: **Aortic insufficiency or incompetence.** (It also causes mitral incompetence).

81. **Most common postoperative** open heart surgery complication: **Respiratory failure.**

82. A **few weeks old** child shows signs and symptoms of **progressively worsening wheezing,** feeding, crying, and **near flexion,** surprisingly is **less** symptomatic when neck is **extended.** Parent also complains of child's vomiting, **brassy cough.**

     MOST LIKELY DIAGNOSIS: Vascular ring compressing on trachea.
     CHEST X-RAY: Normal or mild pneumonia.

DIAGNOSIS CONFIRMED BY: Barium swallow filling esophagus and aortography.
TREATMENT: Surgical correction of anomaly

83. **Anomalous origin** of **(L) coronary artery** and features: Usually from **pulmonary artery** which has **low** perfusion pressure, resulting in **myocardial infarction,** papillary **muscle necrosis** due to infarction causing **mitral valve incompetence,** which present as regurgitant murmur.

     CHEST X-RAY: Cardiomegaly.
     EKG: Inverted T wave in lead I and AVL, **ST elevation.**
     DIAGNOSIS CONFIRMED BY: Echocardiogram, Aortography.
     TREATMENT: Surgical correction.
     Most common cause of death is **cardiac failure.**

84. **Most common** cause of cardiac failure in infective endocarditis: **Vegetation** in **aortic** or mitral valve.

85. **Infective endocarditis** and **emboli:**
    a.   **WITH** VSD: **most common pulmonary** embolism.
    b.   **WITHOUT** VSD: **most** common **CNS** embolism.

86. **Congenital heart** diseases and surgical procedure.

	DISEASES:	PROCEDURE:
a.	Transposition of great vessels with **no** VSD	**Arterial switch is final procedure of choice.** **Rashkind** atrial septostomy is initial procedure. **Mustard operation** has complication.
b.	Transposition of great vessels **with** VSD	**Arterial switch and VSD repair** is the **final** procedure of choice. **Initial pulmonary artery banding** with or without **Rashkind procedure.**
c.	Hypoplastic (L) heart syndrome	**Norwood** operation or Heart transplant.
d.	Congenital aortic stenosis	Aortic valvotomy is procedure of choice.
e.	**Preductal** aortic coarctation	Anastomosis of (L) subclavian to descending aorta.
f.	Postductal aortic coarctation	Anastomosis of (R) subclavian to aorta.
g.	Pulmonary stenosis	Pulmonary valvotomy.
h.	Tetralogy of Fallot	**Blalock-Taussig shunt or** total repair.

DISEASES:		PROCEDURE:
i.	Tricuspid atresia	**First** anastomosis of ascending aorta and pulmonary artery or **Modified Blalock-Taussig shunt or** Rashkind **procedure. Final** operation: Fontan operation (anastomosis of pulmonary artery and right atrium).
j.	Ebstein anomaly	Prosthetic valve in Tricuspid area or Tricuspid valvuloplasty.
k.	Truncus arteriosus	Total repair.
l.	Single ventricle	**First** pulmonary artery banding, **then Fontan operation,** single ventricle function as systemic ventricle.
m.	Total anomalous pulmonary venous return	Total correction.
n.	Atrio-ventricular canal	Total correction.
o.	VSD	Total correction.
p.	PDA	Ligation of PDA.

87. Different cardiac surgical **procedures:**

CARDIAC:		PROCEDURE:
a.	**Arterial switch** in transposition of great vessels	Connect (L) ventricle with aorta and (R) ventricle to pulmonary artery.
b.	**Rashkind** procedure in transposition of great vessels	Balloon atrial septostomy through cardiac catheterization.
c.	**Mustard** operation in transposition of great vessels	Atrial baffle connecting (R) atrium to (L) ventricle and (L) atrium to (R) ventricle.
d.	**Rastelli** operation in transposition of great vessels with VSD	**Ventricular prosthesis** connecting (L) ventricle to aorta, (R) ventricle to pulmonary artery with **valve** prosthesis.
e.	**Norwood** procedure in **hypoplastic (L) heart** Stage I:	Anastomosis of narrow ascending aorta to pulmonary artery.
	Stage II:	Fontan operation.

CARDIAC:		PROCEDURE:
f.	**Fontan** operation in tricuspid atresia and stage II Norwood in hypoplastic (L) heart	Anastomosis of (R) atrium to pulmonary artery.
g.	**Blalock-Taussig shunt in** Tetralogy of Fallot	Anastomosis of subclavian artery to (R) pulmonary artery goretex extension.
h.	**Brook** Procedure in **infundibular pulmonic** stenosis	Transventricular infundibular dilation.

88. **Characteristics** to make the **diagnosis** of **different** congenital **cardiac diseases:**

CARDIAC:		CHARACTERISTICS:
a.	**Tricuspid atresia**	Pansystolic murmur (L) sternal border, (L) axis deviation, **square-shaped** heart.
b.	**Transposition of great** vessels	Lower extremities less cyanotic than upper extremities, **egg**-shaped heart, narrow mediastinum, severe cyanosis.
c.	**Ebstein anomaly**	Massive cardiomegaly, systolic murmur over the whole (L) anterior chest sounds like pericardial friction rub, extra systole present.
d.	**Truncus arteriosus**	No (or mild) cyanosis, **wide pulse** pressure, systolic ejection murmur with thrill in (L) sternal border, single loud 2nd heart sound.
e.	**Single ventricle**	Mild cyanosis, (L) parasternal heave, loud 2nd heart sound with split, **3rd heart** sound, `Q' wave present in most cases.
f.	**Hypoplastic (L) heart syndrome**	Grayish blue skin color, weak or absent peripheral pulses, (R) ventricular heave, **small** (L) ventricular pattern.
g.	**Pulmonary artery-venous fistula**	**Bleeding** (epistaxis, hematemesis), CNS symptom (diplopia, convulsion) due to thrombosis, emboli, **continuous** murmur **over the fistulas** region.
h.	**VSD**	Asymptomatic, pansystolic murmur in (L) lower sternal border and thrill. **Large** VSD due to pulmonary overflow present with dyspnea, poor feeding, poor growth.

CARDIAC:		CHARACTERISTICS:
i.	**Atrial septal defect**	**Systolic ejection** murmur best heard in (L) upper sternal border, **wide split 2nd heart** sound in **all phases** of respiration.
j.	**Atrioventricular canal**	Congestive cardiac failure, harsh systolic murmur with thrill due to VSD, split 2nd heart sound and pulmonary systolic ejection murmur. **EKG:** Characteristics **(L) axis deviation.**
k.	**PDA**	Harsh systolic murmur or grating or swishing type present in (L) upper sternal border near 2nd intercostal space, **bounding** peripheral pulses, machinery murmur in older child.
l.	**Pulmonic stenosis**	**Well-developed, well nourished** child systolic ejection murmur heard best during expiration, split 2nd heart sound.
m.	**Aortic coarctation**	Nose-bleed, cold feet, **diminished** pulse and blood pressure more in lower extremities than upper, systolic ejection murmur in **interscapular region,** high B.P.
n.	**TAPVR**	Oxygen in (R) side of heart **more** than in (L) side of heart, "snow man sign" (figure eight).
o.	**Aortic stenosis**	**Sudden death,** systolic ejection murmur with thrill in aortic area radiate towards neck and apex.
p.	**Mitral valve prolapse**	Rule out Scoliosis, late systolic murmur at apex with click.

89. Prognosis for **fungal** endocarditis: **Poor.**

90. **Most commonly** involved valve in **rheumatic carditis: Mitral valve** (**next** is aortic valve).

91. A child who had open heart surgery seven days **ago,** now develops **fever, pericardial friction rub** and **pleural rub.**

    MOST LIKELY DIAGNOSIS: Post cardiotomy syndrome.

    It may be present even **months after open heart surgery,** may be present with pleural and pericardial **fluid** which might cause cardiac **tamponade.**

    TREATMENT: SYMPTOMATIC PATIENT: Salicylate or indomethacin. Bed rest. If

no response, give **corticosteroid.**
PROGNOSIS: Symptoms might **recur** in **some** patients.

92. **Most common** cause of **organic mitral stenosis: Rheumatic** origin.

93. **Complication** of Rheumatic carditis: **Initial** Mitral **incompetence** due to damaged valve. **Late, after 2 years** Mitral **stenosis,** because symptom does not appear until mitral valve size 25% or less than normal.

94. **Aortic insufficiency** and characteristics: It occurs secondary to Rheumatic heart disease. Patient shows signs of **water hammer pulse** in radial artery and **corrigan pulse** in carotid artery due to reflux of blood in early diastole and peripheral vasodilation. Murmur is hollow, **high-pitched blowing** type over the upper and mid (L) sternal border radiating towards apex and aortic area, presence of presystolic or early diastolic component is called Austin Flint murmur.

95. **Infection causing myocarditis:**

    a.   Diphtheria (due to toxin, occurs in 1st 2 weeks of life present with shock like hypotension, cold clammy skin, arrythmia like A-V block, extrasystole, EKG shows ST depression and T- wave inversion).
    b.   Typhoid (**rarely** occur, T- wave inversion present).
    c.   Rocky Mountain Spotted Fever (present with hypotension, circulatory failure due to **vasculitis.**
    d.   Virus (coxsackie virus A,B; rubella. It is **fatal** in newborns).
    e.   Parasitic (Toxoplasmosis; very rare).
    f.   Fungal (Histoplasmosis; very rare).

96. **Most common site** of cardiac lesion in newborn infant of a **diabetic mother: Ventricular septal** hypertrophy. It also causes **subaortic stenosis.**

97. **Most common** site of **hypertrophic and congestive cardiomyopathy: (L) side of heart** (septal hypertrophy and subaortic stenosis).

98. **Most common** cause of **hypertrophic and congestive cardiomyopathy: Unknown.**

    (**Asymmetric septal hypertrophy** may be transmitted as an **autosomal dominant.**)

99. **First** effect seen when **digoxin** is used: **Reduced heart rate** and then prolonged P-R interval.

100. Congestive cardiac **failure** and management: Patient shows signs and symptoms of dyspnea, exercise intolerance, abdominal pain, examination reveals orthopnea, enlarged liver, rales, dependent edema, and anasarca. **Gallop** is characteristic along with other basic cardiac lesion.

     CHEST X-RAY: Cardiomegaly.
     EKG: (L) ventricular hypertrophy **first** then (R) ventricular.

TREATMENT: Bed rest, **low** salt diet, **diuretics, digoxin,** restrict intake of fluid.

101. **Most important sign** of **digoxin** toxicity **in children: Arrythmia.** Any kind of arrythmia can occur, **but atrial** arrythmia is most common in **infants.** Other signs of toxicity include visual symptoms, vomiting, diarrhea, dizziness, and hypokalemia.

     TREATMENT: First discontinue digoxin.
     a. Potassium for hypokalemia.
     b. Diphenylhydantoin for arrythmia of supraventricular origin.
     c. Lidocaine for ventricular arrythmia of supraventricular origin.
     d. Cardioversion for ventricular flutter and fibrillation.

102. **Drug** that most commonly causes **cardiotoxicity: Adriamycin.**

103. **How** to diagnosis digoxin **toxicity:** It is **mostly a clinical** diagnosis supported by EKG. Do not use serum level as primary means of diagnosis. Level above 2.0 ng/ml cause toxic symptom.

104. Dopamine **different dosages** and **their effects:**

     2 microgram/kg/minute: Renal artery **vasodilation.**
     5-10 microgram/kg/minute: Increased systematic blood pressure.
     11-20 microgram/kg/minute: Renal artery **vasoconstriction,** increase B.P., pulmonary vasoconstriction.

105. Pathogenesis of **viral pericarditis** and **myocarditis: Unknown,** may be due to hypersensitivity reaction. It is a **self-limited** disease, patient who has pericarditis also has myocarditis, and vice versa. **TREATMENT:** Aspirin. Corticosteroid may be needed.

106. **Most common** cause of **purulent** pericarditis:

     Staphylococcus aureus: Other organisms are H. flue type b, N. meningitides. Tuberculosis is common in developing countries. **TREATMENT: Open pericardial drain** and **antibiotics** intravenously.

107. Most common cause of **uremic** pericarditis: End stage renal disease or renal failure. **TREATMENT:** Hemodialysis; if no improvement then pericardiectomy. Pericardial effusion **causes hypotension** when patient **undergoes hemodialysis.**

108. **Most common** cause of **constrictive pericarditis: Unknown,** other cause bacteria, virus, tuberculosis.

     SIGN AND SYMPTOM: Huge hepatomegaly and ascites is out of proportion to other symptoms and signs. LFT is **mildly** elevated. Distended neck veins, **silent** precordium, poor pulses **(poor heart contraction** and **reduce diastolic filling),** pericardial rub, paradoxic pulse. **TREATMENT: Radical pericardial removal.**

109. **Half life** of dopamine and tolazoline:

Dopamine: 2 minutes.
Tolazoline: 6 to 8 hours.
In persistent pulmonary hypertension (PPHN) of newborn, **continue dopamine** infusion even after discontinuation of tolazoline.

110. **Most common site** of cardial involvement in Endocardial fibroelastosis: **Mitral valve incompetence.**

111. **First sign** of pericarditis and **features: Precordial sharp stabbing pain** which radiates to (L) shoulder, pain **increased** by lying down and **decreased** by sitting up, leaning forward. **Late** sign of pericarditis is pericardial **rub. Reliable indicator** of cardiac tamponade is **more than 20** mm Hg of paradoxical pulse.

    EKG: Low voltage QRS complex, ST elevation and T inversion.
    CHEST X-RAY: Water bottle-like picture of heart in effusion.
    DIAGNOSIS CONFIRMED BY: Echocardiogram.

    TREATMENT:
    a.   Supportive and symptomatic.
    b.   Pericardiocentesis in pericardial effusion.

112. **Endocardial fibroelastosis** and features: It affects **(L) side** of the heart.

    Two types: Primary and secondary.
    Primary: **Unknown** cause, no visible cardiac lesion, (L) ventricle **dilated.**
    Secondary: Mostly due to congenital **obstructed** (L) sided cardiac lesion like aortic stenosis, **hypoplastic (L) heart,** (L) ventricle **constricted.**

    Patient usually about 6 months of age **suddenly** becomes sick from **asymptomatic** state, URI symptom present prior to it, presents with (L) **heart failure initially (rales, dyspnea)** then (R) heart.

    CHEST X-RAY: Cardiomegaly.
    EKG: (L) ventricular and (L) atrial hypertrophy.
    DIAGNOSIS CONFIRMED BY: Echocardiogram.
    TREATMENT: Diuretics, digoxin.

113. **Most common endocrine** disorder causing **myocarditis: Hyperthyroidism.** (Hypothyroidism **rarely** causes this problem).

114. Relationship of cardiac output and **hemoglobin;**

    Less than 7 mg/dl: Increase the output.
    Less than 3 to 4 mg/dl: Cardiac failure and enlargement.

115. **Most common** site of cardiac lesion in Hurler syndrome: **Valves,** coronary arteries.

116. **Most common** type of **Glycogen storage** disease causes cardiac failure:**Type II or Pompe disease.** Patient shows signs of **huge** heart, liver, and tongue; **EKG** shows prominent P waves, reduced P-R interval, large QRS, **(L) axis deviation** due to **enlarged (L) ventricle** or biventricular enlargement. Dies before 2 years of age.

117. **Characteristics (L) axis deviation** found in:
    a.   Tricuspid atresia.
    b.   Endocardial cushion defect.
    c.   Pompe disease.

118. **Most common** cardiac problem in **preterm:Sinus arrythmia.** It means different discharge rate of cardiac conduction from the sinus node. Heart rate **slows** down during **inspiration** and **goes up** during **expiration.** Patient is mostly **asymptomatic.**

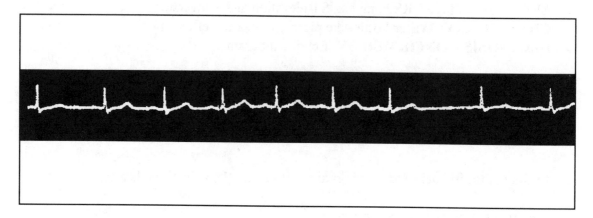

119. **Most common** presentation of **PVC** (Premature Ventricular Complex):**Asymptomatic.** PVC is premature wide abnormal QRS complex not preceded by P wave. It may be **unifocal** or **multifocal.** Unifocal means PVC looks identical, multifocal is not identical in contour. Patient sometimes feels tickle or a skipped beat over the precordium.

MANAGEMENT:

EXERCISE TEST: Most nonsignificant PVC will **disappear after exercise.** If it gets worse, PVC is significant.
TREATMENT: Reassure the family that it is **not due** to structural heart disease; sedation and suppressive drugs used **rarely.**

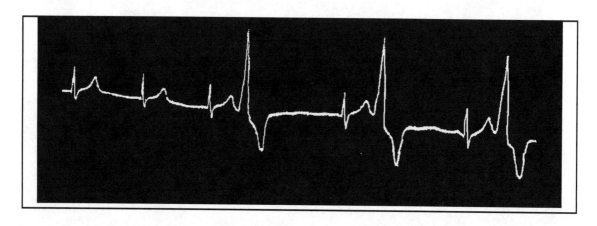

120. **Most common** cardiac problem seen in **athlete:Sinus bradycardia.**Bradycardia means heart rate **less** than **60** per minute, and newborn less than 90 per minute. Patient is mostly **asymptomatic.**

121. Factors which cause PVC: Fever, anxiety, stimulant drugs.

122. **Most common** mechanism of **PAT** (Paroxysmal Atrial tachycardia) **or SVT** (Supraventricular **Tachycardia**): **Re-entry** within the **atrio ventricular node.**

123. A child present with rapid **heart rate** and **palpitation,** examination reveals heart rate **more than 220 per** minute, child was asymptomatic prior to this episode.

    MOST LIKELY DIAGNOSIS: SVT (supraventricular tachycardia).

    In SVT usual rate is **more than 180 per** minute, can go as high as 300 per minute. **Abrupt** beginning and **stop** of the tachycardia may occur. If the heart rate is **very rapid** (close to 300 per minute) or tachycardia persist more than 24 hours or even less, **failure** supervene which present with tachypnea, gray to blue color, hepatomegaly, sick looking child. Increased **temperature** and **high WBC count** is not unusual.

    DIAGNOSIS CONFIRMED BY: EKG.

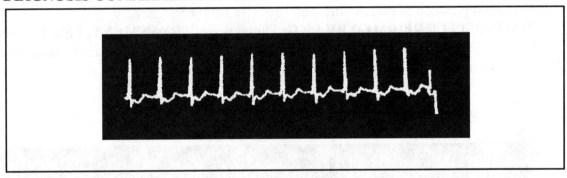

124. How do you manage supraventricular tachycardia **(SVT),** present in newborn? Adenosine is the drug of choice.
    a. Do **not** give verapamil if patient is **less** than 1 year of age.
    b. **First** do Vagal stimulation (give ice pack **over the face** for 30 seconds, do not give carotid sinus pressure if less than 4 years of age, do **not** press over the eyeball because it can cause retinal detachment).
    c. Esophageal override pacing.
    d. Phenylephrine.
    e. Cardioversion.
    f. Digoxin (intravenous).
    g. Propranolol.
    Do **not** give **digoxin** if patient has **WPW** syndrome.

125. Most common complication **fetal tachycardia in utero: Hydrops fetalis.**

126. Side effect of **verapamil** (calcium channel blocker) therapy: **Hypotension.**
    TREATMENT: Intravenous **calcium.**

127. **WPW (Wolff-Parkinson-White) Syndrome: It** presents as **short PR interval** and **delta wave** (slow upstroke of QRS). It is found in **normal** individuals as well as in Ebstein anomaly, cardiomyopathy and corrected transposition of great vessels or ventricular version. WPW due to re-entry circuit is the A-V node and accessory pathway (muscle-bridge) connecting atrium to ventricle. WPW visualization better when tachycardia resolves. WPW.   EKG:

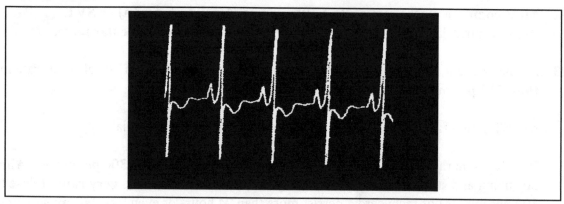

128. **Most common** cardiac complication of newborn to a **mother with lupus:** Heart block.

129. **Atrial flutter:** Heart rate 250-400 per minute. It is **not** common in children. It may occur due to complication of myocarditis, postoperative open heart surgery.
DIAGNOSIS CONFIRMED BY EKG: Flutter wave. **TREATMENT: First** Digoxin (it prolong the conduction form atrium to ventricle) then add Quinidine (which convert to **normal** sinus rhythm) or cardioversion.

EKG:

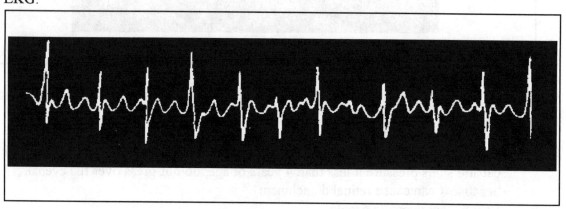

Complication: Congestive cardiac failure.

130. **Atrioventricular** block and **types:**

First degree: **Prolong** PR interval only.
Second degree: **Some** impulses are transmitted to the ventricle.

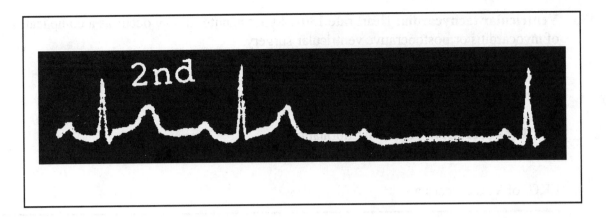

Third degree: **No** impulses goes to the ventricle.

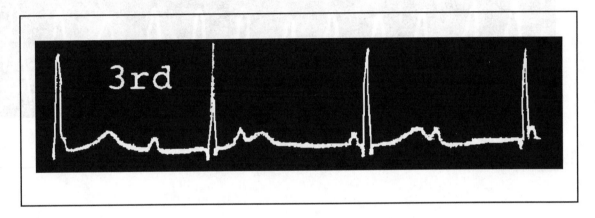

131. **Atrial fibrillation:** Heart rate between **300 to 500 per minute. It is the most common** complication in older children with **rheumatic heart disease. TREATMENT:** First Digoxin then Quinidine.

EKG:

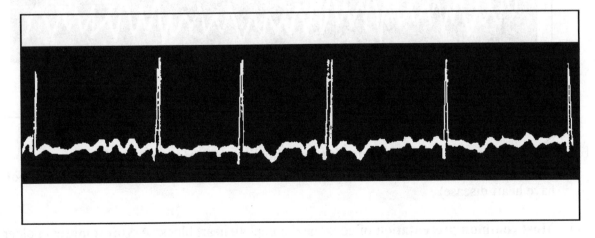

132. **Most common** case of **congenital complete atrioventricular block: Unknown.** Most commonly associated cardiac anomalies are corrected transposition of great arteries (ventricular version), PDA, single ventricle, rarely VSD.

133. **Ventricular tachycardia:** Heart rate 130-240 per minute. It may occur as a complication of myocarditis or postoperative ventricular surgery.

    TREATMENT: Lidocaine (acute onset); for long-term therapy, give Quinidine, propranolol.

    COMPLICATION: Ventricular fibrillation.
    Treatment for ventricular fibrillation: Defibrillator, thump on chest.

    EKG. of V. tachycardia.

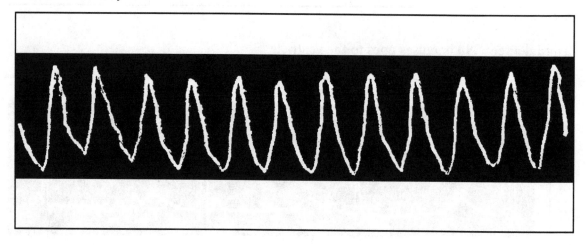

    EKG. of V. fibrillation.

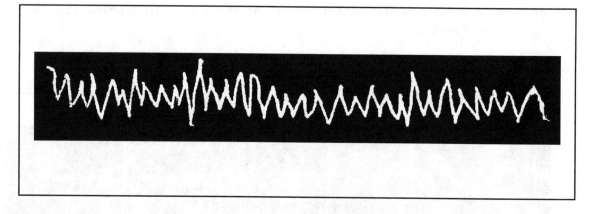

134. **Most common** organism for **infective endocarditis: Streptococcus viridans (second most** common organism is **staphylococci,** which is more common in patients who do **not** have heart disease).

135. **Most common presentation** of congenital complete heart block: **Asymptomatic** in older children. They are sometimes present with **syncope, water-hammer peripheral** pulse due to **huge stroke volume** and peripheral **vasodilation. TREATMENT:**

    a.   ASYMPTOMATIC: None.

b.   SYMPTOMATIC WITH **DIZZINESS AND SYNCOPE:** permanent **pace maker.**

136. **Wenckebach type (mobitz Type 1):** It is a variant of 2nd degree heart block, prolonged P-R interval, constant P-P interval and non conducted P wave.

EKG:

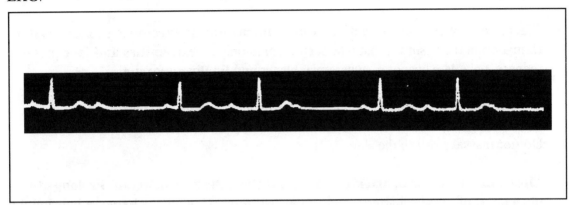

137. Infective endocarditis **most commonly** occur in: **Congenital** and **rheumatic** heart disease.

138. A child present with history **low grade temperature, joint pain,** headache, vomiting. Examination reveals **large spleen, petechiae** over the body, murmur which is **changing** and **new** murmur appearing (due to valve destruction). **MOST LIKELY DIAGNOSIS: Infective endocarditis.**

Infection caused by **streptococci** is **less** serious than by staphylococci which commonly includes **CNS lesion** (emboli, abscess), and **myocardial abscess** formation. **Vasculitis** causes following clinical signs:

Osler nodes: Pea-size tender intradermal nodule in pad of fingers and soles.
Splinter hemorrhage: Linear lesion under the nails.
Janeway lesion: Painless lesion on palm and sole either hemorrhagic or erythematous.

DIAGNOSIS CONFIRMED BY: Blood culture (90% cases organism isolated in 1st two cultures done).

TREATMENT:
a.   BACTERIAL: I.V. antibiotic for 4-6 weeks.
b.   FUNGAL: I.V. amphotericin B.

139. **Most common** site of **venous thrombosis in dehydration: Sagittal sinus of the brain.** Next common site is renal vein with extension to inferior vena cava.

140. **Most common** cause of **post pericardiotomy syndrome:** Unspecific **hypersensitivity** reaction of epi and pericardium due to surgical **trauma.**

Found in approximately **1/6 th** of the patients who have had open heart surgery, present about **7 to 14 days after surgery** with **mild fever, chest pain. Chest x-ray** shows pericardial and pleural effusion.

LAB.: **Anti-heart antibody titre elevated.**
TREATMENT: **Anti-inflammatory** (aspirin **or** corticosteroid) agents used for some time.

PROGNOSIS: Recurrence is **not** unusual, but requires reinstitution of therapy.

141. **Mechanism** of cellular injury in **frost bite: Intravascular thrombosis or ice crystal** formation in the tissues. Frost bite occurs commonly on **extremities and face** present with redness, pale, **less** cyanotic, hyperemia, blister and **finally gangrene.**
   TREATMENT:
   a.   **Rapid rewarming** of skin except for neonate, **gradual rewarming.**
   b.   Analgesic.
   Do **not** massage or rub the skin.

142. **Most common** cause of **arterial** and **venous thrombosis** in newborn: **Prolonged placement** of umbilical arterial and venous **catheter.** Continuous **heparin** infusion through umbilical arterial line **can prevent arterial thrombus formation.** Try to keep catheter for short periods of time.

143. **Most common** complication **(L) atrial myxoma:** Systemic embolism.

144. **Most common** cause of **chilblains** (pernio): **Unknown,** probably due to constriction of **peripheral arteriole.** It shows signs of painful **erythema, blister, ulceration,** swelling, scab formation mostly found in **tip of the fingers and toes, top of the ears.** Lesion usually disappears within 2 weeks.
   TREATMENT:
   a.   Avoid prolonged chilling and protect the areas with woolen clothes, gloves.
   b.   Corticosteroid locally for itching.
   c.   Antibiotics for infection.

145. **Most common** cause of **embolism: Infective endocarditis. Sterile embolism** occur in endocarditis after weeks of adequate treatment with antibiotics other causes of embolism are **fat due to trauma, air** (accidentally introduced into central line). Embolism from leg veins thrombosis is **rare** in children.
   TREATMENT:
   a.   **Remove the source** of emboli.
   b.   **Embolectomy,** sympathectomy, amputation.

146. One of the **most common** complication postoperative **mustard operation: Bradycardia Tachycardia syndrome (sick sinus syndrome).** Malfunction of atria, sinus node, A-V junctional tissue. Patient present with dizziness, syncope, palpitation. **TREATMENT:**

   For tachycardia: Digoxin, propranolol.
   For bradycardia: Demand pace-maker.
   Both medicine and **pacemaker** may be necessary.

147. **Most common cause of venous thrombosis** of children: **Dehydration.** Other causes are

prolonged intravenous central catheter and antibiotic therapy.

148. **Most common** cause for **arterial thrombosis** in children: Polycythemia, cyanotic heart disease.

149. **Most common** cause of **persistent hypertension** in **children:** Renal artery stenosis. Stenosis cause **increased renin** production, then **angiotensin is increased** which causes vasoconstriction. There is **increased production** of **aldosterone** which causes salt and water retention.

150. **Most common** cause of hypertension in **adolescent:** Essential (85-100%). It needs treatment, otherwise develop hypertension in adult. It is **most common** in **Blacks.**

151. **Most common** cause of hypertension in adolescent female: Oral contraceptives. It causes hypertension by **stimulating renin-angiotensin aldosterone** secretion, **increases sensitivity** of vascular smooth muscle to angiotensin II. **Estrogen** causes salt and water retention also; it is found in 15 to 20% cases. Hypertension may persist for **as long as 12 months after stopping** the use of oral contraceptives.

152. Child with **Cushing Syndrome develops hypertension.** The **most common** cause of **hypertension: Adrenal tumor.** Due to **excessive** glucocorticoid, mineralocorticoid activity, **excess** plasma renin, and increase vascular activity.

153. A child with **coarctation of aorta** was diagnosed **late, hypertension** develops for long time, and child had surgery for coarctation. What happenes **usually to the hypertension:**

    Hypertension persists even after surgical correction, so child develops (L) heart failure, cerebral hemorrhage. Coarctation represents only 2% of the cause of hypertension in children. **Pheochromocytoma** represents only 0.5% of the cause of hypertension which is **fluctuating in nature.**

154. **Most common** presentation of primary hypertension in children and adolescent all age groups): **Asymptomatic.**

155. **Most common** presentation of **secondary hypertension:** Manifestation of secondary disease process rather than symptom of hypertension.

156. Symptoms of hypertension in different stages: Most commonly present as headache, blurred vision, dizziness in **older** children; irritability and night wakefulness in **infant and younger** children.

    Hypertensive encephalopathy: Vomiting, high fever, seizure, ataxia, posturing, coma. **Remember:** cerebral bleeding does **not** occur frequently.
    Malignant hypertension: Fundus present with **papilledema,** hemorrhage, exudate, peripheral arterial spasm.

157. When a child is present with **facial nerve paralysis,** what **vital sign** should be checked? **Blood pressure. Hypertension** can manifest as **facial nerve paralysis.**

158. **Mechanism of action of antihypertensive agents:**

a. **Oral diuretic agents:** Chlorothiazide, hydrochlorothiazide, **furosemide,** chlorthalidone, spironolactone, triamterene.

b. **Oral antihypertensive agents:**
   i. **Vasodilator: Hydralazine,** minoxidil, prazosin.
   ii. Central and peripheral inhibitor: **Reserpine.**
   iii. Neuroeffector blockade: Guanethidine.
   iv. **False neurotransmitter: Methyldopa.**
   v. **Beta blocker: Propranolol,** metoprolol.
   vi. Central alpha adrenergic inhibitor: Clonidine.
   vii. Peripheral alpha blocker: Prazosin (minipress), Phenoxybenzamine, phentolamine.
   viii. Converting enzyme inhibitor: **Captopril.**

In addition to above other mechanism of action of drugs:
a. Methyldopa: Direct vasodilator, central vasomotor inhibition.
b. Guanethidine: Depletion of norepinephrine at nerve ending.
c. Reserpine: Depletion of catecholamine stores.
d. Diazoxide: Vasodilator by relaxing smooth muscle.
e. Nitroprusside: Direct vasodilator action on artery and vein.
f. Captopril: Inhibit conversion of angiotensin 1 to angiotensin II.

159. **Diagnosis of hypertension:**

Phase I
a. First, **take history** and **do physical examination.**
b. **Urinalysis,** CBC, **SMA6,** uric acid.
   In older child, do cholesterol and triglyceride level tests.
c. Urine culture should be done in all female patients, and in male patients suspected to have renal disease.
d. Chest x-ray and EKG to be done, but **they are not** very informative.
e. IVP (intravenous pyelography) important in renovascular disease to know the anatomy and physiology of the kidney. Normal IVP does not rule out all kidney disease. It is normal in up to **40% of patients** with disease.

Phase II
   Diagnostic, noninvasive: Scan (renal, adrenal), ultrasound, VCU.
   Plasma (renin, catecholamine, dopamine beta hydroxylase).
   24 hour urine: VMA (vinyl mandelic acid), catecholamine,
   17 keto and 17 hydroxysteroid, aldosterone excretion.

Phase III
   (Specific diagnosis, invasive).
   Arteriography (renal, adrenal), venography (renal vein rein, vena caval catecholamine).

Phase IV
   a.   Renal biopsy.
   b.   Split renal function study.

160. **Most common** cause of hypertension in **newborn:** Thrombosis of renal artery and its branches (second common is coarctation of aorta).

161. **Side effects** of antihypertensive drugs:
   a.   **Sexual dysfunction:** Methyldopa, guanethidine.
   b.   **Ototoxicity:** Furosemide.
   c.   **Gynecomastia, amenorrhea:** Spironolactone.
   d.   **Bronchospasm:** Propranolol.
   e.   **Rebound hypertension:** Propranolol, methyldopa, clonidine.
   f.   **Hypoglycemia:** Propranolol.
   g.   **Positive coombs:** Methyldopa.
   h.   **Lupus reaction:** Methyldopa, hydralazine.
   i.   **Postural hypotension:** Guanethidine, hydralazine.
   j.   **Nasal congestion:** Reserpine.
   k.   **Sedation depression:** Reserpine.
   l.   **Hyperglycemia:** Diazoxide (inhibits insulin secretion).
   m.   **Cyanide toxicity:** Nitroprusside.
   n.   **First dose hypotension:** Prazosin.
   o.   **Hypertrichosis:** Minoxidil.
   p.   **Skin rash, altered taste, proteinuria:** Captopril.
   q.   **Hypokalemia:** Furosemide, chlorothiazide.

162. Treatment of **choice** for hypertension **in neonate:**
   a.   **Mild hypertension:** Lasix.
   b.   **Moderate to severe:** Hydralazine.

163. Treatment for **hypertension** in **children:**
   a.   **Mild:** Lasix.
   b.   **Moderate:** Hydralazine.
   c.   **Severe and impending encephalopathy:** Intravenous diazoxide or sodium nitroprusside.
   d.   **Excess renin angiotensin activity:** Propranolol, captopril.
   e.   **Neural crest tumor:** Alpha blocker (phentolamine, phenoxybenzamine).
   f.   **Chronic renal disease:** Combination of diuretics, sympatholytic, vasodilator. Begin therapy with thiazide, add propranolol, methyldopa, clonidine. If not successful, then use hydralazine.
   g.   Unknown cause: Reserpine, alpha methyldopa, clonidine.

164. **Breast feeding hypertensive** mother, what complication arise if you give reserpine: Reserpine found in breast milk, it is **contraindicated** because of **severe nasal congestion** of the newborn can lead to asphyxia and death. It also cause **gastrointestinal** hypersecretion, bleeding and perforation. It cause **depression** and **sedation** the mother.

165. Which **congenital anomaly mimics** myocardial **infarction?** Anomalous origin of (L)

coronary artery.

166. **Most potent** pulmonary **vasodilator**: **Oxygen.** Other dilators are **alkaline pH, nitric oxide; low CO_2** has no major effect on the vasodilation of pulmonary vessels.

167. **Clinical sign** and **associated cardiac lesion:**

Precordial bulge	Cardiac enlargement.
Substernal thrust	**Right** ventricular hypertrophy.
Apical heave	**Left** ventricular hypertrophy.
Aortic bruit	Aortic stenosis.
Ejection click	Aortic and pulmonary **stenosis.**
Gallop rhythm	Increased third heart sound with ventricular filling.

168. A new-born has medium pitch, **vibratory, short systolic** ejection murmur which is best heard in (L) lower and midsternal border. **MOST LIKELY DIAGNOSIS: Innocent murmur. Most common innocent** murmur is called **"still murmur"** which occurs mostly between 3-7 years of age. Murmur is **vibratory, an ejection murmur, which decreases in sitting** position and increases when patient **exercises or has fever.**

169. `T' wave changes with** disease condition:
    a.   Inverted or flat T wave: Hypothyroidism.
    b.   Tall or tent T wave: Hyperkalemia.

170. A child has **venous hum** (soft humming sound both in systole and diastole) over the **neck or upper chest.** How do you **differentiate** venous hum from murmur? **Light compression** over the hum of jugular venous system results in **disappearance** of the sound in venous hum, but does **not** happen in the case of a murmur. Venous hum is a **benign** condition: changing the position of the head **either decreases or increases** the venous hum.

171. **Vascular thrombosis** (e.g., cerebral veins) occurs commonly in: Polycythemia, and cyanotic heart disease.

172. **Maximum decline** of pulmonary pressure **after birth: First 1-3 days** of life, decline occurs mostly in **the first hour** after birth.

173. Fetal **combined** cardiac output **is approximately:** 220 cc/kg/min.

174. Which **organ** gets the **maximum** blood supply in **fetal** life from **cardiac output? Placenta** (65%). All of the other organs get 35%.

175. **Maximum PO_2** found in which vessel in fetal life? **Umbilical vein** (PO_2= 30).

176. **Most important** factor that causes pulmonary **vasoconstriction? Hypoxia.** Other factors are **acidosis, sepsis** (group B Strep, which releases **thromboxane A2,** which causes

pulmonary **vasoconstriction).**

177. **Time to close functionally:**
Foramen ovale: By 3 **months** of age.
Ductus arteriosus: By 10-15 **hours.**

178. **Most important** factor in ductal closure of **neonate:** Oxygen. (Hyperoxia closes the duct, hypoxia opens the duct.)

179. Factors **closing** the duct: Indomethacin, hyperoxia, alkalosis.

180. Factors **opening** the duct. Hypoxia, prostaglandin E_1, E_2, acidosis.

181. A newborn has **cyanosis** and **respiratory distress.** Initially, how do you differentiate cardiac from pulmonary disease? **Hyperoxia test.** (Give 100% oxygen.) If PO_2 **is more than 100,** then it is probably a **pulmonary disease.** If PO_2 **is less** than 100, then it is probably a **cardiac** disease. **DEFINITIVE DIAGNOSIS:** By **echocardiogram.**

182. A full term newborn has **hypoxia** and **severe respiratory distress, low apgar** and history of **fetal distress,** and is on ventilator with **very high** setting (100% oxygen). This may be due to: **Persistent pulmonary hypertension.**

183. Most common **cause** of **congenital heart** disease: **Multifactorial.**

184. Pulmonary **hypertension** can occur **due** to:
    a. Decreased pulmonary vascular bed (lung hypoplasia).
    b. Congenital cyanotic heart disease (single ventricle).
    c. Pulmonary venous hypertension.
    d. Functional obstruction of pulmonary vascular flow of blood. (Polycythemia.)
    e. Pulmonary vascular narrowing or constriction, with or without pulmonary **vessels' smooth muscles.** (Hypoxia).

185. What happens to **a fetus with cyanotic heart disease** in **utero? Tolerate well** the intrauterine life.

186. **Incidence** of congenital heart disease: 8 per 1000 live births.

187. Which heart disease is most common in **high altitudes:** PDA.

188. When **first** child has congenital heart disease, what is the chance of **the 2nd** child also having it? **2% to 5%.**

189. When **two** siblings have congenital heart disease, what is the chance of **the 3rd** child also having it? **20% to 25%.**

190. **Different syndromes** and **associated cardiac lesion:**
    a. **Trisomy** 21, 13, 18: VSD.
    b. **Deletion** (4p-, 5p-, 13q-): VSD.

c. Apert, Smith-Lemli-Opitz, Seckel, **Treacher Collins:** VSD.

d. Carpenter, Crouzon, Rubinstein Taybi: VSD.

e. **Noonan,** Neurofibromatosis: **PS.**

f. **Marfan, Osteogenesis imperfecta,** Morquio-Ullrich: **A.I.**

g. **Turner: Coarctation; bicuspid aortic valve (most common).**

h. **Kartagener: Dextrocardia.**

i. Friedreich ataxia, muscular dystrophy: **Cardiomyopathy.**

j. **Riley Day:** Episodic or postural hypotension.

k. **Progeria,** alcaptonuria: **Atherosclerosis.**

l. **TAR** (Thrombocytopenia absent radius): **ASD.**

m. **Tuberous sclerosis:** Rhabdomyoma.

n. Homocystinuria: P.I. and A.I.

o. **Pompe disease: Glycogen storage.**

p. Hurler, Hunter: Coronary artery and valve.

q. Ehlers-Danlos: Arterial dilation.

(PS: Pulmonic stenosis; AI: Aortic incompetence, PI: Pulmonic incompetence; ASD: Atrial septal defect).

191. Most common **congenital cardiac lesion** found in **siblings: Pulmonary stenosis.**

192. **Most common** cardiac lesion in **Trisomies:** VSD (ventricular septal defect).

193. **Basic problem** of **Tetralogy of Fallot:** It consists of **pulmonary stenosis,** right ventricular hypertrophy, VSD (ventricular septal defect), overriding of aorta. **Most important** problem is pulmonary stenosis which **reduces** pulmonary blood flow, causing **hypoxia, and metabolic acidosis.**

194. **Difference** in presentation of VSD and Tetralogy of Fallot:
VSD: Child has **murmur,** but **no** cyanosis.
TOF: Child has **murmur and cyanosis,** but murmur is due to pulmonary stenosis, not to VSD.

195. Tetralogy of Fallot, its growth and development: In **severe** cases, there is **delayed growth** and **delayed puberty.**

196. **Different clinical** presentations of **Tetralogy of Fallot: Most of them** do **not** include **cyanosis at birth:**
a. **Severe** Tetralogy of Fallot usually shows itself **at birth or within 1 week, with cyanosis** and **with or without** murmur of short **systolic ejection type in (L) 3rd intercostal space area for** pulmonary stenosis. Hypoxia is due to reduce pulmonary blood flow.

b. **In infants and toddlers** it shows itself **as dyspnea** while exerting themselves during play. (They **need to take a rest** during play). **Squatting position** characteristically **relieves apnea. Cyanosis and murmur** are usually present.

c. **In older children,** shows itself as **dyspnea** when **they walk few blocks,** climb **stairs** or exercise in **gym class. Squatting** position relieves apnea. Cyanosis and murmur are usually present.

d. **'Anoxic blue spell'** or **'Tet spell'** or **paroxysmal dyspnea:** Usually occurs in **first 2**

years, accompanies **dyspnea, cyanosis, gasping, syncope;** common in the **morning,** last **from minutes to hours; severe** cases can cause convulsion, hemiparesis. **Murmur disappears temporarily. ETIOLOGY: Further reduction** of already compromised blood flow, **hypoxia, metabolic acidosis. Hyperpnea** can precipitate the attack by increasing systemic venous return to (R) heart, **(R) to (L) shunt,** hypoxia, acidosis.

197. A child who had **Blalock-Taussig shunt operation one week ago,** had no murmur initially after surgery, but now develops **machinery murmur.** Child is pink and asymptomatic. **MOST LIKELY DIAGNOSIS: Normal,** because it is a **murmur of the shunt** which at first may be **not** heard for several days.

198. Management of **Tetralogy of Fallot spell:**
    a.   **Knee-chest position** on abdomen. **Remove clothing.**
    b.   **Oxygen** by mask corrects hypoxia.
    c.   **Morphine** administered subcutaneously (0.1 mg/kg), relieves infundibular spasm.
    d.   **Sodium bicarbonate** administered intravenously, corrects metabolic acidosis.
    e.   **Propranolol** administered intravenously (0.1 to 0.2 mg/kg), is a beta blocker, so it helps in spell with tachycardia.

199. **Diagnosis** and **treatment** of **Tetralogy of Fallot:**
    DIAGNOSIS: Confirmed by **echocardiogram. (Always remember** that for **any** congenital cardiac lesion, **diagnosis is to be confirmed** by **echocardiogram);**
    CXR: Boot-shaped heart, **diminished** pulmonary circulation. **TREATMENT: Blalock-Taussig shunt that** is anastomosis of subclavian and pulmonary artery of the same side; but **total surgical correction when possible, is always preferred to shunt.**

200. **Most common** complication of **Blalock-Taussig shunt: Blockage** of shunt.

201. **What prophylaxis** is needed after Blalock-Taussig shunt placement: **Prophylaxis for endocarditis.** (Always remember **that prophylaxis for endocarditis** is mandatory for anybody with congenital **organic** heart disease. It is not necessary for those who have only physiologic heart murmur.)

202. In the case of a child with **Tetralogy of Fallot with dehydration,** what is the **most common** complication? **Cerebral thromboses.** It is more common in patients under the age of 2 years.

203. **Most common** association of other cardiac anomalies with Tetralogy of Fallot: Patent foramen ovale, PDA.

204. A child with **Tetralogy of Fallot and PDA.** The child becomes **cyanotic.** What is the **initial** treatment? PGE_1, a synthetic prostaglandin. It keeps the **duct open,** resulting in (L) to (R) shunt from aorta to pulmonary artery, so **it increases** pulmonary circulation.

205. A child with Tetralogy of Fallot and **iron deficiency:** Paroxysmal dyspnea could be **due to low iron,** so give **iron therapy.**

206. Pulmonary **atresia** with **ventricular septal defect:** It is like **a very severe** form of Tetralogy of Fallot. **Cyanosis** is seen at **birth** (unlike most of Tetralogy which present **around 1 year of age). Loud systolic blowing murmur for tricuspid incompetence.**
DIAGNOSIS: Echocardiogram, ventriculography.
TREATMENT: Surgical correction: anastomosis of pulmonary artery with subclavian artery like tetralogy.

207. Pulmonary **atresia** with **intact** ventricular septum: It is a **duct dependent** lesion. Ductus arteriosus **usually closes** in 1st day, then baby becomes **severely cyanotic** because there is no pulmonary blood flow; **single 2nd heart** sound and **no** murmur or murmur of tricuspid incompetence.
TREATMENT: First give PGE_1, to keep the duct open, then perform corrective surgery same as above.

208. **Oxygen saturation and pressure gradient in different cardiac diseases:**

Normal left atrial (LA) saturation	= 94-100%,
pressure	= 4-8 mm of Hg
Normal left ventricle (LV) saturation	= 94-100%,
pressure	= 100/8 mm of Hg
Normal aortic (A) saturation	= 94 -100%,
pressure	= 100/60 mm of Hg
Normal right atrial (RA) saturation	= 74%,
pressure	= 0-3 mm of Hg
Normal right ventricle (RV) saturation	= 74%,
pressure	= 25/3 mm of Hg
Normal pulmonary artery (PA) saturation	= 74%,
pressure	= 25/10 mm of Hg

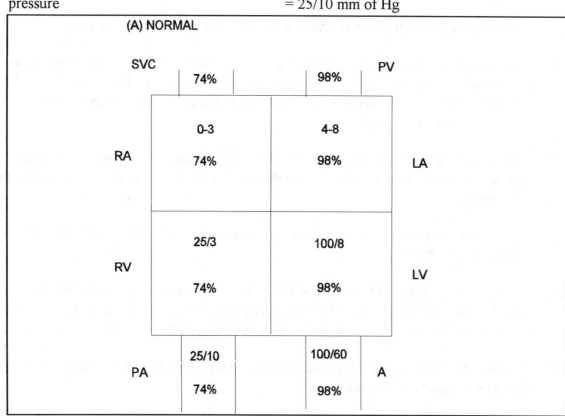

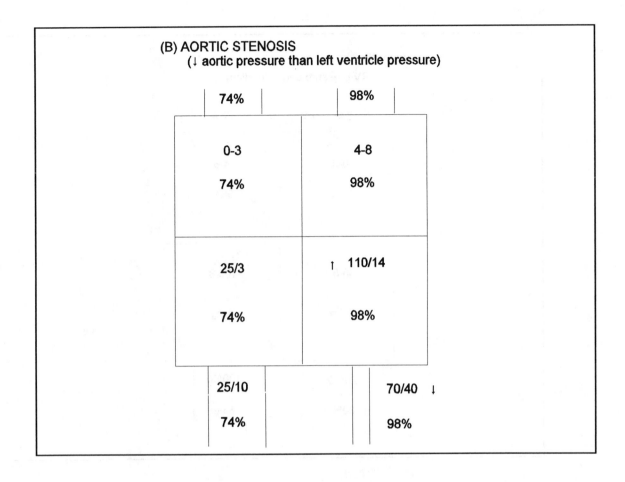

(B) AORTIC STENOSIS
(↓ aortic pressure than left ventricle pressure)

74%   98%

0-3   4-8

74%   98%

25/3   ↑ 110/14

74%   98%

25/10   70/40 ↓

74%   98%

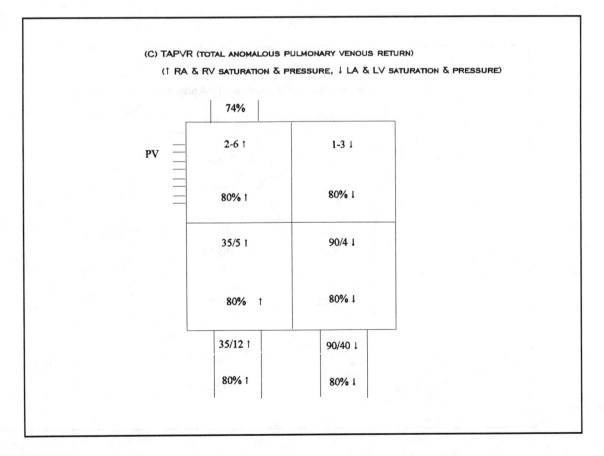

(C) TAPVR (TOTAL ANOMALOUS PULMONARY VENOUS RETURN)

(↑ RA & RV SATURATION & PRESSURE, ↓ LA & LV SATURATION & PRESSURE)

74%

PV

2-6 ↑   1-3 ↓

80% ↑   80% ↓

35/5 ↑   90/4 ↓

80% ↑   80% ↓

35/12 ↑   90/40 ↓

80% ↑   80% ↓

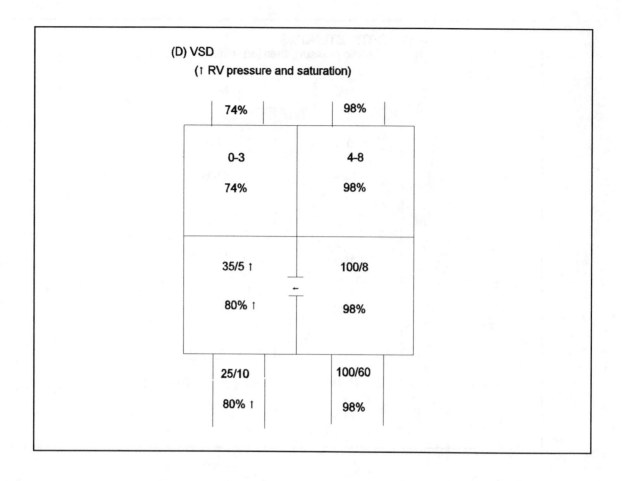

(D) VSD

(↑ RV pressure and saturation)

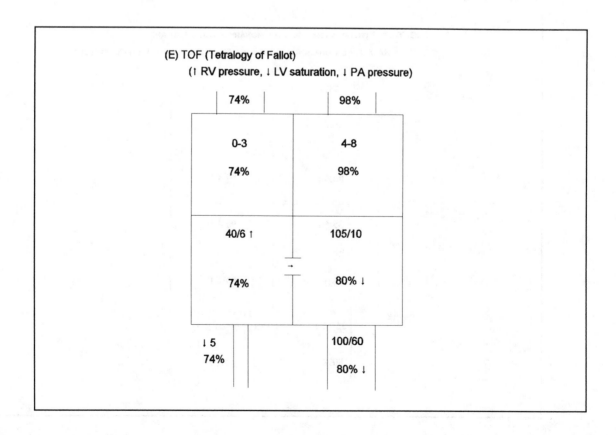

(E) TOF (Tetralogy of Fallot)

(↑ RV pressure, ↓ LV saturation, ↓ PA pressure)

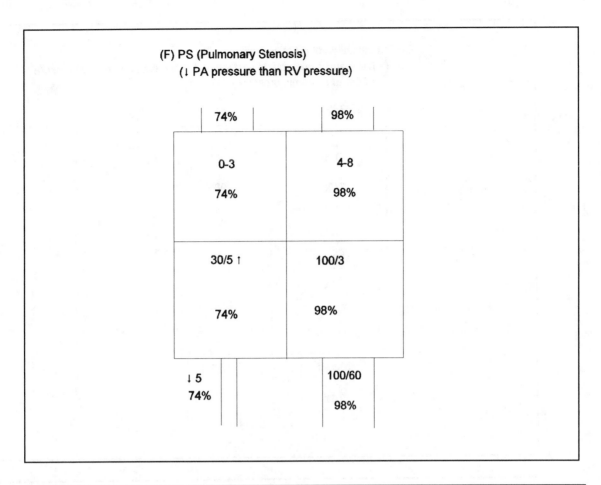

(F) PS (Pulmonary Stenosis)
(↓ PA pressure than RV pressure)

74%	98%
0-3	4-8
74%	98%
30/5 ↑	100/3
74%	98%

↓ 5
74%

100/60
98%

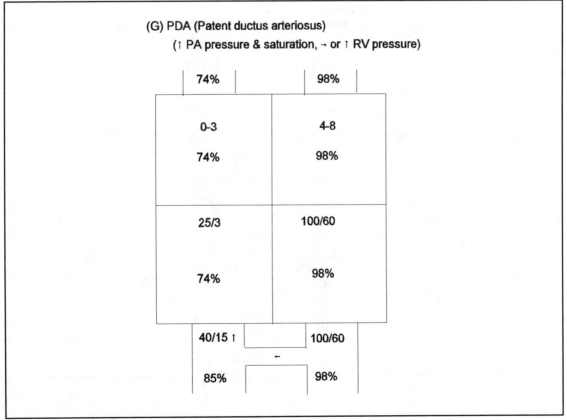

(G) PDA (Patent ductus arteriosus)
(↑ PA pressure & saturation, → or ↑ RV pressure)

74%	98%
0-3	4-8
74%	98%
25/3	100/60
74%	98%

40/15 ↑

100/60

←

85%

98%

(H) Transposition of great vessels
(↑ RV & aortic pressure is systemic ↓ LV & pulmonary artery pressure
< 50% of systemic pressure)

74%	98%
0-3	4-8
74%	98%
100/8 ↑	40/2 ↓
74%	98%

100/60 ↑ 40/2 ↓
A 74% 98% PA

(I) Truncus
(pressure & saturation in both ventricles & truncus
are the same)

74%	98%
0-3	4-8
74%	98%
100/8	100/8
80%	80%

100/8
80%

209. **Calculation of cardiac output (CO) and shunt:**
     Following parameters are provided:
     O_2 consumption : 160 ml/minute. Systemic artery O_2 content: 190 ml/L. Systemic venous O_2 content: 150 ml/L. Pulmonary artery O_2 content: 160 ml/L. Pulmonary venous O_2 content: 190 ml/L. O_2 capacity: 200 ml/L.

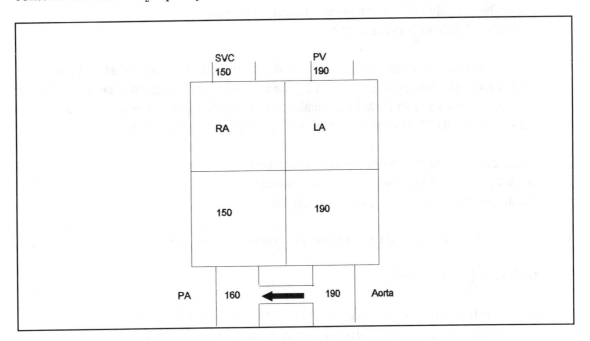

a. Systemic cardiac output:

$$= \frac{O_2\ consumption.}{Systemic\ A\text{-}V\ O_2\ content\ difference}$$

$$= \frac{160}{190-150} = 4L/minute.$$

b. **Pulmonary cardiac output:**

$$= \frac{O_2\ consumption}{Pulmonary\ V\text{-}A\ O_2\ content\ difference}$$

$$= \frac{160}{190-160} = 5.3\ L/minute.$$

c. **Left to right shunt** = 5.3 - 4 = 1.3 L/minute at **pulmonary artery level.**

d. **Right to left shunt** = When systemic cardiac output is higher than pulmonary.

e. **Normal** = Both cardiac outputs should be equal.

210. **Sudden death is the first sign of: Heart diseases.** (Cardiomyopathies, long QT interval/syndrome, coronary artery disease, WPW syndrome, right ventricular dysplasia, rupture of aortic aneurysm in Marfan syndrome, aortic stenosis). CXR, EKG or echocardiogram is **not** routinely done for **all athletes,** but it should be if history and physical examination suggest. Same rules apply to all children.
     Jervell and Lange Nielsen Syndrome: Autosomal recessive, less common type, congenital long QT syndrome with sensorineural deafness.
     Romano-Ward syndrome: Autosomal dominant, more common type, long QT syndrome without sensorineural deafness.

HEMATOLOGY

1. **Blood synthesis** in human **fetus:**

   3rd week after conception: Begin primitive **hematopoietic tissue.**
   2 months: Established in **liver.**
   6 months: Mostly in **liver,** beginning in **bone marrow.**
   By birth: Mostly in **bone marrow.**

2. **Hormone stimulate** the production of **red blood cells: Erythropoietin. Pro-erythropoietin** hormone is secreted by the epithelial cells of **glomeruli,** then activated by the **factor in serum** to form biologically **active erythropoietin** which stimulate the **stem cells** to **form RBC. Hypoxia stimulate** erythropoietin production.

3. Location of hemoglobin **gene** on **chromosome:**
   Alpha polypeptide chain gene: Chromosome **16.**
   Beta, gamma, delta gene: Chromosome **11.**

4. Function of **nucleated RBC in bone marrow:** Active protein synthesis.

5. **Different hemoglobins:**

   a. **Embryonic hemoglobins:** Gower 1, Gower 2 and Portland.
      Maximum 4-8 weeks, **disappear** by **12 weeks.**
   b. **Fetal hemoglobin:** $\alpha 2, \tau 2$.
      Predominate in 8 weeks, maximum at 6 months (90%), **at birth** (70%), by **12 months (less than 2%).** It is **resistent to denaturation by alkali,** so fetal cells can be detected in maternal circulation **in fetomaternal bleeding.**
   c. **Adult hemoglobin:** $\alpha 2, \beta 2$ is **Hgb A.**
      Beta chain hemoglobinopathies: like sickle cell anemia, thalassemia major can be detected by 16 weeks of gestational age, by 6 month (10%), at birth (30%), by 12 months (97%).
      Hgb A2 is $\alpha 2 \, \delta 2$ at birth (less than 1%), by 12 months (2 to 3.4%). Normal ratio of Hgb A to A2 is approximately 30:1.

   Hemoglobin in **fetus** and **newborn:**

   At 6 month gestational age: 90% F, 10% A.
   At birth: 70% F, 30% A, <1% A2.
   12 months after birth: < 2% F, 97% A, 2 to 3.4% A2.

6. **Anemia, Hgb, Hct in children:**

   Hct: Hgb x 3. Anemia when Hgb less than 7-8 mg/dl.
   Normal MCV: 75-100 fl.
   Microcytic MCV: less than 75.
   Macrocytic MCV: more than 100.

7. **Oxygen dissociation curve:** It reflects the **affinity** of hemoglobin for oxygen. **Shift to the right (decrease in affinity, increase of oxygen release to tissue)** occurs in: Acidosis, hyperthermia, increase (CO_2, ATP, ion, adult hemoglobin, 2-3 DPG).

    Shift to the left (increase affinity, decrease oxygen release) occurs in: Alkalosis, hypothermia, decrease (CO_2, ATP, ion, adult hemoglobin), increase (fetal hemoglobin, myoglobin, methemoglobin). It also found in SGA, infant of diabetic mother.

8. **Most characteristic** feature of **Diamond-Blackfan syndrome (congenital pure red cell anemia): Deficiency of precursor of red cells** in a **normal** cellular bone marrow. In this anemia there may be a defect in **tryptophan** metabolism, **increased erythropoietin,** decreased CFUe and BFUe in marrow. It is usually present around 2-6 months of age with **severe anemia** (which is **normochromic, macrocytic),** cardiac failure due to untreated anemia, **increased** Hgb F, platelet and iron. **Decreased** reticulocyte, neutrophil and iron binding capacity. **Spontaneous remission can occur.** Normal RBC survival.
    TREATMENT: Corticosteroid, multiple blood transfusion, chelation therapy.

9. **Hemoglobins** and **different diseases:**

    Increased **Gower** Hgb: Trisomy 13-15.
    Increased **Portland Hgb:** Stillborn with alpha thalassemia.
    Increased **Hgb F:** Beta chain hemoglobin disease like SS, SC; beta thalassemia trait, homozygous thalassemia (cooley anemia), hemolytic anemia, aplastic anemia, leukemia.
    Increased **Hgb A2:** Beta thalassemia trait, megaloblastic anemia (vitamin B_{12}, Folic acid deficiency).
    Decreased **Hgb A2:** Iron deficiency, alpha thalassemia.

10. Function of RBC **without** nucleus: Better oxygen carrying capacity. No protein synthesis.

11. Laboratory finding in **anemia due to chronic infection: Normochromic** and **normocytic. Low** serum iron, **normal** total iron binding capacity, **increased** ferritin, **normal or low** reticulocyte, **elevated** free erythrocyte protoporphyrin (FEP).
    TREATMENT: Treat the **underlying disease.**
    In **iron deficiency anemia: Increase** total iron binding capacity.

12. **Most common factor causing physiologic anemia: Lack of bone marrow stimulation by erythropoietin.** Other factors are **reduced** erythropoietin, **reduced fetal RBC life span, high oxygen** after birth inhibit erythropoiesis. It is found in 6-8 weeks of age in premature and in 8-10 weeks of age in full term. **Anemia in premature** is more than full term, **not** due to low erythropoietin, but due to low respiratory quotient and metabolism.

    TREATMENT: No treatment necessary, **except** in cardiorespiratory compromised patient who needs packed RBC transfusion.

13. Prognosis for **Congenital** pure red cell anemia: **Most common** complication is **hemosiderosis** which causes hepatosplenomegaly and **diabetes mellitus, delayed growth and puberty.** Most **serious** complication is **congestive cardiac failure** due to ischemia and hemosiderosis.

14. **Association** of congenital red cell anemia with and **feature may look like:** Associated with **triphalangeal thumbs.** Feature may look like Turner syndrome, but **normal karyotype.**

15. **Most common** cause of **acquired** pure red cell anemia: **Unknown.** It may be due to **chloramphenicol** therapy or **viral** infection. **Self-limited** disease that last for 1 to 2 weeks. No treatment is required **but in chronic cases,** use **corticosteroid;** if that fails then try immunosuppressive therapy. Chloramphenicol should **not** be used in children.

16. **Effect of transfusion** of adult blood to **premature** newborn: Oxygen dissociation curve shifts to right resulting decrease oxygen affinity to hemoglobin and **increase release of oxygen to the tissues.**

17. **Most common** complication of **goat milk: Folic acid deficiency.**

    It occur around **3-7 months** of age, **earlier than** iron deficiency anemia. It causes **megaloblastic anemia. Folic acid deficiency found in:** Low birth weight, pregnancy (due to increase need), malabsorption syndrome (due to diminished absorption), hemolytic anemia (because folic acid is required for hematopoiesis), congenital folic acid absorption **defect from intestine and defect of transfer of folate** from serum to CNS results in convulsion, calcification and mental retardation; anticonvulsant drug therapy (phenytoin, phenobarbital, primidone causes **malabsorption of folic acid most likely** or **probably due to displacement of folic acid from its carrier).**

    DIAGNOSIS: Serum folate level less than 3mg/ml (normal 5-20).
    TREATMENT: Oral folic acid 2-5 mg/day.

18. **Principal transport** vehicle of vitamin B_{12}: Transcobalamin II. Deficiency of which causes B_{12} deficiency in autosomal recessive manner.

19. **Most common** cause of **vitamin B_{12} deficiency: Inadequate absorption from terminal ileum.**

    Other causes are **rare:** Diminished intake, inability to secrete gastric intrinsic factor, breast-fed infant affected when mother has deficient diet or pernicious anemia. Vitamin B_{12} deficiency present, between 9 month to 5 years of age with smooth red tongue, CNS symptoms (diminished reflex, ataxia, paraesthesia), **surgical ileal resection.**

    DIAGNOSIS CONFIRMED BY: Serum B_{12} level less than 100 pg/ml. Others are **increased** LDH, serum iron and methylmalonic acid in urine. **Hypersegmented large polymorph in smear.**
    TREATMENT: Vitamin B_{12} 1-5 microgram/day, for CNS involvement 1 mg/day I.M. for two weeks. Monthly maintenance of 1 mg I.M. injection throughout the patients's life.

20. **Most common** endocrine abnormality causing **B_{12} deficiency: Hypoparathyroidism.** Hypoparathyroidism with cutaneous moniliasis results in **Familial syndrome** which has **antibody to intrinsic factor.** Abnormal Schilling test. B_{12} deficiency in older child presents with gastric **mucosal atrophy** and **achlorhydria.**

21. **Metabolic** disorder causing **megaloblastic anemia:**

    a. **Orotic aciduria:** autosomal recessive, deficiency orotate phosphoribosyl transferase enzyme, present with mental retardation, responds to treatment with nucleic acid precursor, uridine or yeast.
    b. Lesch-Nyham Syndrome.
    c. Thiamine-dependent megaloblastic anemia, responds to thiamine therapy. It is associated with perceptive deafness and diabetes mellitus.

22. **Most common** hematologic problem in infancy and childhood: **Iron deficiency anemia.** To avoid iron deficiency **0.8 to 1.5 mg iron** must be absorbed daily, **only about 10%** of dietary iron is absorbed, so **diet should** contain 8-15 mg iron daily. It is common **between 9-24 months** of age.

23. **Breast milk** and **iron deficiency:** Breast milk has low iron but **absorption of iron is excellent** from gastrointestinal tract, so it does **not** cause anemia.

24. Most **common clinical** presentation of iron deficiency anemia: Pallor. Other common symptoms are irritability, anorexia, tachycardia, dilated heart and **systolic functional** murmur found when Hgb level is less than 5 gm/dl. **Splenomegaly** found in only 15% cases. **History** of **Pica** in younger children is common. Iron-dependent enzyme (monoamino oxidase) deficiency also causes anemia, diagnosis made by **platelet enzyme** level.

25. **Sequence** of abnormalities found in iron **deficiency anemia:**
    a. **Reduced iron stores** in tissue (hemosiderin in liver).
    b. **Reduced serum ferritin** (less than 10 ng/ml).
    c. **Reduced serum iron, increased total iron binding capacity (TIBC).**
    d. Increased free erythrocyte protoporphyrin (FEP).
    e. Hypochromic, microcytic anemia.
    f. Reduced activity of intracellular enzyme (monoamino oxidase, catalase, peroxidase) containing iron.

    First sign: Reduced hemosiderin.
    Last sign: Reduced intracellular enzyme activity.
    Remember, serum **ferritin level reduced earlier** than iron and TIBC.

26. Causes of **widening of diploe** of the skull: Thalassemia major, hemoglobinopathies, spherocytosis, chronic iron deficiency anemia.

27. A child between 9-24 months present with history of taking **cow's milk** and **carbohydrates. Most likely problem: Iron deficiency anemia.**

28. **Hypochromic microcytic anemia** caused by diseases other than iron deficiency:

    a. **Lead poisoning: Basophilic** stippling of RBC, Increased **lead and FEP** in serum, Increased coproporphyrin in urine.
    b. Thalassemia **trait:** Increased Hgb A2 and F.
    c. Thalassemia **major:** Severe hemolysis and erythroblastosis.

    d.   **Chronic infection and inflammation;Decreased** serum iron and TIBC level, **normal or increased** ferritin level.

29.   **Sequence of response after treatment** of iron deficiency anemia:

    1st day: **Increased appetite, decreased irritability,** increased intracellular iron containing enzyme.
    2nd day: Beginning of marrow response, erythroid hyperplasia.
    3rd day: Reticulocytosis (peak 5-7 days).
    4-30 days: Increased serum Hgb.
    30-90 days: Increased iron storage.
    First sign: Clinical improvement.
    Last sign: Storage improvement.

30.   **Treatment** of iron deficiency anemia and result: Oral **elemental iron 6 mg/kg/day between meals.** Iron more than 6mg/kg/day does not cause rapid hematologic improvement. **Reticulocyte count** rises **after 3-4 days** of iron therapy then **serum iron level increase.** Iron therapy should be given **4-6 weeks after** achieving normal blood values. Milk and tea **inhibit intestinal iron absorption.**

31.   **Sideroblastic anemia** and **characteristics:** It causes **hypochromic, microcytic** anemia. Defect in iron and heme metabolism. Serum iron level increased, **marrow contain ring sideroblast,** which is nucleated RBC with coarse hemosiderin granules around the nuclei. **Normal FEP. Some** are x-linked recessive. **Some** have **deficiency of ALA synthetase enzyme. Some** respond partially to vitamin B_6 (pyridoxine).

32.   **Hemolytic anemias** and **features:** In hemolytic anemia there is increase of serum Hgb which binds with **haptoglobin** and forms a **complex** which is taken up by reticuloendothelial cells. **Serum haptoglobin is reduced** (normal **values 20-200** mg/dl). Like haptoglobin, there is another plasma protein called **hemopexin** which binds with Hemoglobin. **Indirect bilirubin** level increases, **gall stone formation** occurs (15% gall stone formation due to hemolytic anemia), marrow myeloid erythroid ratio **reverses** (**normal** 2:1 to 4:1).

33.   **Most common** cause of **hereditary hemolytic** disease where **hemoglobin is normal: Hereditary spherocytosis.** It is **autosomal dominant, increased sodium** concentration within the cell draws more fluid into the cells to form **spherocyte,** which is **destroyed by spleen.** It can be present in infancy with anemia, jaundice, splenomegaly, sometimes gall stones found in younger child.

    Most serious complication is **aplastic crisis** in children.
    DIAGNOSIS CONFIRMED BY: Osmotic fragility test in which RBC placed on hypotonic solution **cause hemolysis.**
    TREATMENT: Splenectomy after the age of 5 years.

34.   **Most common** diagnostic test for **hereditary elliptocytosis: Peripheral smear showing elliptocytes.** Elliptocytes can be seen in iron deficiency anemia and thalassemia. It is due to **primary abnormality** in **RBC membrane.** It can be present in newborn period with

anemia, jaundice, splenomegaly, bone changes. Gall stone and aplastic crisis occur in older children.

TREATMENT: Splenectomy. Remember: RBC morphology will not change after surgery.

35. A child shows signs of **painful** abdomen, back, and head, mother notices **dark colored urine,** particularly at **night and early** morning, urinalysis shows **large amount of hemoglobin.**

     MOST LIKELY DIAGNOSIS: Paroxysmal nocturnal hemoglobinuria. Due to **intrinsic defect in RBC membrane,** which cause **hemolysis,** and may also cause **low platelet** and **low WBC** count. Infection, thrombosis are serious complications.

     DIAGNOSIS CONFIRMED BY: Positive result in **acid serum** (Ham) **or thrombin test.**
     TREATMENT: Supportive and symptomatic. Bone marrow transplant may be helpful.

36. **Hemolysis** induced in G6PD (Glucose 6 Phosphate Dehydrogenase) deficiency by: **Infection** and **drugs. X-linked recessive,** due to presence of large amount of **abnormal alleles of genes** responsible for G6PD molecule synthesis. Normal enzyme G6PD molecule synthesis. Normal enzyme G6PD B+ found in most of the population, but G6PD A+ common in black Americans. Drugs include sulfur, antipyretics, antimalarials. Fava bean cause **favism** by hemolysis.

37. **Pyruvate kinase deficiency** and **features: Autosomal recessive, disorder due to decreased concentration of ATP** in RBC resulting in rapid **potassium efflux** from RBC causing **hemolysis.** It can be present in newborn with severe **jaundice, anemia.**

     DIAGNOSIS CONFIRMED BY: Spectrophotometric assay showing reduced pyruvate kinase enzyme activity in RBC.
     TREATMENT: Exchange transfusion in newborn if severe hemolysis and jaundice. **Plain transfusion** for anemia. When there is severe anemia requiring multiple transfusions, then do **splenectomy** after 5 years of age. Postsplenectomy **reticulocyte** count may go upto 60%.

38. A **pregnant** mother who took **a sulfur drug** or **naphthalene** gave birth to a newborn who develops **hemolysis** and **jaundice,** but no incompatibility in blood type.
     MOST LIKELY DIAGNOSIS: G6PD deficiency. Blood smear: Heinz body (multiple small round inclusion bodies in RBC).
     DIAGNOSIS CONFIRMED BY: Measurement of reduced G6PD enzyme activity in RBC by direct or indirect method (enzyme activity is **less than 10%** of normal).

39. **Prenatal diagnosis** of **sickle cell anemia:** By **direct DNA analysis** from fetal blood by 16th-20th week of gestation.

40. **Basic** defect in **sickle cell disease: Normal** person has **glutamic acid** in No. 6 position of a beta polypeptide chain. In sickle cell disease, **glutamic acid** replaced by **valine.**

41. **Treatment** for sickle cell disease **with crisis:**

a. Correct dehydration and acidosis.
b. Give antibiotics if infection is suspected.
c. Give blood transfusion if necessary.
d. **Partial exchange transfusion** may be needed to reduce Hgb SS below 40% to reduce the symptoms of **vasoocclusive crisis.**
e. Splenectomy **only** when there is **recurrent sequestration** crisis or **hypersplenism.**
f. Give analgesic for pain.

42. **Peripheral smear** in **hemoglobin cc disease:** Plenty of **target cells** and **spherocytes.** It presents with hemolytic anemia, splenomegaly and reticulocytosis. **Hgb AC** is **trait,** heterozygous, it has no anemia, no symptoms but **target cells are present in smear.**

43. **Aseptic necrosis of femoral head** and **major retinal damage** found in: **Hemoglobin sc disease.** It presents with **less** vasoocclusive crisis than Hgb ss, but **severe anemia** and **splenomegaly, no** growth failure, **longer survival,** may have aplastic and sequestration crisis. **Smear** shows plenty of target cells and irreversible sickle cells. **Electrophoresis confirm the diagnosis:** 49% S, 49% C, 2% F.

44. **Sickle cell disease, growth** and **development:** Most patients are underweight for their age, puberty is delayed, chronic ulcers in legs.

45. **Sickle gene** and **falciparum malaria:** Sickle gene has **resistance** against **falciparum malaria.** Thalassemia has **same feature.**

46. **Diagnostic criteria** for **sickle cell disease:**

    DIAGNOSIS CONFIRMED BY: Electrophoresis (in **early life** because of high fetal hemoglobin, special electrophoretic techniques such as **agar gel in acid pH** or **microcolumn chromatography** are necessary) **shows 90% Hgb S, 2-10% Hgb F, 2 to 3.4% Hgb A2, absent** Hgb A.
    CBC: Hgb 6-8 gm/dl, **sickle cells, target cells,** poikilocytes, nucleated red cells, **Howell-Jolly bodies,** increased reticulocyte (upto 15%) increased WBC and platelet, but **normal ESR.**
    SERUM: Increased LFT and jaundice, increased gamma globulin.
    MARROW: Erythroid cells predominant hyperplastic marrow.
    X-RAY: Osteoporosis, enlarged marrow space.

    Non specific test:
    a. **Sickle cell preparation:** With sodium metabisulfite causes 100% sickling in **both** disease and trait.
    b. **Solubility test:** Reduced hgb s is insoluble and precipitate into turbid solution.

47. **Most common presentation** in **sickle cell trait: Asymptomatic. Sometimes** showed signs of **spontaneous hematuria** usually from left kidney, mild hyposthenuria. Those with this condition **who avoid hypoxic** environment, can have an otherwise normal life style. **Electrophoresis shows HgA 45-55%, HgS 35-45%.**

48. **Sickle cell disease** and **features:** In sickle cell disease, patient is **homozygous** for **sickle**

gene, clinical manifestation does **not** usually occur until the patient is **6 months** to **1 year** of age due to high fetal hemoglobin content of blood.

Most common clinical manifestation is **vasoocclusive crisis,** which is due to **ischaemia** and **infarction.** It shows signs and symptoms of symmetrical pain and swelling of hands and feet which is called "hand foot syndrome" and Dactylitis when fingers or toes are affected . It is also present as large joints involvement (painful swelling), acute surgical abdomen, pulmonary infarction, strokes resulting in hemiparesis.
TREATMENT: Hydration.

Second type is **sequestration crisis,** which is due to significant **amount of blood pooled into liver and spleen** for **unknown** reason, resulting in large liver and spleen with circulatory collapse.
TREATMENT: **Blood transfusion and hydration** will remobilize the cells back to circulation.

Third type is aplastic crisis due to suppression of bone marrow.
TREATMENT: **Blood transfusion**

Fourth type is **hyperhemolytic crisis** which is rarely found in sickle cell disease with G6PD deficiency or infection.

49. **Single gene disorder** diseases diagnosed by **DNA:**
    a. By **direct DNA analysis:** Alhpa 1-antitrypsin deficiency, Duchenne muscular dystrophy, sickle cell anemia, Thalassemia (alpha, beta).
    b. By **RFLP analysis:** Hemophilia (A,B), cystic fibrosis, neurofibromatosis, retinoblastoma, PKU (phenylketonuria), myotonic dystrophy, Huntington's disease, ornithine transcarbamylase deficiency, carbamyl phosphate synthetase.

    * DNA **analysis** also detect **Fragile X syndrome, Lesch-Nyhan syndrome.**

50. **Most common organism** causing infection in sickle cell disease: **Pneumococci.** Due to **functional hyposplenia** and **serum opsonin deficiency** against pneumococci. There is increase incidence of **salmonella osteomyelitis.**

51. Basic genetic **defect** in thalassemia: Processing abnormality in m-RNA, deletion of genetic material.

52. **Most common** type of **thalassemia: Beta thalassemia.**

53. **Increased resistance to malaria** found in: Thalassemia, sickle cell gene.

54. A child shows signs of mild **hypochromic, microcytic anemia,** peripheral blood smear shows poikilocyte, ovalocyte, **basophilic stippling (like lead poisoning),** few target cells.

    CBC shows: Low MCV 65 fl, low MCH (less than 26 pg), slightly low Hgb and Hct.
    Electrophoresis: Hgb A2 3-4 to 7%, Hgb F 2-6%.
    MOST LIKELY DIAGNOSIS: Thalassemia minor (ß Thalassemia trait). **Commonly**

misdiagnosed as **iron deficiency anemia.** Serum iron level is **normal or increases.** **Autosomal recessive:** when both parents have trait, then **there is a 25% chance** of the baby's having the disease. **Prenatal diagnosis** by **direct DNA analysis** from fetal blood.

55.   **Most severe** form of manifestation of **alpha thalassemia: Hydrops fetalis.** Associated with **4 alpha-thalassemia genes,** predominant Hgb is Bart (gamma 4), oxygen dissociation curve is shifted to left resulting in severe tissue hypoxia.

56.   A child shows signs of **severe anemia, enlarged** liver and spleen due to extramedullary hematopoiesis, **hemosiderosis, growth retarded, jaundice. X-ray skill** shows **expansion of marrow space.**

      CBC shows : Hgb less than 4 gm/dl, severe hypochromia, microcytosis, target cells, poikilocytes.
      Serum: Increased bilirubin, LDH, iron.
      Electrophoresis: Hgb F 68%, Hgb A2 less than 3%, ratio of Hgb A2 to Hgb A is very high.
      MOST LIKELY DIAGNOSIS: Thalassemia major (cooley anemia).
      Target cells are **not** specific for thalassemia either major or minor.

      TREATMENT:
      a.   Multiple blood transfusions (hypertransfusion) to keep the Hgb above 10 gm/dl.
      b.   Chelation with deferoxamine to avoid hemosiderosis.
      c.   Splenectomy due to massive size and hypersplenism.

      Complication: Most common complication is **hemosiderosis.** Most common cause of **death** is **myocardial hemosiderosis. Diabetes** is caused by **pancreatic hemosiderosis.**

      Prevention:
      a.   Immunization with pneumococcal vaccine.
      b.   **Prophylactic penicillin.**

      In thalassemia, **distribution of Hgb F** markedly **varies** from **cell to cell.**

57.   A child who is **completely asymptomatic,** electrophoresis shows **Hgb F is 15-30%** and **even** distribution of Hgb F in **all** RBC. **MOST LIKELY DIAGNOSIS: Hereditary persistence of high fetal hemoglobin.**

58.   A child showed signs of severe **hemolytic** anemia, vasoocclusive **crisis, large** spleen.

      CBC shows: Low MCV (70 fl), low Hgb, low Hct.
      Electrophoresis: Hgb S (60-80-%), increased Hgb F, very low Hgb A.
      MOST LIKELY DIAGNOSIS: Hemoglobin S-thalassemia
      In sickle cell disease, **MCV is normal, no** Hgb A, one parent has sickle trait and the other has thalassemia trait in S-thalassemia.
      In **some** cases where beta thalassemia gene is present, electrophoresis may show **absent** Hgb A, Hgb S (90%), Hgb F (10%) which mimics Hgb SS disease.

59. **Most important** cause of **erythroblastosis fetalis** of the newborn: Maternal antibodies cross the placenta and react with antigen on RBC, causing hemolysis.

60. **Drugs** causing **autoimmune hemolytic anemia:**
   a. Penicillin and cephalosporin: drugs attach to RBC membrane, change antigenicity, produce antibodies causing hemolysis.
   b. Alpha methyldopa: Unknown mechanism.
   c. Phenacetin and quinidine: Drugs form immune complex which attaches to RBC causing hemolysis.

61. **Evans syndrome:** A combination of autoimmune hemolytic anemia with immune thrombocytopenic purpura.

62. A child who had history of **URI symptom** for a few days, now shows signs of anemia, jaundice, fever. Examination reveals **large spleen.**

   CBC: Hgb less than 5 gm/dl; **many spherocytes,** polychromasia; approximately 50% of circulating **RBC is reticulocyte** and **high nucleated RBC; strongly positive coombs test; anti 'e' antibody,** presence of **only C3 and C4 are complementary** to RBC.
   MOST LIKELY DIAGNOSIS: Autoimmune hemolytic anemia.
   It also can be present as **chronic** hemolytic process **for months.**

   TREATMENT:
   a. Corticosteroid (Prednisone large doses).
   b. Transfusion of P-RBC if severe anemia.
   c. Splenectomy when corticosteroid fails to improve anemia for long time.

63. **Specific antibody** and **diseases:**

   Anti-i specific antibody: Infectious mononucleosis.
   Anti-e specific antibody: Autoimmune hemolytic anemia.
   Anti-P specific antibody: Paroxysmal cold hemoglobinuria.
   * **Paroxysmal cold hemoglobinuria** is associated with congenital or acquired **syphilis.**

64. **Metal** causing **hemolytic anemia: Arsenic.** (* Phenylhydrazine can cause hemolysis).

65. **Parasite** causing hemolytic anemia: **Malaria,** bartonellosis.

66. **Most important** component of plasma protein responsible for **blood viscosity: Fibrinogen.**

67. **Polycythemia** and **its characteristics:** Increase of total red cells, blood volume, hemoglobin, hematocrit. Venous hematocrit is **more than 65%** when serum viscosity rapidly increases. **Most important** etiologic factor in secondary polycythemia is **hypoxia,** which stimulates **erythropoietin** production from kidneys resulting in polycythemia.

   Most common cause of hypoxia is **pulmonary disease** of (R) to (L) shunt in heart.

68. **Polycythemia** also found in **newborn** due to: Hyperthyroidism, hypothyroidism, hyperfunction of adrenal. **Down syndrome, Beckwith-Wiedemann syndrome** (hyperplastic visceromegaly) develop polycythemia due to increased erythropoietin. **In diabetes,** it is due to delayed switching from gamma to beta chain for unknown reason. **Remember,** cyanotic congenital heart disease does not manifest **immediately at birth** with polycythemia because (R) to (L) shunt within heart does not cause systemic desaturation in utero. Also found in SGA.

69. **Most important** cause of polycythemia in **newborn:** Intrauterine **hypoxia,** transfusion. **TREATMENT:** Partial exchange transfusion with 5% albumin.

70. **Polycythemia rubra vera** (erythremia): Rare, it includes **high count** of RBC, WBC, platelet and **bone marrow hyperplasia.** It has characteristically **high alkaline phosphatase activity** in WBC and **high vitamin B$_{12}$ level** in serum.

71. **Most common** cause of **Acquired Aplastic Pancytopenia: Chloramphenicol.** Other causes are radiation, chemotherapy with methotrexate, 6-mercaptopurine, nitrogen mustard.

72. A child shows signs of **bruises, hyperpigmented skin** with short stature, and absence of thumb.

    CBC shows: Pancytopenia, macrocytosis.
    Bone marrow: Reduced myeloid and erythroid cells precursor.
    Electrophoresis: Fetal hemoglobin increases up to 15%.
    MOST LIKELY DIAGNOSIS: Fanconi syndrome (constitutional aplastic pancytopenia).

    Autosomal recessive, 66% of patients have associated **congenital malformations** (microcephaly, small-eyed, absence of radii and thumb, heart and kidney anomalies). Pancytopenia does not manifest until about 18 months of age. **Chromosomal breaks,** gaps rearrangement has been noted.

    TREATMENT: Blood transfusion, antibiotics, androgenic steroid (testosterone), **bone marrow transplant.**

73. Fanconi anemia with **AML** (Acute Myelogenous Leukemia): **AML** can occur in up to **10% of patients** with Fanconi anemia. Higher incidence also occurs in **relatives** of patients with Fanconi anemia.

    Differential diagnosis from **dyskeratosis congenital:** It is **a rare** form of ectodermal dysplasia that is present with short stature, pancytopenia, hyperpigmentation, **but unlike** Fanconi anemia, there is **no bony or renal** anomaly.

74. **Most common childhood tumor** metastasizes to bone marrow: **Neuroblastoma.** Bone marrow metastasis replaces marrow cells results in **pancytopenia,** which also occurs in **osteopetrosis (or marble bone). Large spleen** found in **osteopetrosis, treatment** of which is **bone marrow transplant.**

75. **Acquired** Aplastic Pancytopenia and **features: First** clinical manifestation is **hemorrhage due to thrombocytopenia.** Elevated fetal hemoglobin, **normal** chromosome (Fanconi syndrome has **abnormal** chromosome).

    TREATMENT: Bone marrow transplant (preferred treatment) antithymosite globulin or dexamethasone.
    Complication: Most common cause **of death** is **pseudomonas** infection. Staphylococcal infection also occurs. May develop paroxysmal nocturnal hemoglobinuria and leukemia.

76. Most common cause of **acute bleeding: Trauma.** Acute significant bleeding causes normochromic, normocytic anemia. Patient may need blood transfusion.
    In **chronic anemia,** transfusion **is only indicated** when patient has **compromised cardiopulmonary status** like tachycardia, tachypnea due to failure, or infection.
    Remember: 10 cc/kg packed RBC transfusion increased Hct by 10. Maximum one-time transfusion to be given up to **15 cc/kg** unless patient has continuous active bleeding.

77. **Platelet transfusion** and features: Spontaneous bleeding occurs when platelet count is **less than 20,000.** Platelet transfusion can be given when platelet count is **less than 40,000,** or patient has **thrombocytopenic active** bleeding. **Transfusion of one unit of platelet** increases the platelet count approximately **100,000/mm3 in newborn** and 10,000/mm3 in adult. Platelets also contain **some RBC** in the infusion bag, so you should **not** give Rh (+)ve donor platelet to Rh(-)ve recipient, **but** Rh(+)ve recipient can take both Rh(+)ve and Rh(-)ve donor blood, because O(-)ve blood is **universal donor.** HLA compatible platelets survive longer. Infusion of **incompatible** platelets **rarely causes** problems.

78. Most common type of hepatitis in blood transfusion: Hepatitis C (non A non B).

79. **Blood transfusion** and **blood typing:** Blood to be transfused to recipient should be the same **blood group** (O, A, B, AB) as donor. **Donor RBC** should be tested for cross match with **recipient plasma** by the Coombs method. Rh(-)ve person should **never receive** Rh(+)ve blood. Rh(+)ve person **should get Rh(+)ve blood first;** if not available, then give Rh(-)ve blood.

RECIPIENT BLOOD TYPE	DONOR BLOOD TYPE
A(+)ve	A(+)ve or O(+)ve or O(-)ve
A(-)ve	A(-)ve or O(-)ve
O(+)ve	O(+)ve or O(-)ve
O(-)ve	O(-)ve

    Type B or AB should be **same as above.** This is **important for examination,** first **mentioned donor** blood is the **best answer.**

80. A child showed signs of malabsorption, diarrhea due to **pancreatic insufficiency.**

    CBC shows: **Neutropenia.**
    MOST LIKELY DIAGNOSIS: Bodian-Shwachman Syndrome.
    It is **familial,** due to atrophy and fatty changes of pancreatic tissues, bone marrow is

hypocellular.
TREATMENT: Give pancreatic enzyme therapy.

Bodian-Shwachman Syndrome has **normal** electrolyte and no pulmonary symptoms (**unlike** cystic fibrosis).

81. A child after vigorous exercise **or** receive epinephrine for asthma, **effect on WBC** count: **WBC count increase** due to mobilization of marginal pool into the circulation.

82. A child develops **fever, chill** during blood transfusion, **the recommended management is: Discontinue blood transfusion immediately** and send the **blood back to bank** for retesting of **donor cells** and **recipient plasma** to **confirm diagnosis** of incompatibility.

    Other signs and symptoms of **hemolytic transfusion reaction** are backache, headache, renal failure, hemoglobinemia, hemoglobinuria, and shock. **Fluid and mannitol** to induce diuresis.

    Three different types of blood transfusion reaction:
    a. **Allergic reaction:** Urticaria is most common presentation, itching ,wheezing (rare), pain in joints.
       TREATMENT: Antihistamine, corticosteroid. If only urticaria is present and blood transfusion is an emergency, transfusion may continue.
    b. **Febrile reaction:** Fever and chill develop shortly after transfusion.
       TREATMENT: Discontinue transfusion immediately.
    c. **Hemolytic transfusion reaction:** Discussed above.

83. Effect of chronic inflammation on **myeloid-erythroid** ratio: Ratio **increased** to 5:1 to 10:1 (normal: from 2:1 to 4 :1).

84. **Increased** eosinophil count due to: **Parasite,** allergy, viral, Hodgkin, familial and genetic.

85. **Decreased** eosinophil count due to: Increase adreno cortical hormone.

86. **Leukopenia:** When WBC count is **less than 5000 mm3.** Most common cause is **viral infection.** It can be due to bacterial infection as well.

87. **Neutropenia:** When absolute neutrophil count is **less than 1500 mm3.** When it is **less than 500 mm3,** then prognosis is usually **worse.** Patient is susceptible to **bacterial infection.**

    Three types of neutropenia:
    a. **Acquired** neutropenia: **Most common** type, usually due to **viral infection,** may be due to **autoimmune disease (here corticosteroid** treatment is effective), acquired copper **deficiency (treat with copper),** malignancy, radiotherapy, chemotherapy, vitamin B_{12}, and folic acid deficiency.
    b. **Chronic neutropenia:** Shows signs of recurrent pneumonia, infection in skin and mouth. RBC and platelet count is **normal, increased eosinophil and monocyte.** It may be due to maturational arrest in bone marrow at myelocyte or metamyelocyte stage. Treat bacterial infection.

c.   **Infantile lethal agranulocytosis:** Autosomal recessive, basic defect is unknown, shows signs of bacterial infection in skin and lung. Treat with antibiotics.

88.   **Leukemoid** reaction **due to:** Infection, intoxication. WBC increased more than **40,000 mm3.** To differentiate from myelogenous leukemia. **Decreased** alkaline phosphatase activity in polymorph in myelogenous leukemia, but **increased** enzyme activity in leukemoid reaction.

89.   A child receiving **aminopyrine** therapy develops high fever, ulcers over skin, mouth, rectum; also develops pneumonia.
CBC shows: Neutrophil count **less than 1100 mm3** and compensatory increase of monocytes, eosinophils.
MOST LIKELY DIAGNOSIS: Drug induced neutropenia (malignant agranulocytosis). Most common cause of death is **sepsis** which occurs within 7 days. It is **a self-limited** disease. **Idiosyncrasies** may be partly responsible for this phenomenon. **Phenothiazine** causes neutropenia by **inhibiting nucleic acid synthesis.** Semisynthetic penicillin **(oxacillin, methicillin)** causes neutropenia also.

TREATMENT:
a.   Discontinue medication immediately.
b.   WBC transfusion in severe neutropenia.
c.   If there is bacterial infection, give antibiotics.

90.   **May Hegglin anomaly:** Rare, autosomal dominant, **neutrophil contains characteristic** irregular blue cytoplasmic inclusion bodies like **Dohle bodies,** which is precipitated **ribosomal material.** Dohle bodies are usually found in severe infections. Here infection may **not** be present. Characteristically **large platelets** and sometimes thrombocytopenia are present. **TREATMENT:** Splenectomy if **thrombocytopenia present.**

91.   A 12-year-old child showed signs of **fever** and **oral ulcer, no** other symptoms.

CBC shows : **Neutropenia** (less than 1500 mm3). Child was re-examined in clinic **after 2 weeks,** repeat CBC was **normal.** Child was then seen after **3 weeks** and again CBC shows **neutropenia.** Bone marrow shows **maturational arrest** of neutrophil formation in first and last visit.
MOST LIKELY DIAGNOSIS: Cyclic neutropenia.

A **benign** condition, which occurs **after 1st decade** of life. Neutropenia occurs for **5-10 days,** then relapse occurs after **2-4 weeks.** Serious complications like perforation of intestine and peritonitis can occur.

TREATMENT: Symptomatic, antibiotic for bacterial infection.

92.   **Transient neutropenia** of newborn: Neutropenia in newborn is due to familial, bacterial infection. **Rarely** is maternal neutropenia due to anti-neutrophil **antibody** crossing the placenta to fetus. Bacterial infection calls for antibiotics, but otherwise **the condition will spontaneously improve** after 2-4 weeks.

93. **Degree** of hemophilia:

    Severe: VIII level less than **1 to 2%** of normal.
    Moderate: VIII level is **2 to 5%** of normal.
    Mild: VIII level is **6 to 30%** of normal.

94. **Von-Willebrand disease: Autosomal dominant, prolonged** bleeding time (**unlike hemophilia** where bleeding time is **normal), decreased both** factor VIII c and **ag level,** usually shows signs of nose bleeding, menorrhagia, prolonged bleeding after trauma or surgery. **TREATMENT: Cryoprecipitate** is **preferred treatment.**

95. **Treatment** for hemophilia:

    a.   Prevention of trauma.
    b.   Avoid aspirin which causes platelet dysfunction and bleeding.
    c.   **Factor VIII infusion** (dose of 25-50 unit/kg will increase VIII level 50-100% of normal). Half life of factor VIII is **8-12 hours.**
    d.   Local care to put cold compress and pressure.

    Complication of Factor VIII infusion:

    a.   **Hyperfibrinogenemia.**
    b.   Factor VIII may contain **anti-A anti-B** isohemagglutinin. Large infusion may cause hemolysis in person with A or B blood group.
    c.   Abnormal liver function test.
    d.   Increased risk of chronic active hepatitis and cirrhosis.

96. To manage **hemarthrosis,** CNS bleed, or major surgery in hemophiliac patient:

    Hemarthrosis: Increase the factor VIII level up to 50%, then keep it above 5% for 3 days.
    CNS bleed or major surgery: Keep the factor VIII level above 75% for 2 weeks by continuous infusion.
    Dental extraction and **mucous membrane bleed:** Give factor VIII and epsilon aminocaproic acid.
    Superficial venipuncture is allowed only.

97. If mother is hemophiliac **carrier,** then what are the chances of **a male fetus** having the disease: 50%. It is X-linked recessive disease, no female has the disease, but females are the only carriers.

98. **Prenatal diagnosis** of the fetus when mother is carrier: Analyze the **fetal blood** factor VIII. C level is reduced, but factor VIII ag level is normal by 16-20 weeks of gestational age.

99. **Factor IX deficiency** or hemophilia B (or Christmas disease): **X-lined recessive, it** contributes 15% of total hemophilia, **prolonged** PT, PTT and thromboplastin generation test. **TREATMENT:** Plasma; **factor concentrate is preferred treatment** (contain factors II, IX, X). Complication of this factor treatment: **Thrombosis.**

100. **Factor XI deficiency,** hemophilia C or PTA deficiency: **Autosomal dominant,** it occurs in **both** sexes, shows signs of mild bleeding (nose), but rarely severe bleeding, **prolonged** PT, PTT and thromboplastin generation test like factor IX deficiency. **TREATMENT: Plasma** infusion for **severe** bleeding.

101. A **3-day**-old newborn on breast feeding shows signs of **bleeding** from umbilical area and gastrointestinal tract.

    MOST LIKELY DIAGNOSIS: Vitamin K deficiency.
    Hemorrhagic disease of the newborn is due to **deficiency** of **vitamin K dependent factors** (II, VII, IX, X), which is 50% of normal in cord blood and reduces rapidly in first 3 days of life. **Breast milk** has **low** level of Vitamin K (cow milk has **good vitamin K level).**
    Most **serious** complication: Intracranial bleed.

    TREATMENT:
    a.   **Vitamin K** 1 mg: bleeding should stop within few hours.
    b.   In severe bleeding or intracranial bleed, give **fresh frozen plasma.**

    Vitamin K is **not** effective in patients with **advanced** liver disease. Vitamin K deficiency **is rarely** found after 1 month of life. It is also found in malabsorption of fat, cystic fibrosis, biliary atresia and prolonged broad spectrum antibiotic treatment.

102. **Aspirin induced thrombocytopenia**: It irreversibly decreases prostaglandin synthesis inside the platelet by **inhibiting enzyme cyclooxygenase,** resulting **reduced** release of **ADP and thromboxane,** which are responsible for platelet aggregation. It is **not** dose-related. It may occur within 1 hour after ingestion of one tablet. **Maternal aspirin** consumption in later part of pregnancy causes neonatal bleeding.
    TREATMENT: Discontinue aspirin; **Give platelets** if **severe** bleeding occurs.

103. Wiskott-Aldrich **Syndrome** and features: **Characteristic** features are **eczema, low platelet count, draining ears,** increased **infection** due to immunologic defect, **X-linked recessive,** defect in **T and B cells, neonate** shows signs of bloody, loose stool and hemorrhage. Bone **marrow** has normal megakaryocyte, but defect in **abnormal platelet formation and release.**

104. Treatment for **Wiskott-Aldrich syndrome:**

    a.   **Treatment of choice: HLA matched bone marrow transplant.**
    b.   If the above is **not** available, then perform T-cell depleted haploidentical bone marrow transplant.
    c.   Splenectomy **cures** thrombocytopenia in 90% of the cases, but overwhelming **sepsis** is the serious problem which need prophylactic **antibiotic** and **gamma globulin.** Rarely, postsplenectomy platelet count is reduced which is self-limited or requires gamma globulin, steroid.
    d.   **Autoaggresive syndrome:** A complication of the disease, present as **leukocytoclastic vasculitis,** which requires **non-steroidal anti-inflammatory drug or steroid.**

105. **Most** common type of malignancy associated with **Wiskott-Aldrich Syndrome: Lymphoreticular malignancy (or reticulo endotheliosis).**

106. **Most common** Thrombocytopenic Purpura in childhood: **ITP (Idiopathic Thrombocytopenic Purpura). It is** sensitized by **viral** infection, **purpura** appears 2 weeks after the infection, and shows signs of bruises, generalized petechial rash, and bleeding which is **asymmetrical** into skin, mucous membrane.

     Most serious complication is intracranial bleed. Liver, spleen, lymph nodes are normal.
     CBC: Low platelet (15000/mm3), **large size platelets.**
     Bone marrow: Normal or increased megakaryocyte, normal erythroid and myeloid series.
     Bleeding time: Prolonged.

     TREATMENT: No specific therapy. Excellent prognosis, most patients **get better within 2 months. By 12 months** of age, 90% of patients will have **normal** platelet count.
     a. Corticosteroid **(prednisone)** is drug of choice. In **severe** cases steroid should be given until platelet is **normal or for 3 weeks.** Steroid **increases the platelet** count in some patients, **reduces** the bleeding symptom, but **neither** reduces duration of disease nor causes true remission.
     b. Intravenous gamma globulin is effective by blocking reticuloendothelial system.
     c. Platelet transfusion is **not effective** except in emergencies.
     d. **Resistant cases,** give vinca-loaded platelets, vincristine, or danazol.
     e. Splenectomy when condition is steroid-unresponsive, or if low platelet count persists more than 1 year.

107. A mother received **dicumarol** by mistake before delivery, so newborn shows signs of active bleeding.

     Recommended drug: **Vitamin K$_1$.** It is the specific antidote for **dicumarol, which** inhibits the synthesis of **factors II, VII, IX, X.**

108. **Most common non-thrombocytopenic** purpura: **Henoch-Schonlein or anaphylactoid purpura.** Due to **inflammation of small blood** vessels of skin, gut, kidney, joints; **rash typically** occurs in **legs and buttocks.** Platelet count is **normal. Other type** is thrombasthenia or thrombocytopathic purpura, where platelet count is **normal** but with **defective** function.

109. **Kasabach-Merritt syndrome: Infant** shows signs of cavernous hemangioma and thrombocytopenia which are due to **destruction of platelets** within the hemangioma. Bone marrow has **normal** platelet count.

     RECOMMENDED TREATMENT: Corticosteroid. External compression of outside hemangioma and excision may cause severe bleeding. **Do not perform** splenectomy.

110. **TAR Syndrome** (Thrombocytopenia Absent Radii Syndrome): Shows signs of **bleeding within 24 hours,** has leukocytosis or leukamnoid reaction with normal hemoglobin. Bone marrow does **not** have megakaryocyte.

111. **Causes** of thrombocytosis (platelet count more than 750,000/mm3). Vitamin E deficiency in premature infants, Kawasaki disease after removal of spleen in ITP. **TREATMENT:** Treat the cause and dispense aspirin.

112. A **newborn** child shows signs of **petechiae few hours after birth,** guaiac (+) stool, hematuria; **normal** liver and spleen. CBC shows platelet count to be less than 20,000/mm3. Maternal platelet count is less than 100,000/mm3.

    MOST LIKELY DIAGNOSIS: Autoimmune thrombocytopenia.
    RECOMMENDED TREATMENT OF CHOICE: Intravenous gamma globulin: if **there is no** response, then perform exchange transfusion or give steroid. Autoimmune thrombocytopenia is due to placental transfer of **antiplatelet antibody** to the fetus. Maternal **idiopathic thrombocytopenic purpura (ITP)** has **low** maternal platelet or **normal count after splenectomy, but remember that in both situations** the baby's platelet count **will be low.** (In **isoimmune or alloimmune** thrombocytopenia, mother's platelet count is **normal,** but it is mostly seen in **PLA (-)ve** mother. (PLA 1 negative is present only in 3% of total population).
    PATHOGENESIS: Baby's platelets go to mother circulation, forming antibodies which go to baby through placenta and cause hemolysis.
    RECOMMENDED TREATMENT OF CHOICE: Washed maternal platelets; or gamma globulin I.V.

113. Neonatal **thrombocytopenia; autoimmune** and **alloimmune:**

    Autoimmune: Maternal **low platelet,** baby's low platelet.
    Isoimmune or alloimmune: Maternal **normal** platelet, baby's **low** platelet.
    Treatment for autoimmune: **I.V. Gamma globulin;** 2nd steroid.
    Treatment for isoimmune: Washed maternal platelet; 2nd gamma globulin.

114. When mother is **PLA 1 negative,** what are the chances that **the baby** will have alloimmune thrombocytopenia? 75%.

115. Most common presentation of DIC (Disseminated Intravascular Coagulation): **Bleeding.** DIC is always associated with systemic serious infection.

    LABORATORY FEATURES: Prolonged PT, PTT, TT; **decreased** fibrinogen, **increased** FSP (fibrin split product), thrombocytopenia, **decreased** factor II, V, VIII and factor C, increased d-dimer > 500.
    TREATMENT: FFP (fresh frozen plasma), treat the underlying cause, platelet if thrombocytopenia.

116. **Most common** precipitating factor of **thrombophlebitis: Trauma.** Other factors are prolonged immobilization, pregnancy, oral contraceptive, nephrotic syndrome. **TREATMENT:** Heparin.

117. **Most common** complication of **deep vein thrombosis:** Pulmonary embolism.

118. Normal **fullterm** infant **at birth** all the coagulation factors are **decreased except:** Factor 1

(Fibrinogen), VIII, VWF (Von Willebrand factor). These three factors are **normal.** All the coagulation factors, **antithrombin III, protein C and S** are decreased at birth.

119. **Most common** clinical manifestation of **hemophilia A** (factor VIII deficiency): **Hemarthrosis** (bleeding into big joints like knee, elbow, ankle). **90% of** the patients with severe disease manifest **this condition by 3 years of age. Newborn** at birth shows signs of **bleeding after circumcision** and **hematoma after vitamin k** or any other injection, because F VIII does **not** cross the placenta.

120. Differentiation of different hemophiliac and Von-Willebrand disease:

	VIII C	VIII ag	Bleeding time	PT	PTT
Classic hemophilia A	↓↓(0-5%)	N	N	↑	↑
Carrier hemophilia	↓(50-60%)	N	N	N	N
Von-Willebrand disease	↓	↓	↑	N	↑
Hemophilia B (↓ IX)				↑	↑
Hemophilia C (↓XI)				↑	↑

121. In Hemolytic uremic syndrome, thrombocytopenia due to: Excessive peripheral destruction of platelets. It usually presents first with episodes of gastroenteritis, then with signs of hemolysis, low platelet count, glomerulonephritis. Peripheral smear shows spherocyte, helmet cells, burr cells, low platelet count. Bone marrow is normal.
TREATMENT: Blood transfusion if there is severe anemia.

122. **Thrombotic thrombocytopenic purpura:** Rare, **mimic** hemolytic uremic syndrome, is due to **embolism and thrombosis** of small blood vessels of the brain resulting in convulsion, blindness, aphasia. Laboratory findings show low platelet count and sign of hemolysis. Treated with **ACTH,** corticosteroid or splenectomy in serious cases.

123. **Accessory spleen** associated with: Most commonly with **intrahepatic biliary atresia.** Accessory spleen commonly located **near hilum.**

124. **Purpura fulminans:** It occurs in convalescent phase of bacterial or viral infection, showed signs of diffuse **symmetrical bleeding into both lower legs and buttock.** Peripheral smear shows **normal or low platelet count,** fragmented RBC, low fibrinogen. **TREATED**

WITH: FFP, corticosteroid, heparin or dextran.

125. **Spleen and hematopoiesis:** Hematopoiesis begins in early fetal life and **ends by 6 months** of gestational age in normal person. **Persistent** hematopoiesis beyond 6 months indicates hemolytic process (thalassemia, osteopetrosis). **In 5-10% of normal cases,** spleen tip may be palpable. Spleen also **removes** pneumococci, Howell-Jolly bodies, sideroblastic granules from circulation.

126. Absence of spleen (anatomical and functional) and blood smear: **Increased** target cells,spherocyte, Heinz body, Howell-Jolly body.

127. Most common diagnostic study of **spleen trauma: CT scan.**

128. **Indication** for splenectomy:
    a. **Surgical:** Traumatic rupture, removal of tumor and cyst, adequate exposure of upper abdomen, surgical shunting, to relieve mechanical distress in Thalassemia, Gaucher disease, to know staging of Hodgkin and other malignant condition.
    b. **Medical:** Hemolytic diseases like spherocytosis, elliptocytosis, pyruvate kinase deficiency. It is responsive to medical treatment in autoimmune hemolytic anemia and ITP, hypersplenism.

129. Most common complication of splenectomy: **Sepsis, mostly due to pneumococci.**

    Other organism Haemophilus influenzae, meningococci. To avoid sepsis, required prophylaxis:
    a. Penicillin.
    b. Immunization to protect from pneumococci, H. flue and meningococci infection. Vaccine is effective after 18 months of age.

130. Most common cause of **acute cervical lymphadenitis: Acute pharyngitis.**

131. **Lymphedema** found in:
    a. Congenital: Milroy disease, gonadal dysgenesis.
    b. Acquired: Post inflammatory, post surgical, post radiation.

ONCOLOGY AND TUMOR

1. **Different cancers** in **different diseases:**

    Leukemia: Down, Bloom, Fanconi syndromes.
    Lymphoma: Wiskott-Aldrich syndrome, IgM deficiency.
    Lymphoma, Leukemia: Ataxia telangiectasia, severe combined immunodeficiency,
    Congenital: X-linked immunodeficiency.
    Wilms tumor: Aniridia, hemihypertrophy, renal dysplasia.
    Retinoblastoma:13 q- syndrome.

Breast cancer: Klinefelter syndrome.
Skin cancer: Xeroderma pigmentosa.
Gonadal cancer: Gonadal dysgenesis.
Thyroid cancer: Multiple endocrine adenomatosis II (sipple syndrome).
Colon cancer: Familial polyposis.
Pheochromocytoma: Neurofibromatosis, sipple syndrome, Von Hippel-Landau syndrome.

2. **Malignancy** and different **causative** factors:
    a. **Intrauterine exposure to diethylstilbestrol.**
        Clear cell adeno-carcinoma of vagina.
    b. **Intrauterine exposure to barbiturate.**
        Brain tumor.
    c. **Intrauterine exposure to dilantin.**
        Neuroblastoma.
    d. **Anabolic steroid.**
        Hepatocellular cancer.
    e. **Asbestos.**
        Mesothelioma.
    f. **Epstein-Barr virus.**
        Burkitt lymphoma (in African children).
    g. **Radiation.**
        Leukemia.

Environmental factors **rarely** cause childhood cancer, but are the most important factors in adult cancer.

3. **Side effects** by **chemotherapeutic agents:**

    Hemorrhagic cystitis: Cyclophosphamide.
    Pulmonary fibrosis: Bleomycin.
    Myocardial toxicity: Anthracyclines (doxorubicin, daunomycin).
    Inappropriate ADH secretion: Plant alkaloid (vincristine, vinblastine).
    Pancreatitis: Asparaginase.
    CNS toxicity: Procarbazine.
    Leukoencephalopathy: Methotrexate.
    Hypotension: Epipodophyllitoxin (VP 16, VM 26).
    Ulcer in mucosa and intestine, liver damage: Methotrexate, 5-Flruoural, 6-Mercaptopurine,
        Alkylating agents, cytosine arabinoside, Actinomycin D.

4. A 3-year-old boy showed signs of history **of URI symptom,** anorexia, **lethargy;**
    examination reveals **paleness, petechiae,** low grade fever, **splenomegaly.**

    CBC: WBC count less than 3000/mm3, low platelet, anemia, leukemic lymphoblast.
    BONE MARROW: Leukemic lymphoblast.
    DIAGNOSIS: ALL (Acute Lymphocytic Leukemia).
    Most commonly found in 3-4 years olds, boys more than girls. **Most common** type is **early
    Pre-B** type (67%), which means a lack of T and B cell marker. **First symptom** is
    nonspecific like URI symptom and **first sign** is **paleness.** It can present itself as **bone pain**

and arthralgia due to periosteal infiltrate and subperiosteal bleeding. It also shows signs of **increased intracranial pressure** (vomiting, headache) due to meningeal infiltrate. WBC count in 50% cases is less than 3000/mm3 and 20% cases is more than 50,000/mm3. Mediastinal mass lesion is common in T-cell type of ALL (25% of ALL).

DIAGNOSIS CONFIRMED BY: Bone marrow examination. Bone marrow failure from **ALL** should be **differentiated** from bone marrow failure from **aplastic anemia,** which is **confirmed by biopsy of bone marrow.**

5. **Most unfavorable** outcome in **ALL** is: B cell **is rarely** cured.

6. Most favorable prognosis in **ALL** is: **Null cell ALL** has **best** prognosis. Remission occurs in 95% of patients, 50% will be in remission for 5 years after onset of therapy. Most patients will be cured.

7. Most common **malignancy** in childhood: **Leukemia** (2nd is CNS, 3rd lymphoma).

    Most common type of leukemia: **ALL** (Acute Lymphocytic Leukemia).
    Most common **subtype** of ALL: **Early Pre-B** type (67%).
    Other subtypes are: Pre-B (18%), T cell (14%), B-cell (0.6%).

8. Most useful **method** of **subtype** of ALL: **Cell membrane marker.** Most common type is **Early pre B.**

9. **Chromosome, ALL** and **prognosis:**
    Presence of hyperdiploidy (increase in chromosome number): **Good** prognosis.
    Presence of Philadelphia chromosome (ph+): **Worse** prognosis.

10. **Treatment** of **ALL in brief:**
    Remission induction (4-6 week): Vincristine, prednisone, aspergenase.
    Intrathecal: Methotrexate, hydrocortisone, cytosine arabinoside.
    Systemic continuation: 6 mercaptopurine, methotrexate.
    Reinforcement: Vincristine, Prednisone.

11. **Chronic Myelocytic Leukemia (CML) and Philadelphia chromosome:** Juvenile type does **not** have Philadelphia chromosome, but adult type does. Adult type causes 3% of leukemia in children.

12. Most common **sites of relapse** in ALL:

    1 CNS: Shows signs of increase intracranial pressure, papilledema, diplopia and strabismus due to 6th cranial nerve.
    2 Testes: It may be the first manifestation of leukemia in extramedullary site. It shows signs of **painless swelling in one testis,** but biopsy should be done in **both testes** to look for leukemic infiltration.

13. **Characteristic** clinical finding of ANLL (Acute Nonlymphocytic Leukemia): **Swelling of the gums** due to leukemic infiltration. Other clinical features include fatigue, repeated

infection, pallor, fever, bone pain, bleeding, hepatosplenomegaly, sometimes lymphadenopathy. It represents 20% of all childhood leukemia.

DIAGNOSIS CONFIRMED BY: Bone marrow examination which shows large irregular nuclei with rod-like structure in cytoplasm (Auer bodies).

Most common site of relapse is CNS (like ALL). Prognosis slightly improves with cytosine arabinoside and daunorubicin. It occurs **typically with chromosomal breakage** like Fanconi anemia and Bloom syndrome.

14. **Non-Hodgkin's lymphoma:** It is more common than Hodgkin's in younger children with Wiskott-Aldrich syndrome, and ataxia-telangiectasia develops in about 10% cases. It shows signs of **painless cervical** lymphadenopathy with anterior mediastinal mass and CNS with 7th cranial nerve involvement. **MOST EFFECTIVE TREATMENT IS:** Chemotherapy.

    Biopsy confirms the diagnosis in both Hodgkin's and non-Hodgkin's. Prognosis is better in stages I and II.

15. Histological characteristic in **Hodgkin's disease: Reed-Sternberg cell,** which has two nuclei, each of which has nucleoli and a nuclear membrane.

    Most common histologic type of the nodular sclerosing variety of Hodgkin's disease is a lymphoma, most common between the ages **of 15-35 years.** Prolonged administration of **hydantoin can cause Hodgkin's disease.**

    Most common clinical presentation is cervical lymphadenopathy. Most typical finding in CBC is neutrophilic leukocytosis with lymphopenia. Always take **chest X-ray** before biopsy to look for disease progression. If chest is involved, then do **CT or MRI to look for airway obstruction.** Prognosis is better in stages I and II. Most of the patients will be cured.

    MOST EFFECTIVE TREATMENT: Combined radio and chemotherapy.

16. Neuroblastoma and features: **Most common site of tumor is abdomen (adrenal). Most of the tumor** gets better spontaneously. Metastasis is more common (70%) over 1 year of age. **Most common presentation** is irregular, firm, nontender **abdominal mass.** It is also present as hypertension or chronic diarrhea.

    DIAGNOSIS: Definitive diagnosis by biopsy. Specific diagnosis: for 24 hours, urine shows increased catecholamine dopa, dopamine, norepinephrine, normetanephrine, vanillylmandelic acid (VMA), homovanillic acid (HVA).

    Most helpful studies for: Abdominal mass CT scan, oral, and I.V. contrast.

    TREATMENT: Surgery, radiotherapy. Prognosis is better if diagnosis is made under 1 year of age, tumor arising from thorax and cervical region syndrome of opsomyoclonus, higher degree of cellular differentiation.

17. **Most common** associated anomaly in **Wilms tumor: Genitourinary** (2nd hemihypertrophy, 3rd aniridia). In **Wilms tumor, chromosomal abnormality is 11 P-, most common site of metastasis is lung, most frequent presentation is asymptomatic abdominal mass. DIAGNOSIS CONFIRMED BY: IVP** (intravenous pyelography). **Surgery to remove kidney is recommended procedure.**

18. **Tumor and calcification:** Pheochromocytoma, neuroblastoma, retinoblastoma. (Wilms' tumor: no calcification)

19. **Most common neonatal renal tumor: Mesoblastic nephroma (fetal renal hamartoma). TREATMENT:** Nephrectomy.

20. Most useful **diagnostic study** in renal cell carcinoma: IVP (Intravenous pyelogram). Patient shows signs of abdominal mass and hematuria.

21. Most common **site** of Rhabdomyosarcoma: **Head and neck** (2nd extremity, 3rd GU system).

22. A **newborn child** shows signs of **grape-like** mass protruding through vagina. **An adolescent boy** shows signs of **swelling in the (R) thigh,** there is **history of trauma** 2 weeks ago, but the swelling **is painful, progressively increasing in size, red.**

    MOST LIKELY DIAGNOSIS in both presentation: **Rhabdomyosarcoma; history of trauma is common.** If it is traumatic lesion, then it **should not increase in size** after 2 weeks.

23. Diagnosis and treatment of Rhabdomyosarcoma:
    DIAGNOSIS CONFIRMED: Biopsy.
    TREATMENT: Radiation, chemotherapy.

24. Most common **site** of origin fibrosarcoma:
    Lower extremities: Metastasis occurs in lung and bone.
    TREATMENT: Surgery.

25. Most common **malignant bone** tumor: Osteosarcoma.

26. Increased alpha feto protein found in : Hepatic caner, Wilms' tumor, neuroblastoma, retinoblastoma, meningomyelocele, omphalocele (decreased in Down syndrome), gastroschisis.

27. **Trismus** is a clinical sign found in: Peritonsillar abscess, rhabdomyosarcoma on face, nasopharyngeal carcinoma.

28. Osteosarcoma and features: Most common site of origin is **long bone, femur** is most commonly affected bone. Most common site of metastasis is **the lung.** Most commonly associated with **retinoblastoma.** Most common clinical presentation is **pain at the site of tumor.** Other findings are limping develop local redness, calor (heat). Bone scan shows increased uptake.

DIAGNOSIS CONFIRMED BY: Biopsy.
TREATMENT: Amputation if feasible, chemotherapy.

29. Most radiosensitive tumor: **Ewing Sarcoma.** Ewing Sarcoma occurs in **2nd decade** of life, **not** found in blacks, **most common site** of tumor is **pelvis,** most common site for metastasis is **the lung,** shows signs of **pain at the site of tumor** with swelling, fever, and tenderness.

    DIAGNOSIS CONFIRMED BY: Biopsy.
    TREATMENT: Radiation, chemotherapy.
    Pelvic tumor has **worst** prognosis.

30. An adolescent girl shows signs of **tumor mass in pelvis,** her history suggests that she was exposed to **radiation therapy.**

    MOST LIKELY DIAGNOSIS: Chondrosarcoma.
    History of exposure to ionizing radiation is characteristic. Most common site is pelvis.
    DIAGNOSIS CONFIRMED BY: Biopsy. It is a radio-resistent tumor.
    TREATMENT: Amputation if possible.

31. **Genetic counseling** for **retinoblastoma:**
    If parent had **bilateral retinoblastoma: There is a 50%** chance that the baby will be affected.
    If parent had **unilateral** tumor: There is a **4-5%** chance that the baby will be affected.
    Uninvolved parent with **one child affected: There is a 4-6% chance that the sibling** will be affected.
    Genetic counseling is therefore very important.

32. Most common clinical sign in **Retinoblastoma: Leukokoria** (yellowish white reflex in the pupil suggests that there is a tumor behind the lens). Other features are squinting, poor vision, pain, hyphema, irregular pupil. Autosomal dominant, chromosome 13 q- location of gene. In 80% of the cases, there are tumors in both eyes. When diagnosis has been made, only 30% of the patients shows signs of bilateral lesion.

    TREATMENT:
    Stage I unilateral: Enucleation of involved eye.
    Stage II unilateral: Chemotherapy.
    Stage III unilateral: Radiotherapy, methotrexate.
    Distant metastasis: Radiotherapy, chemotherapy.
    PROGNOSIS: Stages I and II: 90% survive.

33. Most common **early sign** of **nasopharyngeal cancer: Cervical lymphadenopathy.**
    Other features are nose-bleed, trismus, swallowing difficulty. Local extension to base of skull and hematogenous to bone and lung. **TREATMENT OF CHOICE:** Radiotherapy, rarely chemotherapy.

34. Most common type of **colonic cancer: Mucinous adenocarcinoma.** Most common site of metastasis is **liver. Patient** shows signs of bloody stool, abdominal mass.

DIAGNOSIS BY: Barium enema and confirmed by **colonic biopsy.**
TREATMENT: Surgery, chemotherapy.

35. **Radioresistant** malignant tumors: Chondrosarcoma, liver cancer.

36. Most common type of **liver cancer: Hepatoblastoma.** It is strongly associated with **tyrosinemia. Right lobe of liver** is most commonly affected. **Most common site of metastasis is the lung. Most common clinical sign is abdominal mass. Rarely** due to **gonadotropin** secretion. There may be virilization in boys.

   DIAGNOSIS CONFIRMED BY: **Biopsy.**
   TREATMENT: Surgery.
   PROGNOSIS: Poor.

37. Most common **tumor in area of sacrum, buttock: Sacrococcygeal teratoma or teratocarcinoma. TREATMENT:** Surgery.

38. Most common testicular tumor: **Seminoma.** It occurs in 2nd decade, **painless mass** in scrotum, metastasis to **retroperitoneal lymph nodes** or lung, gynecomastia due to chorionic gonadotropin.

39. **Most common thyroid cancer: Medullary carcinoma.** It is associated with Marfan-like habitus, pheochromocytoma, hyperparathyroid, mucosal neuroma.

40. Most common site for **enchondromas:** Metacarpal and phalanges. Present as deformed mass or pathologic fracture. **TREATMENT:** Curettage.

41. An **adolescent** boy shows signs and symptoms of pain in **tibia or femur,** pain is **severe at night** and **relieved by aspirin.**
   MOST LIKELY DIAGNOSIS: Osteoid osteoma.
   Typically occur in adolescent, pain in femur or tibia, which **worsens at night** and **is relieved by aspirin.**
   X-RAY: Radiolucent nidus of osteoid tissue surrounded by sclerotic bone.
   TREATMENT: Surgery.

42. **Osteoblastoma:** It mimics osteoid osteoma, except osteoblastoma causes more **nerve root pain** due to spinal involvement. **TREATMENT:** Curettage.

43. **First sign** of nonosteogenic fibroma: **Pathological fracture.** Most commonly involved **sites** are the **lower extremities,** long bones at the end of shaft.
   TREATMENT: Not required if it improves spontaneously ; curettage for fracture or weak bone.

44. Bony abnormality with **colonic polyp:** Osteoma.

45. Most common **neoplasm** in infant and children: **Hemangioma.** Usually present by 6 months of age, it grows rapidly in 1st 2 years, then regresses slowly. **TREATMENT:** Resection, prednisone.

46. **Giant cell tumor:** Autosomal dominant, present in patients 3-5 years of age with enlarge mandible.

47. Most common **site for lymphangioma: Head and neck.** Unlike hemangioma, it does **not** regress spontaneously.
    TREATMENT: Excision.
    PROGNOSIS: Excellent.

48. Most common **cardiac tumor: Benign myxomas.** Most commonly found in **left atrium.** Patient shows signs of **fainting spell, systemic embolism,** and **changing character of murmur. 75% of heart tumors are benign.**

49. Most common **malignant tumor** of heart: **Sarcomas.** Most common site is **right side of** heart on **atrial septum.** It is present as obstruction to blood flow, pericardial effusion or tamponade.

50. **Most radiosensitive bone tumor:** Ewing's tumor.

51. Required surgical therapy: **Chondrosarcoma,** osteosarcoma, osteoclastoma.
    (Osteoclastoma is a very rare tumor; not important for examination.)

52. **Most common bone tumor: Osteosarcoma.**
    Second most common is Ewing tumor.

53. History of **night time pain which aspirin can relieve: Osteoid osteoma.**

54. Bone tumor which **responds to antibiotic therapy: Ewing's tumor.**

55. History of exposure to **ionizing radiation: Chondrosarcoma.**

GENITOURINARY

1. Trimethoprim-sulfamethoxazole **(E. coli, proteus, klebsiella).** It does not respond in pseudomonas infection.

2. Prophylaxis for **recurrent UTI: Prophylaxis with nitrofurantoin, bactrim** with 1/3rd of the required doses, once a day for a long period of time. Routinely **urine culture should be done** in one-to three-month intervals for 1-2 years until child improves.

3. Most common cause of **primary** vesicoureteral **reflux: Valvular defect at ureterovesical junction.**

4. **Imaging study for UTI:**

    a. Patient with fever, UTI symptom: **Do sonogram** to rule out hydronephrosis, abscess.

b. When fever subsides and diagnosis of acute pyelonephritis is uncertain: **DMSA** (2,3-dimercaptosuccinic acid) scan. This **scan cannot differentiate** acute from chronic process. CT scan is the **definitive** diagnosis for acute pyelonephritis but is **not necessary.**

c. **After 3 weeks of treatment for UTI:** VCU (Voiding Cystourethrography) to rule out reflux. Some physicians do **not** recommend this for patients under 5 years of age for initial infection because of high radiation. In the male child it is important to see urethral anatomy.

d. If reflux is present, then do IVP (Intravenous Pyelography) to look for renal and ureteral abnormality, but DMSA scan picks up **scars** better than I.V.P.

e. **Don't do** cystoscope because urethral caliber is same for both UTI and non-UTI female.

5. End stage renal disease due to reflux occurs in: 15-20% cases. Because reflux during voiding, it causes high pressure in renal pelvis (normal is less than 10mm Hg) and helps bacteria to go to kidney from bladder.

6. **Secondary** vesicoureteral reflux most commonly found in: **Posterior urethral valve** (more than 50% cases). Other causes are neurogenic bladder, meningomyelocele, sacral agenesis. In 30% of the cases, infection and inflammation, secondary to surgery in ureterovesical junction. **UTI can be present with reflux in 25%** cases which improves spontaneously after proper antibiotics.

7. Grading and treatment of vesicoureteral reflux:
Grade I: Reflux into **lower end** of ureter.
Grade II: Reflux into **upper collecting** part **without** dilation.
Grade III: Reflux into dilated ureter and or calyceal **fornices blunting.**
Grade IV: Reflux with **grossly dilated** ureter.
Grade V: Reflux with ureteral **tortuosity** and dilation.

TREATMENT:
Grade I: Only prophylactic antibiotic, follow up with urine culture study every 3 months; DMSA scan looks for scar, VCU for reflux, sonogram for size of kidney every year.
Grade II: Same as grade I. If antibiotic cannot keep urine sterile, then surgery is needed.
Grade III: Same as grades I and II. More than half of the patients need surgery.
Grade IV: First prophylactic antibiotic, then perform early surgery because scar formation is high in patients younger than 5 years of age.
Surgical treatment results are excellent with some residual reflux which improves spontaneously. Injection of polytef into ureteral orifice for reflux may be helpful.

8. In neurogenic bladder, the best way to control infection other than with prophylactic antibiotics is: **Intermittent self-catheterization:** (Important for Board examination).

9. **Late** complication of reflux or pyelonephritis: **Hypertension** due to segmental renal scar formation.

10. Most common cause of **abdominal mass in newborn: Hydronephrosis.**

11. Mode of spread of tuberculosis to kidney: **Hematogenous. Persistent sterile pus** in urine suggests renal tuberculosis, which also causes **calcification** in kidney. **TREATMENT:** Three to four antituberculous medications like progressive pulmonary disease.

12. Most common cause of **acute non bacterial** cystitis: Adenovirus types 1 and 21. It is present with sudden onset of **gross hematuria.** No treatment is necessary. **Remember: cyclophosphamide** causes hemorrhagic cystitis due to irritation of bladder mucosa.

     TREATMENT : Discontinue the medication, and drink plenty of fluids.
     (2nd most common is multicystic kidney).
     Most common cause of hydronephrosis is ureteropelvic junction obstruction.

13. Most common cause of **renal dysplasia: Early urinary obstruction** (90% of the cases) causes dysplastic kidney that means kidney is **totally malformed,** no difference in cortex and medulla. **Cyst is most common in dysplastic kidney.**

14. Most common **cystic** disorder of newborn: **Multicystic dysplastic kidney.** It is mostly unilateral. When it is bilateral, then it mimics Potter's syndrome. **Initial** diagnostic study is sonogram. Final diagnosis by biopsy shows cyst with no renal tissue. Surgical **excision when infection or hypertension** develops.

15. Most commonly associated abnormality in **autosomal dominant** polycystic kidney disease (ADPKD): **Mitral valve prolapse (remember that it is also found in scoliosis),** MI, TI, AI.
     Prenatal diagnosis in ADPKD with DNA probe, chromosome 16 p. Mostly present in **adult** life. In **newborn it may be asymptomatic** or shows signs of **hypertension, renal failure. DIAGNOSIS:** By **sonogram,** if in doubt do **CT scan, rare** biopsy is needed to differentiate from ADPKD (recessive).
     MI, TI, AI = Mitral, tricuspid, aortic incompetance.

16. Most definitive finding in Potter's syndrome: **Bilateral renal agenesis.**
     "Potter stands" for these disease features:
     P: Pulmonary (hypoplasia, dysplasia), premature presentation (breech), pneumothorax.
     O: Ophthalmic (wide set eyes), oligohydramnios.
     T: Terminal case.
     E: Extremities (deformed due to pressure effect), ears (low set).
     R: Renal (agenesis).
     Death due to pulmonary and renal causes. **Normal child** with **unilateral renal agenesis** can have **normal life.**

17. Most common site and complication of ectopic kidney:
     Site: Pelvis is the most common site for ectopic.
     Complication: **UTI is most common due to reflux.** IVP or VCU showing ectopic kidney in pelvis can be given in Board examination.

18. Most common form of **renal fusion:** Horseshoe kidney. It is common in Turner syndrome and trisomy 18. Patient is usually asymptomatic, but there is an increased chance of **infection and trauma.**

19. Most commonly associated abnormality in autosomal recessive polycystic kidney disease (ARPKD): Hepatic (bile duct hyperplasia, distension, hepatic fibrosis). Most newborn with ARPKD shows signs of **massive abdominal distension due to enlarge kidney.** Severely affected newborns have oligohydramnios and Potter facies, and respiratory difficulty due to pulmonary hypoplasia. Death occurs mostly because of **renal failure** or pulmonary problems. Few patient survive beyond 5 years of age. After that, patients show signs of portal hypertension, enlarged spleen and esophageal varices. Renal involvement includes **cystic dilation of tubule;** glomeruli, interstitium, and rest of the tubules are **normal. (glomerular cyst is common in ADPKD).**

20. Most common presentation of segmental renal hypoplasia: **Hypertension.** If unilateral and hypertensive, then remove that kidney.

21. Renal obstruction and timing:
Early: Form dysplastic kidney (Non-functional).
Late: Form hydronephrosis (functional).

22. A Child shows signs of colicky **abdominal flank** pain, **hematuria,** history of repeated UTI. **MOST LIKELY DIAGNOSIS:Renal stone.**
Most common stone is calcium oxalate and **most common cause** is **idiopathic. Idiopathic** stone consists of **calcium oxalate,** stone after **UTI** with urea splitting organism (proteus, E. coli, pseudomonas) consists of **(struvite) magnesium ammonium phosphate. Metabolic** causes producing stone (cystinuria, xanthinuria, hyperoxaluria, orotic aciduria). **Hypercalcuria** due to secondary hyperparathyroidism, distal renal tubular acidosis, TPN (total parenteral nutrition), prolonged immobilization, corticosteroid therapy. **Uric acid stone mostly forms due to breakdown of nucleoprotein** in treatment of malignancy, sarcoma, leukemia. In thalassemia it is due to increased uric acid excretion.

DIAGNOSIS CONFIRMED BY: X-ray. Radiopaque calculi (except uric acid stone is radiolucent).
TREATMENT: Plenty of fluid and diuresis to keep the urine dilute which prevents stone formation; **alkalinization** prevents cystine and uric acid stone formation **(keeps pH more than 7.5)**; acidification of urine prevents struvite stone; **thiazide** diuretic prevent hypercalcuria, but it may not work on calcium oxalate; **allopurinol** can prevent uric acid stone (**rarely** causes xanthine stone formation due to excretion). **D-penicillamine** binds with cystine and dissolves the stone, but it is poorly tolerated by patient; **mucomist** prevents cystine stone formation; sometimes vitamin B6 is effective. **Lithotriptor** is important to avoid surgery. Stone should be removed if it is struvite, or if there is infection or obstruction.

23. Newborn treated with lasix for long time, complication: **Renal stone** (because lasix cause calciuria without hypercalcemia).

24. In rhabdomyolysis, which constituent causes renal damage? **Tissue thromboplastin,** which is directly toxic to renal tubule. (Myoglobin or hemoglobin is not directly nephrotoxic, but **in dehydration, acidosis or shock they** cause tubular damage and renal failure). Rhabdomyolysis and myoglobinuria caused by use of I.V. amphetamine, viral diseases,

heavy exercise, malignant hyperthermia.

25. Most common clinical feature of diabetic nephropathy: **Proteinuria.**

26. Most common cause of **renal vein thrombosis** and age group:

    Newborn: **Asphyxia,** dehydration, sepsis. (Asphyxia causes endothelial damage).
    After one year of age: Membranous type of nephrotic syndrome.
    Usually shows signs of **sudden onset of gross hematuria** with unilateral or bilateral
    enlarge kidney, renal failure if bilateral. Initial diagnosis with sonogram (enlarged kidney)
    DMSA scan (no renal function), but to **confirm** the diagnosis doppler flow study of
    venacavography of IVC (inferior vena cava) may be necessary. Remember: renal vein
    thrombosis is **not** common in infants of diabetic mother.

    TREATMENT:
    Unilateral: Fluid, electrolyte; antibiotics to control infection. Only use anticoagulant in DIC
    (Disseminated Intravascular Coagulation).
    Bilateral: Thrombectomy or use of fibrinolytic agent.
    PROGNOSIS: Usually kidney becomes **atrophic** due to thrombosis. Remove the kidney if
    there is repeated infection and hypertension is present.

27. Most common cause of **renovascular hypertension: Fibromuscular dysplasia of renal
    artery** and its branches cause renal artery narrowing resulting hypertension. If hypertension
    is **mild** patient is **asymptomatic,** if severe then may develop encephalopathy and
    convulsion. Initial diagnosis of study is IVP which shows asymmetry of kidney sizes.
    DIAGNOSIS CONFIRMED BY: Arteriography; increased renin activity.
    TREATMENT: Antihypertensive drugs. (Captopril alone or with other drugs, is very
    useful).

28. Most common organic cause of enuresis: **UTI.** Enuresis, **nocturnal** more common than
    diurnal, **primary** (child was never dry) is more common than secondary (child had bladder
    control over 1 year), nocturnal is present in 10% of 5-year-old children and 1% of 15-year-
    old children, more in **boys** than girls, 1st born child, lower socioeconomic class and strong
    family history. **Primary** is due to delayed bladder maturation or emotional factors,
    secondary due to some causes like death, birth, separation in family. It is a benign condition,
    and self-limited. Reassurance, support, motivation and encouragement of the child are all
    helpfull and recommended.

29. Toxic nephropathy, most common cause: **Drug induced. Most common offending drug
    is gentamicin.** (Other drugs are aminoglycoside, cephalosporin, penicillin, methicillin,
    rifampin). These are **self-limited. Discontinuation of drugs improves** the clinical
    condition.
    Interstitial nephritis caused by penicillin, rifampin, cephalosporin; **nonoliguric renal
    failure with proximal tubular damage** (Fanconi syndrome); amphotericin B,
    cyclophosphamide; acute allergic interstitial nephritis (lasix, thiazide); vitamin D (calciuria,
    nephrocalcinosis).
    Interstitial nephritis presents with oliguria, hematuria, proteinuria, **eosinophilia,** enlarged
    kidney bilaterally. **Self-limited disease,** but responds to steroids in patients with renal

failure and histologic injury.

30. Most common cause of acute interstitial nephritis in **hospitalized patients: Drugs. Diabetic nephropathy is the most common cause of death** those on insulin for long period of time.

31. **Micropenis:** When stretched penile length is less than 2 cm. in newborn, it is **due to failure of testis** or **pituitary hormonal stimulation** for penile growth. It is found in Prader-Willi, Kallmann syndrome, anencephaly.

32. **Ureteropelvic junction obstruction (UPJ):** It is the **most common** cause of **acute hydronephrosis.** Patient shows signs of **abdominal mass,** hematuria, abdominal pain, vomiting; sometimes **pain increases with large volume of fluid intake** (increase hydronephrosis). It is **bilateral in 20%** of the cases.

    DIAGNOSIS CONFIRMED BY: IVP.
    Most common cause of UPJ obstruction is **congenital stenosis** (kink, fibrous band, abnormal vessel). **Most commonly found by maternal sonogram in utero** which should be confirmed after birth. If **there is no obstruction, sonogram** should be repeated every 3 months for one year.

    TREATMENT: Surgery is treatment of choice.

33. An **IVP showing filling defect in urinary bladder. MOST COMMON DIAGNOSIS: Ureterocele** (lucent area surrounded by contrast material). It is either asymptomatic or cause ureteral obstruction.

34. **Exstrophy** of the urinary bladder: **Mesoderm is unable to invade** cephalic portion of cloacal membrane. It is due to **fetal accident.** Umbilical or inguinal hernia is common, but not found at birth. Other features are: wide separation of pubic rami; exposed bladder; anteriorly displaced anus; epispadias; clitoris duplication;and labial separation. Exposed bladder can cause **adenocarcinoma. TREATMENT:** Surgical repair within 48 hours.

35. Most common anomaly of penis: **Hypospadias. TREATMENT:** Don't do circumcision; total repair **before 18 months** of age.

36. A newborn male showed signs of **distended bladder; weak, dribbling urinary stream;** history of **oligohydramnios.**

    MOST LIKELY DIAGNOSIS: Posterior urethral valve. It is the most common cause of urinary obstruction in the male.
    DIAGNOSIS CONFIRMED BY: VCU which shows elongated and dilated posterior urethra, trabeculated bladder.
    TREATMENT: Transurethral resection of valve.
    PROGNOSIS: Depend on severity of renal damage.

37. **Triad** of Prune-belly syndrome: Occurs only in the **male** child. **Abdominal muscles' deficiency, non obstructive** dilated and dysplasia of urinary tract, **cryptorchidism.** Other

possible features may be pulmonary hypoplasia, posterior urethral dilation, hypoplastic prostate. Dilation of ureter is significant, but **low pressure hydronephrosis. No** treatment is required. Give antibiotics for infection. **Surgery is** indicated if there is **obstruction** or **persistent infection,** in which case urinary diversion is necessary.

38. **Phimosis:** Adhesion between prepuce and glans penis does not clear **until 3 years of** age. If prepuce cannot be retracted after 3 years then it is called phimosis. **TREATMENT:** Surgery.

39. **Paraphimosis:** A complication of phimosis when it is forced to pull out, the constriction band causes pain and swelling of glans penis. **TREATMENT: Firm pressure reduction,** if fail then cut the constricting band.

40. Does urethral meatal stenosis ever cause serious obstruction? **No.**

41. Most common site of undescended testis: **Internal inguinal ring.** Testicular descent occurs during 7 months of fetal life. Spontaneous descent does not occur after 1 year of age. Unilateral cryptorchidism is more common than bilateral. It is most commonly associated **with inguinal hernia. It is either** true undescended testes or ectopic (maldescended) testes. The only **way to differentiate them is by surgical exploration.** Ectopic testis travels through inguinal canal, then end up in subcutaneous tissue. **The most common** site for ectopic testis is lateral to **external inguinal** ring. True undescended testis is found **along the normal path of descent.**

42. Fertility and cryptorchidism: **Unilateral** cryptorchidism has **normal fertility** (same as general population). **Bilateral cryptorchidism** (found in up to 30% of cases) **without treatment: 100% infertile; if treated in childhood:** 30% become fertile, 70% infertile.

43. Complication of **undescended** testis: Tumor, hernia, torsion, psychologic trauma. It can turn into malignancy in 3rd and 4th decade of life in 20-40% cases. **Most common malignant tumor** is **seminoma** whereas seminoma occur in normal testis in 30% cases only.

44. Most common cause of retractile testis: **Exaggerated cremasteric reflex.** Testis was previously present, scrotum is well formed and now testis is absent. Retractile testis can be **brought down by palpation** in relaxed state, warm room, in a squatting position; more than one examination is required. Retractile testis does not have the complication of undescended testis and reaches scrotum by puberty.

45. Surgery and cryptorchidism: **Surgery** should be done at an **early age,** although surgery **cannot change** the malignant transformation. There are, however, few reported cases of malignancy where the surgery was done before the age of 8 years. Undescended testis **at birth** is **histologically normal,** end of 1 year develop **atrophy,** end of **2nd year** loss of germ cells.
    a.   **Extra-abdominal unilateral testis:** Orchiopexy and hernia repair.
    b.   **Intra-abdominal unilateral testis:** First, sonogram to localize the testis; then, if possible, orchiopexy; if not possible, or atrophic, then removal of testis.
    c.   **Extra-abdominal bilateral testis:** Same as unilateral.

d. **Intra-abdominal bilateral testis:** Measure testosterone before and after the stimulation. If testosterone increases then do orchiopexy; if there is no change that does not rule out intra-abdominal testis, laparotomy must still be done. **HCG (Human Chorionic Gonadotropin) cannot replace surgery.**

46. Most common cause **of absent** testis: **Vascular accident occurs prenatally or after birth.** Spermatic cord ends blindly in the inguinal canal or scrotum. It mimics torsion, so the contralateral testis should be fixed with scrotum. Artificial scrotal prosthesis is available when scrotum is removed or missing.

47. Most common type of testicular torsion: **Intravaginal** (torsion of testis only). It is due to lack of posterior attachment of testis with tunica vaginas. It is most common **in patients of less than 6 years of age.** Other type is **extravaginal** (torsion of entire spermatic cord, testis at external inguinal ring). It is mostly found in **newborns.**

48. Glomerular filtration and absorption: Main filtration barrier is **basement membrane. A** molecular weight **of more than 70,000** does **not** filter well. Filtration fraction is 20%. That means 20% of the renal blood flow is filtered, and only a small fraction of filtered material is reabsorbed. **Active reabsorption** occurs in Na, K and **passive reabsorption** occurs in water, chloride, urea.

49. **Renal synthesis: Erythropoietin** hormone (glycoprotein) is synthesized by the kidney in response to anemia or hypoxia. **Prostaglandin** (precursor of arachidonic acid) is synthesized by kidney medullary interstitial and collecting duct. **PGE2 is the most important.** Others are PGF2α and PGD2, PGI2 (prostacyclin), thromboxane A2. PGE1, PGE2 stimulate erythropoietin production. PGE2 stimulates and PGF2 inhibits the production of renin. **Indomethacin inhibits both renin and PGE production. Renin and angiotensin I is secreted by kidney. Angiotensin II is secreted by lung,** and it stimulates secretion of PGE2 and PGF2α. Angiotensin I is **decapeptide,** and II is **octapeptide.**

50. 99% of newborns void urine within: **48 hours.**
    93% of newborns void urine within: **24 hours.**

    Fetal urine formation begins **in the 9th to the 11th week** of gestational age. **GFR increases rapidly after birth** due to decrease of renal arteriolar resistance and increased cardiac output. **Glomerular formation stops** when fetal weight becomes approximately 2500 gm, so **postnatal growth is mostly due to tubular formation. Glomerular function is more mature** than tubular function at birth, which is why they excrete many products filtered through glomeruli.

51. **Hematuria:** It means **more than 5 RBC** per high power field. **Hematuria, particularly microscopic, does not mean renal disease.** It can occur in exercise, fever, gastroenteritis, non-renal infection (respiratory, viral,) contaminated menstrual blood or meatal ulcer in urethra. **Hematuria with proteinuria indicate kidney source.**

52. **Urine color and smell: Pink or reddish** color of urine is found when RBC, free Hgb, myoglobin, urate, porphyrin are present. **Pink color** of urine is due to ingestion of beet, blackberries, candy, soft drinks, vegetable dyes. **Brown or tea color** of urine is found when

RBC and free hemoglobin are present. **Fecal odor in urine** means E. coli infection. **Acetone** smelling means Ketonuria. **Burnt sugar** smell in Maple syrup means urine disease.

53.   **Renal protein loss: Glomerular** damage: loose protein of molecular weight **60,000-500,000; tubular** damage: loose protein of molecular weight **1,500-40,000; overflow** proteinuria is due to excessive production of protein which exceeds the tubular absorption capacity (example: Bence Jones proteinuria, fibrin split product in DIC). **Mild** proteinuria is 150-500 mg; **moderate** is **500-2000 mg; severe** is **over 2000 mg** in 24 hour urine. **Persistent** proteinuria means it occurs everyday 24 hours in any posture. **Transient** proteinuria occurs after fever, exercise, burns, transfusion of blood and plasma. **Orthostatic** proteinuria means protein loss in upright position is **5-15** times higher than in recumbent position. Most of the children are **healthy** in orthostatic proteinuria. Severe protein loss indicates **glomerular damage.**

54.   Glomerular filtration rate (GFR):

$$GFR = \frac{\text{Creatinine excreted (mg/min)}}{\text{Plasma creatinine (mg/min)}} = \text{cc/min.}$$

Normal GFR in children over 1 year is 70 ± 5 cc/min/M^2.
Normal serum creatinine values up to 2 years (less than 0.4 mg/dl),
2 years to puberty (less than 0.6 mg/dl),
Puberty to adult (less than 1.0 mg/dl).

55.   **Renal biopsy:** It is the **most definitive way** to confirm the diagnosis of kidney disease, particularly **that of glomerular** origin. **Closed renal biopsy** is procedure of choice, except **when patient is less than 6 months of age in which case open biopsy is** done in routine screening.

56.   Children in routine screening shows signs of hematuria and proteinuria. Most likely outcome: No renal disease. This is a self-limited condition, so routine screening is not necessary.

57.   A child shows signs of history of **trauma** and **hematuria:**
Most important diagnostic procedure to localize renal lesion: **CT scan** (very important for examination).

58.   **Nephrotic syndrome due to FGS** (focal glomerulosclerosis) or **DMP** (diffuse mesangial proliferation): Both of them have nonspecific histologic changes. **Glomeruli** are affected in **both FGS and DMP.** The latter also causes podocyte fusion, **no immunologic defect is found in Alport disease, heroin addiction and amyloidosis. DMP found in resolving phase of post streptococcal glomerulonephritis. Most common clinical sign is proteinuria,** 2nd is microscopic hematuria. **Prednisone is drug of first choice,** but 50% of the cases are resistent to it. In those cases use cyclophosphamide alkylating agent. Recurrence of nephrotic syndrome is due to FGS which can occur in transplant patient.

59.   **Procedure of choice** and **renal problem:**

   a.   **CT scan: Abdominal trauma.**

   b.   **IVP** (intravenous pyelography): **UTI,** congenital anomaly with functional defect, lower urinary tract problem, ambiguous genitalia, hypertensive renal disease, uncontrolled enuresis, neurogenic bladder, kidney donor for transplant.

   c.   **VCU** (retrograde voiding cystourethrogram: **Posterior urethral valve** or any obstruction.

   d.   **Ultrasound:** Abdominal renal mass, acute pyelonephritis, acute renal failure, polycystic kidney, recurrent abdominal pain when non-renal causes are excluded, newborn sepsis with renal failure, bilateral pneumothorax at birth, renal transplant recipient, before biopsy for kidney location.

Contraindication to IVP: Shock, dehydration. Minor reaction (vomiting, urticaria, flushing) after contrast can occur, but it does not prevent further study.

60.   **Most common cause of nephrotic syndrome in children: MCNS** (minimal change nephrotic syndrome). **Nephrotic syndrome** includes edema (due to low protein), hypoproteinemia (abnormal protein loss through glomerular basement membrane), hyperlipidemia (cholesterol above 220 mg/dl). Primary type is due to renal and secondary type is due to systemic diseases.

61.   **Causes of edema** in nephrotic syndrome:

   a.   Retention of water due to increased ADH (antidiuretic hormone) secretion.

   b.   Reduction of colloid osmotic pressure due to low albumin.

   c.   Reduce excretion of sodium by renal tubule.

62.   Causes of **hyperlipidemia** in nephrotic syndrome: High molecular weight lipid has insignificant loss in urine.

63.   **Clinical characteristics and renal disease:**

   a.   **Chronic renal insufficiency: Most important finding is growth retardation;** polyuria, polydipsia, low calcium, high phosphorous, anemia, metabolic acidosis.

   b.   **Acute renal failure: Most important finding is anuria or oliguria;** hypertension, electrolyte abnormality.

   c.   **Acute glomerulonephritis: Most important finding is hematuria;** RBC cast, hypertension, oliguria, edema, dilutional anemia.

   d.   **Nephrotic syndrome: Most important finding is proteinuria;** edema, high cholesterol, microscopic hematuria rarely hypertension.

   e.   **Mixed** nephrotic and nephritic feature.

64.   Indication for biopsy in MCNS (minimal change nephrotic syndrome) in **atypical features:** Failure to respond to corticosteroid for 1 month, gross hematuria, persistent azotemia, high B.P, prolonged proteinuria, systemic disease, age below 1 year after 10 years.

65.   **Effect of corticosteroid** therapy in MCNS: **(70%) Most of the responsive** patient will **have 1 or 2 relapses.** To avoid relapse therapy **every 48 hours once per day** or **addition of cyclophosphamide is recommended.** Oral chlorambucil is given in frequently relapsing MCNS.

66.   **MCNS (minimal change nephrotic syndrome):** This is **most common cause of**

childhood **(2-7 years) nephrotic syndrome.** Etiology is **unknown,** associated with **HLA B₁₂ antigen,** initially **minimal or no change in biopsy,** so it is called minimal change nephrotic syndrome, change include increase mesangial **matrix or hypercellularity.**

Most common presentation is **edema** which is **periorbital in lying** condition and **pedal in upright** position, in severe cases ascitis and pleural effusion present, blood pressure is **normal or low** unlike other nephrotic syndrome and glomerulonephritis. **Laboratory features** include **low serum** (protein, sodium), **high serum** (ESR; Hgb and Hct due to hemoconcentration), **normal serum C 3.**

DIAGNOSIS CONFIRMED BY: History, clinical and laboratory features. **No** biopsy necessary (**diffuse fusion of podocytes** are characteristic feature).
TREATMENT: Prednisone is drug of choice; cyclophosphamide.
COMPLICATION: Most common **infection is pneumococcus, (peritonitis and sepsis).** Prednisone cause **growth retardation,** cyclophosphamide cause **hemorrhagic cystitis, sterility, increase mortality from chicken pox.** Increase infection due to impaired bacterial opsonization due to low gammaglobulin, loss of C3 proactivator in urine.
Prophylaxis: Penicillin.

67. **Membranous glomerulopathy:** It include 5% of all nephrotic syndrome, **most common cause is idiopathic; thickening and nodule formation** in glomerular basement membrane **due to deposition of immune complex** (mostly IgG; 1/3 cases C3), it is also found in syphilis, SLE, autoimmune thyroiditis, penicillamine therapy, sickle cell disease. Clinical and laboratory finding **same as MCNS** but disease begin after 10 years of age unlike **MCNS (2-7 years). Prednisone is the treatment of choice.**

68. **MPGN** (membranoproliferative glomerulonephritis): **Most common cause is idiopathic.** It occurs in **10%** of all cases of nephrotic syndrome. It is a chronic diffuse **proliferative** disease. Type I is more common than type II.
Type I is due to deposition of 1gG, IgM, C3, CIg, C4, mesangial matrix between endothelial cells and basement membrane.
Type Ii is due to deposition of C3, mesangial matrix within basement membrane.
It occurs commonly in **the adolescent.** Presentation includes (1/3 rd as nephrotic syndrome, 1/3rd as nephrotic-nephritic, and rest as gross hematuria, proteinuria, hypertension). **Type II most** commonly recurs in **transplanted kidney. Prednisone** is the drug of choice and after that azathioprine. 50% patient end up in chronic renal failure.

69. **Most common** type of nephrotic syndrome in first year of life: **Finnish type of congenital nephrotic syndrome** (infantile microcystic disease).
It is a rare, **autosomal recessive disease.** The first clinical sign **at birth is proteinuria;** 2 weeks later, edema develops. There is an increased risk of secondary infection. Etiology is **unknown** but **cystic dilation of proximal tubule is characteristic. Antenatal diagnosis by** amniocentesis (15-20 weeks) shows increased **alpha-fetoprotein.**

DIAGNOSIS CONFIRMED BY: Biopsy.
TREATMENT: Fluid, antibiotics for infection, renal transplant. **(no prednisone)** Syphilis, CMV, toxoplasmosis are important infectious cause of nephrotic syndrome.

70. **Benign asymptomatic persistent proteinuria:** This is **not always a benign** condition: some patients develop persistent hypertension and proteinuria. It presents **only with proteinuria,** otherwise it is asymptomatic. Renal biopsy shows thickening, splitting of basement membrane and fusion of foot process. **Serum C3 is normal. No treatment is necessary.**

71. **Acute post streptococcal glomerulonephritis:** Most common type is **group A** beta hemolytic streptococci. It is the **most common** cause of **all types of glomerulonephritis.** Most common pharyngeal strain is **M 12** and skin strain is **M 49. Most commonly** affected age is **preschool children.** Only **10-15%** of all pharyngitis and skin lesion patients **develop glomerulonephritis.** Prior pharyngeal and skin infection 2-3 weeks before the onset of **dark urine (gross hematuria), periorbital edema, low urine output, hypertension fever.**

    Laboratory: Hemodilutional normochromic anemia, high (WBC, BUN, creatinine), **C3 is low** or normal, low sodium, high potassium.
    Chest X-ray: Later develops pulmonary edema.
    TREATMENT: Penicillin (erythromycin in penicillin allergy), fluid restriction, plenty of carbohydrate for calories, antihypertensive in hypertension. If child feels O.K., encourage **normal** activities, not those that may cause hematuria. **Bed rest is recommended only for a very sick child.**
    PROGNOSIS: Excellent.

    Remember **early antibiotic use** in **streptococcal skin infection** does not prevent glomerulonephritis, but it **does in 50% of cases of pharyngitis.**

72. A child shows signs of **sudden onset of gross hematuria,** otherwise is asymptomatic. History of **URI infection 2-3 days ago,** sometimes precipitated by exercise.

    MOST LIKELY DIAGNOSIS: IgA nephropathy (idiopathic recurrent macroscopic hematuria) **(important for board exam).**
    LABORATORY: Increased serum IgA (50% cases), C3 normal, RBC cast and protein in urine (proteinuria disappears as hematuria disappears). Biopsy is **not** necessary except in persistent proteinuria.
    TREATMENT: None; encourage the patient to lead **completely normal life,** do **not** advise him or her to discontinue exercise.

73. Laboratory features, WHO classification, and treatment of lupus nephritis:
    Laboratory: **Low serum C3, C4, high ANA and anti-DNA,** high BUN and creatinine.
    Urinalysis: RBC, protein, pus cells.
    Most specific diagnostic test: Anti-DNA, because ANA negative lupus also present.

    Remember, **biopsy finding in lupus is nonspecific,and a** similar finding is found in other causes of membranous glomerulonephritis, anaphylactoid purpura, nephritis due to shunt infection or endocarditis. **Biopsy should be done in all patients** to select immunosuppressive treatment.

    WHO classification of lupus nephritis:

a. Class I: No histologic abnormality.
b. Class II-A: Mesangial deposit of immunoglobulin and complement, **mesangial nephritis.**
c. Class III: Focal proliferative lupus nephritis.
d. Class IV: Diffuse proliferative lupus nephritis **(most common and most severe).**
e. Class V: Membranous lupus nephritis **(least** common).

TREATMENT: Prednisone is the drug of choice in all cases of lupus nephritis. Azathioprine should be added to all members of class IV and some members of class III. **PROGNOSIS:** Disease is **controlled,** but **not cured.** Both medical and psychologic support are needed by patient and family members.

74. Glomerulonephritis from infected V-P shunt: Most common organism is **Staph epidermidis,** shows signs of **nephrotic-**like picture. (When glomerulonephritis secondary to bacterial endocarditis, it presents with nephritic picture.) There is deposit of IgG and C3 in both conditions. **TREATMENT:** Antibiotics.

75. Most common type of **lupus nephritis: Diffuse proliferative type** (30% of all lupus cases). Most common **site** involved is **glomeruli.** Most pediatric patients with lupus have **renal involvement.** Other **types are** membranous, mesangial, focal proliferative, interstitial lupus. **Glomerular** sclerosis is the **most common finding** involved in **all lupus** cases and there is deposition of IgG and C3.

76. Causes of **gross hematuria: IgA nephropathy (asymptomatic** patients, **mostly given in Board examination),** acute glomerulonephritis, hemolytic uremic syndrome, Alport syndrome, benign familial hematuria, acute non-bacterial cystitis (viral, cyclophosphamide therapy), nephritis due to Henoch-Schonlein syndrome.

77. **Henoch-Schonlein syndrome nephritis:** Almost 40% of the patients cause nephritis in this syndrome. Nephritis is self-limited. Proliferative changes in endothelial and mesangial cells, deposit of IgA, IgG, IgM, C3. Nephrotic-nephritic manifestation of renal problem, but **most common presentation is characteristic rash** over the lower extremities, joint and G.I. manifestation.

    Laboratory: Normal C3 and platelet; **absence of anti-DNA.**
    Diagnosis is made clinically.
    Biopsy only indicated in nephrotic syndrome, excessive protein loss more than 2 gm/day, diminished renal function.
    TREATMENT: Prednisone and azathioprine.

78. Fanconi syndrome causing **primary RTA:** Characterized by **glucosuria, aminoaciduria, phosphaturia, carnitinuria.** Primary Fanconi syndrome is autosomal dominant or recessive, secondary Fanconi syndrome develops in inherited (cystinosis) or acquired disease (heavy metal, interstitial nephritis, hyperparathyroidism, vitamin D deficiency rickets, outdated tetracycline).

79. **Hemolytic uremic syndrome:** Etiology is **unknown,** precipitating factors are viral (coxsackie, echo and arbovirus), bacterial (Shigella, Salmonella, **E.coli [0157:H7]** Strep

pneumonia), others (oral contraceptive, pregnancy, prolonged high B.P.), **mostly under 4 years of age,** symptoms are **preceded by acute gastroenteritis** (vomiting, bloody stool) or URI symptoms then 5-10 days later showed signs of **pallor, lethargy, oliguria, irritability, dehydration, edema, hepatosplenomegaly, petechiae.**

Laboratory: High WBC, **low platelet,** smear showing helmet, burr and fragmented RBC, coombs negative; urinalysis shows RBC cast, protein.
TREATMENT: Early and repeated peritoneal dialysis, hematologic and renal therapy.
PROGNOSIS: 90% of the patients are cured by aggressive medical therapy. **The symptoms rarely recur.** (This is important for Board examination).

80. Mode of transmission in cystinosis: Autosomal recessive. Cystinosis is due to accumulation of **cystine in lysosome** of kidney, liver, spleen marrow, cornea, conjunctiva and **WBC.** It manifests clinically with polyuria, polydipsia, fever, growth retardation, fair skin and blond hair.

     DIAGNOSIS CONFIRMED BY: Increased cystine content of leukocyte; slit lamp eye examination suggests the disease.
     TREATMENT: Cysteamine.

81. **Principal site** of absorption in renal tubule:
     Na, K, calcium, phosphate: Proximal tubule.
     Magnesium: Ascending limb of Henle.
     Parathyroid hormone **inhibits phosphorous** absorption, **stimulates calcium** absorption.
     Calcium absorption is also **stimulated by thiazide diuretic and reduced ECF** (extracellular fluid) volume; calcium absorption **is inhibited** by saline infusion and furosemide.

82. **Pathogenesis of renal tubular acidosis (RTA): Normally** 85% of $NaHCO_3$ is absorbed by proximal tubule, and 15% by distal tubule.
     In proximal RTA, 60% of $NaHCO_3$ is absorbed by proximal tubule, and 40% reaches to distal tubule, but only 15% is absorbed. **The rest is 25% excreted by kidney.**
     In distal RTA, 85% of $NaHCO_3$ is absorbed by proximal tubule and 5-12% is absorbed by distal tubule. **The rest 3-10% is excreted by kidney.**
     In **proximal RTA,** there is initially a loss of $NaHCO_3$ in urine, serum bicarbonate level falls to 15-18 m Eq/l, then all bicarbonate is absorbed in distal tubule, urine pH is **less than 5.5;** because of huge sodium absorption, K excretion is increased. Loss of ECF volume causes **increased Cl absorption and aldosterone secretion.**

     Serum: **Very low K, low HCO_3, low Ca; high Cl,** high osmolarity.
     Urine: High K, high then normal HCO_3, high Ca, pH low.
     In distal RTA there is a defect in H^+ ion secretion in distal tubule and collecting duct, reduced formation of carbonic acid and CO_2, and urine pH will be above 5.8 to 6.0 for $NaHCO_3$ loss.
     Serum: **Low K, low HCO_3, low Na, low Ca⁻, low pH; high Cl,** normal osmolarity.
     Urine: High K, high HCO_3, high Na, high Ca, high pH; **low Cl.**

83. Mineralocorticoid deficiency causing RTA (renal tubular acidosis): This is due to **reduced**

production of aldosterone and **reduced distal tubular response to aldosterone,** resulting in **high K,** which **inhibits NH4⁺ excretion** in urine.

Serum: **High K, high Cl,** low pH.
Urine: Low K, low Cl, high pH.
It could be due to **a disease of the adrenal gland** (Addison disease, congenital adrenal hyperplasia, primary hypoaldosteronism) **where aldosterone production is reduced,** normal renal function, loss of Na in urine and **increased renin** secretion. **In kidney disease** (interstitial damage and destruction of juxtaglomerular apparatus), there is **decreased** renin secretion and compromised renal function.
In type IV RTA is due to distal tubular unresponsiveness to aldosterone **(Pseudohypoaldosteronism),** plasma renin and aldosterone are high, **normal** renal function and loss of Na in urine.
TREATMENT: Diuretics and or kayexalate (polystyrene sulfonate resin).

Treatment for proximal and distal RTA:
a.   Distal: NaHCO₃ (1-3 mEq/kg) + k (2mEq/kg).
b.   Proximal: NaHCO₃ (5-15 mEq/kg) + k (4-10 mEq/kg).

84.   Characteristic pathologic feature in Hemolytic uremic syndrome: Endothelial cell damage of capillary and arteriole, resulting in the thickening of the wall and narrowing of the lumen. **Microangiopathy in glomeruli and arteriole** (more than 50% of the cases).

85.   **Most common** presentation of sickle cell anemia: **Gross or microscopic** hematuria. Glomeruli is enlarged with dilated capillary loops.

86.   Treatment for renal oxalosis: **Nonspecific.** Pyridoxine and plenty of water.

87.   Clinical manifestation of **different RTA:**
a.   **Isolated** proximal, **distal RTA: Most common feature is growth failure** at the end of the first year.
b.   **Secondary** form for proximal and distal type: Growth failure and clinical picture of other disease.
c.   **Mineralocorticoid deficiency:** Present as kidney disease.

88.   **Basic defect** in Fanconi syndrome: **Failure of reabsorption** of glucose, bicarbonate, amino acid, Na, K, calcium, uric acid in **growth retardation, rickets. osteomalacia, polyuria.**

89.   **Defect in** nephrogenic diabetes insipidus: **Lack of responsiveness of distal tubule and collecting duct to vasopressin.** It is **X-linked recessive** in male child, **present at birth with failure to thrive, constipation,** vomiting, fever, **dehydration due to polyuria,** which results in **dilation** of renal collecting system, ureter, bladder.

Laboratory: Diluted urine (low specific gravity 1002-1006, low osmolarity); serum is high in Na and cl.
TREATMENT: Low solute diet, plenty of fluid, chlorothiazide diuretic; if **no response,** then **indomethacin** which stimulates water absorption in distal tubule and collecting duct.
Genetic counseling: Mother and 50% of sisters are carriers of the disease.

90. **Stag horn kidney stone** is due to: **Cystinuria.** Showed signs of ureteral colic or obstruction at birth, which occurs mostly in the 2nd decade of life. Cystine and uric acid stones form in **acid urine. TREATMENT:** Keep the **urine alkaline, D-penicillamine** which forms cystine-penicillamine complex which is highly soluble.

91. A child shows signs of **episodic gross hematuria, sensorineural deafness.**

    Most likely diagnosis: Alport syndrome (hereditary nephritis, deafness, ocular anomaly like cataract). Most common presentation is **asymptomatic microscopic hematuria.** X-linked dominant, it is the **most common hereditary renal disease,** marked by thickening of glomerular basement membrane and glomerular sclerosis. Urinalysis shows RBC, protein, pus cells.
    Biopsy of kidney confirms the diagnosis.
    TREATMENT: Dialysis or renal transplant.

92. **Benign or idiopathic familial hematuria:** Most common presentation **is asymptomatic microscopic hematuria,** occasionally gross hematuria then only proteinuria found. Electron microscope shows thinning of glomerular basement membrane. Biopsy confirms the diagnosis to rule out other diseases but it is **not** necessary until the occurrence of proteinuria, hypertension and poor renal function. **No** treatment. **Good Prognosis.**

93. **Chromosomal location of adult polycystic kidney:** Chromosome 16 p. **This disease is rare** in children so there is no need to discuss further.

94. **Medullary cystic disease** or Nephronophthisis: **Autosomal recessive,** this cyst is the dilatation of distal tubule and collecting duct. Some children do well until they develop end stage renal disease, or may shows signs of proximal RTA, polyuria, polydipsia, sodium loss.

    Biopsy confirms the disease.
    TREATMENT: Transplantation if necessary.
    Blond or red hair is present.

95. Most common presentation of **Nail-Patella syndrome: Proteinuria.** Autosomal dominant, showed signs of **hypoplastic or absence** of nails and patella. Eye problems include ptosis, abnormal eye pigment, glaucoma. **Duplication** of renal collecting system.

96. **Lipodystrophy:** Shows signs of tall, thin stature, hirsutism. large genitalia, large liver, abnormal glucose metabolism or insulin resistent diabetes mellitus, **hypertension.**

97. A newborn shows signs of **Potter facies,** examination shows **bilateral** renal mass, anuria or oliguria with gross or microscopic hematuria.

    MOST LIKELY DIAGNOSIS: Infantile polycystic kidney (or childhood type). Autosomal recessive, its most **common presentations are bilateral renal mass,** history of oligohydramnios, hypoplastic lungs, hypertension. Death due to progressive renal failure. Initially, do a renal sonogram.
    DIAGNOSIS CONFIRM BY: Biopsy.
    TREATMENT: Is supportive.

98. Most common cause of **acute pre-renal failure** in children: **Renal hypoperfusion.**
    Oliguric renal failure when urine output is **less than 400 cc/m2. Non-oliguric** renal failure output is normal and found in **aminoglycoside nephrotoxicity.**

99. Most common cause of acute **renal and postrenal failure:**
    Renal: Tubular damage.
    Post-renal: Obstruction.

100. Acute renal failure, sign and symptom, laboratory features and treatment: Clinical presentation mostly **due to underlying disease causing the failure,** shows signs of **anuria** (or oliguria), **edema, tachypnea, high K.**
    LABORATORY: High BUN, creatinine, K; low Na, Ca.

	Uosm	Ucr/Pcr	Una	RfI	Fraction Na excretion
Prerenal	>500	>40	<20	< 1	< 1
Renal	<350	<20	>50	>1	>1
Postrenal	<350	<20	>50	>1	>1

RfI (renal failure index) = $\dfrac{UNa\ (mEq/L)}{UCr/PCr}$

FENA (Fraction Na excretion) = $\dfrac{UNa/PNa}{UCr/PCr.}$

TREATMENT: According to the causes of failure.
a. Dehydration: Hydration.
b. Fluid overload:Restrict the fluid to insensible water loss.
c. Hyperkalemia: **Calcium gluconate,** sodium bicarbonate, kayexalate, glucose and insulin.
d. Dialysis: Peritoneal or hemodialysis.
e. Infection: Antibiotics.
*Strict intake and output measure, **body weight** is important.

101. Most common cause of acute renal failure in **newborn:** Congenital **structural** anomaly of kidney and urinary tract or **asphyxia.** Most common sign is **oliguria;** time of presentation is **1st week of life.**

102. Most common cause of **chronic** renal failure in children:**Less than 5 years: Anatomic defect** (dysplasia, hypoplasia, obstruction). **More than 5 years: Glomerular disease** (glomerulonephritis, hemolytic uremic syndrome).

103. End stage renal disease, management: **Ultimate management** is **kidney transplant.** Until the kidney is available, the most useful treatment is **CAPD** which is less effective than hemodialysis. Alternate to CAPD is CCPD (Continuous Cyclic Peritoneal Dialysis). Indication for dialysis is when plasma creatinine level is above 10 mg/dl or over 5 mg/dl in children under 2 years. This patient needs medical, psychological, and social support.

CAPD: Continuous Ambulatory Peritoneal Dialysis.

104. **Most common mechanism of glomerular injury is `hyperfiltration injury'** that means that normal glomeruli increase in size and end up with overfiltration to compensate for damaged glomeruli, one result of which **is that normal glomeruli will be destroyed.** Clinical presentation is nonspecific (growth failure, polyuria, polydipsia, vomiting, lethargy); examination reveals **pale with hypertension.**

> **LABORATORY:** Anemia: high (BUN, creatinine, K, Phosphorus): low (Na, calcium).
> **TREATMENT:**
> a. **Adequate calories for growth** (growth failure occurs when GFR is less than 50% of normal, usually due to inadequate calorie intake).
> b. **Adequate protein** (1-5 gm/kg/d) unless there is nausea, and/or vomiting for high BUN (more than 80 mg/dl).
> c. **Water soluble vitamin.**

105. Renal osteodystrophy in **chronic renal failure:** Chronic renal failure causes ↓ ca, ↑ P, ↑ alkaline phosphatase in serum, and results in secondary hyperparathyroidism which stimulates bone calcium absorption causing osteodystrophy. Hypocalcemia may be due to diminished intestinal absorption due to reduction in 1, 25 (OH)2 cholecalciferol, which normally stimulates gut calcium absorption. 25 (OH)2 cholecalciferol converted to active form 1-25 (OH)2 cholecalciferol in **kidney by 1 hydroxylation.**

> **TREATMENT:**
> a. For hyperphosphatemia: **Low phosphorous milk** (pm 60/40), **oral calcium carbonate** which binds with phosphorous in intestinal tract. Aluminum hydroxide gel can cause **aluminum toxicity (dementia, osteomalacia)** after absorption from intestine. Don't use it.
> b. For hypocalcemia: Oral calcium supplement (Neocalglucon).
> c. **For vitamin D deficiency** in severe renal disease: Give vitamin D3.

106. A child with renal disease with cardiac failure, on digoxin:Digoxin dose should be **reduced to half** because it is mostly excreted by kidney.

107. Gentamicin or other aminoglycoside causing nephrotoxicity: Most common site is **vestibular** damage, next is cochlea.

108. Most common organism for UTI: **E. coli.** Girls are more affected than boys, but when boys are affected that means structural congenital anomaly. Most common presentation of UTI is **asymptomatic,** presenting features are dysuria, urgency, frequency, abdominal pain, enuresis, sometimes hematuria.

> **DIAGNOSIS CONFIRMED BY: Urine culture.**
> Urinalysis shows **more than 5 WBC** in high power field, urine culture positive means growing one organism and more than 100,000 colonies/cc. Blood culture should be done because **pyelonephritis (fever with chill)** may shows signs of sepsis.

109. **Perinephric abscess:** Obliteration of **psoas shadow** in IVP (intravenous pyelography). It

is due to rupture of renal abscess or carbuncle. **TREATMENT:** Surgical drainage, antibiotics.

110. Most common organism in renal abscess: Staph. aureus.

111. Most common cause of **fungal UTI:** Prolonged use of broad spectrum antibiotics. **TREATMENT:** Amphotericin B.

112. **Anterior urethritis: It is a self-limited condition, has a nonspecific** cause, and is accompanied by bloody discharge, and painful urination. **TREATMENT:** Supportive.

113. **Prostatitis:** Most common organism in adolescents is Gonococci. Most common organism in newborns is staph. aureus. Accompanied by dysuria, urgency, and frequency of urination, and nocturia. **TREATMENT:** Antibiotics for both acute and chronic; prostatic massage in chronic only with sitz bath.

114. Most common cause of **neonatal scrotal edema: Unknown. Idiopathic** is most common cause in **early childhood.** A self-limited condition, scrotum is swollen, firm, and pink.

115. Most common association in **epididymitis:** UTI. Treatment of epididymitis: bed rest, **elevate the scrotum,** sitz bath, antibiotics. In acute state, cooling is preferred. Sterility occurs in bilateral cases.

116. Testicular torsion: Most common in children under **6 years of** age, it is accompanied by sudden onset of vomiting, acute **pain and swelling of scrotum, absence of cremasteric** reflex (empty inguinal canal found in torsion, but it is full in obstructed hernia), **blue dot sign** over the testis (torsion of appendices more common in patients between the ages of 7 to 13 years). **Above 13 years, most common cause of testicular pain is epididymitis.** Where there is history of sexual activity or UTI, urinalysis shows WBC. **Diagnosis of torsion** is to be confirmed by **testicular scan, which shows diminished uptake in testicular torsion.**

    TREATMENT: Surgery (detorsion and fixation in scrotum) should be done within 6 hours of torsion, so 90% of testis can be saved. If it is done later, testis will be **infarcted which would require removal and contralateral** orchiopexy. If **torsion of appendices** or epididymis occurs, then **the removal of necrotic tissue** will result in cure. **If neonatal torsion occurs in utero or at birth,** it is impossible to to save testes, and the removal of affected testis and orchiopexy of other testes must be done.

117. Most common site of varicocele: (L) side.

118. Neurogenic bladder, management: **Intermittent self-catheterization is most important** to prevent sepsis.

119. **Most common investigation of choice in renal trauma: CT scan.**

120. **Priapism:** Rare. It occurs in **sickle cell disease, trauma** (perineal), leukemia. **Present with swollen glans penis. TREATMENT:** In traumatic cases, perform surgery. In sickle

cell cases, perform hypertransfusion. In leukemia case, perform chemotherapy with local radiation.

121. **Increased GFR** (glomerular filtration rate): Diabetes insipidus, pyelonephritis, diabetes mellitus. Remember, decreased GFR in congenital nephrosis.

122. Features present in hypertensive retinopathy: **Generalized constriction and narrowing of arterioles,** headache, awake at night , facial palsy.

POISONING

1. Mammalian **bites** and organism:
    Human: Streptococci and staphylococci.
    Dog: Pasteurella multocida.
    Cat: Pasteurella multocida, diphtheroids, staph. epidermidis.

2. **Fetal alcohol syndrome** and characteristics:
    a. **Symmetrical growth deficiency:** length, weight and head circumference less than 5%.
    b. Facial features: **Thin upper lip,** micrognathia, short palpebral fissure, epicanthic folds, maxillary hypoplasia.
    c. **Ventricular septal** defect.
    d. Abnormalities of joints and extremities.
    e. Directly related to amount of **absolute alcohol consumed. Safe** amount of absolute alcohol is **1 1/3 oz (2 drinks/day).**
    f. **In first 72 hours,** newborn develops **hyperactivity,** tremor, seizure; followed by lethargy then normal behavior.
    g. Hypoglycemia, ketoacidosis may present.
    h. Placental transfer of **zinc and amino acids** reduced.
    i. **Severe developmental** delay.

3. A child shows signs of **respiratory depression, has decreased bowel sounds, bullous skin lesion** after ingestion of some pills (unknown):

    DIAGNOSIS: Barbiturate intoxication.
    TREATMENT: First ventilation and oxygenation, then charcoal, alkaline diuresis, dialysis, or hemoperfusion if necessary. (Remember Barbiturate: **Bullous** lesion).

4. Effect of **cigarette smoking** in pregnancy: Baby's birth weight is approximately **200 gm less** than normal. It may increase the incidence of sudden infant death syndrome (SIDS).

5. **Lead toxicity** and **characteristics:**
    a. Earliest symptom is hyperirritability; other features anorexia, abdominal **colic,**

constipation. Patient **later** showed signs of **acute encephalopathy** e.g: vomiting, alteration of mental states, seizure, cerebral edema, lead level is more than 100 ug/dl. Severity of symptom **does not always** depend on the lead level.

b. **Hypochromic microcytic** anemia present.

c. Elevated serum lead and FEP level. (**normal** lead = 5 to 25 ug/dl, FEP = 70 $\pm$ 22).

d. X-ray abdomen: Radio opaque **flecks** indicate recent ingestion.
   X-ray long bone: Increased **metaphyseal density** due to chronic lead storage.

e. **MANAGEMENT** :
   i. **Separate** the child from the source.
   ii. **Calcium EDTA** which initially mobilizes tissue lead level, so serum lead level increases initially. It is used when lead level between 50 to 90.
   iii. BAL: **Very toxic,** it helps in excretion of lead. Used when lead level is more than 90 μg/dl.

f. Side effects of drugs used:
   Ca EDTA: Hypercalcemia, high BUN, kidney damage.
   BAL: Hypertension, vomiting, tachycardia and hemolysis in G6PD deficient patient.

g. Increased incidence of learning disorder.

6. A child shows signs of severe hypotonia, generalized rash, photophobia, diarrhea, rectal prolapse. On exam: Lax ligaments; initially tips of finger, nose, toes are pink with some areas of ischemia.

   Diagnosis: Chronic mercury poisoning (Acrodynia).
   TREATMENT: BAL.
   (*In acute poisoning, child shows signs of severe bloody diarrhea, vomiting, gingivitis, esophagitis).
   TREATMENT: BAL.

7. **An abdominal X-ray of a child showing multiple radiopaque tablets/material: Iron ingestion.** It has 4 phases:

   (6-12 hrs) Phase 1: Local G.I. irritation causes hematemesis, melena, abdominal pain.
   (12-36 hrs) Phase 2: Iron accumulates in liver mitochondria, metabolic effect.
   (12-48 hrs) Phase 3: Hepatic damage, hypoglycemia, increases prothrombin time.
   Phase 4: Pyloric stenosis and scarring.
   TREATMENT: Deferoxamine; emesis, lavage. Deferoxamine should be continued as long as urine color is pink; discontinue chelation, when urine is normal color.

8. **Most common** organ damaged by acetaminophen toxicity: **Liver.**

9. **First sign of liver** damage: Increased prothrombin time.

10. **Alkali or caustics** ingestion: History of caustic ingestion and shows signs of **swallowing** difficulty, **drooling heavily,** chest pain. On exam: **Absence** of oral or pharyngeal lesion **does not** rule out esophageal damage, so esophagoscope is necessary.
    TREATMENT: Mouth lesion needs to be washed with **water.** Keep NPO until esophagoscope is done.
    * If there is no emesis, **no** lavage should be done.

11. Drugs and effects:
    Cholinergic (e.g., Acetylcholine): Miosis, salivation, loose stool, bradycardia.
    Anti-cholinergic (e.g., Atropine): Mydriasis, dry mouth, constipation, tachycardia, and blurred vision.
    Tricyclic antidepressants (Anticholinergic): Drowsiness alternates with agitation; convulsion, premature ventricular contraction plus above mentioned anticholinergic effects.
    TREATMENT: Physostigmine; for premature ventricular contraction, use lidocaine.

12. **Most common** complication of Hydrocarbon ingestion: Hypoxia.

13. **Mushroom** poisoning:
    Cholinergic effect e.g., Increase salivation, miosis, diplopia, abdominal pain, bradycardia.
    TREATMENT: Atropine.

14. **Salicylate intoxication: First respiratory alkalosis then metabolic acidosis.** Respiratory alkalosis is due to **direct effect** of salicylate on respiratory center, and metabolic acidosis is due to **accumulation of lactic and organic acids** secondary to alteration of **Krebs cycle.**

    Sign and symptom: **Hyperpnea** is **most** important; **hyperpyrexia,** vomiting, lethargy.
    Tx: **Sodium bicarbonate;** emesis, charcoal, lavage as indicated.

15. Treatment of acetaminophen toxicity: Acetylcysteine; hemodialysis if necessary.

16. **Shell fish poisoning: Burning sensation** inside the mouth; **numbness** in mouth, extremities; dysphagia, ataxia.

17. **Botulism** food poisoning: Due to **clostridium botulinum. Honey** is important source of infection. Infant showed signs of **floppyness, constipation,** difficulty in sucking, swallowing.

18. **Salmonella** food poisoning: The **most common food** poisoning in U.S.A. **Most common** type is S. typhimurium. **Most commonly** infected animal is **the pig.**

    Signs and symptoms: Begins after 12-18 hours after food ingestion, vomiting, diarrhea contain mucous, **blood, pus.**
    DIAGNOSIS: By positive stool culture.
    TREATMENT: Fluid; antibiotics un-necessary. They only prolong carrier state.

19. **Staphylococcal food poisoning:** This is second most common organism for food poisoning in U.S.A. (* **The first is Salmonella**). Staphylococcus release **enterotoxin.** Symptoms may begin as **early as 1/2 hour,** usually 3-6 hour.
    Signs and symptoms: Abdominal **cramps, diarrhea, vomiting, fever,** and hypotensive **shock.**
    TREATMENT: Fluid.

20. Aluminium intoxication: Causes encephalitis and osteomalacia. Warrants chelation therapy.
    ** P.O. Al(OH)2 gel does not increase aluminium intoxication.

HISTIOCYTOSIS, SARCOIDOSIS, AMYLOIDOSIS

1. Eosinophilic Granuloma or **Histiocytosis X:** Autosomal recessive.
    Three different clinical manifestations in three **different age** groups.
    a. **Eosinophilic granuloma: Older** age group, most commonly involved organ is **bones,** particularly **the skull,** long bones, spine resulting **in osteolytic lesion.**
    b. Hand Schuller Christian syndrome: **Younger** age group, **most** commonly involved organs are **bones (skull,** long bones, spine), **soft tissue** (seborrheic dermatitis, petechial hemorrhage with normal platelet count).
    c. Letterer-Siwe syndrome: In infant, **it is a rapidly progressive and fatal disease.** **The most commonly** involved part is **soft tissue** with or without minimal bone involvement, hepatosplenomegaly, lymphadenopathy, jaundice.

    Other **features** are: Exophthalmos, chronic ear discharge, communicating hydrocephalus, **growth retardation, diabetes insipidus, nodular and** cystic changes in lung.

    DIAGNOSIS MADE BY: Tissue biopsy.
    TREATMENT:
    a. Solitary bone lesion: Curettage.
    b. Disseminated disease: Chemotherapy, Prednisone.
    c. Disseminated disease with symptomatic bone lesion: Radiotherapy.
    PROGNOSIS:
    More than 2 years, nonsystemic disease: Good.
    Less than 2 years, nonsystemic disease: Fair.
    Less than 2 years, **systemic** disease: Poor.

2. A child shows signs of characteristic facies like **sculptured nose, alopecia, short stature, severe growth retardation,** big eyes, looks like **an old person,** but **has normal** motor and mental development.
    Diagnosis: Progeria.
    In **infant, progeria** showed signs of scleroderma, prominent nose and cyanosis in midfacial region. **Normal** growth hormone. Patient **dies** due to **atherosclerosis.**

3. **Most commonly** affected organ in **Sarcoidosis: Lungs** (infiltrate, nodule, hilar lymphadenopathy).

4. **Confirmatory diagnosis** of Sarcoidosis by: **Tissue biopsy.**
    (* Other laboratory test: Kveim test;
    Other laboratory finding: **Hypercalcemia, hypercalcuria,** increased protein and globulin.)

5. Sarcoidosis and complication: **Most common obstructive ling disease:** blindness.

6. **Most common** procedure to diagnose **Amyloidosis:** Rectal biopsy **(first choice).**

7. **Most commonly** affected organ in **Amyloidosis: Kidney** (Nephrotic syndrome, renal failure), (other findings: hepatosplenomegaly, renal vein thrombosis.)

8. **Most common** cause of **death** in Amyloidosis: Renal failure.
    (* Amyloidosis when associated with **myeloma,** then **monoclonal protein,** always present in serum. **Bence Jones Proteinuria** can occur).

SIDS

1. SIDS and characteristics: **Increased** incidence **from 2 to 3 months** of age, **winter** months, **male** child, **during sleep,** between **midnight to 9 am, premature** birth, **low birth weight, apnea, strong family history of** SIDS, **poor socioeconomic** class, **crowded living. Cigarette smoking in pregnancy may increase the incidence of SIDS. Suffocation** may be one important etiologic factor in SIDS, the actual cause is **unknown. No** increased incidence in twins or triplets, monozygotic or dizygotic twins.
    Monitor: Cardiorespiratory monitor, apnea monitor.

EYE AND ENT

1. What should a pediatrician do for a child present with eye trauma? **Patch** the eye and **refer child to ophthalmologist.**

2. Eye injury and features:
    a. Blunt trauma causes fracture of the **orbit.**
    b. **'Blow-out fracture'** means fracture of **floor** of the orbit resulting **extraocular** muscle entrapment causing **diplopia** and **restriction** of eye movement. _upward._

3. **Cherry red spot** found in: **Tay-Sachs disease,** Sandhoff disease, generalized gangliosidosis, Niemann-Pick disease, metachromatic leukodystrophy.

4. A child shows signs of **convulsion** in emergency room. On examination **symmetrical superficial bruises are** noted on the body and on the back. **Denies** history of trauma or any child abuse. Normal growth and history of development is normal.

    MOST LIKELY DIAGNOSIS: Child abuse.
    Eye examination shows bilateral retinal hemorrhage, head CT scan shows **subdural hematoma. MANAGEMENT:** Social service involvement, neurology and neurosurgical evaluation to control seizure and reduce intracranial pressure.

5. **Most common cause** of orbital cellulitis in children: Paranasal sinusitis.

6. **Most common organism** of orbital cellulitis: Staphylococcus aureus.

7. **Most common way to manage** orbital cellulitis: Hospital admission and I.V. antibiotics.

8. **Important clinical findings** in orbital cellulitis: Proptosis (bulging eye), chemosis (edema of conjunctiva).

9. To prevent **eye complication** in diabetes **the most important** factor: To **control the disease well** rather than limit its duration. (Proliferative retinopathy means neovascularization and proliferation, more serious and active than non-proliferative type).

10. Retinal finding in tuberous sclerosis: Phakomata (yellowish, cystic, multiple nodule).

11. A child shows signs of **difficulty in seeing** at night. On examination the child is found to have **loss of peripheral vision.**
    MOST LIKELY DIAGNOSIS: Retinitis pigmentosa (**First symptom** is **difficult night vision).**
    AR, AD, X.
    First sign of Retinoblastoma: Leukocoria or **cat's eye reflex.**
    Retinopathy of prematurity, **most common** important factor: **Hyperoxia.**

12. **Most common cause** of **congenital glaucoma:** Developmental defect and **blockage of angle** of **anterior chamber** with residual mesodermal tissue. **TREATMENT:** Surgery.

13. **Most common tumor of optic nerve** in children: **Optic glioma.** (Associated with **neurofibromatosis;** usual presentation is **loss of vision,** proptosis, but histologically it is **a benign lesion).**

14. **Retinal finding** in **subacute** bacterial endocarditis: **Roth spots** (hemorrhage with white center).

15. **Retinal finding** in **hypertension:** Cotton wool patch flame-shape hemorrhage, papilledema.

16. **Most common** cause of **retinal detachment** in children: Trauma.
    Rubella ⇒ Salt & Pepper

17. **Most common** retinal finding in **Toxoplasmosis: Chorioretinitis.** c macula affected

18. **Upward and outward (posterior)** dislocation of lens: Marfan syndrome.

19. **Downward and inward (anterior)** dislocation of lens: Homocystinuria. (Child shows signs of dislocation of lens in **anterior chamber** with Marfanoid feature means **Homocystinuria).**

20. Subluxation of lens: Ehlers-Danlos syndrome.

21. Characteristics of **lens and different diseases:**

DISEASES	LENS (cataract)
Rubella	Dense, pearly nuclear cataract.
Galactosemia	Oil droplet cataract.

Diabetes mellitus	Snow flake cataract.
Wilson disease	Sunflower cataract.
Steroid induced	Posterior subcapsular cataract.

22. **Most common** cause of **congenital cataract: Congenital Rubella.**

23. **Most common** congenital anomaly in congenital **Rubella: PDA** (Patent Ductus Arteriosus).

24. **Most common** cause of **interstitial Keratitis:** Congenital **syphilis.** → salt & pepper

25. **Most common** cause of **corneal ulcer: Trauma.**

26. **Dendritic Keratitis** characteristic of: Herpes.

27. **Keratoconus** or conical cornea: Down syndrome.

28. **Most common** cause of **ophthalmia neonatorum:** Gonococcal infection.

29. **Inclusion blennorrhea** commonly occurs in: Chlamydia conjunctivitis.

30. **Keratoconjunctivitis** with **preauricular adenopathy** found in: **Adenovirus** type 8.

31. Eye finding in Teacher Collins syndrome: Coloboma (cleft) of eyelid.

32. **Dry eye** (Alacrima) due to: Familial glucocorticoid deficiency. Familial dysautonomia (Riley-Day syndrome). After Steven Johnson syndrome.

33. A **newborn** shows signs of initial **tearing** from one eye with some mucopurulent eye discharge later develops:
    What is the diagnosis: Dacryocystitis (inflammation of nasolacrimal duct mostly due to obstruction in newborn).
    TREATMENT: Massage of the sac and antibiotic eye drop. ointment.

34. Chalazion (Eye). Granulomatous inflammation of meibomian gland. **TREATMENT: Excision.** If warm compress fail

35. **Hordeolum:** Infection of the gland of eyelid; most common organism is Staph, aureus.
    TREATMENT: Warm compress, topical antibiotic; surgical incision and drainage if necessary. (External hordeolum is **stye.** If the child shows signs of **recurrent stye,** rule out **immune deficiency).** Zeiss glands

36. **Congenital Ptosis: Most common** cause is faulty development of levator muscle or its nerve supply. **Autosomal dominant.** Surgical correction can be delayed until 3 yrs. of age.

37. **Opsoclonus** (multidirectional, nonrhythmic eye movement): Most commonly seen in **encephalitis. First sign** in **neuroblastoma.**

38. Nystagmus (Horizontal or vertical, **rhythmic** eye movement): Cause of **congenital** nystagmus is **unknown.** It may be familial. **Acquired** nystagmus requires **immediate** investigation to rule out cerebellar, cerebral, and brain stem diseases.

39. **Spasmus nutans:** A **triad** which includes: Pendular nystagmus, nodding of head, torticollis. **Unknown** cause, **benign, self-**limited disease. Sometimes optic glioma mimics nystagmus of spasmus nutans.

40. Different **syndromes** and **cranial nerves** involvement:

Syndrome	Cranial nerve
Parinaud syndrome	3rd
Moebius syndrome	7th and 6th
Duane syndrome	3rd and 6th
Gradenigo syndrome	5th and 6th

Benign 6th nerve palsy is a **benign** condition, but any **other cranial nerve** palsy **indicates** increased intracranial pressure, tumor, meningitis.

41. **Horner syndrome (oculosympathetic paresis):** Ipsilateral miosis, mild ptosis and enophthalmos. **COCAINE TEST:** It **dilates** the **normal** pupil but in Horner syndrome pupil **will not dilate** or dilate poorly.

42. **Strabismus or squint:**
Esotropia: Inward deviation of eye.
Exotropia: Outward deviation of eye.
Types of strabismus: **Two.**
Paralytic (noncombatant): Less common, indicates increased intracranial pressure.
Non-paralytic (comitant):   **Most common** type of congenital strabismus.
TREATMENT: The goal is to bring the **best possible vision** by lens or by surgical correction. Amblyopia (blindness) needs urgent treatment with occlusion therapy (covering of the eyes).

43. Heterochromia (two irises have different colors, or one iris has two different color): Autosomal dominant, found in **Waardenburg** syndrome **(has white forelock)** in **congenital** type; **acquired** type due to trauma, bleeding, infection.

44. **Aniridia** (absence of iris) found in: Wilms tumor.

45. **Dyslexia** (reading disability due to **cortical** primary or developmental defect): Need ophthalmologic evaluation.

46.   **Amaurosis:** Means partial or total loss of vision.

47.   Retinal changes in syphilis: **Salt and pepper** appearance. like Rubella

48.   Sipple syndrome (mucosal neuroma syndrome): Autosomal dominant, **Marfanoid** features, hypotonia. Higher association with **medullary thyroid carcinoma.**

DERMATALOGY

1.   **Infantile Acne:** Unknown etiology, mostly found in **face,** is due to hypersensitive response of end organ to hormones. Acne usually disappears within weeks or months. No **treatment** is necessary but in severe cases use **benzoyl peroxide gel.**

2.   **Acne vulgaris:** Due to inflammation of sebaceous gland.
     TREATMENT:
     a.   Topical Benzoyl peroxide gel, vitamin A acid.
     b.   Systemic: Tetracycline or erythromycin.
     (Do not use Tetracycline which can cause damage to teeth and deform bones, until the child is at least 8 years old).

3.   **Steroid induced acne:** Folliculitis due to systemic or local application of steroid, usually present **above the diaphragm level** (chest, upper back, neck, face, upper extremity, **except the scalp). TREATMENT:** Discontinue steroid; **may** respond to benzoyl peroxide gel and vitamin A acid.

4.   **Androgen induced acne:** It may present in child with **congenital adrenal hyperplasia.**

5.   **Scabies: Most common** mode of transmission is **direct** contact. Organism is Sarcoptes Scabie, an **extremely pruritic** lesion. Most common site of involvement is **inter-digital space.**
     TREATMENT: 1% Lindane over entire body except head (unless affected), then wash it off after 6 to 8 hours. Treatment may be repeated after 1 week. Safety to use in children is controversial. All family members should be treated, **if affected.** Persistent pruritus **after treatment** does **not** mean inadequate treatment, but shows **hypersensitivity** reaction to the **dead mite.**

6.   Treatment of pediculosis:
     Pediculous capitis: Lindane, **pyrethrin.**
     Pediculous pubis: Lindane.
     DIAGNOSIS MADE BY: Nits on hairshaft than louse.
     Pediculous **pubis** in children (nits attached to body hair if there is no pubic hair) occur through sexual activity. So always **rule out sexual abuse, if possible.**

7.   **Papular urticaria:** Due to insect bite. Usually shows signs of **pruritic hyperpigmented papule,** over the extremities and trunk. There is history of insect bites.

TREATMENT: Antihistamine, soothing lotion; steroid locally in severe cases.

8. **Most common** organism in **folliculitis:** Staph aureus, an infection of hair follicle.

9. **Most common** organism in **Bullous impetigo:** Staph aureus, a bullous skin lesion.

10. **Warts:** DNA virus, showed signs of dome-shaped papule with central umbilication and cheesy material inside. **TREATMENT:** First use **Salicylic and lactic acid** locally; if no response, then try liquid nitrogen or electrocautery, which is painful. It sometimes disappears spontaneously, but spreads.

11. **Candida albicans infection in vagina:** It can occur in adolescent girl who used **antibiotic,** corticosteroid, or oral contraceptive for a long period, or in diabetes mellitus and in pregnant patient. **TREATMENT:** Nystatin vaginal tablet.

12. **Tinea infection, common organism and treatment:**

Tinea capitis	Trichophyton tonsurans and Microsporum audouinii	Oral griseofulvin.
Tinea corporis	Trichophyton rubrum	Topical antifungal; severe cases oral griseofulvin.
Tinea cruris	Epidermophyton floccusum	Topical therapy clotrimazole or miconazole.
Tinea pedis (Athlete's foot)	Trichophyton rubrum	Topical therapy as above.
Tinea's unguium (nail)	Trichophyton rubrum	Oral griseofulvin.
Tinea nigra palmaris	Cladosporium Wernicke	Whitfield ointment.

DIAGNOSIS : Made by **KOH preparation;**
Woodlamp examination in Tinea capitis, **positive florescence in Microsporum,** but negative in Trichophyton.

13. **Swimming pool granuloma:** Formed by **traumatic abrasion** of skin, then infected by **M. marinum** which is **atypical mycobacterium.** It forms papule, nodule around ankle, knee area.
    DIAGNOSIS: Biopsy of the lesion.
    TREATMENT: First antituberculous drugs; if resistant then cycloserine, ethionamide.

14. **Ritter disease** (Staphylococcal scalded skin syndrome): Due to **exotoxin** produced by Staph aureus. Usually shows signs of **flaccid bullae filled with clear liquid,** skin tenderness, erythema, fever. **Positive Nikolsky sign** means separation of epidermis with minimal skin touching. **TREATMENT:** Nafcillin.

15. **Most common** organism in **Blistering distal dactylitis:** Beta hemolytic Streptococci, an

infection in **palmer** aspect of **distal** finger.

16. **Most common** organism in **Ecthyma:** Beta hemolytic Streptococci which resembles impetigo.

17. **Impetigo contagiosa:** Caused by **group A beta hemolytic** Streptococci, usually shows signs of erythematous macule, vesicle, pustule with **crust formation.** Streptococci colonize in skin. **Different strain** of Streptococci cause **skin** impetigo and **pharyngeal** infection. Superimposed infection with **Staph.** is common.
TREATMENT: Penicillin for streptococci; If Staph. infection, then dicloxacillin; Penicillin allergic patients use erythromycin. Early initiation of treatment for impetigo caused by nephritogenic strain does not reduce **acute glomerulonephritis.**

18. **Mucocele or mucous retention cyst:** When present on the floor of the mouth it is known as **ranulas. TREATMENT:** Excision.

    A child shows signs of **small midline mass** on the **floor of the mouth always suggests** of **ectopic thyroid.** It may be the **child's only functioning** thyroid.
    DIAGNOSIS: Thyroid scan.
    TREATMENT: Keep **that mass for the rest of the patient's life.**

19. **Aphthous stomatitis** (canker sore): Recurrent multiple painful ulcers in mouth. Severe form results in **periadenitis aphthae. TREATMENT:** Xylocaine, benadryl, corticosteroid **administered locally.** (Xylocaine may cause convulsion.)

20. **Twenty nail dystrophy:** Fragility, notching, and discoloration of nails, caused by **lichen planus; a self-limited** disease. **No treatment** is required.

21. **Alopecia areata: Idiopathic, round or oval patches** of hair loss. In alopecia **totalis** there is total hair loss. **TREATMENT:** Fluorinated steroid, intradermal injection of systemic steroid.

22. **Most common** cause of **alopecia in newborn:** Positional (place of contact of head with bed.)

23. **Trichotillomania:** Due to compulsive **pulling, breaking** of hair. **Most common** site is crown of head. **Hairs** have **different length's** and **blunt end. Sometimes** diagnosis is difficult then do biopsy. **TREATMENT:** Try to persuade the **patient to stop it.** Sometimes the patient needs psychiatric consultation.

24. Toxic alopecia: Due to radiotherapy and chemotherapy. Hair loss **is diffuse,** hairs are **dystrophic,** and breakage of **hair shaft occurs.**

25. **Traction alopecia:** Due to **tight braiding** or **pony tail It is reversible. TREATMENT:** Try to persuade the patient not to braid hair or wear it in a pony tail.

26. **Most common** cause of **localized** hypertrichosis: Familial.

27. **Drugs** causing hypertrichosis: Minoxidil, diazoxide, androgen, corticosteroid, dilantin.

28. Metabolic causes of alopecia: Homocystinuria, acrodermatitis enteropathica.

29. **Most common** form of mastocytosis in children: Urticaria pigmentosa.

30. Miliaria or prickly heat: Due to retention of **sweat gland** due to hot and humid weather.
    TREATMENT: Cooling the patient.

31. Subcutaneous fat necrosis: Due to **inflammation of adipose** tissue due to trauma,
    asphyxia, hypothermia. Usually present in buttock, back, upper extremities, thigh, face. It is
    irregular, farm nodule with violet color. It is **a self-limited, benign condition.**
    TREATMENT: None.

32. **Scleroderma neonatorum: A serious** manifestation of disease like sepsis, pneumonia.
    There is **a sudden onset** of **diffuse hardening** of **cold and nonpitting skin.**
    TREATMENT: Treat the underlying cause.

33. **Ehlers-Danlos syndrome: A connective tissue** disorder. The skin is **hyperextensible**
    when pulled and **snaps back** to normal position. Fragility of the skin causes bleeding,
    ecchymosis.

34. **Granuloma annulare:** Not a scaly lesion (like **tinea)** but are firm, **erythematous,**
    papulonodules which enlarge to form **a ring** with a central **atrophic** area occurring **mostly**
    on dorsum of hands feet, as well as trunk, scalp. **Etiology:** Unknown.
    TREATMENT: Corticosteroid (topical or injection into lesion).

35. **Most common** light-induced photosensitivity in children: Acute sunburn reaction.

36. **Essential fatty acids deficiency:** Found in newborn or child who is on **total parenteral**
    nutrition (fat free diet). It is due to deficiency of linoleic, linolenic, and arachidonic acids.
    Most common presentation is **generalized scaly dermatitis;** increased bacterial infection.
    TREATMENT: Give essential fatty acids (intralipid).

37. Syndromes associated with lcthyosis:
    a. **Refsum syndrome: Autosomal recessive,** deficiency of enzyme alpha decarboxylase
       which cannot breakdown the phytic acid which is present in chlorophyll (present in
       green plants). Usually appears as **retinitis pigmentosa,** anosmia (no smell),
       polyneuritis, paralysis, bony abnormalities.
       TREATMENT: Avoid green vegetables.
    b. **Sjogren-Larssen syndrome: Autosomal recessive. Three** major presentations are
       mental retardation, ichthyosis, spastic diplegia; also degeneration of retinal
       pigment. Most patients are **wheel-chair bound.**
    c. **Rud syndrome:** Shows signs of **sexual infantilism, epilepsy,** ichthyosis, mental
       retardation.
    d. **Chondrodysplasia punctata:** Pathognomonic defect is **stippled epiphyses** in
       cartilage of skeleton; **short femur, humorous,**

Conradi Hunermann syndrome: Autosomal dominant.
Rhizomelic dwarfism: Autosomal recessive.

38. **Photosensitivity** and **deferent disease: Due to sunlight** or **artificial light. Avoidance of sunlight** is **the best** management.

   a. Acute sunburn reaction: Erythematous lesion, severe tenderness, pain, edema, blisters over the **exposed** part of the body. Child does **not** look sick.
   TREATMENT: Cool tap water, lotion topical, corticosteroid.
   Harmful effect of sunburn: Carcinoma, melanoma, premature aging, actinic keratosis. Physician should advice the family to use **sun screen lotion** to avoid those problems.

   b. Congenital erythropoietic porphyria: **Autosomal recessive,** shows signs of **bullous** eruption, skin **fragility,** increased pigmentation and keratosis; **hemolytic anemia, red urine,** enlarged spleen.

   c. Erythropoietic protoporphyria: **Autosomal dominant,** shows signs of itching, burning followed by erythema, edema, vesicle **(not bullous).** Increased **protoporphyrin** in RBC, serum and urine.
   TREATMENT: Of both porphyria. Avoidance of sunlight, beta carotene lotion.

   d. **Cockayne syndrome:** Autosomal recessive, **photosensitivity skin reaction, eye** (cataract, optic atrophy, abnormal retinal pigment), premature aging, dwarfism, mental retardation. (It **mimics** progeria which has **no** skin or eye problems).

   e. **Xeroderma pigmentosa:** Autosomal recessive, DNA damage by ultraviolet light, showed signs of scaling, bullae, crust, erythematous skin lesion over **exposed** areas, eye (photophobia, lacrimation). When associated with dwarfism, hypogonadism, microcephaly and retardation is called **De Sanctis-Cacchione syndrome.** Xeroderma pigmentosa is a serious disorder. Genetic counseling and amniocentesis should be done for the appropriate family. **Early malignancy** detection is very important.

   f. **Bloom syndrome:** Autosomal recessive, showed signs of erythema and telangiectasia over the **face in butterfly** distribution, photosensitivity, dwarfism. **Normal** mental status. **Lymphoreticular malignancy** is common sequelae.

   g. **Hartnup disease:** Autosomal recessive showed signs of aminoaciduria, **pellagra-like skin lesion,** cerebellar ataxia, mental retardation.
   TREATMENT: Nicotinamide, avoidance of sunlight.

   h. **Rothmund-Thomson syndrome:** Autosomal recessive, occurs in **infancy,** shows signs of erythema, edema, then increased pigmentation and **telangiectasia,** bullae; short stature, hypogonadism, **cataract,** retardation, bone and dental anomalies.

39. **Pityriasis rosea: Christmas tree pattern** of **herald patch** (solitary oval) skin lesion over the **trunk** (back); **may be** preceded by pharyngitis, joint pain, fever. Rash disappears in few weeks. **TREATMENT:** None.

40. **Seborrheic dermatitis: Cradle cap** (scaly, crusty) lesion **over scalp,** is **most common** manifestation. Lesion also involves face, neck, axilla, diaper area.
Leiner disease: Seborrheic dermatitis with 5th component of complement defect.
Histiocytosis X: Histiocyte infiltrate cause seborrhea-**like** lesion. **TREATMENT:** Topical corticosteroid.

41. **Psoriasis:** Multifactorial, unknown etiology, positive family history and more in girls. Usually shows signs of erythematous papules which combines to form plaques. When treatment fails then plaques become white or silvery scales which upon removal causes pinpoint bleeding **(Auspitz sign). TREATMENT:** Corticosteroid (topical).

42. Nummular **eczema: Rare;** shows signs of **coin-shaped** lesion over the **extensor** surface of extremities. **TREATMENT:** Fluorinated corticosteroid.

43. **Allergic contact dermatitis:** T-cell mediated, shows signs of **characteristic distribution** of lesion **only in the area of contact.** Lesions are **itchy, eczematous, vesicobullous. Poison ivy** or oak or Rhus dermatitis: Due to poisonous plant touching the skin, **linear distribution of vesiculobullous** lesion. Spread of lesion **comes not** from ruptured vesicle, but from **antigen** present under nails, clothing, animal fur.

    TREATMENT: Basically **avoid contact with poisonous plant.**
    a.　Acute contact dermatitis: Corticosteroid (topical), cool compress.
    b.　Chronic contact dermatitis: Fluorinated steroid (topical).
    c.　Bullous lesion of poison ivy: Oral corticosteroid for few days.

44. **Chronic bullous dermatosis of childhood (IgA dermatosis):** Multiple large tense bullae with clear or hemorrhagic fluid over trunk, legs, genitalia etc. **TREATMENT:** Oral sulfapyridine, oral corticosteroid.

45. Dermatitis herpetiformis: Unknown etiology, associated with **celiac sprue. Symmetric** distribution of group of papulovesicular small, tense, itchy, erythematous lesion **over the joints** (knee, shoulder, elbow), scalp and mucous membrane. **TREATMENT:** Oral sulfapyridine.

46. Pemphigus vulgaris: **First** manifestation is oral painful ulcers, then develops **large flaccid bullae on non-erythematous skin.** (In herpes: bullae on **erythematous** base). **Positive** Nikolsky sign: avulsion of epidermis by gentle pressure. **TREATMENT:** Oral corticosteroid.

47. **Acrodermatitis enteropathica:** Autosomal recessive, due to **zinc** deficiency. It occurs when **changing from** breast milk to cow's milk. **Symmetric** distribution of vesicobullous and eczematous **skin** lesion **perioral, acral, perineal, cheeks** area; **eye** findings are photophobia, conjunctivitis; **G.I.** findings are **diarrhea,** stomatitis, glossitis; growth retardation; superimposed bacterial and fungal infection. It is **most likely** due to **diminished absorption** of zinc from **intestine** or deficiency of zinc binding ligand. **TREATMENT:** Zinc sulfate, acetate, gluconate.

48. **Steven-Johnson syndrome:** A serious manifestation of erythema multiforme. Presents with **symmetrical** distribution of skin lesion over **extensor** surface of hands, feet, arms, legs, palm, sole **except the scalp.** Characteristics of **lesion** are macular, papular, nodular, urticarial, central vesicular and **intradermal bleeding. Target or iris** lesion is diagnostic. **TREATMENT:** Systemic or local corticosteroid, mouthwash, glycerin swab in mouth, topical anesthetic (benadryl).

49. **Toxic epidermal necrolysis (Lyell disease):** It is due to **hypersensitivity** reaction to drug, vaccination, infection, radiotherapy. Showed signs of **flaccid** bullae with **positive Nikolsky** sign, **oral lesion,** unable to eat and drink results in **dehydration,** shock due to secondary infection. **TREATMENT:** Antibiotics, hydration.

50. **Erythema multiforme:** Unknown etiology but **most likely** due to **hypersensitivity** reaction to **drugs** (sulfur, penicillin, barbiturate, aspirin, phenacetin, tetracycline), **infections** (mycoplasma, echo-virus, influenza, mumps, **tuberculosis,** diptherea, salmonella), collagen disorder, polio vaccine.

51. **Waardenburg syndrome: White forelock,** deafness, hypopigmentation, heterochromic iris. Autosomal dominant.

52. **Tuberous sclerosis: Autosomal dominant. Most reliable** cutaneous **sign is white leaf macule,** most commonly seen skin mark is **adenoma sebaceum, periungual fibromas; other** findings **are mental retardation,** epilepsy, calcification of brain, **cyst** (of kidney, bone, lung), rhabdomyoma of heart. Adenoma sebaceum is not sebaceous gland tumor but it is **angiofibromas. Cafe-au-lait** spot is present.

53. Chediak-Higashi syndrome: **Autosomal recessive. Photophobia, bluish skin** and hair color, nystagmus, increased liver and spleen, increased susceptibility to infection.

54. **Incontinentia pigmenti acromions (Hypomelanosis of Ito):** Presents with **hypopigmented macule** distributed in a sharply demarcated whorl, streaks, matches over the body. It also presents with **seizure, mental retardation,** asymmetry of extremities, scoliosis.

55. **Vitiligo (hypopigmentation of skin):**
It is found in: hyperthyroidism, hypofunction of adrenal gland, diabetes mellitus, pernicious anemia. **TREATMENT:** Psoralen.

56. **Albinism:** Autosomal recessive. Different types:
    a. Hermansky-Pudlak syndrome: Tyrosinase negative, **bleeding** disorder, low platelet.
    b. Tyrosinase-negative: **White** hair, **white** skin.
    c. Tyrosinase-positive: **Brown** hair, **pink** skin.
    d. Cross-Mckusick-**Breen** syndrome: Tyrosinase positive, **microopthalmia,** spasticity, retardation.
    e. Tyrosinase-variable: **White** hair, **pink** skin.

    In albinism there is **lack of melanin** which protect the skin, so increased chances of **carcinoma** and actinic **keratosis. TREATMENT:** Sun screen lotion.

57. **Incontinentia pigmenti** (Bloch-Sulzberger disease): **X-linked dominant.** Three stages of skin presentation: First erythematous streaks over the extremities, second **vesicle** formation and third **pigment** formation. Other features includes seizure, **microcephaly, retardation, dental** problem and **alopecia.**

58. **Neurofibromatosis** (Von Recklinghausen disease): **Autosomal dominant, cafe-au-lait**

(**hyperpigmented,** macular) spots are **significant** when:
Prepubertal: at least 5 spots and each over 5 mm in diameter.
Postpubertal: at least 6 spots and each over 15 mm in diameter.
Cafe-au-lait spot may not be apparent at birth. At that time look for **crowe sign (freckling in axilla)** and hyperpigmentation over the upper part of chest, groin area.

59. **Leopard syndrome (multiple lentigines syndrome). Autosomal** dominant. **Pulmonary stenosis,** perceptive deafness, **hypertelorism,** genital abnormality.

60. **Ataxia Telangiectasia: Autosomal recessive. Progressive ataxia** indicates **vestibular defect; telangiectasia** (dilated blood vessels) of conjunctiva. Cafe-au-lait spots present, gray hair, scleroderma, nystagmus.

61. **Cutis Marmorata** of newborn: A **benign** condition, present as dilatation of superficial capillaries and veins at birth. **TREATMENT:** None required.

62. **Osler-Weber-Rendu disease** (Hereditary Hemorrhagic Telangiectasia). **Autosomal dominant,** show signs of recurrent epistaxis and, later, **massive bleeding,** which is **the most serious** complication. Bleeding is due to **dilation and rupture** of blood vessels; **normal clotting time. TREATMENT:** Cauterization (chemical or electric).

63. **Klippel-Trenaunay-Weber syndrome: Triad: Hypertrophy** (bone, soft tissue), venous **varicosity, port** wine nevus.

64. **Ectodermal dysplasia:**
Types
a. Anhidrotic or Hypohidrotic: Triad defect
Absence of or reduced **sweating,** abnormal **dentation** (peg shaped teeth), **hypotrichosis** (absence of or less hair in eyebrows and/or eyelashes). Diminished **lacrimation. X-linked recessive disorder.**
DIAGNOSIS CONFIRMED: By **biopsy of palm (or sole).**
Absence of sweat pores which is **decreased** in **carrier** female. Palm has **maximum** concentration of sweat glands.
TREATMENT: Artificial tears for eyes, early dental evaluation, wig when grows up. Do not expose children to high temperatures, because their bodies cannot lose heart.
b. **Hidrotic ectodermal dysplasia (clouston type):** Normal dentition, normal sweating; **hypoplastic nails, hyperkeratosis of palm and sole. Autosomal dominant.**

65. **Port wine Nevus (nevus flammeus, flat hemangioma):** Present at **birth, permanent defect** in development of matured capillaries results in **macular, well-defined, pink or purple color lesion** in skin.
Sturge-Weber Syndrome: Includes port wine nevus in trigeminal area, **seizure, hemiparesis** in opposite side of skin lesion, **same sided** brain **calcification.** It may shows signs of glaucoma. It is also found in **Trisomy 13.**
TREATMENT: Cryosurgery, excision and skin graft.

66. **Kasabach-Merritt syndrome (Thrombocytopenia with cavernous hemangioma). Hemangioma,** which is rapidly progressive, with **thrombocytopenia** due to **destruction**

and sequestration of platelets. Thrombocytopenia and decreased level of consumed clotting factors cause **bleeding** either externally or internally into the organs. **TREATMENT: Corticosteroid orally;** surgery if anatomically feasible.

67. **Strawberry Nevus (capillary hemangioma):** It is bright red, well defined, compressible skin lesion found **mostly** on the **face,** scalp, back, chest. It might present at birth or appear in first few months of life. **Initially** it **increases** in size, then remains the **same** size, finally **reduces** in size. It disappears **in 50% of cases by 5 years, 70% of cases by 7 years, 90% of cases by 9 years** spontaneously. **TREATMENT:** Not required.

68. **EEC syndrome:** Ectrodactyly, ectodermal dysplasia, cleft (lip and palate).

69. **Focal dermal hypoplasia** (Goltz syndrome): Hernia of **fat** through the defective dermis, **X-linked dominant. Most common** bony defect is syndactyly.

70. **Amniotic constriction Band:** A band formed after rupture of amnion, this band **constricts the fetal** parts and can lead to the need for amputation.

71. Name the important tissue structure that can be present in **Thyroglossal cyst: Aberrant thyroid tissue.** It is very important to save thyroid tissue.

72. **Neonatal benign pustular melanosis:** A benign condition in newborns, mostly in blacks, usually present initially as a pustular, then a macular lesion. It disappears within a few days. Gram stain shows **polymorph,** but **no** bacteria. No **treatment** is required.

73. **Mongolian spot:** It has a bluish or slate gray color due to **melanin** containing melanocyte which has stopped migration from neural crest to epidermis. **Most common** site is **presacral** area. Usually **disappears in the first few** years of life.

74. **Cutis Marmorata:** It is **a lacy reticulated** red or blue vascular lesion in the skin of a newborn. **Mostly due** to **hypothermic** environment. It is due to **vasomotor** response. It usually disappears with age maturity. **Persistent** cutis marmorata can be seen in **Trisomy** 21, 18; cornelia de lange syndrome.

75. A newborn shows signs of **pearly white color papular rash** 1-2 mm diameters over the face and on midline of **palate. DIAGNOSIS: MILIA;** called **"Epstein pearls"** when on the palate. Milia can occur at any age.

INFECTIOUS DISEASES

1. In newborns the most **common mode** of transmission of gonococcus: Direct contact in vaginal delivery. (Other mode of transmission through fomites.)

2. In **Tzanck smear** if you see:

      a.   Multinucleated giant cells and balloon cells: Herpes virus infection.

      b.   Acantholytic epidermal cells: Pemphigus.

3.   Most commonly reported infectious disease in U.S.A.: Gonorrhea.

4.   **Most common** presentation of Gonorrhea: Asymptomatic.

5.   **Most common** site of gonococcus infection in newborn: Eye (ophthalmia neonatorum).

6.   **Primary** site of infection with Gonorrhea in **male:** Urethra.

7.   **Primary** site of infection with gonorrhea in female.
      Vulva and vagina: Prepubertal.
      Cervix: Post pubertal.

8.   **Most common** presentation in **male** gonorrhoea urethritis: Purulent urethral discharge and dysuria.

9.   Most common presentation in **female** gonorrhea infection:
      Prepubertal: **Vaginal discharge,** swollen erythematous vulva. May be dysuria.
      Post pubertal: Purulent discharge, dyspareunia, dysuria.

10.   **Most common** presentation in **newborn** gonorrhea: Purulent eye discharge (unilateral or bilateral). **(Sometimes** gonorrhea can present as **mild** discharge, and **chlamydia** can present as **purulent,** so type of discharge will **not** determine the diagnosis.)

11.   **Most common** site of infection involved in **disseminated** gonorrhea infection: **Joints** cause arthritis. (Other infections are carditis, meningitis, dermatitis).

12.   **Most common** site of **cardiac gonococcus** infection: Aortic valve.

13.   **Definitive diagnosis** of gonorrhea: By culture. Gram stain showing gram negative intracellular diplococci in **male** suggests gonorrhea, but in **female that** is **not** enough, because **Mima polymorpha and Moraxella** (normal vaginal flora) have identical appearance.

14.   **Fitz-Hugh-Curtis Syndrome:** The spread of gonococci from uterine tube into peritoneum and over the liver causes right **upper quadrant pain** with acute or subacute **salpingitis.**

15.   **Most frequent** complication of gonorrheal **urethritis in male:** Prostatitis (by local extension).

16.   **Most common** cause of **blindness in newborn:** Gonococcal ophthalmia neonatorum. (Gonorrhea also causes corneal ulcer, opacity, and blindness).

17.   **Prevention** of Gonococcal ophthalmia neonatorum: 1% **silver nitrate** eye drop, erythromycin eye ointment locally into both eyes. It should be given **within 1 hour** after birth.

18. Treatment for Gonococcal infection: Ceftriaxone (because gonocooci are penicillin-resistent). (It is also used in ophthalmia neonatorum.)

19. Patient **allergic to penicillin, treatment** for gonorrhea: **Spectinomycin.**

20. What **other disease** should be ruled out when person has gonorrhea: Syphilis: **conduct serology test immediately.**

21. H. influenzae **types and site of infection: Type ' b'** causes all **serious** diseases (meningitis, epiglottitis). **Nontypable** causes otitis media, chronic lung disease.

22. **Increased H. influenzae** infection occurs in: Day-care center, black child, sickle cell anemia.

23. H. flue vaccine: **when to administer it and what it protects against:** Given around 2 years of age. It only **protect** against H. flue **type b,** which causes meningitis, but **not** against **nontypable** infection, like otitis media and chronic lung disease. H. flue infection occurs mostly in **winter** months.

24. **Most common** cause of **bacterial** meningitis:
Newborn (neonatal age): Group B streptococci.
2 months to 12 years: H. influenzae type b.
Over 12 years: Strep. pneumonia.

25. **Most common complication** of meningitis: Hearing loss. (Always **do a hearing** test after meningitis).

26. **H. flue** meningitis, epiglottis and **antigen-antibody: Cellular antigens** are **genetically different** in two diseases. **Antibody titre** goes up **considerably after epiglottitis,** but **not** in meningitis.

27. **Most common** cause of **septic arthritis and cellulitis** under **2 years of age:** H. influenzae type b. (It is **not** the most common organism for osteomyelitis in this age group).

28. **Most common** type H. influenzae infection in **newborn: Non-typable.**

29. **Prophylaxis for H. influenzae type b** infection: Rifampin prophylaxis should be given to:
    a. Child with the primary **infection** to eradicate nasopharyngeal carrier which was not done by usual antibiotic therapy.
    b. All other children, family members, parents exposed to the infected child.
    c. Children and personnel in day-care center being exposed.
    Dose: 20 mg/kg for 4 days.

30. **Most common** complication of **pertussis:** Pneumonia.

31. Does **newborn** get immunological protection against pertussis from mother **transplacentally: No.**

32. When **newborn** is exposed to pertussis in nursery: Give oral **erythromycin** to prevent infection.

33. **Pertussis and antibiotics** (erythromycin) therapy:
    a. Does **not** shorten paroxysmal stage.
    b. Does **eliminate** or **stop** the disease in **catarrhal** stage.
    c. **Reduces** the **period** of communicability by eliminating nasopharyngeal carrier.

34. **Most common** cause of **death** in pertussis: Pneumonia.

35. **Pertussis:** Organism is B. pertussis which is non-motile, gram negative organism. It is **a highly contagious** disease, most common in patients under 5 years of age, immunization (DPT) helps to reduce the incidence and mortality, but it is protective **only in 70-90% of cases** and **there is no permanent** protection.

    Three **stages** of the disease:
    a. Catarrhal (1-2 week): URI symptom.
    b. Paroxysmal (2-4 week): **Whooping** cough.
       (5 to 10 coughs in one expiration followed by one massive inspiration which causes whoop when air passes through narrow epiglottis.) It is **not** present in all cases of croup.
    c. Convalescent (next 1-2 week): Getting better from whooping cough and vomiting, but cough persists sometimes for months.
    Laboratory: Increased WBC (20,000-40,000) with increased lymphocytes. It is most prominent in end catarrhal and early paroxysmal stages.

36. **Most common** type of E. coli **diarrhea in neonate:** Enteropathogenic E. coli.

37. **Most common** type of E. coli diarrhea in **visitors to Mexico: Enterotoxigenic** E. coli. Not common in U.S.A. It releases enterotoxin.

38. Diarrhea in different types of E. coli infection:
    a. Enteropathogenic: Watery mucous stool, low grade fever, **no blood** in stool, resolves spontaneously.
    b. Traveler's diarrhea Enterotoxigenic: Severe watery stool with **crampy abdominal pain,** vomiting, fever, **no** blood in stool.
    c. **Enteroinvasive: Bloody** mucous diarrheal stool, tenesmus, sudden onset of fever.

39. A **student** expecting to visit **Mexico,** what diarrhea prophylaxis should you advise: Trimethoprim and sulfamethoxazole BID.

40. **Treatment** for E.coli diarrhea: **Most important** is oral or parenteral **hydration.** Do **not** use "over-the-counter" antidiarrheal medicine. **Only infants** with **enteropathogenic** E. coli may be treated **with oral neomycin** therapy. **No antibiotic** necessary in all other conditions.

41. One of the **most common** cause of **bacterial** diarrhea in U.S.A: Salmonella enteritidis; type **E** most common in U.S.A.

42. When salmonella causes **diarrhea** in **large gathering** (e.g. picnic), who is the **carrier:** One of the people(not the food).

43. **Most commonly infected animal** who **is also carrier** of salmonella : Chicken.

44. **Acidic** stomach pH 2.0 can **kill salmonella.**

45. A group of students went to the park for **picnic** in **summer** vacation. **From 8 to 48 hours** after eating (cheese, mushroom, mayonnaise, chicken), most of the students came down **with acute abdominal pain, vomiting, watery loose** stool, in a few instances blood and mucous, **fever (up to 102 degrees).**

    Most likely cause of this episode: **Salmonella food poisoning.** which is most common in late summer and early fall, incubation period **from 8 to 48 hours.** Fever and **chills mean septicemia.** G. I. symptoms.
    TREATMENT: Hydration only. Do not give antibiotic: it does not eliminate Salmonella from G.I. tract.

    Indication of antibiotics: Administer only to those who **can spread** the disease to others, e.g., those **less than 3 months of age, immunodeficient** child, **severely ill child.**
    In **Salmonella septicemia, typhoid (enteric) fever,** or **metastatic infection, antibiotics should be used:**
    Antibiotics: **Chloramphenicol (preferred);** ampicillin, trimethoprim, sulfamethoxazole. (Those who are **resistent** to ampicillin are usually **sensitive** to **chloramphenicol.** Those **resistant to chloramphenicol [less** likely in U.S.A.] **are sensitive to ampicillin and bactrim). Amoxicillin 100 mg/kg/d Q.6.H. is as good as chloramphenicol and better than ampicillin. Chloramphenicol resistant strains should be treated with ceftriaxone and cefoperazone. Some authorities prefer to use ceftriaxone as the initial treatment of choice.**

46. Typhoid bacillus **only infects** people.

47. What is the **most common** source of typhoid fever in U.S.A.: **Chronic human** carrier.

48. **Symptoms** produced by Salmonella typhosa due to: **Endotoxin.**

49. **Salmonella and arthritis:** Salmonella reactive arthritis usually occurs **about 2 weeks** after the **Salmonella diarrhea,** with **polyarticular migratory arthritis in knee or ankle** which is swollen tender. Recurrence, regression, and **sudden exacerbation** of symptoms.
    DIAGNOSIS: Salmonella reactive arthritis.
    CBC: **Elevated ESR,** mildly increased WBC.
    Joint fluid: No pus and no organism.
    Blood: HLA B27 antigen present.

50. A child shows signs of **gastroenteritis, fever (up to 106 degrees),** seizure.
    On examination: **Enlarged liver** and jaundice; **maculopapular rash** over the abdomen and lower part of the chest. **High temperature and low pulse** may be seen together (which seems paradoxical).

MOST LIKELY DIAGNOSIS: Typhoid fever.
Complication: First intestinal **bleeding, then perforation. Septic arthritis** and **osteomyelitis** occur **more in hemoglobinopathies.** Others are pneumonia, encephalopathy, pyelonephritis, meningitis, carditis.

51. Usual **laboratory** features of **typhoid fever:**
Blood: **Blood culture** is positive in **early** part of disease.
Stool and urine culture: Positive in **later** part of disease.
(* In abscess formation, there is **high WBC** count and **low platelet count).**

52. **How to detect** Salmonella **enteric carrier:**
   a. **Positive stool culture,** because such patients excrete a lot of Salmonella in stool (approximately 10^6 - 10^9/gram of stool).
   b. If **negative** stool culture, then do **duodenal aspirate culture** to find out **about biliary excretion of Salmonella.**

53. **Complication** of **chloramphenicol (preferred)** in typhoid fever:
   a. Increase relapse of the disease.
   b. Cannot prevent chronic carrier state.

54. **How to treat chronic carrier:**
   a. High dose of ampicillin for plus probenecid 4-6 weeks.
   b. Cholecystectomy.
   c. Norfloxacin or ciprofloxacin may also be used.

55. **How to control** salmonella infection:
   a. Hand washing, proper sanitary practice for everybody (particularly those carriers who work in the kitchen) and taking care of the patient to prevent person-to-food and person-to-person transmission.
   b. Do **not** give prophylactic antibiotic to those who are exposed to the disease, because it does **not** prevent the disease.

56. **Most common type** of **Shigella infection** in U.S.A.: Shigella flexneri. Most common in American Indian.

57. **Major** source of infection of Shigella: Human. **No** animal carries Shigella. (**Salmonella** source is **chicken).**

58. **Most common mode of** transmission in Shigella: **Fecal-oral route.** Other mode of spreads through contaminated water, food, flies and inanimate objects.

59. **Indication** of giving **typhoid vaccine:**
   a. Close contact of household carrier.
   b. Typhoid outbreak in the community and institution.
   c. Living in or visiting a region where typhoid is endemic due to **contaminated water.**
   (Do not give vaccine to child going either to summer camp or to endemic region.) Dose is 0.5 cc subcutaneously.

60.   **Symptoms** produced by **Shigella** due to: Enterotoxin (diarrhea); endotoxin (systemic symptoms but are **not** common in U.S.A.).

61.   Children between **the ages of 1-4 years** initially **have crampy abdominal pain** and **high fever** for 2 days, then develop **severe diarrhea** (16 stools/day) with **blood and mucous, no vomiting.**
       On examination: **Non-specific lower** abdominal pain.
       Most likely cause of diarrhea: **Shigella.**

       [**Newborn with Shigella** can show signs of it in **three** different ways:
       a.   Asymptomatic carrier.
       b.   Meningitis or sepsis.
       c.   Bloody stool and diarrhea.]
       DIAGNOSIS CONFIRMED: Positive stool culture.
       (Stool contains RBC, leukocyte: **not** diagnostic.
       Leukocyte in stool can be present in salmonella, enterotoxigenic E. coli).

62.   **Treatment of Shigella infection (Gastroenteritis):**
       a.   **Ampicillin** is the **drug of choice.** (Amoxicillin is **less** effective than ampicillin, but better absorbed.) If Shigella **is resistent** to ampicillin, then give **trimethoprim and sulfamethoxazole.**
       b.   Fluid and electrolyte.

63.   What **an antibiotic does** when it is used for Shigella gastroenteritis:
       a.   It **removes Shigella** from intestinal tract (**not** in **Salmonella).**
       b.   Long-term **carrier state** usually **not found as it is** (found in Salmonella).

64.   Effect of **lactulose** (synthesize from lactose) on **salmonella** in intestinal tract;
       a.   **Reduces excretion** of Shigella transiently.
       b.   **Inhibits the growth** of Shigella.
       Normal gut flora metabolizes lactulose to form short-chain fatty acid and reduces the stool pH, resulting in inhibition of Shigella growth.

65.   Prevention of Shigella infection: Strict hand washing.

66.   **Third world countries** and **Shigella infection:** Hemolytic uremic syndrome (renal failure, low platelet count, anemia) and coagulopathy occur due to endotoxin. Not common in U.S.A.

67.   **Reiter syndrome and Shigella:** Shigella with **positive HLA B27** associated with Reiter syndrome.

68.   **Cholera (not important for examination): Very rare** in U.S.A., cholera is caused by vibrio cholerae due to **contaminated water and food.** Most common site of infection is jejunum. Enterotoxin produces symptoms such as sudden onset of rice water stool, abdominal pain; in severe cases it causes shock. Definite diagnosis by **isolation of V. cholerae.** Strict hand washing is important. Tetracycline is effective with patients 8 years or older; erythromycin with hydration is effective with those younger.

69. **Most common** organism causing bacterial **pneumonia:**
Less than 1 month: Group B streptococci.
1 month to 1 year: Staph. aureus.
1 year to 4 year: Pneumococci.

70. A child whose foot had been punctured by nail while wearing sneakers, develops green or blue pus, **Most** likely organism: **Pseudomonas.**
Since it is gram-negative bacilli, present in **water** and **soil,** newborn child on **mechanical ventilator** is susceptible to this infection because of **distilled water,** which should be changed frequently. It releases **endotoxin** which causes the symptoms. It can cause meningitis, orbital cellulitis, pneumonia, UTI, endocarditis. It is also found in neutropenia (congenital or acquired) and in malfunction of neutrophil. This infection is most common in **cystic fibrosis** and **leukemia,** then in burns.

71. **Most common** bacterial infection in **cystic fibrosis** and **leukemia** patient: **Pseudomonas.**

72. Brucellosis infection to **human** being from **direct contact** with the following **animals (infected):** Cow, dog, goat.

73. A child with **leukemia** receiving chemotherapy suddenly becomes **very sick,** develops **fever.**
On examination: **Bluish, ecchymotic necrotic** central **skin** lesion surrounded by **bright areolae** is called **ecthyma gangrenosum. Progressively** develops respiratory failure and bradycardia and is placed on a mechanical ventilator.
What is the **most common** organism: **Pseudomonas.**
DIAGNOSIS: Positive blood culture.
TREATMENT: Gentamicin, carbenicillin, ticarcillin.
PROGNOSIS: Poor.

74. **Epidemic** of brucellosis and **food** products: Mostly due to **contaminated** milk and dairy products (butter, cheese, cream, ice-cream containing B. abortus and B. melitensis).

75. **Most common** complication of Brucellosis in humans: **Osteomyelitis,** mostly involves vertebrae and intervertebral disc results in suppurative spondylitis.

76. A child with history of contact with **animals** (like cows, goat, dog) or whose father has **dairy farm gradually comes down with constipation, myalgia, evening rise of very high fever (up to 108 degrees F)** with sweating, chills, abdominal pain, and **epistaxis.**

On examination: **Enlarged** liver, spleen, lymph nodes (cervical, axillary).
Most likely diagnosis: * **Brucellosis or Goat's milk fever.**
TREATMENT: Tetracycline (more than 8 years of age), Trimethoprim and sulfamethoxazole (less than 8 years).

77. Complication of **antibiotic** treatment in **Brucellosis:** Herxheimer reaction. (* It also occurs in Syphilis treated with penicillin).

78. Tularemia: **Ulceroglandular** type **most** common, found in U.S.A., caused by Francisella

tularensis a **gram negative** bacillus. The organism directly penetrates **the skin** (bite of an infected arthropod or animal contact) or **pharyngeal mucosa** (infected **rabbit** or squirrel meat). Tularemia shows signs of **ulcer** on the feet, hepatosplenomegaly, lymphadenopathy **or fever (high), chills,** joint pain, muscle pain, photophobia, **maculopapular rash.**

DIAGNOSIS: By characteristic **history** and **clinical** finding.
TREATMENT: Streptomycin.
Death due to pneumonia. Develop life-long immunity.

79. **Listeria infection** in the **Newborn:** One of the **most common** neonatal infections, **the most common** type is type IV, which cause **sepsis, meningitis, pneumonia** in newborn. Pregnant mother is **asymptomatic.**
    DIAGNOSIS: Positive blood culture.
    TREATMENT: Ampicillin.

80. **Most frequently** affected **cranial** nerve in **Tetanus; 7th** cranial nerve **(facial).** (* Other cranial nerves involved: 3rd, 4th, 9th, 10th, 11th).

81. **Most common** cause of **Tetanus in newborn:** Contamination of umbilical cord.

82. **Prophylaxis** against tetanus: Tetanus toxoid 0.5 c.c. I. M. (**active** immunization).

83. Clostridium tetany, **spores** and **vegetative** form: It **enters** the site of infection as **spores** which then convert to **infective form** which is called **vegetative** and releases **exotoxin.**

84. How to administer tetanus prophylaxis to a child who is **over** 6 years of age and **never** received immunization and has a history of injuries or cuts?
    Three doses of Td (tetanus-diphtheria): First dose stat, 2nd dose **after** 1 to 1-1/2 month of 1st, 3rd dose **after** 1/2 to 1 year of 2nd.

85. Treatment of tetanus: Penicillin, tetanus immunoglobulin (human) I.M. (**don't** give I.V.).

86. **Risus sardonicus** and tetanus: Risus sardonicus due to **spasm of facial** muscles.

87. **Pseudomembranous colitis and antibiotics: Most common** organism is **clostridium difficile. Most commonly,** the antibiotic causing this is **clindamycin (other antibiotics** are penicillin, ampicillin, amoxicillin, cephalosporin, chloramphenicol, tetracycline). Antibiotics **alter the intestinal** floras resulting in growth of **C. difficile** which releases toxins which cause **diarrhoea with mucous and blood,** abdominal pain.
    DIAGNOSIS: Positive stool culture.
    TREATMENT: Vancomycin; discontinue antibiotic which causes the problem.

88. A child shows signs of **diplopia, dysphagia, dysarthria, vomiting, constipation, urinary retention,** postural hypotension. Examination reveals **normal** sensory; but **also ptosis, dilated pupils, paresis of extraocular muscles, and dry mouth.** CSF is normal.
    MOST LIKELY DIAGNOSIS: Botulism. C. Botulinum is gram-**positive** organism.

Three types of infection can occur:

a.   Food botulism: Food contaminated with **toxin.**
b.   Wound botulism: Wound contaminated with **organism.**
c.   Infant botulism: **Spores and release toxin** in intestinal tract of infant.
Toxins prevent release of **acetylcholine** at **prejunctional** level of terminal neurone.

DIAGNOSIS CONFIRMED:
a.   Identification of **toxin in food** in food botulism.
b.   Identification of **toxin in serum** in wound botulism.
c.   Identification of **toxin in feces** in infant botulism.
EMG: May or may not be positive, usual characteristics Brief Small Abundant motor unit Potential (BSAP).
TREATMENT: Penicillin, antitoxin, supportive.
PROGNOSIS: Excellent for infantile type.

How to differentiate from:
a.   Guillain-Barre syndrome: **Increased** CSF protein.
b.   Myasthenia Gravis: **Response to Edrophonium chloride** (Tensilon) or neostigmine.

89.   **Bacteroides, anaerobe and infection;** Bacteroides is a gram-**negative** bacilli **which are not** spore forming. Two kinds of gram-positive bacilli are: CLOSTRIDIUM, which is spore-forming; and ACTINOMYCES, which is not spore-forming.

Bacteroides infection **is mostly due to:**
a.   Newborns with maternal **prolonged rupture membrane.**
b.   Newborns or others with intestinal obstruction and **perforation.**
Bacteroides infection **characteristically involves a foul smell** and the **soft tissue** in **any part** of the body:
Example: On tonsils it forms ulcers with brown foul smelling exudate by fusobacterium which is called **Vincent angina.** In sublingual and submandibular region, it forms cellulitis which spreads rapidly and is called **Ludwig angina.** In newborns, it appears as **Necrotizing enterocolitis.** It causes infection after **animal, or human bite or** long term **use of aminoglycoside.**
DIAGNOSIS: There is a history of **foul smell, wound culture** should be taken appropriately; blood, CSF, or any other body fluid culture should also be taken.
TREATMENT: For **all** gram-positive and gram-negative **bacilli, penicillin G** is **preferred drug except** B. fragilis which responds to **clindamycin** and carbenicillin. **Metronidazole** is also effective.

90.   Pseudomembranous colitis, **food:** Clostridium **perfringens** type A is **the most** common organism, which is found in food contaminated with spores which convert to infective **vegetative** form and release **toxins** which cause diarrhea and abdominal pain.
PREVENTION: Cook the food well.
TREATMENT: Fluid and electrolyte; **no** antibiotic.

91.   A **newborn** infant shows signs of **poor** sucking, poor swallowing, **hypotonia, ptosis, dilated pupil.** CSF examination is **normal.** The most likely diagnosis: **Infantile Botulism.**

92.   **Most common organism** in different **infections:**

Organism	Infection.
Staph. aureus	Burn.
Staph. epidermidis	Ventriculoperitoneal shunt, central venous catheter, dermal sinus tract, surgery (cardiac, general).
Strep. viridans	Cardiac disease (congenital, acquired).
E. Coli	Urinary catheter.

93. How to **diagnose** ventriculoperitoneal shunt **infection: Erythema of skin or scalp** over the shunt is **diagnostic, fever is always present.** To **tap the shunt** is helpful when patient is on antibiotic.
    Treatment for shunt infection:
    a. **Remove** the shunt.
    b. Administer antibiotic.

94. How to **diagnose** ventriculoperitoneal **shunt obstruction. No** fever **or** redness but history of increased intracranial pressure which induces **lethargy, vomiting. Diagnosis** made by **pressing** the shunt reservoir which **remains depressed even after releasing the pressure** (normally the reservoir should be filled when pressing is stopped).

95. **Most common organism** responsible for infection in certain diseases:

Organism	Diseases
Pseudomonas:	Malignancy, immunosuppressive condition.
Strep. pneumonia:	**Nephrotic syndrome, sickle cell** disease, **splenic malfunction,** C3 complement deficiency, exudative enteropathy.
Staph aureus:	**Cystic fibrosis,** G6PD, **chronic granulomatous** disease, diabetes, job syndrome.
Candida.	Polyendocrinopathy, **myeloperoxidase deficiency.** This disease requires **corticosteroid** therapy (collagen disease, inflammatory bowel disease).

96. A child shows signs of **fever, and foul smelling, profuse** diarrhea develops **bloody stool, crampy periumbilical** abdominal pain 2 days later.
    Most likely organism causing this problem: **Campylobacter enteritis.**
    Surgeons often think of **intussusception or appendicitis** and take the patient to O.R. for laparotomy. Mesenteric adenitis is the common finding in campylobacter infection.
    Campylobacter sepsis brings on **fever, sweating, chills but not** diarrhea.

    TREATMENT:
    a. Sepsis: Gentamicin.

b.   Enteritis: **Oral** tetracycline or erythromycin.

97.   **Campylobacter and the Neonate:** Maternal campylobacter infection causes **abortion and prematurity. Neonatal** campylobacter infection causes **sepsis and meningitis.**

98.   A child shows signs of history of respiratory distress (due to **pneumonia), chest pain, high fever,** chill, **diarrhoea.**
CBC: **Increased** ESR, normal WBC.
LFT: Slightly **elevated.**
SMA6: **Mildly increased** BUN and creatinine.
CXR: Patchy, nodular **infiltrate.**
Diagnosis: Legionnaires disease (legionellosis).

It is gram-negative bacilli, and one of the **leading causes** of **hospital acquired pneumonia. The most** commonly involved organs are the **lungs (pneumonia).** It is common in **immunodeficient** patient or one receiving **corticosteroid. TREATMENT: Erythromycin.** If **no** response then rifampin.

99.   **Bites of different mammals** and **most common** organism involved:

Bites of mammals	Organism
Humans	**Staph. aureus,** anaerobe.
Cats	Pasteurella multocida.
Dogs	Pasteurella pneumotropic. (Also found in cat).
Skunks, foxes, raccoons, wolves, coyotes, dogs, cats, bats, squirrels, weasels, **mongooses, opossums, muskrats.**	Rabies virus.

100. **Most common** type of **actinomycosis: Cervicofacial.** Actinomycosis is gram-positive bacilli. It appears as areas of suppuration surrounded by fibrosis and sinus tract formation. It contains sulfur granules. **TREATMENT:** Penicillin.

101. Pittsburg pneumonia (PPA): Common in immunocompromised patients which show signs of **pneumonia,** chest pain, fever, cough, sputum. It does **not** respond to usual antibiotics or to antituberculous treatment.

TREATMENT: Erythromycin; if no response, rifampin.
PROGNOSIS: Poor.

102. Different **organisms** carrying PPA and the corresponding **treatment:**

Organism	Treatment
Anaerobe, pasteurella, streptococci, Gonococci, Pneumococci, Clostridium	Penicillin (if resistant, choose sensitive antibiotic).

Bacteroides	Clindamycin.
Staphylococci	Nafcillin, dicloxacillin.

103. Characteristics of **discharge** of a given **organism:**

Organisms	Discharge
Anaerobe	**Foul odor** and or crepitation.
Pasteurella	Purulent, no foul smell, gram-**negative** rod.
Clostridium	Purulent, gram-**positive** rod with spores.
Streptococci	Purulent, gram-**positive** cocci in chain.
Staphylococci	Purulent, gram-**positive** cocci in cluster.
Pneumococci	Gram-**positive** diplococci.
Gonococci	Purulent, gram-**negative** intracellular diplococci.
Bacteroides	Purulent, gram-**negative** rod.

104. A late adolescent **immunocompromised boy shows signs of dyspnea, chest pain,** fever, **productive cough,** weight loss.
CXR shows **bronchopneumonia,** cavity, **effusion,** and **empyema.**
Diagnosis: **Nocardiosis.**
MEANS OF DIAGNOSIS : Sputum culture, gram stain.
TREATMENT: Sulfonamide, abscess drain.

105. A child shows signs of **weight loss, cough, evening rise of temperature.**
CXR shows **enlarged lymph nodes** in hilar, pulmonary region.
Most likely diagnosis: **Tuberculosis.**
Most important screening test: **Tuberculin test.**
Most important **definitive** diagnostic test: **Culture** of sputum, gastric material (not gram stain) showing of isolation of **mycobacterium tuberculosis.**
Most common presentation in children is conversion to **positive tuberculin test** from previous negative one.
Miliary T.B.: **Most common** in **infant and young** children usually shows signs of **dyspnea, cyanosis, hepatosplenomegaly.** Tuberculin test **is positive** in **90%** and negative in 10%, of the cases of symptomatic patients.
Most common site of T.B. of superficial lymph nodes: Cervical region.
Most common cause of **death** in T.B.: Meningitis. It occurs most frequently in patients younger than 6 months of age.

Meningitis develops in three stages:
a. Nonspecific symptoms.
b. Definite neurologic sign (positive nuchal rigidity, cranial nerve and brain stem involvement resulting in ptosis, strabismus, exaggerated deep tendon, and absent

superficial reflexes),

c. Comatose condition.

CSF shows **increased protein** and **decreased glucose.**

Most common neurologic outcome in T.B. meningitis is **mental retardation.**

106. **Most common** site of T.B. in **female genital tract:** Fallopian tube.

107. T.B. of **urinary system** and **its symptoms:** Initially, it is **asymptomatic,** then **its only presentation** is **pyuria,** but negative culture; after that, dysuria, frequency and urgency of urination.

108. **Most common** cause of **T.B. intestine: Swallowed infected sputum** (from pulmonary T.B.). T.B. intestine presents itself as abdominal pain, diarrhea (sometimes alternate with constipation), weight loss.

109. **Most common** mode of spread of **T.B. from mother to newborn or fetus: Hematogenous** through placenta.

110. **Most common organ** involved in **transmission of T.B. from mother to newborn or fetus:** Liver.

111. Most common **clinical sign** of T.B. of fetus or newborn: Jaundice. (Other signs: hepatosplenomegaly, anemia, pneumonia, low platelet count).

112. How to **make diagnosis** of newborn T.B.: **Most** commonly made by **study of history of maternal T.B.** In newborn T.B., PPD is negative, sometimes tuberculous **bacilli are seen in gastric aspirate,** liver, or lung **biopsy.**

113. **First** sign of **streptomycin toxicity:** Vertigo (or ataxia).

114. **Anti-T.B. drugs** and **their txicity:**

Ethambutol	Optic neuritis.
Streptomycin	**Vestibular** and cochlear damage.
Rifampin	Body fluid turns **red.**
INH	Hepatotoxicity and peripheral neuritis are **uncommon** in children. **Benign** drug.

115. **Indications** to use **INH:**
   a.* For **a newborn** born to a mother with **positive CXR or active** T.B.
   b. Anybody who was exposed to **active T.B. (INH for 9 m).**
   c. Anybody who is **a recent converter** (i.e., becomes positive from negative) and has never been treated **(INH for 9 m.).**
   d. **Recent converter** receiving immunosuppressive therapy e.g. corticosteroid (give INH only during **therapy).**

e.   **Recent converter** with history of H. influenzae, pertussis, and rubeola; or receiving rubeola vaccine (give INH for 1 month).

* **In category (a) mentioned above:** First give INH for 3 months, then check PPD; if positive, then continue **only 9 months when CXR of the child is negative.**

116. Newborn child is born to a mother who has **recently tested positive for PPD** and chest **X-ray negative:**
How do you manage the child: **Don't do anything to child at birth;** follow up in clinic when child is around **6 weeks** of age and **place PPD.** If PPD **is negative,** then do tuberculin test every 3 months for 1 year; if PPD **is positive,** do CXR; if CXR is **negative,** give INH for 9 months; if CXR is **positive,** give **three antitubercular** drugs for 6 to 9 months. Asymptomatic child of HIV (+) mother should receive INH for 1 year. Patient who is resistence to INH should receive rifampin for 9 months.

117. Newborn child's mother has **PPD and chest X-ray both positive** that means **active T.B.**
How do you manage the newborn: First, do CXR of the baby to rule out congenital T.B. If active T.B., give **three anti-T.B.** drugs. If **no** active T.B. then give INH **for 9 months** only. Same management if mother has advanced pulmonary or extra pulmonary T.B. or disseminated condition.

118. **Most common** disadvantage of **INH prophylaxis in newborn:** Non-compliance by parents.

119. **Advantages** of **BCG** vaccination: **Only one** injection, more effective, less toxic.

120. **Disadvantage** of BCG vaccination: **False** positive PPD **result is difficult to interpret,** so separate mother and infant after BCG until skin test is positive and protected.

121. When mother has **active T.B.** and has started antituberculous **therapy, how long** do you want to separate the mother from the newborn: About **2 weeks after** treatment begins, because by then mother should be **non-infectious.**

122. Can you give BCG when INH prophylaxis already started? No, because INH **prevents** BCG multiplication.

123. **Most frequent site** of involvement by **nontuberculous** mycobacterium: Cervical lymph nodes.
"Swimming pool granuloma" is caused by this organism, by penetrating the swimmers' abraded skin and forming **granuloma and ulcers** in the **foot.**

124. **Non-tuberculous** mycobacterium and PPD: It causes weaker reaction to PPD (less than 10 mm diameter).

125. Treatment for **non tuberculous** mycobacterium infection:
a.   **No** prophylaxis given to any children.
b.   Only active disease person should be treated with **INH or ethambutol** and add **rifampin** if **no** response, then give ethionamide, cycloserine, capreomycin.
c.   **Most useful** treatment is **surgical intervention** of the local lesion which is most

effective in swimming pool granuloma caused by M. maximum. **No chemotherapy** is given before and after surgery.

126. **Most common** presentation of **newborn syphilis: Asymptomatic.**

127. What does **"passive transfer** of syphilis from mother" means? It means **that the newborn does not have syphilis.** It is due to maternal antibody (IgG) transfer through placenta, resulting in positive serology in baby. In this case, newborn's titre is either **less or equal** to mother's. Do **not** treat the baby for syphilis.

128. What does **"active infection in newborn"** mean? It means that the baby is infected and that its titre will be **more** than mother's. Baby should be **treated with penicillin for 10 days.**

129. When mother received penicillin **during her last month** of pregnancy what happened to baby's treatment? Baby was **not** treated adequately, and so has to be **treated again.**

130. Full-blown congenital syphilis **usually accompanies:** Erythematous **maculopapular rash** over the hands and feet which **desquamate** later, **hepatosplenomegaly,** jaundice, snuffles, interstitial-keratitis, osteochondritis, metaphysitis of long bones.
CBC shows **leukemoid** reaction of increase WBC count with **low platelet count.**
Hutchinson teeth: peg-shaped, **upper central incisors (permanent teeth)** appear around 6 years of age.
Higoumenakis sign: Thickening of sternoclavicular portion of the **clavicle** bilaterally.
Mulberry molar: Excessive number of **cusps** in first lower molar teeth.
Diagnosis of congenital syphilis:
Definitive Treponemal tests: FTA-ABS, MHATP, TPI.
Non-definitive non-treponemal test: RPR, VDRL.

In syphilis, treponemal test results **remain positive for rest of patient's life,** but non-treponemal test results become **negative** 1 to 2 years after treatment.
In neurosyphilis, CSF = VDRL and FTA-ABS is positive even when there is no symptom of neurosyphilis. Therefore, to make diagnosis, **blood and CSF** treponemal and non-treponemal tests should be done.
TREATMENT: Penicillin G crystalline, Penicillin G procaine.

131. What is **incubating syphilis** to newborn: Baby is **infected,** but serological test **is negative.** It occurs when mother is infected in **last month** of pregnancy. Mother's titre is very low and baby's is negative. Baby should be **treated.** Baby's titre will be positive a few weeks later if not treated.

132. If a syphilitic mother is treated with **erythromycin** for penicillin allergy, what happens to baby's treatment? Baby is **not** treated, because erythromycin does **not** cross the placenta well because of high molecular weight. Baby should be **treated with penicillin.** (Newborns do not have penicillin allergy).

Cephalosporin has cross-sensitivity to penicillin, so **it cannot be given** to penicillin-allergic patient.

133. **False positive** FTA-ABS:
    Very rare, but found in:
    a. Normal pregnant women.
    b. **Diseases like** cirrhosis, collagen vascular disorder, drug addiction, lymphoproliferative disease.

134. **Jarisch-Herxheimer** reaction: It is the development of **fever** and **systemic reaction** when syphilitic patient is treated with penicillin. Mechanism is **unknown,** but may be due to sudden lysis of treponema.

135. **Non-venereal** diseases and **treponema:**
    Bejel: Treponema pallidum.
    Yaws: Treponema.
    Pinta: Treponema pertenue.
    These diseases are **not** found in U.S.A.
    DIAGNOSIS MADE BY: serological test same as for syphilis.
    TREATMENT: penicillin.

136. Rat bite fever and organism: Spirillum minor. History of rat bite, shows signs of indurated, suppurative, and erythematous. Treated with **penicillin,** tetracycline.

137. **Most common** cause of **conjunctivitis** and different timing:
    First 24 hours: Chemical due to silver nitrate.
    2 to 5 days: Gonococcus from the mother.
    6 to 14 days: Chlamydia from the mother.

138. Newborn between **3 and 16 weeks** old, has mild **tachypnea, cough,** vomiting, **cyanosis** and **conjunctivitis bilateral.** Child has history of normal spontaneous vaginal delivery which was uneventful. Mother's cervical culture for **bacteria** is negative, but has history of vaginal discharge prior to delivery. Chlamydia culture was not done.

    Chest X-ray shows **hyperinflation** and **patchy infiltrate.**
    CBC shows **increased eosinophil** count.
    MOST LIKELY DIAGNOSIS: Chlamydia pneumonia.
    DIAGNOSIS MADE BY: Chlamydia culture.
    TREATMENT: Erythromycin **orally.**
    Local application of eye preparation will cure conjunctivitis only. In order to eradicate nasopharyngeal **carrier, oral erythromycin is necessary.**

139. Most common **malformation** in congenital rubella: **Cataract. (Most common cardiac** lesion is **PDA.)**

140. **Most** characteristic **sign** of **acquired** rubella: Lymphadenopathy (**retroauricular,** posterior cervical, and posterior occipital).

141. Child, between **10 and 15 years** old, has of **persistent cough** for 2 to 3 weeks, sore throat, and low grade fever. Physical examination was unremarkable.

Chest X-ray shows pneumonic **infiltrate** in **lower lobe.**
PROBABLE DIAGNOSIS: Mycoplasma pneumonia.
DIAGNOSIS CONFIRMED BY: Isolation of organism.
TREATMENT: Erythromycin, Tetracycline.
Mycoplasma has **no** cell wall. **Most common** in school age children. **Most prominent** symptom is **persistent cough,** rales occasionally present, cold agglutinin **titre 1:64** or more, helps in the diagnosis.

142. A child with **hacking cough,** conjunctivitis, **runny nose,** fever, **maculopapular blotchy rash** mostly over face, neck, upper part of chest. Examination reveals **Koplik spot** (gray white dots on cheek opposite the lower molar), enlarged posterior cervical lymph nodes. Definite diagnosis is **measles** because Koplik spot **only found** in measles.

     Complications of measles: Pneumonia, encephalopathy, otitis media, Guillain-Barre syndrome. Remarkably, there is **no** correlation between severity of measles and neurologic manifestation.
     Immunization: MMR (active immunization) or measles vaccine **before** the disease.

143. **Only** natural host of Rubella: Human.

144. **Congenital rubella** and **diabetes:** Rubella virus damage the pancreas cause **diabetes mellitus.**

145. **Definitive diagnosis** and **TORCH** infection:

Toxoplasmosis	IgM specific for toxoplasma by **ELISA**
Rubella	Isolation of virus by culture
CMV	Urine CMV culture
Herpes	Isolation of virus by culture

146. **Contraindication** to Rubella **virus vaccine:**
     a.   **Most important not** to give during **pregnancy.**
     b.   Fever, hypersensitivity to vaccine, immunodeficiency.
     c.   Patient taking steroid or other anticancer drugs.

147. If a pregnant woman **is exposed to Rubella** for the first time, how do you manage her treatment:

     HI (Hemagglutination-inhibition) test should be done **immediately** to know the immune status. If antibody present, the baby is protected and pregnancy may continue, if **no** antibody is present, the baby is **not** protected then give the mother **two** options:

     a.   If mother does not want abortion, then give passive immunization with **ISG** (immune serum globulin) immediately, **or**
     b.   follow up the antibody titre. If it is **rising,** the baby is **susceptible** for infection, so **do abortion.**

148. What is the **infective form** of Toxoplasmosis? **Oocyst** (found in cat feces).

149. What is the **Triad** of **Toxoplasmosis?** Hydrocephalus, chorioretinitis, calcification of brain.

150. Brain **calcification** and **Toxoplasma, CMV:**
Periventricular: CMV
Diffuse: Toxoplasmosis.

151. **Most common** clinical manifestation and TORCH infection:

Toxoplasmosis	Asymptomatic.
Rubella	Cataract.
CMV	Asymptomatic.
Herpes	Vesicular rash over the scalp and behind ears, **sick** child.

152. **Usual presentation** of **any TORCH** infection: Small for gestation age (SGA), hepatosplenomegaly, micro-or normo-or macrocephaly, lymphadenopathy, thrombocytopenia.

153. **Most common outcome or sequelae** of TORCH infection: **First psychomotor** retardation; then vision loss; hearing loss.

154. Most common **symptomatic** patient with Toxoplasmosis has: Chorioretinitis.

155. Causes of death in TORCH infection:
Herpes, Toxoplasmosis: CNS disease.
CMV: Bacterial infection.

156. **Pseudoparalysis** occurs in: Syphilis, scurvy.

157. **Rash** in **TORCH** infection:

Rubelliform rash	CMV.
Blue-berry muffin	Rubella, CMV (neuroblastoma).
Polymorphic rash	Syphilis.
Vesicular rash	Herpes.

158. **Mode of transmission** and TORCH infection:
Toxoplasmosis: **Oral** (meat, soil), placental.
Rubella: **Respiratory** (droplets, contamination), placental.
CMV: **Respiratory,** sex, breast milk, blood, urine, sperm, placental.
Herpes: **Direct contact,** sex, breast, blood, and placental.
(CMV infection **most commonly** occurs **at or near the time of delivery**.)

159. **Placental characteristics:**
     Large placenta and edematous: Hydrops (due to Rh disease).
     Large placenta, but **not** edematous: Syphilis.

160. **Intranuclear** inclusion body: Herpes.
     Paranuclear inclusion body: Chlamydia.

161. **Type of herpes infection** in newborn and different sources:
     From mother, type 2 (75%) more than type 1 (25%).
     From nursery personnel, type 1 (25%) more than type 2 (9%).
     Type 2 is common in **genitalia,** type 1 is common in **mouth.**

162. A child shows signs of **high rise of temperature** (up to 105 degrees) for few days, then **a sudden drop** of temperature and the appearance of **generalized maculopapular rash** all over the body.
     MOST LIKELY DIAGNOSIS: Exanthem subitem (Roseola infantum).

163. A child shows signs of **low** grade fever, **slapped cheek** (livid erythematous) appearance, maculopapular rash with central clearing, results in lacy **reticulated** appearance.
     Diagnosis: Erythema infectiosum (fifth disease).
     Most common complication of erythema infectiosum: Arthritis.
     Organism causing erythema infectiosum: Parvo virus B 19.

164. A pregnant mother infected with **parvo virus B 19.** What is the impact on the **fetus?**
     Hydrops fetalis.

165. A child with known hemoglobinopathies (e.g., sickle cell disease) infected with **parvo virus B 19,** what is the result? **Aplastic crisis.**
     It **also occurs** in acute hemolytic anemia, hereditary spherocytosis, pyruvate kinase deficiency, and thalassemia.

166. Most common **site** of herpetic gingivostomatitis: **Tongue** (cheek).
167. **Primary site** of herpes infection in adult female: **Cervix.**

168. **Most common** type of **non-epidemic encephalitis** in U.S.A.: Herpes.

169. **Mode of spread** of **different herpes** to central nervous system:
     Type 1 is spread by **nerves.**
     Type 2 is spread by **blood.**

170. A pregnant women who has positive primary herpes type 2 in genitalia, and is about to deliver a child:
     If mother's membrane rupture **less than 4 hours** old or **intact,** then **do cesarean section.**
     If membrane rupture is more than 4 hours, then there is most likely **an ascending** infection, so cesarean section is **not** indicated.

171. A newborn child born with **a few clusters of vesicular** lesions over the scalp, **jaundice, and sick looking.**

MOST LIKELY DIAGNOSIS: Neonatal herpes.
TREATMENT: Acyclovir parenteral.
Herpes in newborn is **a very serious** disease, but herpes in adults is a self-limited disease. **A maternal** herpetic genital lesion is **a usually painful,** multiple superficial ulcer. Any newborn shows signs of **cluster of vesicle** should always be considered **to have herpes** until **proven otherwise.**

172. Neonate with **herpes** shows signs of **convulsions:- Most common** site of CNS epilepsy: **Temporal lobe.**

173. **Most common** complication of chicken pox: Secondary bacterial skin infection.

174. Most common **CNS** complication of chicken pox: Encephalitis.

175. Patient receiving corticosteroid or immunosuppressed with chicken pox: Fatal lesion with complications.

176. **Newborn** infant and **mother with** chicken pox: Baby **needs VZIG** (varicella zoster immunoglobulin) when mother develops chicken pox **5 days before or 2 days after** delivery, because in that period baby got the virus from the mother but not the protective antibody.

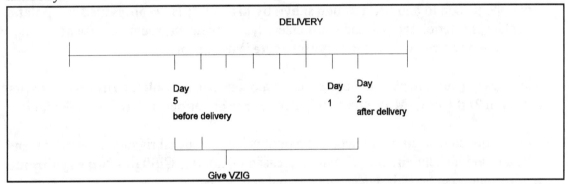

   Other indications for giving **VZIG:** Immunodeficiency, malignancy, leukemia.

177. **Most commonly** involved organ in **congenital CMV** infection: Central nervous system. (It is less involved in **acquired** infection except in immunocompromised patient).

178. A child shows signs of **severe** pain and tenderness **along the dermatome** develops **vesicular rash.**

   MOST LIKELY DIAGNOSIS: Herpes zoster.
   DIAGNOSIS: Clinical.
   Chicken pox occurs after herpes zoster infection. Patient should be **isolated** in the ward and away from immunocompromised household.
   TREATMENT: Symptomatic; in the case of immunocompromised patient, give Acyclovir.

179. Name a **virus** which has the electron microscopic and physicochemical **similarities** of **CMV:** Herpes virus.

180. **Ramsay-Hunt syndrome:** Paralysis of the **facial nerve** and **vesicle** formation of **external auditory canal** due to infection with **herpes zoster** affecting facial nerve or geniculate ganglia.

181. **Examination finding** in **certain diseases:**
   a.   Chorioretinitis: Usually CMV and toxoplasmosis.
   b.   Salt-and-pepper fundus of retina: Usually rubella and syphilis.
   c.   Microopthalmia: Usually toxoplasmosis.
   d.   Hydrocephalus: Usually toxoplasmosis.

182. Name **one** of the TORCH infections which, when acquired **after** birth, **resembles infectious mononucleosis:** CMV.

183. A **sexually active** adolescent shows signs of **tonsillopharyngitis with exudate,** fever, sore throat. Examination reveals **petechiae** at the junction of soft and hard palate, **hepatosplenomegaly,** enlarged lymph nodes particularly **posterior cervical** and **epitrochlear.** He said he has been taking **ampicillin** from an other doctor and developed a rash over body after taking antibiotic.

   MOST LIKELY DIAGNOSIS: Infectious mononucleosis.
   The Epstein-Barr (E-B) virus, which belongs to herpes virus group causes it. It transmits from one person to another through **saliva by kissing. It is accompanied by palatal** petechiae, posterior cervical and epitrochlear lymph node enlargement, rash after ampicillin due to unknown reason. **Atypical lymphocyte** is usually present.

184. Most **dangerous** complication of infectious mononucleosis: **Splenic rupture.** (Occurs mostly in **2nd week. Most common**ly due to **trauma** or occur during examination.)

185. **Neurologic** complication of infectious mononucleosis: Nuchal rigidity, convulsion, and ataxia found initially; **meningitis** with increased monocyte, **Guillain-Barre syndrome, Bell palsy,** transverse myelitis, encephalitis found subsequently.

186. **Laboratory** diagnosis of infectious mononucleosis:
   a.   **CBC** shows increased **atypical lymphocyte** which is almost 20-40% of total lymphocyte of 75%.
   b.   Increased heterophil antibody titre.

187. **Negative** heterophil antibody titre found in:
   a.   Infectious mononucleosis **without** antibody formation.
   b.   Hepatitis A.
   c.   Toxoplasmosis.
   d.   CMV.
   Atypical lymphocyte present in **all** of these conditions, as well as **in** mycoplasma, tuberculosis, typhoid, malaria.

188. **Treatment** of **infectious mononucleosis:**
   a.   If spleen is enlarged: Stop athletic activity to avoid splenic rupture.
   b.   If positive group A beta Strep: Give penicillin treatment.

c. No specific treatment.

d. If edema is obstructing airway (upper): Give corticosteroid to reduce the edema.

189. Newborn **infant** and **maternal mumps:**
   a. If mother had mumps **before** this pregnancy: Baby is **protected** up to 8 months of life from passively transfered maternal antibody.
   b. If mother develop mumps **1 week before** delivery: Baby may develop mumps at birth or within its first month.

190. **Diagnosis of mumps: Clinical diagnosis. (CBC shows leukopenia, but also lymphocytosis; there is increased serum** amylase).

191. **Most common** complication of mumps in **children: Meningoencephalitis. (Mumps virus** can cause aqueductal stenosis and hydrocephalus.)
   In **adolescent boys, orchitis and epididymitis** are common complications. This **results in reduce** fertility, but total infertility is **rare. In females** it cause oophoritis, but does **not** cause infertility. In mumps meningoencephalitis, **CSF** showed **increased lymphocyte only.** Unlike **enterovirus, aseptic** meningitis **polymorph** predominates early.

192. **Treatment of mumps:**
   a. Only symptomatic.
   b. If there is headache due to meningoencephalitis: Do spinal tap.
   c. In orchitis: Bed rest and support for the testes.

193. **Most** common **symptom** of parainfluenza virus infection: **Cough** (In 80% of patients, cough presents as URI symptom).

194. **Most common** cause of **croup.** Parainfluenza virus. (RNA virus, which belongs to paramyxovirus group). Types 1, 2, and 3, of this virus cause symptoms, but type **4 is asymptomatic.**

   Type 1**: Commonly** causes laryngotracheitis.
   Type 3 **: Commonly** causes **bronchitis, bronchiolitis, pneumonia.**
   Most common disease caused by **parainfluenza virus** is **croup.**

195. **Most common** cause of **bronchiolitis:** RSV (Respiratory syncytial virus).

196. **Most common** disease caused by **RSV: First bronchiolitis** (then pneumonia, then croup).
   (**Newborn** is **not protected from RSV** by placental transfer of maternal antibody, but breast milk **may offer** some protection.)

197. **Most common** mode of transmission of **hepatitis B:** Through **serum,** so-called "serum hepatitis" (other modes are: **sex,** through **body fluids** like saliva, feces. Incidence is **very high** among those who **live in institutions** because of living condition).

198. A **2-month-**old child showed signs of **runny nose, cough,** low grade fever. Examination revealed **pharyngitis,** diffuse **rhonchi,** wheezing. Chest X-ray showed **air trapping (hyperexpansion).**

MOST LIKELY DIAGNOSIS: Bronchiolitis.
Most common organism causing bronchiolitis is RSV, second most common is parainfluenza virus.
DEFINITIVE DIAGNOSIS: Virus isolation from nasopharynx.
TREATMENT: Humidified oxygen.

199. **Most common** symptom of **RSV** infection: Runny nose.

200. **Most common** clinical symptom of **adenoviral** infection: Pharyngitis.

201. A child shows signs of **bilateral conjunctivitis, pharyngitis,** fever, runny nose, **posterior cervical lymphadenopathy.**
PROBABLE DIAGNOSIS: Pharyngoconjunctival fever due tn adenovirus (DNA).
Adenovirus can cause intussusception, hemorrhagic cystitis, pertussis-like symptom diarrhea, pneumonia.

202. **Most common** disease caused by **Rhino virus:** Common cold.

203. **Infectious hepatitis** (Hepatitis A) and **features:**
    a. Transmitted mostly from **person to person, rarely** from contaminated **food and water.**
    b. Most commonly found in **children** (without jaundice mostly). Jaundice develops after 4-6 weeks.
    c. **Homosexuals** and **day care center** employees have **high** infection rate.
    d. Newborn for **first few months protected** by maternal antibody.
    e. If mother develops **hepatitis during pregnancy or around delivery,** then there is **no infection, no abortion,** and **no teratogenicity** to fetus.
    f. **In stool** hepatitis A, antibody titre is **maximum** even **before** the jaundice develops.

204. Mother with hepatitis **B surface antigen positive** in **first month** of pregnancy. What happened to the fetus? **Prematurity.** (No abortion, **no** malformation.)

205. In **acute** hepatitis A or B, viral damage to **hepatocyte** showed signs of **mostly:** Balloon degenerative changes and necrosis of hepatocyte in the center of lobule. Regeneration begins in hepatocyte; usually after 3 months, liver morphology becomes **normal;** if not, that means **chronic hepatitis.** In **fulminant** hepatitis, parenchyma is **totally destroyed.**

206. **Gianotti-Crosti syndrome** and **hepatitis B:** This syndrome represents papular **acrodermatitis** of childhood caused by hepatitis B.

207. Liver transaminase and different hepatitis:
    a. Hepatitis A: It reaches **high peak** quickly then **drops rapidly.**
    b. Hepatitis B: Peaks **lower** than hepatitis A and goes down more slowly than hepatitis A.
    c. Non-A, non-B (Hepatitis C): Intermittent elevation for long period of time.

208. A child with **hepatitis suddenly** comes down with bilirubin **more than 20 mg/dl, bleeding, ascites** and edema, then develops **drowsiness, stupor,** and **coma.**

PROBABLE DIAGNOSIS: Acute fulminating hepatitis due to complication of hepatitis. It is mostly due to **hepatitis A** and **non A-non B** (hepatitis C).

209. A child with **hepatitis** slowly develops **anorexia, vomiting, weight loss.** Examination reveals **enlarged liver and spleen, joint pain, low grade fever, clubbing,** ascites.

    PROBABLE DIAGNOSIS: Chronic active hepatitis due to complication of hepatitis. It presents **with increased** liver enzymes and prothrombin time and decreased platelet count. Hepatitis B surface antigen **is usually negative.** It represents **increased** gamma globulin in serum and the presence of antinuclear, antiglomerular, antimitochondrial and anti-smooth-muscle antibodies.

210. A child with **hepatitis** has **low WBC count or ecchymosis,** which is a dangerous sign. Bone marrow shows **aplastic** anemia, and marrow replaced by fat.
    PROBABLE DIAGNOSIS: Aplastic anemia due to complication of hepatitis.

211. **Prophylaxis** of **hepatitis A** with **immune serum globulin:** Hepatitis A **endemic area** where person **wants** to **stay there for long time (months).** (Do **not** give to person who is going to **endemic** area for **few** days).

212. **Most** common type of hepatitis through **blood transfusion: Hepatitis C** (non-A- non-B).

213. Hepatitis B infection **may occur** through: Blood, fibrinogen, Factor IX concentrate, antihemophilic globulin, contaminated needle.

214. Mother with **positive** HBsAg and HbeAg. What happened to newborn? When HBeAg is positive, the chances of infecting the baby are **much higher.**

215. Mother with positive HBsAg (hepatitis B surface antigen). How do you manage the **newborn?**
    a. **First,** baby should be **washed thoroughly** to remove all maternal blood from body surface.
    b. **Second,** baby should receive Hepatitis B **immunoglobulin** within 12 hours of birth and **hepatitis B vaccine** within 7 days of birth but vaccine can be given with immunoglobulin, injection should be given in **two different sites.** Hepatitis profile of the baby should be drawn **before** immunoglobulin is given.
    c. **Fluid and secretion precaution** is necessary, but isolation is not.

216. Mother with positive HBsAg, complete prophylaxis schedule of the newborn should be and interpretation:
    a. **At birth** hepatitis B immunoglobulin and hepatitis B vaccine within 12 hours of birth (vaccine can be given up to 7 days of age) in two different sites.
    b. At 1 month, hepatitis B vaccine should be given.
    c. At 6 months, hepatitis B vaccine should again be given.
    d. At 9 months, repeat baby's hepatitis profile:
        i. If **antibody to hepatitis B is positive** that means the baby is **protected** and immunization is successful.
        ii. If **antigen** to hepatitis B is **positive** that means the baby is **infected** and

immunization is **not** successful.

iii. If **both** antibody and antigen are **absent,** then **another dose** of hepatitis B **vaccine** should be given and the baby should be retested for hepatitis profile and interpretation should be same as that above mentioned.

PROGNOSIS: About 90% of infants with HBsAg positive due to perinatally acquired infection will become **chronic carriers of hepatitis B virus,** and **25% of chronic** carrier babies will develop **cirrhosis or hepatocellular carcinoma** usually in 3rd and 4th decade of life.

217. **Most common** presentation of hepatitis in **newborn:** Asymptomatic.

218. **Most common** site of **neuronal lesion in polio: Anterior** horn cells of spinal cord.

219. Mother with **positive non A non B hepatitis.** During **which trimester** of pregnancy is the fetus **mostly** affected? Third trimester.

220. When newborn has received **hepatitis B vaccine,** blood has been drawn within **24 hours,** and it is found to have **positive HbsAg.** What is your interpretation of the baby's status? Hepatitis B surface antigen can be **positive within 24 hours after vaccine is given** and it is due to vaccine which is antigen but if it is positive any other time that means immunization failure.

221. Mother is HBsAg positive. How do you advise her sexual partner and others in the household? First, they should be **screened** for hepatitis status. If there is no evidence of previous hepatitis infection, then give immunization.

222. **Most common** presentation and management of newborn of a mother who has **non-A-non-B hepatitis:**
Asymptomatic: may be mild elevation of liver enzymes after 1 to 2 months.
Immunization to newborn: Immune serum globulin 0.5 c.c. is recommended within 24 hours.

223. **Hepatitis D, or delta hepatitis, of mother and newborn:** Delta hepatitis **virus (RNA)** is a delta antigen which is **covered by HBsAg.** It can cause infection either **with** hepatitis B or superinfection to **chronic carrier** of hepatitis B. Transmission mode is the same as Hepatitis B.

DIAGNOSIS MADE BY: Detection of delta antigen and antibody. Newborn who has positive HBsAg can be infected. No prophylaxis is available yet.

224. **What** is the natural host for **enterovirus** infection? Only human beings.
(Enterovirus is coxsackie, echo, and polio virus).

225. **Histologically,** polio virus does not affect the following areas:
a. Cerebral cortex **except** motor area.
b. Cerebellum **except** vermix and deep midline nuclei.
c. White mater of spinal cord.

226. **Most common** disease involved in **coxsackievirus B:** Myocarditis. Enlarged heart with dilation of chambers, mostly **B5.** Among echoviruses **type 6** mostly involves the heart.

227. **Most common** presentation when infected with **polio virus** and **other enteroviruses** (e.g., echo and coxsackie). **Asymptomatic.**

228. **Most common among enterovirus** causing **cardiac** problem is: Coxsackie virus B.

229. **Most common** cause of **neonatal** myocarditis:Coxsackie virus B.

230. **Prophylaxis schedule** for **Rabies:**
     First day:
     a.   Human rabies immunoglobulin (HRIG) (half at the site of injection and half by intramuscular) and human diploid cell vaccine (HDCV) intramuscularly.
     b.   **On days 3, 7, 14 and 28:** Only HDCV.
     (Pregnancy is **not** contraindication to vaccination because rabies is fatal.)

231. A child who plays with his **cat** at home is found to have **painless, non-itchy erythematous papule** and **pustule** over the upper extremities. His axillary and epitrochlear lymph nodes were enlarged.

     MOST LIKELY DIAGNOSIS: Cat scratch disease (Benign lymphoreticulosis, Felinosis). It is a self limited disease **of unknown** etiology. It may be caused by chlamydia-like organism, history of scratch by cat, dog, monkey.
     DIAGNOSIS MADE BY: History or **intradermal skin** test with antigen.
     CBC showed **increased** eosinophil and ESR.
     TREATMENT: Nonspecific, aspiration of nodule, which is sterile.

232. Which **enterovirus** causes **the common cold? Only** coxsackievirus **A21.**

233. **Most common** causative organism in **hand, foot, mouth syndrome: Coxsackievirus A16.**

234. **Arthropod vector** and **diseases:**

Tick	Rocky mountain spotted fever; Q fever (rarely).
Mite	Rickettsial pox, scrub typhus.
Louse	Epidemic typhus; murine typhus (rat, flea).

235. The Rickettsial diseases are usually present with fever and rash **except:** Q fever **(has fever).**

236. Treatment of all Rickettsial diseases: Tetracycline or chloramphenicol.

237. A child shows signs of **history of tick bite** while playing in **the woods,** has discrete maculopapular rash which **begins in lower extremity (ankle or wrist)** then spreads all over the body, including palm and sole. **His spleen is enlarged, and thrombocytopenia** present.

What is the most likely diagnosis? **Rocky mountain spotted fever.**
DIAGNOSIS MADE: Clinically.
Control: Use tick repellents. **Remove the tick immediately** from the skin.

238. **Most common** presentation of **Q fever:** Severe frontal headache.

239. **Blastomycosis** and features: **Usually the** patient is **asymptomatic.** When symptomatic **the most common** involvement is **pneumonia.** In disseminated disease, **the most common** extra pulmonary site involvement is **skin.** It is a self-limited disease.
     TREATMENT: Amphotericin B **used only** in disseminated and **chronic** progressive disease.

240. **Most common** organ involve in **aspergillosis:** Lung (Pneumonia). Aspergillosis is a fungus. Infection occurs by **inhalation** of **spores** present in **soil.** It can cause life-**threatening pneumonitis.**

241. An **immunocompromised** child who has **a pigeon** in his house, shows signs and symptoms which mimics **influenzaes** (e.g., cough, fever, rales, pleuritic chest pain).

     Chest X-ray shows granuloma, cavity, or infiltrate
     CBC is normal.
     MOST LIKELY DIAGNOSIS: Cryptococcosis.
     DIAGNOSIS BY: Positive culture sputum, bronchial wash, or biopsy of body specimen or fluid.
     It is a fungal infection caused by **cryptococcus neoformans,** which is a soil saprophyte. Humans are infected by **spores** through **birds (e.g., pigeons),** influenza-like symptoms are characteristic.
     Most common serious complication: Meningitis.
     Most common sign of cryptococcal meningitis: **Headache.** (Plus **usual signs** of meningitis).
     CSF in meningitis: **Increased (**protein, pressure and monocyte), **decreased** glucose.
     TREATMENT: Amphotericin B.

242. Sporotrichosis and its characteristics: **It is a rare,** fungal infection. **Spores** is its infective form. **The most common** site is **the skin** (painless papule with ulcer). Systemic infection **is uncommon** in children.
     TREATMENT: For skin lesion, oral potassium iodide. For systemic lesion, amphotericin B.

243. **Malt workers** lung and its features: It is caused by aspergillus and repeated exposure to **organic dust,** which causes **allergic alveolitis,** which shows signs of cough, rhonchi (**no** wheezing) a few hours after **exposure.** CXR shows **diffuse** infiltrate.
     CBC and sputum are **normal.**

244. A child who lives in **California, Arizona, or Texas** comes down with **influenza-like symptoms,** like cough, fever, night sweat, chills, chest pain. Examination reveals **erythema nodosum,** generalized maculopapular rash **mostly over the groin.**

MOST LIKELY DIAGNOSIS: Coccidioidomycosis (San Joaquin fever).
It is a fungus infection which occurs through inhalation of **spores**. It can cause **abscess** formation in skin and bone, **meningitis**, and massive pulmonary effusion. **Intrauterine** infection has been noted.
Most serious complication is **meningitis, which mimics tuberculosis.**
DIAGNOSIS: By biopsy or isolation of fungus by culture.
TREATMENT: Amphotericin B.
This medicine does **not** cross the blood-brain barrier **well**, so intrathecal administration is usually required. **Intrathecal** administration causes transverse myelitis and arachnoiditis.

245. **Most common infective form** of toxoplasma: **Oocyst.**

246. **Allergic bronchopulmonary aspergillosis and its features:** It is found in **asthmatic** children showed signs of wheezing; pulmonary **infiltrate is** found in chest X-ray, and CBC shows **increased eosinophil.**
DIAGNOSIS BY: Positive sputum culture for aspergillus.
TREATMENT: Steroid.

247. A group of children who went **to the park** to play came down with influenza-like symptoms like **dry cough,** fever, malaise, headache and body ache. Physical examination reveals **hepatosplenomegaly,** lymphadenopathy and **rales** over the chest.

    MOST LIKELY DIAGNOSIS: Histoplasmosis.
    It is a fungus infection which occurs due to contamination of **soil** through avian and **bird feces,** is found **throughout the U.S.A.,** and is most common in Tennessee and Kentucky.
    Definitive diagnoses: Identification of organism by culture or biopsy.
    TREATMENT: Usually **no** treatment is necessary because it is a self-limited disease. In case of severe disseminated infection, give amphotericin B.

248. **Most common** presentation of **Amebiasis:** Asymptomatic.
    Amebiasis is caused by Entamoeba histolytica. Infection occurs by **cyst** through contaminated **water and food. Not common in U.S.A.** Usually causes **flask-shaped** ulcer in large intestine, resulting in mucous with blood in stool. **Its most serious** manifestation is **hepatic amebiasis,** which **most commonly** causes **single cavity** in right lobe of liver. **Man is the reservoir.**
    DIAGNOSIS: Demonstration of organism in stool.
    TREATMENT: Metronidazole.
    PREVENTION: Proper sanitation and hand washing.

249. **Most common** site of **pulmonary aspergilloma:** Upper lobe.
    It is more common in leukemia and other immunocompromised children. **Invasive** pulmonary aspergillosis is treated with **amphotericin.**

250. **Giardiasis and features:** It is caused by **Giardia lamblia.** Infection is caused by **cyst** through contaminated **food and water, commonly found in immunocompromised children in U.S.A. Man** is the reservoir.
    Usual presentation is **weight loss, diarrhea, malabsorption** of sugar, fat, and fat soluble vitamin (A,D,E,K).

DIAGNOSIS: By **duodenal aspiration** (because cyst excretion in stool is irregular).
TREATMENT: Metronidazole.
PREVENTION: Proper sanitation, hand washing, **identification of** the **carrier** and **treat them.**

251. **Mode of infection** of toxoplasmosis to human:
    a.   **Fecal oral transmission** of contaminated cat feces containing oocyst.
    b.   Ingestion of contaminated **improperly cooked meat** containing cyst.
    c.   Human to human transmission occurs **only:**
        i.   Mother to fetus.
        ii.   Rare, organ transplant or transfusion related.

252. Severity of infection of Toxoplasmosis and **gestation age of fetus:** When infection occurs in **later** part of pregnancy then **less** chance and **less** severity of infection.

253. **Diagnosis** of Toxoplasmosis:
    a.   Mother: **IgG specific toxoplasma (progressively increasing titre),** IgM for toxoplasma.
    b.   Newborn: IgM specific for toxoplasma.

254. Management of **insect bites: First wash** with **soap and water immediately; calamine lotion** locally. **Corticosteroid ointment** may reduce some pain and inflammation. In **the case of a severely ill child** with systemic effect (e.g., caterpillar), **bed rest and sedation** (mild) are needed.

255. **Prevention** and **treatment** of Toxoplasmosis:
    Prevention:
    a.   Dispose cat litter everyday.
    b.   **Women** who do **not** have protective antibodies should eat meat only if it is thoroughly cooked and should avoid cats.
    c.   All meat should be **thoroughly cooked.**
    d.   Treat the mother and **prevent intrauterine infection.**
    TREATMENT: Sulfadiazine and pyrimethamine but also folinic acid because pyrimethamine is **an antifolinic** agent. Mother should be treated during pregnancy with **spiramycin** which has no major side effects to fetus.

256. **Trichinosis** and **its features:** Due to Trichinella spiralis. Infection is caused by **larvae** present in **meat,** showed signs of **characteristic periorbital and facial edema,** diarrhea, abdominal pain.

    DIAGNOSIS BY: Muscle biopsy.
    TREATMENT: Thiabendazole; corticosteroid used in myocarditis and CNS symptoms.

257. Echinococcosis (Hydatid disease) infection caused by: Dog.

258. **"Swimmer's itch"** due to : **Schistosomiasis.** Caused by Schistosoma **haematobium. Human beings become** infected by **contact with water.** Man is the **definitive host.** Swimmer's itch is **a papulopruritic rash** found in swimmers, which is also accompanied by

fever and chills. Examination reveals **enlarged** liver, spleen, and lymph nodes. CBC shows **an increased eosinophil** count. In **severe** cases, it can cause **hematuria, dysuria.**

DIAGNOSIS:
S. haematobium: eggs found in urine.
S. mansoni, S. japonicum: eggs found in stool.
TREATMENT: S. haematobium: Metrifonate.

259. Arcanobacterium haemolyticum infection: It is a gram positive bacillus. A human being is the primary reservoir. It appears with acute pharyngitis mostly in adolescents and young adults. pruritic exanthem first appears in extensor surface of distal extremities, then spreads centrally, but there is no petechiae, strawberry tongue, or complications. Diagnosis is confirmed by culture. Erythromycin is the drug of choice. Pharyngitis mimics group A streptococcal infection.

260. Astrovirus infection: It is an RNA virus, incubation period is 1 to 2 days, and mostly affects children younger than 4 years. Appears with gastroenteritis and fever, but resolves spontaneously in a few days. No confirmatory test is available but antibody detection can confirm the diagnosis. Virus can be cultured and electronmicroscopic detection of virus from stool can be done. Enteric precaution due to fecal oral transmission. Only supportive treatment is required.

261. Do not give oral acyclovior under the following conditions:
    a. Pregnant woman with uncomplicated varicella.
    b. Immunocompromised children (who needs I.V. acyclovior).
    c. To prevent varicella in an exposed person.
    d. Healthy child with uncomplicated varicella.

262. I.V. acyclovior is recommended under the following conditions:
    a. Pregnant woman with complicated varicella.
    b. Immunocompromised patient.

263. Oral acyclovior is recommended in the following conditions:

    a. Healthy persons with increased risk of moderate to severe varicella infection. e.g., a person receiving corticosteroid (P.O., I.V., aerosolized), chronic lung or skin infection, older than 12 years.
    b. Some experts recommended for secondary household cases with severe infection except in infants (less than 12 months because of insufficient data for safety and efficacy).

264. Prevention of STD (sexually transmitted diseases): Counsel the adolescent to abstain from sexual intercourse or at least use condoms.Discuss with and educate the adolescent. Primary prevention is much more effective than treating the disease.

265. **Tick paralysis** and its features: Due to tick bite that causes **flaccid ascending motor paralysis** which begins in **lower** extremities. **Management:** Search entire body for ticks. Remove ticks **immediately,** using **petrolatum** or heat to remove them completely.

OROFACIAL AND GASTROINTESTINAL

1. Newborn shows signs of **micrognathia, pseudomacroglossia** (tongue size is **normal,** but looks big due to hypoplasia of mandible), with **respiratory distress** at birth, and high, arched, palate. Newborn looks **less distressed** when in **prone** position.

    MOST LIKELY DIAGNOSIS: **Pierre-Robin syndrome.** Due to **hypoplasia of mandible** which grows spontaneously in first few months of life, so respiratory difficulty increases. **Normal** mandibular size is achieved around **4 to 6 years** of age. **Severe respiratory distress** cases which do **not** improve when child is in prone position may require fixation of tongue on the floor of mouth or tracheostomy. **When the child is in prone position, the tongue falls forward** and breathing is improved.

2. **Most common** cause of **lower eyelid coloboma: Treacher Collins** Syndrome or Franceschetti-Klein Syndrome or Mandibulofacial dysostosis.

3. A **newborn** child shows signs of **deformed pinna, coloboma of lower eyelid,** narrow palpebral fissure **slanting downward and outward,** micrognathia, hypoplastic mandible. **MOST LIKELY DIAGNOSIS: Treacher Collins Syndrome.** It is an autosomal dominant, **only conductive hearing loss** found, dental malocclusion and high arch palate present.

4. **Total anodontia** in a child found in: **Ectodermal dysplasia.** ("Anodontia" means "absence of teeth").

5. **Initiation** of **primary teeth formation** occurs during: 12th week of fetal life.

6. **Initiation** of **permanent** teeth formation occurs during: 5th month of fetal life.

7. **Partial** anodontia (absence of teeth) due to: Cleft palate or genetic or familial.

8. **Supernumerary teeth:** They always impede the **eruption** of adjacent teeth, so that the latter are **displaced. Mostly found** maxillary central incisor. **Management:** Should be **removed.**

9. Newborn child born with **loose natal teeth.** How do you manage this condition? Remove the teeth because they can cause aspiration.

10. **First primary** (milk) teeth appear: **Lower central incisor** at **6 months** of age.

11. **First permanent** teeth appear: **Lower central incisor** at around **6-7 years** of age. (First molars, both upper and lower, appear at the same time).

12. **Discoloration of teeth** is due to:
    a. Foreign material.
    b. Tetracycline. Its use produces brownish-yellow discoloration. Enamel hypoplasia **affects both primary and permanent teeth.**
    c. Erythroblastosis fetalis. (Blue-black color of primary teeth and of tip of 1st molar of

permanent teeth is due to **hemolysis).** Do **not** use tetracycline on patients younger than **8 years of age.**

13. **Most common** cause of **premature eruption** of **permanent** teeth: **Early loss** of the primary teeth of that area.

14. A child with signs of **dentition** of all teeth that is advanced for its age. **MOST LIKELY ENDOCRINE CAUSE: Hyperpituitarism.**

15. Causes of **delayed** eruption of **permanent teeth: Nutritional** disorder, rickets, **hypopituitarism,** hypothyroidism, cleidocranial dysostosis.

16. **Most common** benign tumor of the jaw: Ossifying fibroma.

17. Different **systemic diseases** and **their dental** characteristics:
    a. Congenital syphilis: **Hutchinson teeth** (screw-driver-shaped **permanent** incisor teeth).
    b. Ectodermal dysplasia: **Total or partial absence** of teeth because alveolar bone did **not** develop; **conical teeth.**
    c. Osteogenesis imperfecta: Dentinogenesis imperfection (**hereditary opalescent** teeth).

18. **Most common** site of **osteomyelitis** of the mandible and maxilla: Newborn: Premaxillary suture of maxilla. Children: Mandible.

19. **Most common oral problem** in children: **Dental caries** (common in children from 4 to 8 years old and from 12 to 18 years old).

20. **Most common** organism for **dental caries:** Streptococci.

21. **How flouride protects teeth:**
    a. Prevents dissolution of teeth by acid.
    b. Reduces acid production by bacteria.
    c. Mineralizes damaged teeth.

22. **Normal fluoride** requirement for **breast-fed newborn:** 0.25 mg/day.

23. **Most common** cause of **malocclusion of teeth:** Genetic. (Other causes include sucking of thumb, and acromegaly).

24. **Thumb-sucking: What causes it,** and **when should** it stop? Most likely due to stress. It should stop **by the age of 5 years.** If it does not, it will cause **displacement of permanent** teeth. **Motivate the** child to stop and reward him or her for his or her efforts to stop.

25. **Times to repair** cleft lip and palate: Cleft lip: **1-2 months** of age. Cleft palate: **12 months or earlier,** because child starts learning to. To avoid nasal intonation, let maxilla grow for up to 12 months.

26. **Most common** complication of cleft palate: **Recurrent otitis media.**

27. **Contraindication** to adenoidectomy:
    a. Submucous cleft palate. After adenoidectomy, child develops **speech defect.**
    b. Palatopharyngeal incompetence.

28. **Most common** site of**, and how to manage, impacted teeth: Most common** site is **maxillary canines** (mandibular 3rd molar). Extraction of impacted teeth is required.

29. **Most common** site of, and how to manage **dentigerous cyst:** Most common site is **mandibular 3rd** molar (maxillary canine). **Extraction** of the teeth is required. Due to **prolonged staying of impacted teeth in alveolar** bone, **or to cystic degeneration** of epithelium of enamel.

30. **Epstein pearls** (Bohn pearls): This is **an epithelial retention cyst** on the palate on each side of median raphe. It disappears after a few weeks.

31. A **bluish** cyst inside the mouth near salivary gland area. **MOST LIKELY DIAGNOSIS: Mucocele** or mucous cyst. If it forms after traumatic rupture of duct of salivary glands. **TREATMENT:** Excision.

32. Cluster of **yellowish white granules** in **oral** mucosa or lips. **MOST LIKELY DIAGNOSIS:** Fordyce granules (normal sebaceous gland). **TREATMENT:** None.

33. Newborn shows signs of **tumor**-like growth on **gum: MOST LIKELY DIAGNOSIS:** Epulis. It may, or may not, have peduncle: most of them are reactive rather than neoplastic. **TREATMENT:** Removal. (Will **not** cause metastasis.)

34. Newborn shows **white flaky plaques** all over inside the mouth: **MOST LIKELY DIAGNOSIS:** Candida albicans. It is **normal** for newborn and might appear after antibiotic therapy. **Persistent** oral candidiasis may be a **sign of immunodeficiency syndrome.** Candida lesion, when removed, leaves the **red surface** underneath. **TREATMENT: Oral nystatin.**

35. Child shows signs of **multiple,** small, **and painful** ulcers surrounded by **red margin. MOST LIKELY DIAGNOSIS: Aphthous ulcer** or canker sore. It is due to **stress. TREATMENT:** Local tincture benzoin to reduce pain.

36. A **chronically ill and malnourished** child has a **foul-smelling** mouth, and a small ulcer with **a gray, necrotic membrane** and hyperemic base. **MOST LIKELY DIAGNOSIS: Necrotizing ulcerative gingivitis** or vincent angina or vincent infection. It is **not** found in a normal child. **TREATMENT:** Mouth wash.

37. **Most common** example of **chemical burn** in children is due to: Holding aspirin directly on buccal mucosa or teeth.

38. Complication of **chronic dilantin therapy:** Gingival hyperplasia.

39. **Most common** type of **Tracheo-esophageal fistula:** Upper esophageal end is blind, and lower end is connected to trachea **(in 87% of cases).**

40. **Types of tongue** and **the diseases they are symptomatic of:**

Fissured tongue	Down syndrome.
Black hairy tongue	Prolonged antibiotic therapy.
White strawberry tongue	Early scarlet fever.
Red strawberry tongue	Late scarlet fever.
Taste bud reduced or absent	Riley-Day syndrome.
Atrophic glossitis	Niacin deficiency.
Atrophic glossitis with pale salmon color	Pernicious anemia, hypochromia anemia, sprue, achlorhydria.
Geographic tongue	Cold, chronic systemic infection.

41. **Most common** cause of **recurrent parotitis: Idiopathic.** It can occur in **normal** child, unilateral swelling with little pain of parotid gland. It resolves spontaneously. **No** treatment is required.

42. A child shows signs of **bilateral painless swelling of both parotid, and lacrimal** glands, **no** tears and **dry mouth. MOST LIKELY DIAGNOSIS: Mikulicz disease. Idiopathic.**

43. A child shows signs of **frog's belly**-like **cyst** on **floor of mouth** in sublingual area. Cyst is large, soft, and mucous inside. **MOST LIKELY DIAGNOSIS: Ranula. TREATMENT:** Excision.

44. A **newborn** in the delivery room has a **profuse esophageal secretion** and a maternal history of **polyhydramnios;** or, baby might show signs of **choking and cyanosis** after **first feeding. MOST LIKELY DIAGNOSIS: Tracheoesophageal fistula. DIAGNOSIS:** It should be made in the **delivery room.** Most significant is the **inability to pass the catheter** into the stomach or an X-ray shows coiling of nasogastric tube at the neck. (Do **not** give contrast material.) **TREATMENT:** NPO (nothing per oral), and drain the esophageal secretion constantly. Surgical repair.

45. **Most common** cause of **external** compression of esophagus: **Enlarged lymph nodes** in subcarinal area, which may be due to tuberculosis, lymphoma, histoplasmosis.

46. **Most common** cause of **suppurative parotitis: Staphylococcus aureus.** It is unilateral, and accompanied by redness, swelling, **and severe pain.** Needs antibiotic treatment.

47. **Moebius syndrome;** Includes facial diplegia, flaccid bulbar palsies with lower motor neurone disease.

48. In **achalasia,** what is the defect in **lower esophagus? Ganglion cells** are **decreased** and surrounded by inflammatory cells. Achalasia is **less common** in children, usually accompanied by dysphagia, regurgitation of food, or failure to gain weight. **TREATMENT: Dilate** the cardioesophageal junction.

49. **Most common** type of **Hiatal hernia: Sliding type.** It is mostly congenital and associated with gastroesophageal reflux. **TREATMENT:** It should be directed towards gastroesophageal reflux, but not towards hernia.

50. A **newborn vomits** excessively after feeding, otherwise does not look sick, **and sucks vigorously. MOST LIKELY DIAGNOSIS: Gastroesophageal reflux. DIAGNOSIS CONFIRMED: By 1st pH probe of lower esophagus;** 2nd Barium **study. TREATMENT: Thick, frequent, and small feedings, and elevation of head.**

51. What is the **outcome** of medical management of gastroesophageal reflux:? **65%** of those afflicted become **asymptomatic** by age 2 years. 30% of them retain symptoms that persist for up to 4 years, but no esophageal stricture. 5% develop esophageal stricture. <5% death, die due to aspiration.

52. Child with **gastroesophageal reflux** has been on intensive medical **treatment for the last 6 weeks,** but is still **very symptomatic.** How do you manage: **Operative repair.** Operation is definitely indicated in stricture.

53. An infant age between **the ages of 6 to 12 months** shows signs of **growth retardation** and history of **regurgitation.** Examination reveals mother was divorced and is **depressed.** Most likely diagnosis of the child: Rumination (Merycism). Etiology: Unknown, psychological factor disturbs **the mother-child relationship. TREATMENT: If loving relationship** between mother and child cannot be established, then **surgically** treat the gastroesophageal reflux.

54. **Most common** cause of **corrosive esophagitis: Household cleaning material ingestion.**

55. **Site of perforation** of esophagus:
In neonate: Perforation of **right** side.
In children: Perforation of **left side** of **distal** esophagus.

56. **Side effects** of cimetidine (H2 receptor antagonist). Gynecomastia and, rarely, coma.

57. **Mallory-Weiss Syndrome** and **management:** Tearing of **distal esophageal mucosa and submucosa** by violent retching results in **hematemesis. DIAGNOSIS:** Esophagoscope. **TREATMENT: Blood transfusion** usually stops the bleeding because of the self limited nature of the disease.

58. **Common complication** of **portal hypertension: Esophageal varices.** It usually accompanies **recurrent hematemesis** of bright, red blood with tarry stools.

59. A child suffering from **coughing** and **choking refuses to eat solid food,** but will drink some liquid. **MOST LIKELY DIAGNOSIS:** Foreign body in esophagus. **X-ray shows coin** in **coronal plane,** which means it is in esophagus. **TREATMENT: Removal** of the foreign body by direct esophagoscope.

60. **Time of appearance** of intestinal structures and their functions.

10th week	Na^+ - K^+ - ATP ase activity.
12th week	Pyloric muscle, true villi, beginning of disaccharidase activity.
14th week	Parietal and chief cells.
20th week	Peyer patches.
24th week	Sucrase activity.
32nd week	Maltase activity.
36th week	Lactase activity.

61. **Sites of absorption** of **food** components **in intestine.** Carbohydrates, Protein, Fat: Upper half of small intestine. Water: Large intestine. Bile salts and vitamin B_{12}: Distal ileum. Iron: Duodenum and proximal jejunum.

62. **Most common site** of **peptic ulcer** in **different age** groups:
Newborn: Gastric.
After newborn period to 2 years: Gastric and duodenal with equal frequency.
Between 2 to 6 years: Duodenal and gastric with equal frequency.
After 6 years: Duodenal.

63. **Most common** site of **stress** ulcer in **children: Gastric.** Stress means sepsis, trauma, shock, burn etc. In **head injuries,** ulcer is commonly found in distal stomach and duodenum; in burns, ulcer present in duodenum and **proximal** stomach.

64. **Most common** sign of peptic ulcer: **Painless bleeding.**

65. **Most common** cause of **peptic ulcer** in **newborns up to 5 years** of age: Stress ulcer.

66. **Most common site** of intestinal **obstructive** lesion (atresia or stenosis): **First ileum,** second duodenum.

67. **Zollinger-Ellison syndrome:** Rare occurs **with multiple recurrent ulcer** in duodenal and jejunum, accompanied by increased gastric acid secretion and acidity. It is due to massive elevation of **gastrin-like activity** from **tumor or for hypertrophy of islet cells.** TREATMENT: Cimetidine.

68. A child had surgery for pyloric stenosis (pyloromyotomy, Ramstedt), then **started to vomit after feeding.** How do you **treat** the patient? Stop feeding for 4 hours, then resume. **Persistent** vomiting indicates **incomplete surgery** or hiatal hernia or chalasia.

69. Certain **features** of pyloric stenosis: It occurs commonly **in the first born** male infant, with a higher incidence in **monozygotic twins. Projectile vomiting, olive mass** palpable in abdomen, **and hypochloremic metabolic alkalosis also accompany pyloric stenosis. Most commonly** diagnosis is made by clinical examination and **confirmed** by **sonogram.** Barium is **not** necessary for diagnosis, but if it is done, then note `string sign' (fine, elongated, pyloric canal). SMA6 shows **low Na, low** Cl, low K, **high** pH, **high** CO_2.

Differential diagnosis from **adrenal insufficiency** reveals **high K, low** pH (metabolic acidosis), **low** Na in SMA6.

70. What do you **expect after pyloromyotomy? Vomiting should stop completely,** but radiologically mild narrowing of pyloric canal may persist for months in asymptomatic patients.

71. **Initial** presentation of **site of intestinal** obstruction:
High obstruction: Vomiting.
Low obstruction: Abdominal distension.

72. **Most common** intestinal obstructive lesion in **Down syndrome: Duodenal atresia.**

73. A newborn suffers from **abdominal distension, and bilious vomiting,** X-ray of the abdomen shows **calcification** or **typical ground glass** appearance in **right, lower** quadrant.
MOST LIKELY DIAGNOSIS: Meconium plug syndrome.

74. **Radiological sign** in Intestinal **obstruction:**
Double-bubble sign: Duodenal obstruction.
Triple-bubble sign: Jejunal obstruction.
String sign (barium): Pyloric stenosis.
Corkscrew sign(barium): Malrotation
Cobblestone sign: Crohn disease.
Ground glass appearance: Meconium plug syndrome.

75. A full-term newborn who suffers from **bilious vomiting,** but **has no abdominal distension** after feeding, shows **abdominal tenderness upon being examined.**

   MOST LIKELY DIAGNOSIS: Malrotation of the intestine. It could be due to **sepsis,** but abdomen should **not be** tender. It could be due to NEC (necrotizing enterocolitis), which is **less** frequent in **fullterm** newborn, but abdomen is **tender.** It could be due to **paralytic ileus** for any reason. In malrotation, cecum **fails to move to the right, lower quadrant,** but rather remains in the **left side** of duodenum. There is also a **band** connecting cecum to the posterior right, upper abdominal wall which **crosses over the duodenum** and causes duodenal obstruction. This band is called Ladd's band.
   TREATMENT: Removal of the band and fix the cecum in correct position. This is a surgical emergency.

76. Meconium ileus or meconium plug syndrome **most commonly** found in: **Cystic fibrosis.** In the case of any newborn with meconium plug syndrome **always rule out cystic fibrosis.** Only 10% of cystic fibrosis patients develop this complication.

77. **Meconium plug syndrome:** its diagnosis and treatment: **DIAGNOSIS CONFIRMED BY: Gastrografin enema.** Plain X-ray is characteristic like **ground glass or bubbly appearance.** Intra -bdominal **calcification** means intrauterine **perforation,** but perforation **closes spontaneously** before birth, so **no** intervention is necessary.
TREATMENT:
a.　　**Uncomplicated: Gastrografin enema** can reduce meconium plug; it can be

repeated after 8-12 hours; if that fails, then **perform laparotomy.**

b.   **Complicated with perforation:** Do not administer enema; **only** perform laparotomy.

78.   **Most common** cause of **colonic obstruction** in newborns: **Congenital megacolon or Hirschsprung disease.** Due to presence of **aganglionic segment** ,which is **most commonly** found in, **rectosigmoid junction.** It usually accompanies acute obstruction in newborn and chronic **constipation,** sometimes **alternating with diarrhea** as in the case of older children.

79.   **Most common** cause of **paralytic ileus** in **infants: Pneumonia.**

80.   **Most common** cause of paralytic ileus in **older children: Perforated appendicitis.**

81.   **Hirschsprung disease: its diagnosis and treatment: Rectal biopsy** (punch or suction) demonstrates absence of ganglion cells. **TREATMENT: Colostomy,** proximal to site of lesion and, later, do definitive **end-to-end anastomosis** around 6-12 months of age. In case of **total colonic aganglionosis, ileal-anal anastomosis,** is preferred treatment. **Delayed toilet training** is a common problem after surgery.

82.   **Most common** sign of **Meckel diverticulum: Painless rectal bleeding (usually dark red blood; bright red when profuse).** Meckel diverticulum is the **partially** atretic **vitello intestinal duct** which connects the intestine to yolk sac. It is present in **2%** cases, **2** inches long and situated **2** feet proximal to the ileocecal valve. It contains gastric and pancreatic tissues in about a third of the cases. **Little hernia:** When meckel diverticulum herniates through inguinal canal. **Diagnosis** of meckel diverticulum: **Meckel scan. TREATMENT: Excision** of diverticulum.

83.   **Most common** cause of **mechanical** intestinal obstruction in infants: Incarcerated inguinal hernia due either to meckel diverticulum or intussusception.

84.   **Colonic polyp** and **features:** Usually accompanies **painless rectal bleeding,** 80% of colonic polyps are **single** and occur in **rectosigmoid region,** They do **not** become malignant, and usually **disappear spontaneously** due to necrosis from twisting.

85.   **Management** of foreign body in the stomach:
a.   If foreign body went **beyond pylorus,** then **only observe** and **check every stool** and look for foreign body. Give **normal diet,** no laxative at all.
b.   If it is **a sharp** object (needle, hair pin, bobby pin), then it is dangerous, because it might perforate the intestine. **Remove** the **foreign body** either by scopy or laparotomy.

86.   **Most common** cause of intestinal **obstruction** between the ages **of 2 months and 6 years. Intussusception.** Intussusception is **mostly ileocolic in type, of unknown** etiology, and may be an adenovirus **or,** more likely, due to **hypertrophic** peyer patches in the ileum which stimulate intussusception. Patient **suddenly** looks **very sick,** persistently **vomits, is lethargic, suffers** paroxysmal abdominal pain initially, **has bile-stained vomitus, and current jelly** stool (with mucous and blood). Examination might reveal **sausage-shaped**

mass in right abdominal area. **DIAGNOSIS CONFIRMED:** By barium enema.
TREATMENT: Barium **enema is also therapeutic** and this can reduce intussusception. **If it does not,** then do surgery (laparotomy).
Contraindication to **barium enema:**

a.   When duration of intussusception is more than 48 hours, because chances of perforation are high.

b.   In the case of ileoileal intussusception, it is not effective.

87. Characteristics of **campylobacter jejunal** enteritis: **Chronic bloody diarrhea,** crampy lower abdominal pain.

88. **Most common** organism causing **diarrhea in children** in U.S.A.: **Rotavirus.** It is more common in the **winter and is a self limited** disease. It causes **diarrhea** by **releasing enterotoxin or impairing absorption of sodium and chloride** in the **small intestine** through **cyclic AMP, or epithelial** cells of intestine fail to differentiate.
TREATMENT: Fluid and electrolyte.

89. **Bezoars, its types** and **their management:**

Trichobezoar: From hair ball. Lactobezoar: From milk card.
Phytobezoar: From fibrous material. A mildly **retarded** child with history of **swallowing unusual material** gives evidence of abdominal pain, vomiting, and other signs of intestinal obstruction.
MOST LIKELY DIAGNOSIS: Bezoar. It could be any of the above-mentioned types depending on the patient's history.
DIAGNOSIS: By Barium study: barium will **surround the bezoar.**
TREATMENT: Surgical removal, then evaluate psychologic status.

90. **A tall, thin, asthenic teenaged girl** has history of bilious vomiting **and losing weight.** Examination reveals she has **lumbar lordosis. Barium** study shows **dilated duodenum** as well as dilated stomach. **MOST LIKELY DIAGNOSIS: Cast syndrome** or superior mesenteric artery syndrome, or chronic duodenal ileus. Due to **compression of the third** part of duodenum between aorta (behind) and superior mesenteric-artery (front).

TREATMENT:

a.   First conservative: **Prone knee-elbow position** after meal helps relieve pressure on duodenum, **or nasojejunal** tube feeding to provide enough nutrition.

b.   **LAST SURGICAL:** If conservative management fails, then perform **L**add **procedure.**

91. **Characteristics** of **yersinia** enterocolitis: Diarrhea, arthritis, **periumbilical pain,** right lower quadrant pain, erythema nodosum.

92. An **adolescent** boy with history of **crampy, lower abdominal pain followed by** fecal urgency **and diarrhea with fresh blood.** Examination reveals presence of anal fissure, **diffuse** abdominal pain, tenderness, and distension. Stool contains **mucous, blood, and leukocyte. MOST LIKELY DIAGNOSIS: Ulcerative colitis.** It is due to **an unknown** cause, affects the **large intestine,** more common in **Jews, and those with strong family**

history among first degree relatives. It is also common in **patients with ankylosing spondylitis** and **HLA B27 antigen** positive.

TREATMENT:
a. **Medical:**
    i.   Mild cases-Hydrocortisone enema.
    ii.   Moderate cases-Oral Prednisone.
    iii. Severe cases-I.V. Hydrocortisone.
b. **Surgical: Indication:** unresponsive to medical treatment, massive bleeding, perforation, malignant changes.
PROCEDURE: Subtotal **colectomy** at first, then **permanent ileostomy.**

93. **First sign** of necrotizing enterocolitis: Abdominal distension and gastric residual.

94. **Most common long-term** complication **after medical** management of severe necrotizing enterocolitis: **Stenosis or stricture** of intestine.

95. An **adolescent** boy with history of **fever,** joint pain, **weight loss,** anorexia; **or,** with crampy abdominal pain, diarrhea. Barium study shows **cobblestone**-like pattern, thickened bowel with segmental distribution. **MOST LIKELY DIAGNOSIS: Crohn disease. Remission and exacerbation** are characteristics of this disease. It affects **mostly the distal ileum** and colon, and forms **non-caseating** granuloma with **fistula in intestine. Etiology in unknown.** More common in **Jews, and those with strong positive family history** of **first degree relatives. It** is found in patients with ankylosing spondylitis and HLA B$_{27}$ positive. Malignant changes are fewer than in ulcerative colitis. **DIAGNOSIS CONFIRMED BY: Rectal biopsy** showing granuloma. **TREATMENT: Prednisone.**

96. A **premature** newborn shows signs of abdominal **distension** and **guaiac positive stool** after few feedings **with milk.** Abdominal X-ray shows **bubbly appearance** in right lower quadrant area. **MOST LIKELY DIAGNOSIS: Necrotizing enterocolitis (NEC). DIAGNOSIS CONFIRMED: By abdominal X-ray showing pneumatosis intestinalis** (air within the muscle wall). **TREATMENT:** NPO, I.V. fluid and electrolyte, antibiotics. **Surgery** is indicated when there is **perforation or** child has low platelet, neutropenia, low pH and progressive deterioration.

97. **Most serious** complication of **active necrotizing** enterocolitis: **Perforation** of the intestine.

98. **Definitive surgical indication of** necrotizing enterocolitis: Perforation of the intestine.

99. **Most common** cause of **pseudomembranous** enterocolitis: **Clostridium perfringens** producing **enterotoxin** in large intestine.
Most common antibiotics causing pseudomembranous enterocolitis: **Clindamycin,** next ampicillin.

100. **Treatment of choice** for **cow's milk protein intolerance: Prolonged breast feeding.**
50% of children who have an **intolerance to cow's milk** also have **it to soy milk.**

101. A 10-month-old, child was doing fine until mother gave cow's milk to the child, who then

developed vomiting, **and diarrhea with occasional blood in stool. MOST LIKELY DIAGNOSIS: Cow's milk protein intolerance. DIAGNOSIS CONFIRMED:** Depending on patient's history, symptoms **should improve** after **discontinuation of milk** within 48 hours in acute cases and within 7 days in chronic cases. Milk protein intolerance is a **transient** phenomenon and most patients improve by the age of 2 years. **Some older** patients can suffer generalized edema, hypoproteinemia, and anemia due to **protein and blood** loss in intestine. Symptoms improve after stopping milk. **Some older** children show signs of **chronic diarrhea, mostly** in European countries.

102. **Recommended treatment** for pseudomembranous enterocolitis: Oral vancomycin.

103. **Most common** complication of **oral ampicillin:** Diarrhea.

104. A child who is known **to be an asthmatic** or **is an atopic dermatitis** patient with history of **vomiting, diarrhea,** abdominal pain and **is not** gaining weight. Child has not taken any asthma medicine for the past few months. **CBC** shows **high eosinophil** count with normal WBC count, SMA12 shows **low albumin. MOST LIKELY DIAGNOSIS: Eosinophilic gastroenteritis. DIAGNOSIS CONFIRMED: Biopsy** by endoscopy. **Endoscopy** shows inflammation of stomach and duodenum. **Biopsy** shows increased eosinophil in lamina propria and shortening of villi. **TREATMENT: Corticosteroid.**

105. A child with **failure to thrive, and abdominal distension,** upon examination reveals **wasting** of **proximal muscles; foul bulky pale stool is found. MOST LIKELY DIAGNOSIS: Celiac syndrome** or **malabsorption syndrome.** In this syndrome, **the most important** relationship is that between **food and presenting symptom** (e.g., having a history of **gluten** intake can cause **celiac disease** or celiac sprue).

106. **Tissue** diagnosis of malabsorptive syndrome by **small bowel biopsy: Suction** biopsy helps in the diagnosis of: celiac disease, abetalipoproteinemia, lymphangiectasia, viral and giardial enteritis, gamma globulin deficiency, tropical sprue, cow and soy milk intolerance, mucosal disease, disaccharide deficiency, and congenital anomalies.

107. In **malabsorption syndrome, the most important** part of initial physical examination: **Rectal examination.**

108. Laboratory diagnosis of **malabsorption syndrome:**
    a.   For fat:
        i.   Patient should take **more than** 20 gm fat per day for 4 days. In **normal** cases **fecal** fat excretion should **not** exceed **15%** of intake in an **infant** and 10% in **an older** child.
        ii.   **Fasting serum carotene level:** In normal child, level should be **more than 100 mg/dl.** In this syndrome, level is **less than 50 mg/dl.**
    b.   **For carbohydrate:**
        i.   **Random stool test** for **reducing substance:** A result of **more than 0.5% suggests** the presence of the disease. **Normally,** sugar should not be present in stool except for breast-fed infants. Test is done with the **tablet (clinitest)** mixed with random stool sample. The presence of reducing substance is abnormal. Most sugars are reducing substances **except sucrose. The pH** of the stool is

usually **less than 6.0** when sugar is present in the stool, because of the organic acid produced by bacterial action on sugar.

    ii.   **Breath hydrogen concentration test:** Give sugar orally 2 gm per kg or maximum 50 gm, and in first two hours measure breath hydrogen. **More than 10 ppm** is abnormal. Normally, sugar is absorbed in upper intestine, if it is not then enteric bacteria is acting on sugar in large intestine and ileum is forming hydrogen, which is excreted by lung.

  c. **For protein:**

    i.   Give intravenous injection of 51 CrCl and measure it in stool for 4 days. More than 0.8% of injected dose in stool is abnormal.

    ii.   Fecal excretion of alpha 1 antitrypsin: More than 15 cc per day measured for 48 hours is abnormal.

  d. **For folic acid:** Measure **RBC folic acid** level (more accurate than serum).

  e. **For vitamin B$_{12}$:**

    Schilling test: Tracer dose of vitamin B$_{12}$ is given orally. Measure urine for next 24 hours. Urinary excretion **of less than 0.5%** indicates **malabsorption,** which also found in resection of major portion of distal ileum.

109. What is the basic problem of **only giving parenteral** nutrition: Intestinal mucosal **mass and absorptive** surface is **reduced** significantly when oral intake is **withheld** completely, but reverses if the oral intake resumes soon. It is **very important** to **resume** oral nutrition as soon as possible.

110. **Which organic functions does chronic malnutrition usually affect? Pancreatic exocrine function. 90%** of the functioning tissue should be damaged before significant clinical presentations occur. Kwashiorkor: Intestinal villi are **flattened, atrophic.** Marasmus: Villi **normal,** but **microvillous changes.**

111. **Steatorrhea** found: When bile flow from liver to duodenum is interrupted, as **in biliary atresia** or **hepatobiliary disorder.** It also cause malabsorption of fat soluble vitamins A, D, E, K.

112. **Most common** cause of **diarrhea** in immunodeficient children: **Unknown.** Giardiasis is common in these children.

113. **Most common** cause of **primary immune** deficiency: **Isolated IgA deficiency.** This deficiency does **not** cause diarrhea itself, but when **superimposed infection or disease** occurs, then diarrhea is manifest (e.g., giardiasis, crohn, ulcerative colitis, celiac disease).

114. What is the **intestinal biopsy** finding in X-linked chronic granulomatous disease: **Granulomas** consist of multinucleated giant cells and lipid histiocyte.

115. **Most common** presentation of **hypogammaglobulinemia. Diarrhea.** This disease accompanies **disaccharidase** deficiency and sometimes **shortening** of intestinal villi.

116. In **Bruton disease,** common superimpose infection: Giardiasis. Burton disease or congenital X-linked Panhypogammaglobulinemia shows signs of mild, intermittent diarrhea which improves after 2 years of age. Biopsy of intestine **confirms the diagnosis** which shows

crypt abscess.

117. **Most common organism** present in intestine for months in **severe combined immune deficiency: Rotavirus.** Severe combined immune deficiency (Swiss type) present **itself early** in life. **Severe diarrhea** and **malnutrition** are mostly due to **disaccharidase** deficiency. **Intestinal biopsy confirms** the diagnosis which showed **PAS positive granule** and **atrophic villous.**

118. A child with history of **upper intestinal surgery** and who now shows sign of partial obstruction like vomiting, distension, also **emits foul smell and bulky stool** suggestive of **steatorrhea.** CBC showed **megaloblastic anemia** due to vitamin B_{12} deficiency.

     MOST LIKELY DIAGNOSIS: Blind loop syndrome or **stagnant loop syndrome.**
     TREATMENT:
     a.   **Definitive operative correction** for partial obstruction.
     b.   Small dose of **trimethoprim-sulfamethoxazole** to stop bacterial floral infection.

119. What causes **Blind loop syndrome besides** postoperative partial obstruction? Congenital intestinal obstruction, like duodenal band, malrotation, or stenosis.

120. A child shows signs of **diarrhea** after feeding and **malabsorption.** History reveals baby was born premature and had **intestinal resection** for NEC (necrotizing enterocolitis).

     MOST LIKELY DIAGNOSIS: Short gut syndrome or short small intestine. Intestinal length in **normal** newborn is about **250 c.m.** Short gut syndrome usually occurs when more **than 25%** of the gut is removed **surgically, or** it is due to **developmental** anomaly like malrotation, atresia; **loss** of ileum **(particularly ileocecal valve)** is **a most dangerous** and difficult situation for newborn, because jejunum **cannot** compensate for ileal loss. Ileum **absorbs vitamin B_{12}** and **bile salts exclusively. Ileocecal** valve prevents the colonic **bacteria** from going to small intestine. **Bile salts** causes diarrhea when they reach the **colon.** Increased gastric acidity is also noted.

     TREATMENT:

     a.   **Medium chain triglyceride** which is absorbed directly through vein.
     b.   **Monthly vitamin B_{12} injection** (100 micrograms; **clinical manifestation of B_{12} deficiency takes** almost **2 years).**
     c.   Give vitamin A, D, E, K.
     d.   **No antidiarrheal** agent.

121. What is **celiac disease** and its association with **antigen?** Due to intolerance of **gliadin** fraction of **gluten** which is **the protein** present in **wheat and rye. Mostly** associated with **HLA B_8 antigen.**

122. **Most common** mode of transmission of **celiac disease: Mendelian dominant** with **incomplete** penetrance.

123. What are the typical and atypical presentations of **celiac disease:**

Typical: Chronic **pale, foul-smelling** diarrhea, **weight loss,** anorexia, **wasting of muscles,** particularly **proximal group.** Symptoms begin around 1 year of age.
Atypical: May be accompanied by vomiting and diarrhea, or by constipation.
Constant features: Weight loss, growth failure.

DIAGNOSIS CONFIRMED: By biopsy of duodenum of jejunum **which shows short and flat villi, deepened crypts,** and vacuolated epithelium with lymphocytes.
TREATMENT: Gluten-free diet that is, no wheat or **rye for the rest of** life. Give **oat meals, vitamin A, D, E, K, and folic** acid. If lactase deficiency develops don't give lactose.

124. What happens **to most children** who suffer **from chronic diarrhea** and mild absorptive defects: They usually **become normal.**

125. A child between 6 months and 3 years of age experiences an **acute diarrheal episode** which is watery, induces vomiting, and may or may not be associated with fever. **Chronic loose stool,** which usually **gets worse** after **drinking fruit juice, follows.**

    MOST LIKELY DIAGNOSIS: Post-enteritis malabsorption. It usually get worse after **drinking sugar** or **hyperosmolar fruit juice.**

    TREATMENT:
    a.   **Reassure** the parents because they get frustrated.
    b.   **Avoid** fruit juice and milk.

126. **Tropical sprue: Not** found in U.S.A. Its etiology **is unknown.** Fever usually precedes diarrhea, wasting of muscles, and abdominal distension. Biopsy of the intestine confirms the diagnosis which shows short villi, increased crypt depth, and red cell infiltration.
    TREATMENT: Antidiarrheal agent, oral antibiotics, vitamin B_{12}, folic acid, nutrition.

127. What is the **etiologic** agent in **Whipple disease?** Rod-shaped bacilli. **Whipple disease** mostly affects the small intestine and is accompanied by **diarrhea, joint pain** fever.
    DIAGNOSIS CONFIRMED: By duodenal biopsy which shows bacilli and PAS positive macrophage.
    TREATMENT: Antibiotics, nutrition.

128. What is **the preferred treatment** for intestinal lymphangiectasia? **Medium chain triglyceride.** It does **not need** lymphatic to be absorbed. It is absorbed **directly through vein. Intestinal lymphangiectasia patient most commonly** shows signs of **edema** due to loss of protein in intestine. It is also accompanied by lymphocytopenia, steatorrhea.

129. What is the basic defect in Wolman disease? **Lipid accumulation** in intestine and other organs. It is rare, is accompanied by both enlarged liver and spleen, and vomiting due to **obstruction of** lymphatic.

130. Mode of inheritance of **Abetalipoproteinemia:** Autosomal recessive.

131. **Characteristics of Abetalipoproteinemia: Mental retardation, acanthocytes in blood smear, retinitis pigmentosa, ataxic neuropathy, malabsorption. DIAGNOSIS:** Made

by **acanthocytes** in peripheral blood smear, **low** cholesterol, and **low** beta-lipoprotein level.

132. **Treatment** of Abetalipoproteinemia: **Nonspecific** treatment only. Give vitamin A, D, E, K in large doses. A large dose of **vitamin E may prevent neurologic degeneration.**

133. **Defect in amino** acids absorption and associated diseases:

AMINO ACID	DISEASE
Tryptophan	**Hartnup disease** (ataxia, pellagra like rash, retardation), **Blue diaper syndrome.**
Methionine	Retarded white child **whose urine has a sweet odor.**
Cystine	Cystinuria.
Lysine	Hyperlysinuria.

134. Where is the location of **disaccharidase enzyme** in intestine? **Brush border.**

135. **Diagnosis** made **in disaccharidase** deficiency: Confirmed by mucosal **biopsy of intestine.** Breath hydrogen test is also helpful.

136. How **disaccharidase** enzyme deficiency **causes diarrhea:** It causes accumulation **of sugar** in the intestine which draws **water** into the lumen, thus causing **diarrhea.**

137. **Types** of disaccharide deficiency, **its characteristics** and **management:**
       a.   **Lactase deficiency:** Most common in premature babies and children older than 3 years appears with **abdominal distension, and loose** stool in premature **babies. Crampy abdominal pain** accompanies diarrhea in older children.
             MANAGEMENT: Discontinue lactose.
       b.   **Sucrase-isomaltose** deficiency: Mostly congenital, and appears with abdominal distension, watery stool, excoriated buttock. **MANAGEMENT:** Discontinue sucrose-isomaltose.
       c.   **Glucose-galactose** deficiency: Very rare.
             TREATMENT: Discontinue glucose-galactose.

138. What is the defect in **Juvenile pernicious anemia? Intrinsic factor production in stomach is** defective, resulting **in vitamin B$_{12}$ malabsorption** and megaloblastic anemia. Structure and function of stomach are **normal. Proteinuria** is commonly **associated** with megaloblastic anemia which manifests around 1 year of age. **TREATMENT** for megaloblastic anemia: Vitamin B$_{12}$ injection.

139. **Mode of inheritance** of **vitamin D-dependent rickets:** Autosomal recessive.

140. A **newborn child** comes down with **severe watery diarrhea,** has maternal history of **polyhydramnios,** and SMA6 shows **low k, low chloride, high pH (alkaline). MOST LIKELY DIAGNOSIS: Chloride-losing diarrhea. A rare** disease with **congenital defect of chloride-transport of ileum,** resulting **in accumulation of chloride in the intestine and diarrhea.** Stool has **high chloride. TREATMENT:**

a. **Give Potassium supplementation.**
b. **Restrict chloride** intake.

141. What is the **defect** in **primary hypomagnesemia?** Defect in intestinal transport of magnesium. Hypomagnesemia secondarily causes hypocalcemia and tetany. **TREATMENT: Give magnesium.**

142. A child comes down with **chronic diarrhea, and skin rash around mucocutaneous junction** of mouth, **hands and feet. MOST LIKELY DIAGNOSIS: Acrodermatitis enteropathica.** Due to **zinc deficiency** caused by **malabsorption. DIAGNOSIS:** Made clinically and **confirmed** by **low serum zinc level. Biopsy of intestine** shows paneth cell inclusion, which is reversible with treatment. **TREATMENT: Zinc sulfate orally.**

143. **Most common** cause of **irritable bowel syndrome: Unknown,** but physical and emotional stress can aggravate the problem.

144. **Menkes (kinky hair) syndrome** and relationship to **copper:** In this syndrome, **serum** copper and ceruloplasmin are **low,** but tissue **copper** is **high.** It is rare, **autosomal recessive, and due** to **defect in intestinal copper transport, resulting** in abnormal hair, reduced growth, cerebellar **degeneration,** and premature death.

145. Different **drug** use and **defective** absorption:

Phenytoin	**Hypocalcemia, rickets.**
Cholestyramine	Hypocalcemia, steatorrhea.
Sulfasalazine	Reduce folic acid absorption.

146. An **infant or toddler** has history of **watery stool for several days. Mother** stated that stool is usually **formed in the morning,** followed by bouts of watery stool. On examination, the child looks normal, is not dehydrated, drinks very well. Physician admits the child for further investigation, but child improved immediately after admission. **MOST LIKELY DIAGNOSIS: Irritable bowel syndrome.**

147. A **school age** child suffering from **recurrent abdominal pain** in **epigastric or periumbilical** region, **denies any relationship** of pain to his food. On examination, child passes **flatus few** times, **has increased intestinal sound,** passes **pellet-like** matter or **soft** stool, **and shows diffuse tenderness** in abdomen, with some **guarding in lower abdominal region** in both sides. Upon further questioning, the child stated that she does not want to go to school because she feels insecure with her friends and concerned about **her brother** who has been **sick for few months.**

MOST LIKELY DIAGNOSIS: Irritable bowel syndrome.
The clinical presentation may depend on **stressful situations** like **illness, or death.** It can **mimic** appendicitis. Proctoscopic finding shows **pale areas with hyperemia in** between dilated rectal vault. Child also can show **autonomic** nervous system disturbances like dizziness, pallor, and blurred vision. This child **talks** like **a mature child.**

TREATMENT:

a. **Strong supportive** and **sympathetic attitude of physician** toward **patient and family members.**

b. Nutrition with fibre diet.

c. Antispasmodic may or may not work.

148. **Most common** reason for **childhood surgery: Acute appendicitis.**

149. **Most common** cause of **acute appendicitis: Obstruction of the lumen,** but obstruction could be from different causes like appendicolith, twisting, torsion, **or infection the causes hyperplasia** of submucosal lymphoid tissue. Non-obstructive type is rare.

150. **Most important physical sign of appendicitis:** Persistent, localized pain in right lower quadrant.

151. **How does obstruction** cause **appendicitis? Obstruction** of lumen causes **increased** intraluminal **pressure** due to continuous mucous secretion, resulting **in compression** of mucosal **blood vessels, necrosis, ischemia,** then **perforation, fecal contamination, peritonitis, and abscess** formation.

152. When **in doubt** whether patient has appendicitis, CBC, abdominal X-ray, and urinalysis are **inconclusive. HOW DO YOU MANAGE: Admit the patient and observe** him, but do **not** give antibiotics. Appendicitis patients usually **get worse with time.**

153. **Management** of **acute appendicitis:** Definitive management is **appendicectomy.** Antibiotics **(ampicillin, gentamicin, clindamycin together,** or cephalosporin) should be given **prior** to surgery when appendix is **perforated or there are signs of peritonitis.**

154. **Post-operative appendicectomy complications:**

a. **Infection of the wound is most common.**

b. Another complication is **abscess** formation, which is **diagnosed by ultrasound. All pelvic abscesses** usually rupture and **resolve spontaneously,** but **abscesses below diaphragm** require **surgical drainage.**

c. Another complication is **obstruction.** If it occurs **within 1 month** of surgery, then **try non-operative** treatment. **After a month** has passed since the surgery, **first try non-operative** like nasogastric suction and drainage for short period. If that fails do **laparotomy.**

d. In females, **uterine tube obstruction** can result from complication of pelvic peritonitis.

155. What **other** diseases can **mimic** acute appendicitis? **Acute mesenteric lymphadenitis.**

156. **Treatment** for **anal fissure: Warm sitz bath,** which **relaxes anal sphincter.**

157. **Prolapse and procidentia: Prolapse** means descent and/or protrusion of **mucous membrane** of rectum through anus. Procidenta means that all layers of rectum protrude through anus.

158. A child passes bloody stool only painfully, and so **refuses to do so at all. MOST LIKELY DIAGNOSIS: Anal fissure. DIAGNOSIS MADE: By inspection only.** Most fissures occur **dorsally** in **sagittal plane,** and may have **tag** at the **end.** Pain is due to **spasm of lower fibre** of **internal sphincter.**
    TREATMENT:
    a. **No** treatment required as it heals spontaneously in **most cases.**
    b. **Soften** the stool with appropriate **diet.**
    c. **If there is no response** to medical management, then do **surgery** which includes stretching of anus, or excision of fissure, or sphincterotomy of internal anal sphincter, or all of the above together.
    COMPLICATION: It rarely recurs.

159. What is the **preferred treatment** for anal **fistula? Incision and removal of fistulas tract completely.** It **never** closes spontaneously.

160. **Most common** cause of **pruritus ani: Enterobiasis.**

161. Treatment for **postanal dimple: None** required.

162. **Pilonidal sinus** and its characteristics: It is **an acquired** condition, **and has no** relation to anal dimple. When **it is obstructed** it forms a pilonidal **cyst or abscess.**

163. **Procidentia** means that all **layers of** the rectum protrude through anus: It is common in **infants,** because the rectum lies in **the lowest** plane of the pelvis structure, and **a vertical** sacrum predisposes one to this problem. It is common in **malnutrition** because of **reduced ischiorectal fat,** mostly in cystic fibrosis. It should be distinguished from intussusception.
    TREATMENT: For prolapse:
    a. Constipation should be corrected by **diet.**
    b. **Mineral oil** to soften the stool.
    c. Push it **back** inside.
    d. **Insert sclerosant agent** into **rectal ampulla** if medical treatment fails.
    For procidentia; for rectum and sigmoid:
    e. **Abdominal sigmoidopexy: Surgery.**

164. **Most common** treatment for **dermal sinus: Excision. Dermal sinus** connecting postanal dimple with sacrum or coccyx, is attached to **duramater,** so **there is a chance** of **recurrent meningitis.** Dermal sinus is **congenital.**

165. An adolescent shows signs of **redness, swelling, heat, and tenderness** over the **sacrococcygeal area. MOST LIKELY DIAGNOSIS: Infected pilonidal cyst or sinus. TREATMENT: Excision and drainage.** If infection comes from the infected sinus, **pus** will come out.

166. **Familial polyposis syndrome: Rare. It is a premalignant** condition.

167. An **infant** experiences **painful defecation, and is not able to sit comfortably.** Examination reveals diaper rash with **a few pustules, swelling** around the anus, **but no** fever. **MOST LIKELY DIAGNOSIS: Perianal abscess.**

TREATMENT:
a. **Incision and drainage** immediately under anaesthesia.
b. Hot sitz bath after surgery.
c. Antibiotics are not effective.

In **older** children with **ischiorectal** abscess, always **rule out** crohn or ulcerative colitis. The most common organism in **both** abscesses is E. coli. **TREATMENT: Surgical drainage.** In **these kinds** of abscesses, surgery should be done **immediately,** unlike **in the case of cervical lymphadenitis,** where one may wait **until fluctuation. COMPLICATION:** Fistula formation.

168. Which kind of intestinal polyp is **most common** and can turn into **a malignancy: Familial adenomatous polyposis coli.** It is **autosomal dominant, and mostly** present in **distal large intestine.** In patients aged **10-20 years,** there are initially **no** symptoms but later returns with **blood loss, diarrhea, abdominal pain,** and shows evidence of strong **family history. DIAGNOSIS CONFIRMED:** By **biopsy** after **colonoscopy. TREATMENT: Pancolectomy; genetic counselling.**

169. **Most common intestinal malignant tumor** in children: **Lymphosarcoma in small intestine.**

170. Which polyp is **both non-malignant** and found in **small intestine: Peutz-Jeghers syndrome. It is autosomal dominant, and appears with mucosal pigmentation** of lips and gums. **TREATMENT:** Removal of polyp in symptomatic patient, genetic counselling.

171. **Most common** tumor of the intestine in **childhood: Juvenile colonic polyp. It is a hamartoma** that usually occurs in patients **1-15** years of age. It is usually (80%) located in **distal large intestine.** It is usual presentation is **painless rectal bleeding, and occurs in a non-malignant** form. **DIAGNOSIS CONFIRMED: Fiberoptic colonoscopy and biopsy. First rectal examination.**
TREATMENT:
a. **This is a self-limited disease.**
b. When polyp is **visualized by colonoscopy, remove** it.
c. When polyps are **multiple** and **proximally** located and so cannot **be assessed, then only** perform laparotomy and removal.

172. Which polyp is **pre-malignant,** found in both **small and large intestine,** and is associated with **osteoma and soft tissue tumor? Gardner syndrome.** It is a rare disease, **is autosomal dominant,** and is found in **early adult age. TREATMENT: Aggressive surgical management.**

173. **What** is the most common **site** for **carcinoid tumor: Appendix. Very rare** in children, and shows symptoms **like** those of appendicitis. **DIAGNOSIS:** High urinary concentration of **5-hydroxyindole acetic acid, which** is metabolite of serotonin **produced by tumor.**

174. **What kind of tumor** causes **diarrhea?** Neuroblastoma or ganglioneuroma causes diarrhea **due to increase of VIP** (vasoactive intestinal peptide). (Pheochromocytoma: **No** diarrhea).

175. **Inguinal hernia is most common** in which **age group? Premature infants.**
TREATMENT: Repair to **avoid incarceration,** which is more common in **younger** than in older children.

176. A newborn shows signs **of upper intestinal obstruction** (vomiting, no distension), and has maternal history of **polyhydramnios. BARIUM X-RAY** shows **obstruction** of **2nd part** of duodenum. **MOST LIKELY DIAGNOSIS: Annular pancreas.** It is associated with **Down syndrome,** atresia, imperforate anus, malrotation.

177. **Most common** cause of **viral pancreatitis: Mumps.** (Other causes are hepatitis A and B, rubella, coxsackie B, influenza A, Reyes' syndrome).

178. **Shwachman syndrome** and **features:** It includes **pancreatic insufficiency, neutropenia** (constant or episodic or cyclic), thrombocytopenia, hypoplastic anemia, **short stature** (less than 3rd percentile), **and metaphyseal dyschondroplasia of bones.**

    Etiology is unknown. **It is autosomal recessive.** Pancreatic acini replaced by **fat.** It usually seen **in infant** suffering malabsorption and **recurrent infection. X-RAY LONG BONE:** Bone age is **appropriate** for height. **TREATMENT: Pancreatic enzyme supplementation. Patients** improve with age. Sweat chloride test: Normal.

179. An adolescent with **epigastric pain** which **radiates to the back, vomiting,** lying quietly. **MOST LIKELY DIAGNOSIS: Acute pancreatitis. Most ominous** sign is **high fever.** Bluish discoloration around **umbilical area** means **bleeding.**

    DIAGNOSIS MADE: Increase amylase level (it increases during first 12 hours, then **returns** to **normal** after 24 hours); hypocalcemia, hyperglycemia; use sonogram to rule out pseudocyst; in **recurrent** pancreatitis, rule out **obstruction** by **endoscopic retrograde cholangiopancreatography.**
    TREATMENT:
    a. **Bed rest** and **support** for the patient, **NPO, nasogastric suction.** Sedation for severe pain.
    b. **Cysts** which persist **for more than 6 weeks or increase in size** need surgical drainage.

180. Liver enzyme **most specific** for **liver disease: SGPT. (ALT = Alanine aminotransferase).**

181. A mother brought **her two children** to your office for physical examination. The younger child, who is **an infant** has **2 to 3 cm** palpable liver, while the other, older child has **1 to 2** cm palpable liver: How do you manage the patient? These signs are **normal** for their age and do **not** need any further investigation.

182. What is the **grave prognostic** sign of **severe hepatocellular failure like** fulminant hepatitis? Rapid rise of **total** bilirubin, **mostly in the indirect** component, so **the ratio** of direct and indirect decreases.

183. Liver enzyme **most specific** for **obstructive** liver disease: Direct bilirubin. (Alkaline

phosphatase **increases** in **both** obstructive and inflammatory diseasess. In **sepsis, first indirect** bilirubin, **then direct** bilirubin increases. In **hypothyroidism, indirect** bilirubin increases which is also found in **pyloric stenosis.**)

184. **Important clinical presentations in different diseases:**
Cataract: Galactosemia.
Kayser-Fleischer ring: Wilson disease.
Carotenemia: Hypervitaminosis A.
Pruritus: Chronic cholestasis.
Retinitis pigmentosa and posterior embryotoxin: Watson-Alagille syndrome (Arterio-hepatic dysplasia).

185. **Most common cause** of **malformation** of **biliary tree: Biliary atresia.** (The second most common is **choledochal cyst.**)

186. **Liver biopsy:** It is **the most important diagnostic procedure of choice for the treatment of most liver** diseases like storage disease, enzyme defect, metallic toxicity (copper in Wilson disease). **Contraindication to liver biopsy:**
a.   Prolonged PT (more than 16 seconds).
b.   Thrombocytopenia (less than 40,000).

187. **Imaging** procedure for **obstructive** jaundice:
First: ultrasonography the **procedure of choice** for the treatment of gallstone, choledochal cyst, dilated bile duct, biliary atresia.
Second: PIPIDA scan after administering **phenobarbital** to stimulate bile flow.
Final biopsy of liver if first two procedures are **not** conclusive. First **laboratory test** should be **direct bilirubin.**

188. Causes of **severe cholestasis** during **first** month of life: TORCH infection. Alpha antitrypsin deficiency.   Galactosemia. Hereditary fructose intolerance.

189. **Most important** cause of direct **jaundice** around **6 weeks of age: Biliary atresia. TREATMENT:**
a.   **Kasai procedure**, prognosis for the child is **better** if the procedure is done **before he or she 2** months of age. Kasai procedure includes anastomosis of intestine with the liver at porta hepatis.
b.   **Medical: Diet**
Low fat, high protein, MCT oil; vitamin A, D, E, K in water soluble form.

190. Histologic features of **extrahepatic biliary atresia: Periportal fibrosis** and proliferation of **interlobular ducts.**

191. Syndrome associated with **intrahepatic biliary atresia: Watson-Alagille syndrome.** This syndrome is found in **early infancy. Characteristic facial features include:** Hypertelorism, **downward slanting** of **palpebral** fissure, flat nose, **prominent frontal head, pulmonary stenosis, anterior vertebral arch defect.**

192. **Most common** association of **polycystic liver disease is: Polycystic kidney** (in about 50%

of the cases).

193. **Most common metabolic** dysfunction of **parenteral nutrition** (TPN): **Liver dysfunction (increased SGPT, SGOT,** direct bilirubin).

194. **Most common cholestatic** jaundice of **newborns** (mostly premature) **around 2 weeks** of age: TPN. TPN-induced **cholestatic jaundice** is **reversible** after discontinuation for TPN. **TPN** is the **most common** cause of increased **direct** bilirubin in the **NICU.**

195. **Most common** cause of **indirect** hyperbilirubinemia in **newborns:** Physiologic jaundice (90% of newborns).

196. **Most common hemolytic** disease of the newborn: 'ABO' incompatibility. Remember, coomb's test is positive in only a third of the cases of 'ABO'. Set up (mother is `O' and baby either `A' or `B'), then do **Elution test (wash RBC,** remove **covering layer** over antigen on RBC. Antibody contact with antigen causes hemolysis).

197. **Laboratory differentiation** between **cholestatic** jaundice and **hepatocellular** jaundice: Cholestatic: **Very high alkaline phosphate;** mildly high SGPT, SGOT. Hepatocellular: **Very high SGPT, SGOT;** mildly high alkaline phosphatase, **low prothrombin (increased PT).**

198. **Drug-induced hepatotoxicity** and **its features:** It is a **transient** phenomenon that corelates with a history of **drug ingestion** (acetaminophen, antimetabolite), fever, rash, **and eosinophilia. TREATMENT: Discontinue the drugs.** There should be clinical improvement within a few days and biochemical improvement within weeks.

199. A child who has a **history of** either influenza-like symptoms or chicken pox **suddenly develops vomiting, initially hyperactive** behavior followed by **somnolence** and coma. Blood test shows normal bilirubin, **increase SGPT, SGOT, ammonia, PT. MOST LIKELY DIAGNOSIS: Reye syndrome.**
ETIOLOGY: Unknown. It is most likely due to **mitochondrial** swelling, pleomorphism, dense body loss.
TREATMENT: PICU admission, vitamin k to correct prothrombin time, **mannitol** if intracranial pressure is **more than 20,** phenobarbital. **Monitor intracranial pressure** and other vital signs.

200. **Most common** type of hepatitis in **childhood:** Hepatitis 'A'. Hepatitis A usually **disappears spontaneously** and does **not** develop into chronic hepatitis.

201. **Most common diagnostic** test for **hepatitis: Liver biopsy.**

202. **Urea cycle defect** and **Reye syndrome:**

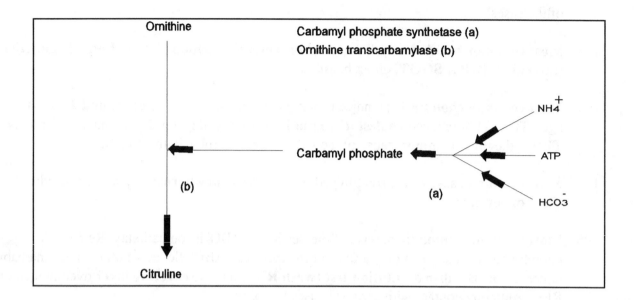

Normally the above reaction occurs **within mitochondria.** In **Reye syndrome,** there is **a defect in both enzymatic** reaction in (a) and (b), resulting in **increased ammonia** and **orotic acid.** Orotic acid interferes with synthesis of lipoprotein, resulting in fatty liver.

203. **Most common** type of hepatitis in **newborns:** Hepatitis 'B' Hepatitis B usually **persists** for **months or years, but rarely** develops into chronic hepatitis. Newborns infected by **vertical** transmission become **carriers mostly.** Very **few** cases of **chronic active hepatitis** are hepatitis B antigen **positive.**

204. **Liver function test** and **different** types of hepatitis:
    a. Acute hepatitis B: In both, **mild elevation** of SGPT, SGOT, bilirubin.
    b. Chronic persistent hepatitis: In both, **mild elevation** of SGPT, SGOT, bilirubin.
    c. Chronic active hepatitis: Increase **(SGPT, SGOT, Bilirubin), normal** (Alkaline phosphatase and albumin).
    d. Fulminant hepatitis: All are very high.

205. **Outcome** of different types of **hepatitis chances of complete recovery:**
    a. **Acute hepatitis B: 90% chance (most common) of complete recovery.**
       Chronic **persistent** hepatitis: less than 10% chance.
       Chronic **active** hepatitis: less than 1% chance.
       Fulminant hepatitis: less than 1% chance.
       PROGNOSIS: Good mostly.
    b. Chronic **persistent** hepatitis:
       Complete recovery: 100% chance (most common).
       PROGNOSIS: Excellent.
    c. Chronic **active** hepatitis:
       Cirrhosis: more than 60% chance (most common).
       Complete recovery:less than 40% chance.
       PROGNOSIS: Not good.
    d. **Fulminant hepatitis:**
       Death: 90% (most common).

Recovery: 10%. **PROGNOSIS: Worse.**

206. **Histologic features** of different **types of hepatitis:**
   a.   Chronic **persistent** hepatitis: **Normal** hepatic cord, but lack of uniformity in hepatocytes. Presence of **councilman bodies.**
   b.   Chronic **active** hepatitis: Both hepatic cords and hepatocytes are **damaged.** Presence of **pseudoacini** and **ballooning** of hepatocytes.

207. Treatment for different types of hepatitis:
   a.   Chronic **persistent** hepatitis: Reassure the family and do LFT every month.
   b.   Chronic **active** hepatitis:
      i.   Surface antigen negative (most common type): **Prednisone.**
      ii. Surface antigen **positive:** Prednisone use is **controversial.**
   As most children have **negative** type, give **prednisone.**

208. **Wilson disease** and **its features: Autosomal recessive,** it is due to **excess copper deposits** in liver, kidney, brain, and cornea, due to **defective biliary excretion of copper. Triad** of clinical features:
   a.   Cirrhosis.
   b.   Kayser-Fleischer.
   c.   **Low** serum copper and **high** tissue copper, **low** ceruloplasmin (copper binding protein).
   In kidney, copper **deposits in proximal** tubule results in loss of glucose, phosphate, amino acid, uric acid, and **renal tubular acidosis. DIAGNOSIS CONFIRMED BY: Liver biopsy** which shows macronodular cirrhosis, fatty degeneration and Mallory bodies (alcoholic hyalin).

   Excess copper content (more than 400 microgram per gram of dry liver tissue) **is the most reliable** indication of disease, but it **can be found** also in **chronic active hepatitis** in advanced disease condition.
   TREATMENT:
   a.   **D- penicillamine** for chelation.
   b.   **Corticosteroid** to prevent recurrence.
   c.   Vitamin B_6 as penicillamine is used.

209. **Most common** type of chronic **active** hepatitis with hepatitis B surface antigen: 95% of hepatitis B surface antigen is negative, the rest (5%) is antigen positive.

210. **Side effects** of **D-penicillamine therapy:**
   a.   **More common:** Low **WBC** count, increase lymph nodes, fever, rash.
   b.   **Most serious:** Aplastic anemia, membranous glomerulonephritis.
   TREATMENT FOR COMPLICATION: Discontinue penicillamine.

211. Prognosis of **Wilson disease** with or without treatment:
   a.   All **untreated** patients: Die of neurologic, hepatic, renal, hematologic problems.
   b.   Patients with chronic **active** disease: **They respond poorly** to therapy and end up with cirrhosis.
   c.   Patients with **acute liver** failure and neuromuscular involvement: **They do not**

respond to therapy.

d.　**Early** treatment: Better outcome with **therapy.**

212.　**How do you manage** a sibling of **patient with Wilson disease? Normal siblings** should **receive** D-penicillamine therapy to **prevent the disease completely** or **cure them.**

213.　**Chronic inflammatory bowel disease is most commonly** associated with which **kind** of hepatitis? **Chronic active hepatitis.**

214.　**Sclerosing cholangitis is most commonly　associated with which kind of bowel disease: Ulcerative colitis.**

215.　**Most common** complication of **cirrhosis:　Hemorrhage** from ruptured esophageal varices **due to portal hypertension.** (Other complications are ascites and coma.)
Treatment for esophageal bleeding:
a.　Whole blood transfusion.
b.　I.V. **vasopressin.** If bleeding doesn't stop, then **balloon** (Sengstaken-Blakemore) tube is inserted and inflated to stop bleeding.
Treatment for ascites:
a.　**Low sodium, low protein** (due to cirrhosis), starch vitamin supplement.
b.　Abdominal paracentesis can be done for **diagnostic purposes.**
c.　**Avoid therapeutic** paracentesis until acute respiratory distress occurs.

216.　**Management** of **hepatic coma:** Exchange blood transfusion. Steroids have **no** value. **Lactose** is a non-absorbable synthetic disaccharide which **reduces** the formation of **ammonia** by **inhibiting colonic flora.**

217.　**Most common** cause of portal hypertension in children: **Extrahepatic portal vein obstruction. Its etiology** is **unknown** in 66% of cases, but **umbilical venous catheter** is the cause in 33% of cases.

218.　**Most common** clinical manifestation of portal hypertension:　**Massive hematemesis. DEFINITIVE TREATMENT:**
a.　**Splenorenal shunt** to reduce portal hypertension.
b.　**To stop hematemesis:** Whole blood transfusion, I.V. vasopressin, NG (nasogastric) tube, **Blakemore** tube in gastroesophageal junction.

219.　**Most frequent** cause of **fatty infiltration:　Obesity.** Other causes are diabetes, starvation, galactosemia, familial hyperlipidemia. **Normal** fat content of liver (3-5%) and it goes up **to 40%** in **infiltration.** But in fatty degeneration, total hepatic **fat content** remains the **same,** and there is **an alteration in ratio** between hepatic cholesterol and other lipid.

220.　**Most common** clinical manifestation of fatty infiltration:　**Hepatomegaly** but it is asymptomatic.

221.　**Treatment** for fatty infiltration:　**Reduce** the fat and give **more** protein.

222.　**Most common** cause of **cholecystitis** in **the older child:** Cholelithiasis (gall-stone).

223. **Most common** cause of cholecystitis in **infants:** **Sepsis (Streptococci,** Salmonella, Giardiasis).

224. A child has pain in **right upper quadrant,** and fever. Examination shows palpable **mass** in that region. **MOST LIKELY DIAGNOSIS:** **Cholecystitis. DIAGNOSIS: First cholecystography,** but I.V. cholangiogram if cholecystography is not helpful. **TREATMENT OF CHOICE: Cholecystectomy.**

225. **Most common** cause of ascites in **children:** **Renal (Nephrotic syndrome).** An other cause is cardiac in origin.

226. **Most common** organism causing **primary peritonitis:** **Pneumococcus.** Other organisms are Group A Streptococci and gram negative organisms.
     Clinical symptom and sign of peritonitis: Vomiting, abdominal pain, fever (or **hypothermia** in very sick patients). Examination reveals **rebound tenderness, guarding or** doughy feeling.
     LABORATORY FINDING: Leukocytosis with increased polymorph.
     X-RAY ABDOMEN: Dilated intestine and edema.
     TREATMENT: Antibiotics.

227. Causes of **true** chylous ascites: Congenital anomaly, injury (postoperative), obstruction. **TREATMENT: High protein** diet and **MCT. PROGNOSIS: Not good.** Patients rarely recover, and whether they do depends on etiology.

228. **Most common** cause of **neonatal** peritonitis: Infection acquired **during and after birth** (less through placenta).

229. **Most common** cause of **secondary peritonitis** in **children:** Ruptured appendix.

230. **Different hepatitis and transmission.**

     Transfusion of blood and blood products: Hepatitis (B and Non A, Non B).
     Immune serum globulin: Hepatitis (B, Non A Non B, A).
     Breast milk: None.
     Transient episode: Hepatitis A. [* Non A, Non B = Hepatitis C]
     Sexually transmitted: Hepatitis (A,B).
     Newborn affected: Hepatitis (B).
     Dialysis: Hepatitis B.

231. **Most common** cause of **secondary** peritonitis in **newborns,** particularly **premature newborns:** NEC (necrotizing enterocolitis).

232. **Most common** sign of **perforation** of intestine: **Free air** in peritoneal cavity.

233. **Localized** peritonitis due to **ruptured** appendix: **Abscess** formation is a common complication. **DIAGNOSIS OF ABSCESS:** Sonogram. **TREATMENT: Surgical drainage** with appendicectomy and **antibiotics.**

234. A newborn child shows **severe respiratory distress, and cyanosis** at birth. Examination reveals heart sounds coming from **right side, close to sternum, and scaphoid abdomen.**
MOST LIKELY DIAGNOSIS: Diaphragmatic hernia (congenital).
DIAGNOSIS CONFIRMED:
a.   **Before** birth: sonogram.
b.   **After** birth: **chest and abdominal X-rays show intestine in the chest.**
MOST COMMON SITE: Posterolateral segment of (L) side of diaphragm or Bochdalek triangle defect.
TREATMENT: First, **elevate head** and neck, then **insert nasogastric tube,** then intubation and ventilation, then **corrective surgery.**

235. **Difference between ulcerative colitis and Crohn's disease:**

Ulcerative colitis	Crohn's disease
Large intestine	**Small and large intestine**
Ulcerative lesion	Granulomatous
Superficial lesion	Deep lesion (all layers).
Diffuse lesion	Segmental lesion
↑ Tenesmus, ↑ pain	↓ Tenesmus and pain, sometimes massive bleeding.
Extraintestinal involvement is less	**More involvement** (arthritis, clubbing).
(ESR, Hgb, albumin) normal	↑ ESR, ↓ Hgb, ↓ albumin
Biopsy: Poly. and crypt abscess	Granuloma
↓ Fistula, ↓ perianal abscess	↑ (Fistula and abscess)
No cure	No cure
Operation: colectomy	Not possible
Prednisone, sulfasalazine	**Prednisone, azathioprine**
↓ Recurrence	↑ Recurrence
Constant pattern	**Exacerbation and remission**
↓ Obstruction (intestine)	↑ Obstruction
↑ Cancer (very high)	↑ Cancer (mildly high)
Diagnosis confirmed by biopsy of rectum	**Confirmed by barium (upper G.I.), rectal biopsy.**

236. Most common **complication of diaphragmatic** hernia (congenital): PPHN (persistent pulmonary hypertension).
TREATMENT:

a.   **Ventilator management** to keep the pH 7.45 to 7.55, CO_2 35-45, PO_2 80-100.

b.   **Drug management:** Tolazoline or priscoline.

It is a **pulmonary vasodilator** that **dilates all the blood** vessels of the body **except in kidney** which gets constricted.

Most common complication of Tolazoline: **gastric hypersecretion.** Other complications are gastric bleeding, gastric rupture, bleeding from any site, low platelet count, **hypotension.**

Management of **Tolazoline complication:**

    i.   **Cimetidine** to prevent gastric complication.

    ii. **Dopamine** to prevent hypotension.

    iii. **Blood, FFP, vitamin K** for bleeding.

    iv. **Most important: discontinue** tolazoline.

    v.   Platelet count for thrombocytopenia.

c.   High frequency ventilator.

d.   ECMO (extra corporeal membrane oxygenation) when other management fails.

237. Gastric acid secretion and ages:

    a.   At birth: Neutral pH (gastric).

    b.   Within few hours after birth: Gastric pH ↓ 1.5 to 3.0.

    c.   First 10 days: ↑ gastric acid secretion and ↓ pH.

    d.   10-30 days: ↓ gastric acid secretion and ↑ pH.

    e.   At 3 months: Reach lower limit of **adult values.**

DIABETES

1.   Most common endocrine metabolic disorder of childhood: **Diabetes mellitus.** Type 1 (insulin dependent or juvenile diabetes): **Diminished insulin secretion** may be due to **autoimmune destruction of pancreatic beta cells.** The peak age is 5-7 years and at puberty. **There is an increased frequency** with HLAB8, DR-3, DR-4, BW 15, properdin factor b. Homozygous **absence of aspartic** acid at 57 position of HLA-DQ beta chain **(non Asp/non asp)** will increase the **risk of diabetes by 100%.** HLA typing is **not use** for genetic counseling, because there is no way to prevent it. **Risk to sibling of a diabetic patient is 6% if the proband under 10 years, and 3% if older.** Risk to offspring is **2 to 5% if mother is diabetic, higher (6%) if father is diabetic. Risk to identical twin is 30-50%** to become diabetic, but environmental or genetic factors may also be important. **Most important triggering factors for diabetes are mumps, rubella, coxsackievirus (important for board examination).** These viruses cause diabetes by **destroying pancreatic beta cells or by triggering immune response to endocrine tissue.**

2.   **Glucosuria** in diabetes occurs when renal threshold exceeds: **180 mg/dl.**

3.   Most common cause of Type 1 diabetes: **Autoimmune phenomenon or auto aggression:** here autoantibodies, along with T cells and complement, cause destruction of pancreatic beta cells. It **mimics Hashimoto thyroiditis.** Islet cells antibody (ICA) shows up in 80-90% of patients. This **ICA disappears after removal of pancreas** but **reappears** when new pancreas is transplanted. **ICA usually manifests months or years before the clinical**

manifestation of diabetes, which occurs after the destruction of 80% of beta cells. Anti insulin antibody is also present.

4. First (or initial) and last (or late) clinical manifestations of diabetes:
First: Post-prandial hyperglycemia.
Last: Fasting hyperglycemia.

5. **Stress hormones, insulin and type 1 diabetes:** Stress hormones are epinephrine, cortisol, growth hormone, and glucagon. All enhance diabetes by different mechanisms:
   a. Impair insulin secretion: epinephrine.
   b. Antagonize insulin secretion: epinephrine, cortisol, growth hormone.
   c. Increase all of the following: glycogenolysis, gluconeogenesis, lipolysis, ketogenesis.
   d. Decrease glucose utilization and increase glucose clearance: epinephrine, growth hormone, cortisol.

6. Formula to calculate serum osmolality (mOSM/kg):
$$(\text{Serum sodium} + \text{Serum potassium}) \times 2 + \frac{\text{Glucose (mg/dl)}}{18} + \frac{\text{BUN(mg/dl)}}{3}$$
$$\text{(mEq/l)} \quad \text{(mEq/l)}$$

7. **Lipid metabolism** and **diabetes:** Low insulin and high stress hormones cause **increased lipolysis** and inhibit lipid synthesis, resulting in **increase total lipid, cholesterol, triglyceride, free fatty acids.** Free fatty acid forms **ketone bodies** (betahydroxybutyric acid, acetoacetic acid) which cause **metabolic acidosis.** Body compensates by **respiratory alkalosis** i.e., increase respiration (Kussmaul respiration). Acetoacetic acid converts to **acetone which causes fruity smell** in breathing. **Ketone excreted in urine** causes loss of water, and electrolytes cause dehydration, acidosis, **and diminished cerebral oxygen utilization,** which causes coma.

8. Usual presentations and weight loss associated with diabetes: Usual presentations are polyuria, polydipsia, polyphagia and weight loss. **Weight loss is** due to **loss of 50% of total calorie intake in urine** i.e., 1000 calories lost in urine in the **form of glucose.** No matter how much child eats, he loses weight due to catabolic state. **25% of children show signs of ketoacidosis. Abdominal pain** is also present.

9. **Diagnosis of diabetes:** History of **polyuria, polydipsia, hyperglycemia, glucosuria with or without ketoacidosis.** If there is any doubt, do glucose tolerance test.

10. **Renal glycosuria:** Glucose excreted in urine, but **no hyperglycemia** (unlike diabetes). Along with glucose, **galactose, pentose, and fructose appear** in urine. It is found in cases of Fanconi syndrome, cystinosis, and the use of outdated tetracycline.

11. **DKA means:** Serum glucose **is more than 300 mg/dl, ketonemia, metabolic acidosis with a pH less than 7.30 and bicarbonate less than 15 mEq/l, plus glucose and ketone found in urine.**
Precipitating factors for DKA: Stress (trauma, vomiting, infection, psychologic factors).

12. A child known to be diabetic and on insulin develops DKA frequently. Most likely cause: **Inadequate insulin doses** or **stress.**

13. **Non-Ketotic hyperosmolar coma:** It represents serum glucose **of more than 600 mg/dl, absence or mild ketosis, nonketotic metabolic acidosis,** severe dehydration due to glucosuria, altered sensorium, and finally coma. **Neurologic signs are very common** (convulsion, hemiparesis, hyperthermia, positive Babinski signs). **Rarely** do patients have Kussmaul respiration for lactic acidosis. First manifestation is polyuria, or polydipsia; later, thirst disappears because of **hypothalamic thirst center alternation due to osmolarity** or preexisting hypothalamic defect. Hyperosmolarity inhibits ketone production and inhibits lipid breakdown.
    TREATMENT: Correct vascular volume deficit by adequate hydration (half normal saline initially), then start **insulin therapy.**

14. **Immediate goal** of therapy in DKA: Expansion of intravascular volume. Work up should include CBC, SMA6, EKG (rule out hyperkalemia), strict intake and output measurement. **Remember: catheterization of bladder is not recommended routinely (important for Board examination).**

15. During the treatment of DKA with insulin, which parameter improves **fast? Serum glucose.** Serum glucose **improves faster than pH and bicarbonate. Insulin infusion must be continued as long as the acidosis persists,** even when serum glucose is **below 300 mg/dl,** then add D5 0.2 N saline to prevent hypoglycemia. If the **acidosis still persists** even with the above therapy, consider **gram negative infection. Insulin infusion should be stopped and changed to S.C. insulin** when acidosis is corrected, but glucose is around 300 mg/dl. Remember, when acidosis is corrected, ketonuria may persist for another day or two. **Ketonuria** does **not indicate** poor therapeutic response.

16. **Major complication** of therapy in **DKA and therapy:** One life-threatening complication of DKA therapy is **cerebral edema** which is due to the rapid decline of serum osmolality, so don't give a hypotonic solution. **Initially a 0.9% saline** (20cc/kg) should be given (50-60% of the deficit in 1st 12 hours, remaining 40-50% in next 12 hours). When serum glucose is close to 300 mg/dl, start D 5-0.2 N saline. **In acidosis, K goes out of** the cells. In DKA serum, k may be normal, but total body K is depleted, so resume k early. In alkalosis, K goes inside the cells, so after hydration K goes into the cells, and this can cause severe hypokalemia (low T wave and U wave in EKG). **In DKA, degree of dehydration varies, but it is usually close to 10%.** In DKA, there is also **low phosphate,** which is a component of **enzyme 2,3 DPG** (diphosphoglycerate). A deficiency of phosphate causes a deficiency of 2,3 DPG, which shifts the **oxygen dissociation curve to left** (i.e., less oxygen release to tissue). At the same time, **acidosis** of DKA shifts that **curve to right, resulting in more oxygen delivery to tissue and correct acidosis. Sodium bicarbonate** therapy is indicated only when pH is less than or equal to 7.2 (between 7.1 to 7.2, $NaHCO_3$ 40 mEq/m^2; less than 7.1, 80 mEq/m^2 over 2 hours infusion).
    Insulin: Initial dose of 0.1 u/kg of regular insulin, then continuous infusion of 0.1 u/kg/hr is the **most accepted method of therapy.**

17. A child with DKA has been receiving treatment with fluid and insulin. **With respect to his chemistry, the patient is improving** (acidosis corrected, glucose reduced in serum). **A few hours after treatment has started,** however, child comes down with headache, vomiting, altered consciousness, delirious outburst, and unequal pupillary reaction.
    MOST LIKELY DIAGNOSIS: Cerebral edema.

TREATMENT: Mannitol and hyperventilation can save the child's life. (**Remember, subclinical cerebral edema** occurs in **most** patients with DKA receiving insulin and fluid therapy). **Polyuria might occur due to diabetes insipidus** (erroneously interpreted as osmotic diuresis due to glucose) **which might coexist with diabetes mellitus. Cerebral edema due to excessive fluid given** (restrict intake up to 4.0 L/m²/24 hour), **excessive use of bicarbonate** (try to prohibit it), **large doses of insulin,** or compensatory response to intracellular acidosis.

18. What is the **most important reason** for **not using NaHCO₃ in DKA therapy:** NaHC0₃ metabolizes to CO_2 and H_2O; CO_2 diffuses throughout the blood-brain barrier faster than does bicarbonate, resulting **in severe cerebral acidosis and cerebral depression.** Other reasons are **alkalosis,** the shift of the oxygen dissociation curve to the left, causing hypokalemia.

19. **Aim of therapy** in **postacidotic** phase or transition period (usually after 36-48 hours): Adjust **insulin** doses, treat infection, give advice for **proper nutrition,** educate parents and patient.

20. **Advantage of human insulin over pork insulin:** Human insulin is **less allergenic** and **shows less antibody formation** than pork insulin, but otherwise they are the same. Human insulin (synthetic) is synthesized in bacteria via DNA recombinant method or by chemical modification of pork insulin (semisynthetic).

21. **Nutritional advice** to a diabetic patient: No special nutritional requirements other than what is **necessary for optimal growth and development.** Distribution of calories is same as for a normal person (55% carbohydrate, 30% fat, 15% protein). 70% of **total carbohydrate intake should be complex carbohydrates (starch,** which takes a long time to metabolize in the gut, lessens swing in glucose level). **Avoid sucrose and refined sugar (beverages), sorbitol, xylitol, saccharin.** Recommend high fibre, high polyunsaturated fat.

22. **Distribution of calories** in diabetes: 20% breakfast, 20% lunch, 30% dinner; **10% each** at midmorning, mid-afternoon, and evening snacks.

23. Management of **hypersensitive reaction** to insulin: **Change it to other type of insulin.** The reaction includes urticaria, erythema, **but rarely** angioedema. Allergic reaction due to IgE.

24. **Antibody formation** to insulin therapy in diabetes: It develops after **several months** of treatment. While it does **not** interfere with metabolic response, it may **create instability** by forming a reservoir of insulin and an unpredictable release of it. **Rarely,** antibodies form true resistance to insulin and require higher doses.
    TREATMENT: Pure pork, pure beef, or human insulin resolves the problem; **rarely** requires steroids or desensitization. It is due to IgA and IgM.

25. Reliable index for **long term** metabolic control of diabetes: Hemoglobin A1c (glycosylated hemoglobin).
    Glucose is non-enzymatically attached to hemoglobin. The higher the glucose level and the longer the duration of exposure to hemoglobin with glucose, the higher the fraction of

HbA1c which is a percentage of total hemoglobin. It reflects serum glucose level for the last 2-3 months. Normal HbA1c value is less than 7%. In diabetes, values of 6-9% indicates very good control, 9-12% fair control, over 12% poor control.

26. Most common complication in diabetic patient **active in sports: Hypoglycemia.** Due to **increased absorption of insulin from injection site.** Regular exercise increases insulin reception and metabolic control. In poorly controlled patient, vigorous exercise causes ketoacidosis, because exercise increases counter-regulatory hormones. **TREATMENT: Glucose** (before exercise to prevent hypoglycemia, or during and after exercise) in the form of orange juice or carbonated beverages. **Reduce insulin dose by 10-15%** and give **injection in abdomen** (not in legs).

27. Why residual beta cells **cannot** prevent DKA: **Not clear,** but may be due to increased catecholamine secretion (due to stress) which prevents insulin secretion from beta cells.

28. Honey-moon period in diabetes (residual beta cell function): Residual beta cell function is directly proportional to C-peptide, i.e., **high insulin secretion means high C-peptide level.** 75% of newly diagnosed diabetic patients, after initial control with insulin, require **progressively lower insulin doses. First clinical manifestation is hypoglycemia.** Honey-moon period lasts from weeks to months, up to 2 years maximum. This is **due to high C-peptide response, which means a residual active beta cells function.** TREATMENT: Reduce the insulin doses.

29. A child who is a known diabetic on insulin suddenly comes down with **sweating, pallor, tremor, tachycardia (due to increase catecholamine), drowsiness, confusion, and seizure (due to cerebral glucopenia).** **MOST LIKELY DIAGNOSIS:** Insulin-induced hypoglycemia. **TREATMENT: Glucose** (candy, carbonated beverage) or **glucagon in unconscious patient.** It can occur when serum glucose level suddenly drops (not necessarily less than 60 mg/dl in normal person). * **Hypoglycemia** is **the sudden onset,** but **DKA (hyperglycemia) is a gradual process.** Hypoglycemia is mostly due to increase insulin, low calories, honey-moon phase. Most important is for the patient and family members to understand the problem.

30. **Infection and diabetes:** Infection among diabetics occurs in **same frequency as in the nondiabetic population. During infection, the insulin dose should be increased** because of stress hyperglycemia, which present **as vomiting.** If vomiting does not stop even after increasing insulin, then admit the patient to the hospital.

31. **Growth and diabetes:** Puberty may be **delayed,** but eventually the patient will attain normal adult height range. His or her height, however, will be less than his/her genetic potential would predict.

32. **Surgery and diabetes:** The goal is to avoid **hypoglycemia.** In elective surgery patient should be admitted 24 hours before surgery. Give only regular insulin Q6 hour and nutrition. In the morning of operation, keep NPO and I.V. D5 0.45 N saline, K 20 mEq/l. Add 1 unit of insulin with each 4 gm of glucose. The rate of infusion is determined by maintenance fluid and fluid lost in surgery. Keep Gl level between 120-150 mg/dl.

Postoperative, **resume oral intake of food** and adjust the insulin doses.

33. **Somogyi, Dawn phenomenon,** and **Brittle diabetes:**
Somogyi phenomenon: Hypoglycemia precedes hyperglycemia. Hypoglycemia is due to insulin, while hyperglycemia is due to secretion of counter regulatory hormones.
Hypoglycemia occurs in **late night or early morning** accompanied by sweating, and terror. Within 4-6 hours, **hyperglycemia, ketosis, glycosuria, and ketonuria develop.**
Dawn phenomenon: **Hyperglycemia in early morning (5-9 a.m.) without previous** hypoglycemia. Blood sugar should be done 3,4, and 7 a.m.
Dawn: 3 and 4 a.m. (Gl = 80→), 7 a.m. (Gl = 140 ↑) = ↑ intermediate acting insulin P. M. dose by 10%, or give PM injection later.
Somogyi: 3 and 4 a.m. (Gl = 50 ↓), 7 a.m. (Gl = 140 ↑) = ↓ intermediate insulin P.M. dose by 10%.
Brittle diabetes: Blood glucose level fluctuates even with the increase of insulin doses. Most common causes are Somogyi and Dawn phenomena.

34. **Most common long term** complication of diabetes: **Retinopathy.** Other complications are nephropathy, neuropathy, and atherosclerosis. Mauriac syndrome: diabetes, dwarfism, glycogen-filled enlarged liver. It is due to under-insulinization.

35. Management of child with impaired glucose tolerance test: No special management except in obese children to reduce their weight. Impaired glucose tolerance test means that when one is fasting, one's blood sugar is less than 140 mg/dl and after 2 hours is more than 140 mg/dl.

36. In case of diabetes with Hashimoto thyroiditis (chronic lymphocytic thyroiditis), **always look for: Adrenal insufficiency.** Accompanied by hyper pigmentation, asthenia, and salt craving. Type 1 diabetes mellitus occurs in cystic fibrosis (exocrine pancreatic defect) and multiple endocrine neoplasia syndrome.

37. **Diabetes in Prader-Willi syndrome:** In this syndrome there is obesity and increased insulin secretion, but **increased resistance to insulin** and carbohydrate intolerance. Defect lies either in insulin receptor or anti insulin antibody.

38. **Transient diabetes** mellitus in a newborn **is most common** in: SGA. **Insulin level is normal,** but its response to glucose is low, resulting in **hyperglycemia. TREATMENT: Insulin for short period is mandatory. PROGNOSIS: Excellent.**

39. **Hypoglycemia in a newborn:** Most common presentation is **asymptomatic** or irritability. At birth, full term below 35 mg/dl, preterm below 25 mg/dl, and after 3 days below 45 mg/dl. After birth, blood glucose level reaches the lowest level **after 2 to 3 hours.**

40. **Hyperinsulinism:** When hypoglycemia associated with insulin level is more than 10 µu/ml.

ENDOCRINOLOGY

1. **Hypoglycemia and Nesidioblastosis:** The latter is **not** an islet cell tumor, but **a diffuse**

proliferation of islet cells throughout the pancreas due to inappropriate control of early development of pancreatic endocrine cells. Its etiology not known. The child shows signs of uncontrollable hypoglycemia despite medical treatment. **TREATMENT: Pancreatectomy (total) is the final.** Medical treatment includes glucose, glucagon, diazoxide, hydrocortisone.

2. **Panhypopituitarism causing hypoglycemia:** Due to **hyperinsulinism.** A newborn male with microphallus and hypoglycemia shows the symptoms of panhypopituitarism.

3. Erythroblastosis fetalis, Beckwith syndrome, and hypoglycemia due to: **Pancreatic cells hyperplasia.**

4. **Leprechaunism (Donohue syndrome) and hypoglycemia** due to: Defect in insulin receptor.

5. Most common form of hyperinsulinemic hypoglycemia: Type 1 diabetes mellitus.

6. **Ethyl alcohol and hypoglycemia (Important for Board examination):** (History of alcohol intake either in the party or left over alcohol taken by children or received alcohol bath). Patient shows signs of **hypoglycemia and convulsion,** but when pregnant mother consumes alcohol, her newborn does not develop hypoglycemia, usually because of the immaturity of enzyme alcohol dehydrogenase.

7. Most common cause of hypoglycemia in childhood: **Ketotic hypoglycemia.** It occurs between **18 months to 5 years,** common in low birth weight babies, present in the **early morning** with **episodes of vomiting, illness, hypoglycemia, ketonuria.** Children with this disease are otherwise in **good health,** but are lean and thin. Fasting **precipitates this disease.**
   TREATMENT: **Frequent feeding** with high carbohydrate and protein. Mechanism of hypoglycemia is **unknown,** but during hypoglycemia, there is **a diminished response of epinephrine** (which is **elevated in normal persons with hypoglycemia and increased glucose level).** It is also found in hypofunction of adrenal and pituitary gland.

8. **Drugs causing hypoglycemia: Propranolol; salicylate and acetaminophen** (through enzyme system, with no effect on insulin); **sulfonylureas** (causes life-threatening hypoglycemia in newborns at birth when their mothers consume in last trimester); Jamaican vomiting sickness derives from bush tea.

9. **Reye syndrome:** Accompanies encephalopathy, fatty, degeneration of the viscera, hypoglycemia (hepatic damage causes **decreased glucose production;** insulin level is **normal; no** response to glucagon). Hypoglycemia responds to glucose.

10. **Most commonly** affected organ with hypoglycemia: **Central nervous system (CNS).** The CNS having a shortage of glucose,uses it only for metabolism, needing a constant supply of glucose to function. CNS learns to utilize amino acids, and ketone **only in patients with prolonged** hypoglycemia.

11. Chromosomal location of:

Growth hormone: 17.
Prolactin: 6.

12. Most common cause of **hypopituitarism: Idiopathic.** In the idiopathic type, **there is usually no lesion** in pituitary, though more in **male than in female.** A history of maternal bleeding, breech or forceps delivery results in **damage or hypoxia of the hypothalamus (mostly),** and pituitary. It is mostly autosomal recessive (some dominant). Initially there is a GH (growth hormone) deficiency and later TSH and ACTH deficiencies. Other types of **hypopituitarism are congenital defects** of pituitary (anencephaly, holoprosencephaly, septo-optic dysplasia), and **destruction of pituitary (most common are craniopharyngioma,** histiocytosis, tuberculosis, toxoplasmosis, sarcoidosis, and hypothalamic tumor).

Septo-optic dysplasia (de Morsier syndrome): Visual defect (due to optic nerve hypoplasia), short stature, absent septum pellucidum.
Aplasia of pituitary: Microphallus in male with hypoglycemia (typically at birth).
Craniopharyngioma: Calcification (intra and suprasellar).
Histiocytosis: Mostly associated with diabetes **insipidus.**

13. **Clinical presentations of hypopituitarism:**
   a. **Without pituitary lesion: Normal** at birth (height and weight) but develops growth retardation around 12 months of age or may **at birth** evidence apnea, hypoglycemia, cyanosis, **microphallus (male), or** may evidence certain **facial features** (frontal bone prominence, saddle-depressed nose, bulging eyes), **high-pitched cry,** small hands and feet, **underdeveloped genitalia with delayed puberty. Normal** intelligence is present.
   b. **With pituitary lesion: Most common is craniopharyngioma,** where **first manifestation is growth failure,** then neurologic manifestations (papilledema, loss of vision, optic atrophy, cranial nerve palsy). Patients appear **normal at birth, but then develop growth failure,** asthenia, absence of sweating, **regression** of genital growth, and become susceptible to cold **due to atrophy of pituitary, adrenal cortex, and thyroid gland.**

14. **Laboratory diagnosis of hypopituitarism:**
   a. Random serum growth hormone less than 10 ng/ml.
   b. **Provocative test** (with L-dopa, glucagon, insulin-arginine): GH level **less then 7 ng/ml** (test done twice). **Confirm the diagnosis.**
   c. Decreased somatomedin C level (IGF 1).
   d. Once GH deficiency is established, **look for deficiency of hypothalamic-pituitary-adrenal axis:** hypothalamic defect (by TRH, stimulation test shows positive response), thyroid (by TSH level low, low T4, T3), adrenal (low serum and urine steroid level).

15. **X-ray finding in hypopituitarism:**
   Craniopharyngioma: **Enlarge** sella turcica.
   Pituitary aplasia: **Small** sella turcica.
   In hypopituitarism: Delayed ossification centers, presence of **Wormian bones (bones in between sutures).**

Head CT scan and MRI are very important and recommended for all patients.

16. **Sleep, exercise, and GH:** GH level increases during sleep and exercise.

17. Hypopituitarism due to emotional disturbance: Does **not** respond to GH, **so treat the underlying cause.**

18. **Treatment for hypopituitarism:**

Idiopathic	GH (growth hormone) stimulates growth in 80% patient.
Craniopharyngioma	Surgery (removal and biopsy).
With adrenal deficiency	Hydrocortisone.
With thyroid deficiency	Thyroid hormone.
Microphallus	Testosterone enanthate.

Maximal response to GH occurs during first year of treatment.

19. **Somatomedin C (IGF 1)** level in **constitutional** delays primary hypopituitarism:
Constitutional delay: **Slightly reduced.**
GH deficiency: **Severely reduced,** but improved within 16-28 hours of hGH administration.

20. Differential diagnosis of hypopituitarism:
Other causes of short stature:
a. **Laron syndrome:** End organ resistance, i.e., cells do not response to GH; ↑ GH level.
b. **Turner syndrome:** GH → (normal), 45X0.
c. **Emotional disturbance:** GH ↓ (low), does not respond to GH. Ideal management is to avoid disturbed atmosphere. (Child grows rapidly after that. They then evidence pseudotumor cerebri, which means a separation of cranial sutures for rapid brain growth. This is a normal phenomenon.)
d. **Primordial dwarfism:** GH →, growth retardation begins in utero and shows itself at birth.
e. **Silver-Russell syndrome:** GH →, low birth weight, present with short stature, **triangular face,** frontal prominence.
f. **Constitutionally short stature: chronological age is more than skeletal age,** which is same as height age. Usually grows around puberty. GH →.
g. **Genetically short stature:** chronological age is **same as** skeletal age? Skeletal age is more than height age. **They remain short for the rest of their lives. GH →.**
h. **Beta thalassemia:** Somatomedin C (IGF 1) is ↓ due to hemosiderosis.
i. **Hypothyroidism (primary):** ↓ T4 and T3, ↑ TSH and clinical features of hypothyroidism.

21. **Most common cause of diabetes insipidus (D.I.): Craniopharyngioma.** Other causes are optic glioma, basal skull fracture, histiocytosis, reticuloendotheliosis, Wolfram syndrome (it includes diabetes mellitus, insipidus, optic atrophy, perceptive deafness). **In newborns it is due to asphyxia,** intraventricular hemorrhage (IVH), sepsis (due to listeria and group B strep.). It is rarely hereditary, autosomal dominant, or **x-linked recessive.**

DNA study shows defect in AVP-NP II gene on chromosome 20. D.I. due to damage of neurohypophyseal tract or supraoptic-paraventricular nuclei, resulting in **diminished secretion of vasopressin** (which acts directly on distal tubule and collecting duct to absorb water).

22.   **Most common symptoms** of diabetes insipidus: **Polyuria and polydipsia.** Other manifestations are **infant who cries all the time** for milk but is never satisfied, also evidenced by **hyperthermia, weight loss, dehydration,** vomiting, **and constipation.** Children develop **secondary enuresis,** and anorexia, but **prefer high carbohydrate** food, **they do not sweat and have dry and pale** skin. In tumor, they show signs of **sexual precocity,** emotional problems, and growth disturbance (cachexia or obesity).

23.   **Diagnosis of diabetes insipidus:**
      Urine: ↑ **volume 4-10 or more** liters, **Sp. Gr. 1001-1005** ↓
               ↓ osmolality (50-200 mOSM/kg water).
      Most confirmatory test: plasma vasopressin level **less than 0.5 pg/ml.**
      Water deprivation test: 3 hour period of dehydration increases serum osmolality, but **urine osmolality remains below** plasma level.
      X-ray skull: in tumor, there is **calcification,** enlarged sella turcica, and clinoid process erosion. MRI and head CT to be done for tumor and reticuloendotheliosis.

24.   **Treatment** for diabetes insipidus: First treat the underlying cause. **The preferred drug is desmopressin (dDAVP) which is given through nasal mucosa.** Use intravenous preparation only after transsphenoidal surgery. **In postoperative patient, D.I. is transient,** use of dDAVP should be monitored daily. **dDAVP** can be used in **enuresis** in slightly higher doses. It also acts on **V2 extrarenal receptor,** releasing factor VIII and Von-Willebrand factor, so it can be used in hemophilia A (mild or moderate) and Von-Willebrand disease with **15 times more** doses than when treating for **neurogenic diabetes insipidus (5-15 μgm).** Children **less than 2 years** need **lower** doses.

25.   Most common problem in arginine-vasopressin (AVP) secretion: **Inappropriate secretion of antidiuretic hormone (SIADH).**

26.   Why it is called **inappropriate** secretion of ADH? Normally, ADH is secreted when serum is more concentrated or hyperosmolar (that is, **an appropriate secretion of ADH)** to keep water inside the body to maintain serum osmolality normal. When ADH is **secreted even with normal serum concentration** (as in **meningitides, brain tumor,** Guillain-Barre syndrome), it is called **an inappropriate** secretion of ADH.

27.   **Increased ADH secretion: Most common complication of meningitis.** Remember, **oat cell carcinoma of lung, Ewing sarcoma, tumor** of pancreas, duodenum or thymus **produce (synthesize) ADH, causing increased secretion of ADH.** Removal of tumor usually solves this problem. It also occurs in **pneumonia, perinatal asphyxia, postoperative condition, encephalitis,** subarachnoid bleeding, and the use of vincristine and vinblastine.

28.   **Most common presentation** of SIADH: Asymptomatic (other findings **are a reduced** ↓ urine output, ↑ body weight, irritability, convulsion).

29. **Laboratory diagnosis of SIADH:**
Serum: ↓ Na, ↓cl, →HCO$_3$, ↓ osmolality.
Urine: ↑ Sp.Gr, ↑ osmolality.
Renal and adrenal functions are **normal.**

30. **Treatment of SIADH:** Treat the underlying cause, **restrict fluid intake (treatment of choice), fursemide;** demeclocycline (experimental).

31. **Reticuloendotheliosis and D.I.:** D.I. spontaneously resolves in some cases.

32. **Histiocytosis and D.I.:** D.I. does not show up at the time that diagnosis of histiocytosis been made, but it **may appear within 4-5 years.**

33. **Differential diagnosis of disease with polyuria, polydipsia and diabetes insipidus:**
    a. **Nephrogenic D.I.:** It does **not** respond to vasopressin or desmopressin **due to end-organ resistance to kidney. X-linked dominant,** it mostly occurs in **male.**
    b. **Primary renal disease:** high BUN and creatinine; **normal or high urine osmolality.** (In **D.I., low** osmolality).
    c. **Psychogenic polydipsia:** affected person **usually has concentrated urine** when fluids are withheld. Urine osmolality is usually **higher in dehydration** than in vasopressin administration, so if urine osmolality is **significantly higher after vasopressin, then** vasopressin is deficient. This holds both in high and low urine concentrations.
    d. **Adipsia or hypodipsia:** rare, most commonly seen in hypothalamic tumors glioma, germinoma, histiocytosis. It is an **isolated defect in thirst centers;** vasopressin and thirst centers are closed. It accompanies low thirst, increased urine output due to ↓ ADH secretion.
    e. **Familial syndrome:** intermittent polyuria, seizure, ↑ phosphorous in serum.

34. **Hyperpituitarism: Increased pituitary hormones secretion due to:**
    a. **Primary hypofunction** of thyroid, adrenal and gonads (testis or ovary) resulting in decreased hormonal feedback from those target organs to pituitary, causing ↑ pituitary hormone secretion, i.e., **secondary hyperpituitarism.**
    b. **Primary hyperpituitarism:** Due to pituitary tumors secreting hormones like eosinophilic adenoma (GH), basophilic adenoma (ACTH), and chromophobe adenoma (prolactin). Remember, any pituitary tumor can compress normal pituitary tissue, causing **pituitary hypofunction. Normally** it causes **hyper-function of respective hormones secreted.**

35. **Most common cause** of pituitary gigantism or acromegaly: **Eosinophilic adenoma.** Occurs rarely. Most commonly occurs in pubertal age group, but can occur in early childhood. Symptoms are **enlargement** of the whole body **especially hands and feet,** coarse facial features, large tongue, teeth separated due to excessive mandibular growth, large head, **lethargy, and fatigue.** May accompany hypogonadism and delayed sexual maturation. Sign of increased intracranial pressure occurs **late.**

DIAGNOSIS CONFIRMED: ↑ GH (400 ng/ml), ↑ IGF 1 (somatomedin C). ↑ **prolactin.**

X-ray: enlarged sella turcica and paranasal sinuses, but normal bony maturation.
TREATMENT: Surgical removal of tumor, bromocriptine (dopamine agonist binds with pituitary dopamine receptors), **octreotide (somatostatin analog) is more effective,** but expensive.

36. **Sotos syndrome (cerebral gigantism):**
Etiology: **unknown,** but may be due to hypothalamic defect. **Characteristic presentation:** At birth baby is LGA with macrocephaly (>90%); by 1 year of age, height (>97%). **Experiences accelerated growth for first 5 years then growth becomes normal. Clumsiness and awkward features in walking are specific for this disease, and child has lot of difficulty in sports.** Puberty occurs by normal time or early. **Mental retardation is present.**
Laboratory: No definite features. GH →, no endocrine abnormalities.
EEG: Abnormal (dilated ventricle in CT scan).
X-ray: Enlarged skull, high orbital roof, bone age **is same** as height age.
PROGNOSIS: ↑ risk of neoplasm (hepatic carcinoma, Wilms tumor, ovarian and parotid tumor).
Remember: LGA, ↑ growth up to 5 years, clumsiness, mental retardation, abnormal EEG with dilated ventricles.

37. An adolescent present with **Tanner stage 1** in breast and **stage 5 in genitalia: Adrenal cortical tumor.** (Important for Board examination).

38. An adolescent evidences having **Tanner stage 5 in breast and stage 1** in genitalia: **Prolactinoma is the diagnosis (pituitary tumor).**

39. **Hyperprolactinemia and primary hypothyroidism:** In primary hypothyroidism, there is pituitary hyperplasia causing increased prolactin secretion. **TREATMENT:** Thyroid hormone.

40. **First sign** of puberty in boys: **Testicular growth.**

41. **First sign** of puberty in girls: **Breast bud.**

42. Prolactinoma: Most common tumor of pituitary **in adult. Rare** in children, it is the presenting feature in type 1 MEN (multiple endocrine neoplasia). Evidences **gynecomastia and galactorrhea,** but **also delayed puberty and growth, and amenorrhea.** Delayed puberty is due to **multifactorial** causes (may be due to ↓ GH, ↓ gonadotrophic hormone, ↓ LHRH, direct gonadal inhibition by prolactin). ↑ Prolactin and MRI help in the diagnosis.

DIAGNOSIS CONFIRMED BY: Biopsy after surgery.
TREATMENT: Surgical removal of tumor. Bromocriptine reduces tumor size. **Micro adenoma is treated conservatively** because it does not change to macro **adenoma.**

43. **Precocious puberty:**

TRUE	PSEUDO
Isosexual	Isosexual or **heterosexual.**

Precious gonads and secondary sexual character	Premature gonads and precocious secondary sexual character.
Normal activation of pituitary-hypothalamic-gonadal axis	No activation of that axis.

44. **Peak height velocity:**
    Boys: **After puberty,** maximum growth 14-16 years.
    Girls: **Before menarche, 2 years earlier** than boys.
    In girls: Breast bud formation 10-11 years, onset of menstruation 2-2.5 years (maximum 6 years) after breast bud formation.

45. **Precocious puberty means:**
    Boys: Onset of secondary sexual character **before 9 years.**
    Girls: Onset of secondary sexual character **before 8 years.**

46. **Most important determinant factor to predict onset of puberty** within a year or two: **Nocturnal LH pulses,** which means sleep stimulates LH secretion in a pulsatile fashion due to stimulation by LHRH from hypothalamus. It means **puberty will begin** in a year or two **(important for examination).**

47. **Turner syndrome, anorchia and gonadotrophin level:** In both the conditions gonadotrophin level is **higher** than in normal population. Because of hypoplastic gonads, there is no feedback inhibition to **gonadotrophin (FSH, LH).**

48. **Hormones** which rise **before any other hormone and any sign of puberty: DHEA and DHEAS** (Dehydroepiandrosterone and **sulfate**) rise around 6 years of age. They appear before gonadotrophin (FSH,LH), testosterone, estradiol. DHEAS is the most predominant adrenal C 19 steroid.

49. **LH, estrogen,** and **adolescence:** Normally, **LH** from pituitary **stimulates** secretion of **estrogen** from ovary, then **estrogen inhibits LH secretion** by feedback (negative) mechanism. In **mid-or late adolescence, in mid-menstrual cycle estrogen** actually stimulates LH secretion by positive feedback. It is **not** found in **early** adolescence.

50. **Earlier onset of menstruation in the present** generation than in previous is due to: **Better nutrition and good health.** Athletes, swimmers, runners have **delayed puberty** because of leanness and strenuous physical activities. Blacks have more advanced secondary sexual character than whites.

51. **Most common cause of true precocious puberty** or precocious puberty without other pathologic findings (constitutional): **Unknown.**

52. **Clinical manifestations** of true precocious puberty:
    Girls: First breast develops then pubic hair, then axillary hair and menstruation (anovulatory, irregular), early pregnancy.
    Boys: First testes and penis, then pubic hair, deepening of voice, erection and ejaculation; spermatogenesis is in progress, interstitial cells are present early.

Height: Final height is **short** because of advanced bony maturation (bone age **more than** chronological age).

Mental age and dental: **Normal** as chronological age.

53. **Diagnosis** of true precocious puberty:
Serum: ↑ FSH, ↑ LH; ↑ pulsatile secretion of gonadotrophin **particularly LH during sleep**; LHRH causes brisk increase of LH secretion as in normal person (severely elevated LH level, **hCG secreting tumor should be ruled out,** because hCG and LH cross-react in assay). ↑Testosterone (boys), ↑ estradiol (girls).
Sonogram: Pubertal size ovary.
   CT and MRI: Rule out intracranial lesion.

54. **Treatment** of true precocious puberty: **Analog of LHRH** (leuprolide acetate) which is more potent, long acting IM injection Q.1 month. It **reduces** (breast development, bony maturation) so ↑ final height. Discontinuation of drug **resumes normal puberty.**

55. **Differential diagnosis** of true precocious puberty:
   a.   Gonadotrophin-**dependent:** rule out cerebral lesion by MRI, CT scan.
   b.   Gonadotrophin-**independent: Male:** congenital adrenal hyperplasia, adrenal and leydig cell tumor, hepatoma-producing gonadotrophin, familial. **Female:** ovary (cyst, tumor), feminizing adrenal tumor, McCune-Albright syndrome, exogenous estrogen supply.

56. **Precocious puberty due to organic brain lesions:**
Etiology: It is due to **postencephalitic scar,** T.B., meningitis, tuberous sclerosis, hydrocephalus, severe head injury. All of them **activate hypothalamus,** causing precocious puberty by **unknown** mechanism, but they cause **scarring, or invasion of, or put pressure on, hypothalamus.**
Most common pineal tumor causing precocious puberty is **germinomas or astrocytomas.** It stimulates hCG secretion which stimulates Leydig cells in boys. **In girls it** does **not** cause precocious puberty, because FSH is necessary for complete ovarian function.
Hypothalamic hamartoma diagnosed by CT or MRI causes precocious puberty. LHRH is secreted sometimes.

57. Most common cause of **rapidly progressing** precocious puberty in **young children:** **Hamartoma of tuber cinereum.**

58. **Diagnosis of organic precocious puberty:** Same as idiopathic. Head CT and MRI must be done in all patients.

59. Treatment of **organic** precocious puberty: Depends on the lesion. Pedunculated hamartoma can be removed surgically. **LHRH analog treatment same as idiopathic.**

60. **Hypothyroidism and precocious puberty:** Usually hypothyroid causes **delayed puberty,** but precocious puberty is **not** uncommon. It is common in **Down syndrome.** Male shows enlarged testes **without** virilization; female, enlarged breast and menstruation.
MRI: Enlarged sella turcica due to compensatory large pituitary.

Serum: ↑ **TSH,** ↑↑ FSH more than ↑ LH, ↑ Prolactin.
Male: Testes enlarged **without** Leydig cells (unlike true precocious puberty).
Female: In ovary, ↑ estrogen, but **normal** androgen.
TREATMENT: Thyroid hormones.

61. Most common hepatic tumor causing isosexual precocious **puberty by secreting gonadotrophin: Hepatoblastoma.**
Present with **enlarged liver** which **secretes** ↑ **hCG,** ↑ **alpha feto protein,** ↑ **testosterone,** ↓ FSH, ↑LH as it cross-reacts with hCG ↑.
TREATMENT: Same as cancer liver. **High mortality.**

62. Most common **site of tumor** in Klinefelter syndrome: **Mediastinal tumor secretes hCG.**
Other tumors that secrete hCG are: choriocarcinoma, teratoma, teratocarcinoma; more in boys than girls.

63. **McCune - Albright syndrome** (precocious puberty, polyostotic fibrous dysplasia, abnormal pigmentation);
Most common cause of this syndrome: **autonomous hyper-function of involved glands.**
Most common in girls. **Most common showing is with precocious puberty** (earliest 6 m.), vaginal bleeding (earliest 4 years).
Serum: ↓ LH, ↓ FSH, no response to LHRH, ↑↑ estradiol.
Sonogram: **Ovarian cyst. Iuteinized follicle cyst** causes precocious puberty, **independent of gonadotrophin** and unresponsive to LHRH in **young girls; in pubertal age,** gonadotrophin secretion begins in normal response to LHRH, then pregnancy occurs.
Hyperthyroidism in this syndrome: multinodular, equal in male and female (unlike Graves disease).
Cushing syndrome in this syndrome: bilateral adrenocortical nodular hyperplasia, ↓ ACTH, cortical function not suppressed by dexamethasone. ↑**GH can** be found in some patients of Albright syndrome.
TREATMENT: Ovarian cyst disappears spontaneously, so there is no need for surgery or aspiration;
Cushing syndrome: Remove adrenal gland.
Hypersomatotropism: **Octreotide** (somatostatin inhibitor).

64. A child **more than 2 years** old shows **isolated thelarche.** Most likely cause: True or pseudo-precocious puberty (not a benign condition). **In a child less than 2 years** of age, **it is mostly benign condition.**

64. **Clinical presentation** of organic precocious puberty: **Hypothalamic hamartoma: unnatural laughing or crying (gelastic seizure)** occurs. **In some cases the first** manifestation is **precocious puberty.** Radiological findings may appear one year later, or it may show itself as diabetes insipidus, hyperthermia, obesity, or cachexia. Remember, **sexual precocity is isosexual.** Intracranial tumor may be found (40% boys and 10% girls).

65. Gonadotrophin-**independent** precocious puberty: **Autosomal dominant, and only in boys, precocious puberty occurs around 2 years of age,** showing advanced osseous maturation; initially gonadotrophin independent, it later becomes dependent.
Biopsy of testis: **Mature Leydig cells.**

Serum: ↑ Testosterone; LH →, **no** response to LHRH.
TREATMENT: Ketoconazole (antifungal drug) inhibits c-17, 20 lyase and testosterone synthesis. In older child, LHRH agonist can be used.

66. **Partial precocious puberty:**
Only premature thelarche: Isolated breast development by 2 years of age, unilateral or asymmetric bilateral. **Normal** genitalia, growth, and bony maturation. Breast **usually decreases** in size but never increases. Normal reproduction and menstruation time. Mostly **sporadic** cases.
Serum: ↑ **FSH** and ↑stimulation to LHRH; ↓LH; ↓estradiol.(Remember, in **true precocious** puberty: ↑ LH).
Sonogram: Ovarian cysts.
It may be due to **imbalance of FSH-LH secretion from pituitary axis.** It is **benign,** but it may be the **1st sign of true or pseudo-precocious puberty.**

67. Partial (incomplete) precocious puberty:
a. **Premature adrenarche:** More in **girls** than boys, **it first shows hair in labia majora,** then pubic, finally **axillary hair with axillary odor** like adult. Advanced osseous maturation and height. It is most likely due to early adrenal androgen production from maturation of zona reticularis. It can be **confused** with adrenal hyperplasia because of ↑ DHEAS, ↑ 17 hydroxy progesterone level due to diminished activity of enzymes (3 beta - hydroxy steroid dehydrogenase, C 17, 20 lyase) in adrenal gland. It is a **benign condition. ACTH stimulation test should be done when** it is combined with enlarged clitoris, acne, increased bone age.
b. Premature menarche: Rare, accompanies menstrual bleeding, **but no** other problem, ↑ **estradiol only** due to ovarian overactivity.

68. **Exogenous** estrogen and **color of areola of breast: Dark brown color.** (* Endogenous estrogen does **not** produce this color.)

69. **Premature adrenarche:**
Normal child: ↑ HT, ↑ Bone age; ↑ (Testo, DHEA C 19); FSH and LH →.
Cerebral damage: ↓ HT, ↓ Bone age,; same as above.

70. **Functions** of thyroid hormones: Increased tissue oxygen consumption, stimulated growth and protein synthesis, also carbohydrate, lipid and vitamin metabolism. Free T4; T3 binds to cytosol receptor, then transported to **nucleus,** which is the site of active transcription; nucleus thyroid hormone receptor is C-erb A proto-oncogene.

71. **Most of the physiologic** action of thyroid is done by: **T3.** T3 is 3-4 times more potent than T4. **20% circulating T3 is secreted by thyroid gland** and **the rest (80%)** is formed from deiodination of T4 in liver, kidney, peripheral tissue by type **I-5' deiodinase;** in brain and pituitary, 80% of required T3 is formed from T4 by enzyme type II 5' deiodinase.

72. Most of the thyroid hormones **binds with: TBG** (thyroxine binding globulin) 70%, TBG synthesized in **liver.**

73. TSH has two subunits **alpha and beta.** Which one gives **specificity** of hormone? **Beta.**

74. **Steps of stimulation** of thyroid hormone: TRH from hypothalamus → to TSH from pituitary → to T4, T3 from thyroid (acts on **adenyl cyclase**). TRH is tripeptide, the **first peptide synthesized and is used in clinical medicine.** It is found in places other than the hypothalamus.

75. **Daily** recommended doses of iodine: Infant **40-50 μg,** children **70-120 μg,** adolescent and adult **150 μg.**

76. **Most sensitive laboratory indicator** for primary hypothyroidism: **TSH** (thyrotropin). Normal level after neonatal period is less than 6 ug/ml. In **normal** person TRH administration **increases** TSH secretion within 30 minutes, but in **hyperthyroidism, there is no** response, because high T4, T3 block TRH action in pituitary.

77. Most commonly used material in thyroid scan: **Technetium** (99m Tc). It is better than iodine because it is taken up by thyroid but **not** organified. It has a half-life 6 hours.

78. **Acute release of TSH** in newborn: **Within 30 minutes of birth in fullterm,** TSH level peaks up to 70 μu/ml which goes down **mostly in first 24** hours and becomes **normal after 48 hours. T3 level** peaks up to 300 ng/dl in **4 hours.** (T3 formed from peripheral conversion of T4), declines and becomes **normal after 1 week, but reverses T3** maintained high level (200-ng/dl) for 2 weeks and normal after 1 month. Remember, T4 crosses the placenta in **very small** amounts, so it does **not** interfere the diagnosis. **Don't do newborn screen in first 48 hours after birth.**

79. **TBG level and factors:**
    ↑ TBG: Pregnancy, newborn, estrogen, heroin, perphenazine.
    ↓ TBG: Anabolic steroid, androgen. glucocorticoid, L-asparaginase.

80. Drugs causing abnormality in Thyroid function test:
    Phenytoin:↓ T4 level in serum (↑ hepatic degradation and ↑ tissue utilization), **displaces T4, T3 from** TBG.
    Phenobarbital: ↓ T4 level in serum.

81. Does low or high level of TBG, manifest clinically? It **never manifests** clinically and **does not require** treatment. Both TBG deficiency and excess are **X - linked dominant.**
    ↓ **TBG deficiency:** ↓ **total T4,** → **free T4 and TSH,** ↓**TBG** ↑ **RT3.**
    ↑ TBG excess: ↑ total T4, T3, → free T4 and TSH, ↑ TBG, ↓ RT3.
    These situations may show up in newborns and can confuse neonatal screen.

82. Most common cause of **congenital hypothyroidism: Thyroid dysgenesis (90%),** showing either complete absence of thyroid (33%) or more usually, an **ectopic thyroid** (from tongue base along the anterior neck up to thyroid area).

83. Most common presentation of hypothyroidism at birth: Asymptomatic (even with aplasia of the gland).

84. Thyroid dysgenesis, **is most likely** due to: Thyroid growth-blocking and cytotoxic antibody.

85. Radio iodine, pregnancy, and lactation: Radio iodine is absolutely contraindicated in pregnancy and lactation; **so do pregnancy test before giving** it. It causes **hypothyroidism in newborn.**

86. Patient with hypofunction of both thalamus (↓ TRH) and of pituitary (↓TSH) gives evidence of: Hypofunction of thyroid (↓ T4, T3).

87. **Isolated deficiency of TSH** and DNA: **Point mutation in DNA** in TSH beta subunit gene.

88. Defect in thyroid hormone synthesis: It causes **congenital** hypothyroidism:
    a. Defect in iodine transport to thyroid.
    b. Defect in organification (oxidation to form reactive iodine is an example). **(Pendred syndrome:** goiter and sensorineural deafness).
    c. Defect in Thyroglobulin synthesis (bind with mono, diiodotyrosine).
    d. Defect in deiodination (release of mono, diiodotyrosine from thyroglobulin.

89. **First sign** of neonatal hypothyroidism: **Prolonged physiologic jaundice** is due to defect in glucuronide conjugation. Other sins are **heavy at birth, lethargy poor feeding,** edema, **constipation, umbilical hernia, large protruding tongue,** apnea, **large** anterior and posterior fontanelle. **Later shows growth retardation, except for enlarged head.**

90. A newborn present with **midline mass** anywhere from tongue base up to thyroid region of neck. **MOST LIKELY DIAGNOSIS: Ectopic thyroid.** This is the **only** functioning thyroid tissue. Diagnosis **is confirmed by thyroid scan. Never** remove that mass.

91. Mother with **Hashimoto thyroiditis on antithyroid medicine and newborn:** Newborn showing **hypothyroidism.** It is the **most common cause of Graves disease** in the mother. TBIAb (TSH binding inhibitory antibody) from the mother crosses the placenta and blocks TSH receptor in newborn thyroid, causing **neonatal hypothyroidism. DIAGNOSIS CONFIRMED:** TBIAb level in mother and in baby. Thyroid scan: shows **no** uptake in thyroid, so physician might treat the patient mistakenly.

92. Mother with Graves disease, and Hashimoto thyroiditis, but **not taking any antithyroid medicine,** has a newborn showing signs of: **Hyperthyroidism,** because of transplacental transfer of thyroid stimulating antibody.

93. Most common complication of untreated congenital hypothyroidism: Mental retardation. Early diagnosis and treatment can prevent it.

94. Mother with Graves disease and Hashimoto thyroiditis had **thyroid surgery in the past** and she is **normothyroid** now. What will happen during this pregnancy to newborn? Newborn can develop **hyperthyroidism** (because of thyroid stimulating antibody crossing the placenta).

95. Newborn on breast feeding and congenital hypothyroidism: Clinical manifestation may be **delayed** because breast milk contains a good amount of thyroid hormone (particularly T3), but it does **not** protect the newborn completely.

96. LGA (large for gestational age) newborn: all the organs are large **except: Brain.**

97. SGA (small for gestational age) newborn: all the organs are small **except: Brain** (except in symmetrical SGA when brain is small also).

98. Carotenemia and jaundice:
Carotenemia: Yellow skin, white sclera.
Jaundice: Yellow skin, yellow sclera.

99. Picture of Down syndrome and congenital hyothyroid child: Difficult to distinguish, **look at the picture section.** Protruding tongue present in both.
Down syndrome: **Upward slanting** of palpebral fissure.
Hypothyroidism: **Normal** palpebral fissure.
(Important for Board examination).

100. Pseudohypertrophy of calf muscle, jaundice and hypotonia: Kocher-Debre-Semelaigne syndrome.

101. **Thyroid function test and different diseases:**
a. Primary hypothyroidism: ↓ T4, ↓ T3, ↑ TSH.
b. ↓ TBG or laboratory error: ↓ T4, ↓ T3, → TSH.
c. Secondary hypothyroidism (hypopituitary or hypothalamic): ↓ T4, ↓ T3, ↓ TSH (or ↓ TRH). Do TRH stimulation test: ↑ TSH in hypothalamic and ↓ TSH in hypopituitary).
d. Primary Hyperthyroidism: ↑ T4, ↑ T3, ↓ TSH.
e. Secondary hyperthyroidism (hyperpituitary or hyperthalamic): ↑ T4, ↑ T3, ↑ TSH or (↑ TRH).

102. X-ray finding for newborn with suspected congenital **hypothyroidism:** X-ray of **distal femoral epiphysis:** normally present at birth, but will **be absent** in hypothyroid. Skull X-ray: **Wormian bones** (between sutures); wide sutures. Delayed dental bud formation and eruption.

103. **Confirmatory diagnosis** of congenital hypothyroidism: ↑ **TSH** along with ↓ T4, ↓ T3. Do **not** hold treatment for thyroid scan.

104. Cardiac problem in congenital hypothyroidism: Enlarged heart and pericardial effusion. EKG: Low (P, T wave and QRS complex) voltage.

105. Treatment of choice for congenital hypothyroidism: **Sodium L thyroxine.** Complication of thyroxine: **Pseudotumor cerebri.** Keep the level of T4 and TSH normal. **Improvement in growth indicates** adequate treatment.

106. **Prognosis of** congenital hypothyroidism: **Earlier** the treatment is started **the better** the outcome. Thyroid hormone is absolutely necessary for development of **CNS in infant.**

107. Most common cause of **acquired** hypothyroidism (juvenile): **Lymphocytic thyroiditis (Hashimoto or autoimmune).** Other causes are postoperative thyroid surgery, cystinosis,

irradiation to thyroid, drug (amiodarone), congenital defect of thyroid present in childhood.

108. **First clinical sign** of juvenile hypothyroidism: **Growth deceleration. (Most patients are asymptomatic)** Other signs are myxedematous skin, constipation, feeling cold and sleepy, delayed osseous maturation; visual defect, precocious puberty or galactorrhea. **Surprisingly, school grades and work do not suffer even when the disease is severe. Few show signs of hyperthyroidism.**

109. Most common site and organism of **acute suppurative** thyroiditis: **(L) lower lobe; Eikenella corrodens is most common organism.** It is accompanied by swelling, redness, and tenderness in thyroid gland. Treatment with incision, drainage, antibiotics.

110. **Goiter** (enlargement of thyroid gland): It could be euthyroid, hypo-or hyperthyroid.
    a. **Congenital: sporadic, maternal intake of antithyroid medicine or iodides** during pregnancy causes neonatal goiter and hypothyroidism which requires thyroxine treatment for a few months only. **Severely enlarged thyroid** may cause respiratory distress due to pressure. Its effect is treated with partial thyroidectomy.
    Hyperthyroidism in infant is almost always accompanied by mild goiter due to maternal Graves disease. Iodine deficiency in **early** pregnancy causes **intrauterine brain damage** without goiter. In cases of a lobulated, asymmetric, firm, large thyroid mass, rule out **teratoma.**
    b. Endemic: most common is **the result of iodine** deficiency. Mild iodine deficiency does not cause goiter until puberty when demand is more; moderate to severe deficiency causes goiter. **Nervous syndrome** shows up ataxia, spasticity, deafness, fetal retardation in mother who had **iodine deficiency in 1st trimester.**
    Myxedematous syndrome evidences a delay in growth and sexual development, and retardation when maternal iodine deficiency occurs in **last trimester.**
    c. **Sporadic:** most common cause is **lymphocytic thyroiditis.**
    d. **Iodide goiter:** iodide preparation causes goiter in a few patients **Wolff-Chaikoff effect:** acute iodine administration causes goiter. **Lithium carbonate causes goiter.**

111. Hyperthyroidism: Due to **excessive secretion of thyroid hormone.**
    Two types: **Graves disease, and congenital hyperthyroidism.**

    Graves disease: enlarged thymus, spleen, and lymph nodes; **lymphocyte and plasma cell infiltration** in retro orbital tissue and thyroid glands. Thyroid gland is infiltrated by T helper cells (CD 4+), T cytotoxic cells (CD 8+), and B lymphocyte. B cells are responsible for **antithyroid antibody.** TSIB (thyroid stimulating antibody) and TBIAb (TSH -inhibiting antibody), clinical presentation depends on the **ratio** of the two antibodies.
    Most common in adolescent girls, **its earliest signs are emotional disturbances,** restlessness, tremors, poor school performance, exophthalmos, and tachycardia.
    Thyroid "crisis" or "storm": hyperthyroidism, tachycardia, hyperthermia, restlessness, progress to coma, death.

    "Apathetic" or "masked" hyperthyroidism: hyperthyroidism, lethargy, apathy, cachexia.
    Combination of both forms: Possible.

DIAGNOSIS CONFIRMED: ↑ T4, ↑free T4, ↑T3, ↑ free T3, ↓ TSH; scan for thyroid antibodies is rarely necessary.

TREATMENT: Medical treatment (propylthiouracil, methimazole) is preferred to surgical. Methimazole **is more potent than propylthiouracil.** Both are toxic drugs that can cause SLE-like picture, ↓ WBC, hepatitis, and failure due to vasculitis.

Toxic patient: propranolol to control tachycardia.

Surgery: give KI for 2 weeks to make euthyroid, then **perform subtotal thyroidectomy (procedure of choice).**

Most common complication of surgery: hypoparathyroidism (transient or permanent), vocal cord palsy.

112. Diagnosis and treatment of acquired hypothyroidism: Same as congenital. During the first 18 months of treatment, skeletal maturation **is faster** than linear growth, resulting in a loss of 7 cm in final adult height. **Complication of treatment (thyroxine):** School performance deteriorates, restlessness, short attention span, less sleep; all of these occur in first year of therapy, and are **transient** phenomena, so assure **the family.**

113. **Definitive diagnosis** of lymphocytic thyroiditis: **Biopsy.**

114. Presence of **antithyroid antibody** found in **(nonspecific finding):**
    a.   Lymphocytic thyroiditis (antimicrosomal antibody present in 90% cases).
    b.   50% of **normal** siblings of affected patient.
    c.   **Mother** of a child with Down or Turner syndrome.
    d.   20% patient of diabetes mellitus and 23% in rubella.
    People in last three categories do **not** have thyroid disease.

115. A child exposed to ionizing radiation. Most common thyroid complication: solitary thyroid nodule (benign or malignant).

116. **Congenital hyperthyroidism:** Most common cause is maternal **Graves disease** (lymphocytic thyroiditis). Maternal transfer of (stimulatory) **TSAb** causes severe symptoms of hyperthyroidism. Transfer of **TBIAb** (inhibitory) reduces the symptoms. Infant with tachycardia shows restlessness, fever, and weight loss with ravenous appetite.

    Serum:↑↑ T4; Skull X-ray: Craniosynostosis. **TREATMENT:** Emergency. **lugol iodine or propylthiouracil;** in **toxic** period give **digoxin, propranolol.** Remember, **intrauterine administration of propranolol** to mother causes **respiratory depression in newborn.**

117. **Thyroid cancer:** Rare, **first** clinical manifestation is **painless nodule on thyroid gland. Most common site of metastasis are the lungs.**
    Type of cancer: Papillary, follicular.
    Thyroid scan:↓ uptake by nodule;
    DIAGNOSIS CONFIRMED: By biopsy. TREATMENT: Perform thyroidectomy, then **use Sodium L-thyroxine** to suppress TSH.

118. **Medullary carcinoma of thyroid:** Arises from parafollicular cells (C cells) of thyroid gland. **Most common** symptom is **goiter;** metastasis occurs in lymph nodes and liver. **DIAGNOSIS CONFIRMED: By biopsy.** Always **look for** tumor, specifically

pheochromocytoma. TREATMENT: Total thyroidectomy.

119. Multiple endocrine neoplasia (MEN), type IIa (sipple syndrome). Medullary carcinoma of **thyroid** with **adrenal** medullary hyperplasia, or pheochromocytoma and parathyroid hyperplasia, is called MEN, type IIa. Gene location on chromosome 10, and DNA testing can be done for family. **TREATMENT:** Thyroidectomy.

120. Multiple endocrine neoplasia (MEN), type II B: **Medullary carcinoma** with **multiple neuroma, pheochromocytoma.** Patient looks like one with Marfan syndrome (tall, long fingers), and scoliosis. In infancy it is accompanied by diarrhea, constipation, and failure to thrive. **TREATMENT:** Thyroidectomy.

121. **Action of PTH (parathyroid hormone):**
    a.   ↑ absorption of calcium from intestine.
    b.   ↑ absorption of calcium from bone.
    c.   ↓ renal excretion of calcium.
    Calcitonin has **opposite** effect of (b) and (c). Calcitonin is secreted by **parafollicular or C cells** of thyroid gland. Its action is **independent** of PTH and vitamin D. It causes **inhibition of reabsorption of bone** by decreasing the number and activity of **osteoclast,** so it is used in **Paget disease.** It also acts as neurotransmitter to inhibit cellular function. Calcitonin is also secreted from brain, pituitary, G.I. and pancreas.

122. Hyperparathyroid mother and **newborn** infant: Hyperparathyroid mother causes **hypercalcemia** which crosses the placenta to fetus and suppresses fetal parathyroid gland, causing **hypocalcemia (transient).** When cause of **hypocalcemia in newborn** is **not known,** measure maternal level of Ca, P, and PTH.

123. Humoral **hypercalcemia syndrome of malignancy** due to: **Elevated PTH P (PTH related peptide).** It is a recently isolated **protein** which has structural similarity to PTH. **It acts** like PTH and **activates PTH receptors on bone and kidney, resulting in ↑ production of 1, 25 (OH)2 D in kidney,** results in ↑ bone resorption of calcium ↑ serum **Ca and ↓ phosphorus** (by stimulating phosphaturia). It is widely distributed in the body tissues (placenta, gastric cells, fetal tissues, lactating mammary tissues). Very **high level is found in breast milk and pasteurized bovine milk.** Location: chromosome 12; location of PTH: chromosome 11.

124. **Hypoparathyroidism:** PTH level is **low** in cord blood and reaches **normal** by 6th day of life. **Hypoparathyroidism causes following problems.**
    a.   Early neonatal hypocalcemia (first 3 days): primi, asphyxia, IDM.
    b.   Late (3-7 days) hypocalcemia: type of feeding is most important.
    c.   Transient idiopathic (first through 8th week) hypocalcemia: very low PTH level.

125. **Di George syndrome: Hypoplasia or aplasia of parathyroid gland** and defective development of 3rd and 4th pharyngeal pouch.
    Most common cardiac anomaly is truncus. Most common association is aplastic or hypoplastic thymus.   CXR should be done.
    Hypocalcemia and absence of thymus indicate this syndrome. Location: chromosome 22.Tetany may be **transient.** It is also found in IDM (diabetes), CHARGE syndrome, fetal

alcohol syndrome.
CHARGE : coloboma, heart defect, atresia choanae, retarded growth and development, and ear anomaly.

126. Mother who took **retinoic acid** in **early** pregnancy for acne, has what effect on fetus? **Di George syndrome.**

127. **Familial congenital hypoparathyroidism:** **X-linked recessive,** 2-week to 6-month-old child evidences afebrile seizure. Autopsy shows **defect in embryogenesis** causing hypoparathyroidism. Serum: ↓ Ca, ↑ P, ↓ PTH.

128. **Surgical hypoparathyroidism:** **Found after thyroidectomy** due to damage (blood supply, edema, fibrosis or accidental removal) of parathyroid gland, so **parathyroid function should be checked** after thyroidectomy. It can manifest with **immediate** postoperative tetany or develop **cataract formation gradually** after month or more.

129. Pigment deposition in parathyroid and hypoparathyroidism:
Iron deposition: Thalassemia.
Copper deposition: Wilson disease.

130. Idiopathic hypoparathyroidism: Etiology is **unknown.** May be due to **autoimmune** phenomenon. Manifests in first 2 years of life. Very few will have **incomplete** Di George syndrome.

131. **Autoimmune hypoparathyroidism:** It is associated with **Addison disease** (hypofunction of adrenal) and **chronic mucocutaneous candidiasis.** If **two of** the above three conditions manifest, then it is called polyglandular autoimmune disease type I. 33% of patients have all three features, and 66% has two features. **1st feature is candidiasis.** 2nd is hypoparathyroid. **3rd** is hypoadrenal.

132. **Clinical presentation** of hypoparathyroid: **Muscular pain, cramp** occur early, then tingling, numbness of the hands and feet, (+)ve Chvostek or Trousseau sign, **very soft teeth,** dry skin, **fungal infection in mouth, nail, Cataract** develop in long standing cases. Delayed treatment can cause **physical and mental retardation.**

133. **Laboratory features** and treatment of hypoparathyroidism:
Serum: ↓ Ca, ↑ P, ionized Ca (45%), alkaline phosphatase → ↓ ; ↓ vit D3, ↓ PTH.
X-ray skull: Calcification in basal ganglia.
EEG: Slow activity.
In hypoparathyroidism with Addison disease, serum Ca is normal, but after treatment of the Addison disease, Ca becomes low again.
TREATMENT: I.V. calcium gluconate, vit D2, then P.O. neocalglucon. Avoid high phosphate food (milk, cheese, eggs).

134. How ↓ Mg, cause ↓ Ca: ↓ Mg inhibits release of PTH ↓ and causes **resistance** to the effects of PTH.

135. **Kenny Caffey syndrome:** Symptomatic hypocalcemia, short stature, medullary long bone

stenosis, idiopathic hypoparathyroidism and abnormal PTH.

136. **Defect** in pseudohypoparathyroidism (Albright hereditary dystrophy): At the PTH **receptor** site - adenyl cyclase system. Here parathyroid gland and its secretion are normal, but PTH cannot raise serum calcium because of the defect at the receptor site.

137. Types of pseudohypoparathyroidism (PHP): Most common type Ia. (Others are Ib, II).

    Type Ia: Genetic defect in **alpha subunit of guanine (Gsa) nucleotide binding** protein, which is important for hormone receptor **to activate cAMP.** Autosomal dominant. Decrease of **fertility** in male. Children show **short, stocky built, round face** (2nd metacarpal and metatarsal bones are **not** affected, so **index finger is bigger than middle finger), calcium deposits in subcutaneous tissue,** mental retardation, basal ganglia calcification, lenticular cataract.
    Serum: **Ca →, P →, ↑ PTH**
    This variant is **pseudopseudohypoparathyroidism.**
    Along with resistance to PTH, there is **resistance to TSH,** gonadotrophins, glucagon. No clinical hypothyroidism. ↑ **TSH, ↓ thyroxine can diagnose type Ia PHP in newborn** by newborn screen.
    DEFINITIVE DIAGNOSIS: ↓ **urinary phosphate and cAMP** after infusion of synthetic 1-34 fragment of human PTH.

    Type Ib: Normal G protein, normal-looking child, only resistance to PTH (**no** resistance to other hormones).
    Serum: Ca →,P →, ↑ PTH (immunoreactive), → **PTH (bio active).**
    Defect is **unknown,** but may be due to inactive hormone, inhibitory PTH peptide, defective PTH receptor, or adenyl cyclase catalytic subunit.

    Type II: Normal cAMP activity, but no response to cellular level. ↑ urinary excretion of cAMP (but **not** the phosphate) after PTH stimulation, the only difference from type I.

138. Most common cause of **primary** hyperparathyroidism:
    Newborn: Parathyroid gland **hyperplasia.**
    Children: Parathyroid gland **adenoma** (single, benign).
    Secondary hyperparathyroidism: **most common cause is vitamin D deficient-rickets,** malabsorption syndrome due to hypocalcemia resulting in increased parathyroid activity.
    Tertiary hyperparathyroidism: **most common cause is, after renal transplant,** parathyroid gland continue to secrete PTH for months or years.

    MEN type I (hyperparathyroidism): **3 P's** (pancreas, pituitary, parathyroid). Pancreatic islet cell hyperplasia or adenoma (secrete insulin, gastrin, pancreatic polypeptide, rarely glucagon), anterior pituitary (secret prolactin), parathyroid (PTH). Occurs in **adults.** Carrier can be detected by DNA probe. Location: chromosome 11. (Not important in Board examination).

    MEN type II: 3 P's and medullary carcinoma of thyroid and pheochromocytoma.
    Zollinger-Ellison syndrome: 2 P's (parathyroid, pancreas), hyperparathyroidism, peptic ulcer due to pancreatic islet cell tumor.

Ectopic PTH production (hyperparathyroidism): hormone is **PTHrP (not** the PTH). Remember this.

Transient neonatal hyperparathyroidism: Most common cause is maternal hypoparathyroidism (idiopathic, surgical) or pseudohypoparathyroidism. Maternal hypocalcemia (undiagnosed) causes chronic fetal exposure to ↓ Ca, which causes ↑ parathyroid activity. (Important for Board examination).

139. Hypercalcemia (↑ Ca) **due to any other causes except** hyperparathyroidism.
     Serum PTH level is → (normal), but in other conditions PTH ↑.
     Treatment for ↑ Ca when PTH is → (normal): corticosteroid; it does **not** reduce Ca in hyperparathyroidism.

140. **All other causes of hypercalcemia:**
     a. Familial hypocalcuric hypercalcemia: Autosomal dominant, asymptomatic patient. Hypercalcemia is an accidental finding. **There is a normal** parathyroid gland, so **parathyroid surgery does not control hypercalcemia.**
         Defect: **unknown,** insensitivity of kidney and parathyroid to hypercalcemia means unresponsiveness to ↑ Ca.
         Serum: ↑ Ca, ↑ Mg, PTH →.
     b. **Granulomatous diseases:** Most common is **sarcoidosis** (less common T.B.).
         Serum: ↑ Ca, ↓ **PTH,** ↑ vit D3.
         Granulomatous lesion contains plenty of T. lymphocyte which secretes interferon alpha which stimulates macrophage, which secretes vitamin D3.
     c. **Malignancy:** Due to ↑ **PTHrP.**
         Serum: ↑ Ca, → PTH, ↑ **PTHrP,** → vit D3.
         Example: malignant rhabdoid kidney tumor, mesoblastic nephroma.
     d. **Miscellaneous causes:**
         i.   Subcutaneous fat necrosis.
         ii. Hypophosphatasia.
         iii. William syndrome (idiopathic hypercalcemia).
         iv. Vitamin D toxicity.
     TREATMENT FOR ALL OTHER CAUSES: prednisone (corticosteroid).

141. Clinical manifestations of **hyperparathyroidism:** All clinical manifestations **are due to hypercalcemia** accompanied by **muscle weakness, constipation,** vomiting, **polyuria, polydipsia,** fever, weight loss, nephrocalcinosis, renal stone and colic, pain in back, **and reduced height due to** vertebral compression.
     Parathyroid crisis: It occurs when **serum Ca is more than 15 mg/dl,** present with oliguria, ↑ BUN and creatinine, stupor, coma. In infants **hypotonia,** retardation (physical and mental), seizure, and blindness occur.

142. **Diagnosis and treatment** for hyperparathyroidism:

     Serum: ↑ Ca, ↓ P, ↓ Mg, ↑ PTH. (→ calcitonin chronic and ↓ level in acute).
     X-ray: Most characteristic findings are resorption of periosteal bones of the phalanges. In advanced cases, generalized rarefaction, cyst, tumor, and fracture occur. Rickets are found in 10% cases.
     TREATMENT: Surgical exploration of parathyroid gland for inspection. If this is a case

of adenoma or a neonate with severe ↑ Ca, **remove the parathyroid glands;** postoperative I.V. calcium, then P.O. high Ca and P diet for few months. Implantation of a portion of parathyroid in forearm helps maintain postoperative calcium blood level. Neither CT scan, nor sonogram is required routinely to localize adenoma and then differentiate adenoma from hyperplasia. Such procedures may, however, be indicated in persistent or recurrent hyperparathyroidism. Arteriography or selective venous sample is replaced by CT scan, sonogram, and scan to localize the tumor.

143. **Hormones secreted** by adrenal glands:
    a.   Medulla: Dopamine, epinephrine, and norepinephrine are all catecholamine.
    b.   Cortex (from outside inward):
        i.   Zona glomerulosa: Aldosterone (↑ Na, ↓ K).
        ii.   Zona fasciculata: Glucocorticoid, androgen.
        iii.   Zona reticularis: Sex hormones.
    Principal glucocorticoid is **cortisol, or compound F, or hydrocortisone. ACTH stimulates zona fasciculate,** secretes cortisol which produces negative feedback to **ACTH, which is also controlled by CRH (corticotropin releasing hormones).** Medulla is formed by ectoderm (neural), and cortex is formed by mesoderm.

144. Size of adrenal and kidney in fetus and newborn:
    2 months of fetal life: Adrenal **is bigger** than kidney.
    4 months of fetal life: Kidney grows rapidly.
    6 months of fetal life: Kidney is **double** the size of adrenal.
    Full term at birth: Kidney is **triple** the size of adrenal.

145. Proportion of cortex and medulla of adrenal:
    Fullterm at birth: Cortex is 80% of whole gland.
    2 weeks after birth: Cortex size is reduced by 50%.
    6 months of age: Cortex is very small.

146. Most important hormone produced by fetal adrenal cortex: DHEA and DHEAS (dehydroepiandrosterone sulfate).

147. In **fetal adrenal hyperplasia,** maternal **urine shows: High estriol** (this is the major estrogen found in maternal urine). Remember, **low** estriol level occurs in **hypoplasia.**

148. Cortisol converted to cortisone at: **Peripheral tissue** by 11 beta-hydroxysteroid dehydrogenase. Deficiency of this enzyme causes heritable form of mineralocorticoid excess.

149. Glucocorticoid has catabolic effect in all tissues **except: Liver.** (Glucocorticoid increases protein and glycogen content, stimulate neoglycogenesis and enzyme activity in liver.)

150. Potency of various steroids:
    a.   Betamethasone and dexamethasone produces 25 times **more potent anti-inflammatory** activity than does cortisol; has very little effect on salt and water.
    b.   Halogenative derivative (fluorohydrocortisone) is 15 times **more anti-inflammatory** than hydrocortisone and 20 times more active in **salt and water** retention.

c.   Prednisone and prednisolone have 4 times **more anti-inflammatory** activity and act on carbohydrate metabolism as natural steroids. They are less active in salt and water.
Most potent anti inflammatory steroid: Beta-and dexamethasone (next, fluorohydrocortisone; then prednisone).
Most potent salt and water retention activity in steroid: Fluorohydrocortisone (second, prednisone; third beta-and dexamethasone.)

151.   Enzyme that is **absent** from fetal adrenal **until term: 3 beta-hydroxysteroid dehydrogenase.** It is needed to form progesterone, so fetus borrows **placental pregnenolone** to form **DHEAS,** cortisol, and aldosterone; placenta borrows fetal DHEAS to produce **estrone and estriol.**

152.   **Most potent** adrenal androgen: **DHEAS** (dehydroepiandrosterone sulfate). It is formed either from adrenal gland or after sulfation of DHEA in peripheral tissue. It is low in children, but increases before any other hormonal changes in puberty, resulting **in adrenarche. It does not** initiate puberty, but **forms axillary and pubic hair.** It is **not** controlled by ACTH. Adrenarche mostly due to **Z. reticularis. Maximal** rise of DHEA occurs in adrenal tumor, **moderate** rise in precocious adrenarche, **mild** rise in adrenal hyperplasia.

153.   Mechanism of **aldosterone** (mineralocorticoid) secretion:
Salt and water loss, hypovolemia, hypotension
  ↓
↑ Renin secretion (by juxtaglomerular kidney apparatus)
  ↓
Binds with alpha 2 globulin (formed in liver)
  ↓
Angiotensin I (inactive **decapeptide formed in kidney)**
  ↓ (by converting enzyme)
Angiotensin II (active **octapeptide formed in lungs)**

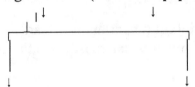

Pressor agent: Aldosterone (from adrenal cortex)
                                              ↓

(50 times more active   (salt, and water **retention in distal tubule**
than norepinephrine;   and K excretion in kidney, so correct
maintains blood   electrolytes and blood volume).
pressure.)
Aldosterone secretion is stimulated by:
a.   Hyponatremia (↓ Na)
b.   Hyperkalemia (↑ K)
c.   Renin-angiotensin pathway
d.   ACTH (**minimal** effect in normal person, **maximal** effect in anephric person).

154. Most important catecholamine **excreted in urine: VMA** (3 methoxy-4-hydroxy mandelic acid), metanephrine, normetanephrine.
     All catecholamines (dopamine, epinephrine and norepinephrine) are secreted mainly from adrenal medulla, but also secreted from brain, sympathetic nervous system, and chromaffin tissues outside the adrenal gland. In fetus, there is no epinephrine; at birth, mostly **norepinephrine;** but in adult, **mostly epinephrine.**
     Epinephrine: ↑ systolic B.P., ↓ diastolic B.P. (by decreasing peripheral vascular resistance), ↑ heart rate, ↑↑ serum glucose.
     Nor-epinephrine: ↑ both systolic and diastolic B.P. (by increasing peripheral vascular resistance), **no** change in cardiac output, ↑ serum glucose (mild).
     ↑ Glucose: By glucocorticoid, glucagon, catecholamine, Cushing syndrome.
     ↓ Glucose: By androgen, insulin, Addison disease.

155. Most common association of hypoplasia of pituitary gland (corticotropin or ACTH deficiency): Secondary hypoplasia of adrenal, other hormonal deficiency.

156. Most common cause of corticotropin or ACTH deficiency: **Idiopathic** or destructive (craniopharyngioma) lesion of pituitary. Other cause is hypothalamic hypofunction.

157. Primary adrenal aplasia/hypoplasia causing insufficiency: X-linked recessive disorder, **disorganization and cytomegaly** of hypoplastic adrenal cortex (not found in hypoplasia due to ACTH deficiency), associated with glycerol kinase deficiency and **Duchenne muscular dystrophy, DNA analysis** can diagnose diseased child and carrier mother (microdeletion in X p21 region), together with **mental retardation and delayed puberty due to hypogonadotrophic hypogonadism.**

158. Adrenal hypofunction in **familial glucocorticoid deficiency:** Autosomal recessive, atrophy of cortex except Z. glomerulosa, accompanied by **hypoglycemia,** convulsion, **absent tears, pigmentation,** and achalasia of cardia.
     Serum: ↓ glucocorticoid, → aldosterone, ↑ ACTH.

159. Most common cause of adrenocortical insufficiency **in infant** (important for Board examination): **Salt losing form of congenital adrenal hyperplasia,** mostly due to **21-hydroxylase deficiency.**

160. Adrenal hypofunction due to **isolated aldosterone defect:** Defect in enzyme P450C11, which inhibits aldosterone formation from 18 hydroxycorticosterones, together with **dehydration and newborn's failure to thrive.**
     Serum: ↓ Na, ↑ K, metabolic acidosis, ↑ renin.
     TREATMENT: 9 alpha-fluorocortisol;
     Autosomal recessive, prenatal diagnosis and detection of carrier are possible.

161. **Adrenal hemorrhage:** In newborns due to asphyxia or difficult delivery. Death occurs from severe hemorrhage due to exsanguination or hypofunction of adrenal gland; calcification occurs later. Meningococcal infection with shock causing adrenal hemorrhage is called Waterhouse-Friderichsen syndrome.

162. **Defect** in pseudohypoaldosteronism: **End organ resistance (renal tubule) to**

aldosterone.

Serum: ↑ aldosterone, ↑ renin, ↓ Na, ↑ K due to increase activity of **renin-angiotensin system.**

Infant with salt losing dehydration.

TREATMENT: Give **dietary salt** until the condition resolves spontaneously around 2 years of age.

163. **Most common cause** of Addison disease: **Autoimmune destruction** of gland (adrenal cortex).

Atrophic cortex infiltrated with lymphocytes, medulla is intact; shows **first** manifestation of **cortisol** deficiency, **2nd aldosterone** deficiency and salt loss, finally, **all** cortical function is **lost.**

Serum: Anti-adrenal cytoplasmic antibody, immunoglobulin inhibit the effect of ACTH by **unknown** mechanism.

It is found in two syndromes:

Type 1 autoimmune polyendocrinopathy (or autoimmune polyendocrinopathy-candidiasis-ectodermal dystrophy, APECD): First manifestation is **mucocutaneous candidiasis.** Second, **hypoparathyroidism.** Third, **Addison disease.** Rarely type 1 diabetes and hypothyroidism. Other presentations are alopecia, vitiligo, gonadal failure, chronic active hepatitis, nail dystrophy. The presence of anti adrenal and steroid cell antibodies predict **future development** of Addison disease or ovarian failure.

Type II autoimmune polyendocrinopathy: It includes Addison disease, autoimmune thyroid disease, or type 1 diabetes; HLA-D3 and HLA-D4 found in this patient.

164. Adrenoleukodystrophy causes adrenal failure: Only 33% of cases and usually after 4 years.

165. **Drugs** causing hypoadrenalism: Ketoconazole (inhibit adrenal enzyme); phenytoin, phenobarbital, rifampin (by inducing enzymes in liver which enhance steroid metabolism).

166. **Clinical presentation** of hypofunction of adrenal:
    a. **Newborn period:** Salt loss (↓ Na, ↑ K), vomiting, dehydration, hypoglycemia, lethargy (occurs in defect in steroid formation, pseudohypoaldosteronism, adrenal hypoplasia).
    b. **Children (Addison disease):** Muscle wasting, weakness, **hypotension, craving for salt, hyper-pigmentation (in mouth, face hand, genitalia, axilla),** sometimes **vitiligo which does not disappear with suntan.**
    Adrenal crisis: Present with tachycardia, tachypnea, cyanosis, cold skin, hypotension. It is precipitated by infection, trauma, drugs (barbiturate, morphine, laxative, insulin thyroxine).
    c. **ACTH (corticotrophin) deficiency:** **No** pigmentation; present with ↓ glucose; salt is normal because of residual secretion of aldosterone.
    d. **Familial glucocorticoid deficiency:** Pigmentation, seizure, ↓ Glucose.

167. **Diagnosis and treatment** of hypoadrenalism: **MOST DIAGNOSTIC TEST: Serum cortisol level is low before corticotrophin (ACTH) and does not increase after that.**
    Serum: ↓ Na, ↓ Cl, ↑ K, ↑ Renin; ↑ BUN (dehydration).
    Urine: ↑ Na, ↑ Cl, ↓ K (excretion).
    ↓ Serum aldosterone: Salt-losing congenital adrenal hyperplasia, adrenal hypoplasia,

Addison disease, isolated defect in aldosterone synthesis.

↑ Serum aldosterone: Pseudohypoaldosteronism, familial glucocorticoid deficiency.

Anti-adrenal antibody: Indicates autoimmune phenomenon.

↑ ACTH level: Primary cortisol deficiency (adrenal).

↓ ACTH level: Hypothalamic or pituitary hypofunction causing secondary hypofunction of adrenal.

CRH (corticotrophin releasing hormone) given: ↑ ACTH , indicates **hypothalamic** defect.

CRH given: ↓ ACTH, indicates **hypopituitarism.**

CRH stimulation test can localize the site of defect.

TREATMENT:

a. **Acute hypoadrenalism:** 5% glucose with 0.9% saline to correct hypoglycemia and hyponatremia; Hydrocortisone hemisuccinate; salt-retaining hormone DOCA (deoxycorticosterone acetate).

b. After acute episode: Discontinue I.V.; oral cortisol, DOCA.

c. Chronic patient: Oral cortisol.

d. Only glucocorticoid deficiency: Cortisol.

e. Only mineralocorticoid deficiency: DOCA.

f. Adrenal hemorrhage: Whole blood, vitamin K and C.

168. Investigation needs to be done:

    a. Congenital adrenal hypoplasia: Chromosome analysis for deletion of Xp21 region.

    b. Duchenne muscular dystrophy: CPK ↑↑.

    c. Glycerol kinase deficiency: Triglyceride ↑.

169. **Most common cause** of congenital adrenal hyperplasia: 21-hydroxylase deficiency (95%).

170. **Most common type** of congenital adrenal hyperplasia:
Salt-losing type = 75%.
Non-salt losing type = 25%.

171. Most of the **mutation** in 21-hydroxylase deficiency is due to: Recombination (gene conversion or deletion) between active gene (CYP 21 B) and pseudogene (CYP 21 A).

172. **Most characteristic presentation** of congenital adrenal hyperplasia: **Virilization of genitalia (isosexual).**

173. Most characteristic presentation of **11 hydroxylase deficiency: Hypertension.** Virilization shows up in all the patient, gynecomastia in prepubertal children.

174. Clinical manifestations of congenital adrenal hyperplasia:

    a. **Salt-losing type:** Symptoms begin at birth.
Male: **Normal** genitalia, but vomiting, dehydration, weight loss like pyloric stenosis or obstruction, salt loss.
Female: **Virilized** external genitalia, vomiting, dehydration, weight loss, salt loss.
3 beta-hydroxysteroid dehydrogenase defect: Mildly virilized, more salt loss; in male, hypospadias with or without cryptorchidism or bifid scrotum; in female, mild labial fusion and enlargement of clitoris.
Lipoid adrenal hyperplasia: Normal genitalia, salt loss.

b. Non-salt losing type:

Male: **Normal** at birth, symptoms appear from 6 months to 5 years, present with isosexual precocity. **Enlarged** penis, scrotum, prostate pubic hair, acne, deep voice, advanced bony maturation and epiphyseal closure resulting in short stature, developed muscles.

Remember, normal testes mostly, and rarely ectopic. Hyperplastic adrenal tissue cause enlarged testes. Normal mentation and abnormal physical growth cause behavioral problems.

Female: **Masculine features at birth (female pseudohermaphrodite),** labial fusion, common opening of vagina and urethra (urogenital sinus), enlarged clitoris that looks like a penis, **premature development of pubic and axillary hairs,** deep voice, well built-muscles, **tall for her age,** progressively enlarged genitalia, **normal breasts, no** menstruation, but **normal female internal organs.** Some reared as a male who had go on to have normal heterosexual relations.

175. **Laboratory** diagnosis:

a. **Classic form (21 hydroxylase ↓): Most confirmatory test is (17-OHP) 17 hydroxy progesterone level in serum.** It is **high in first 3 days** of life, even in normal child, then it falls, but in **diseased child it rises.** Serum cortisol is **low in salt-losing** type and **normal** in non-salt-losing type. **Serum level of steroid can be measured in all types of adrenal hyperplasia,** so 24 hour-urine test is not done, but rather ↑ 17-ketosteroid and ↑ pregnanetriol in urine.

b. **Late onset type:** Serum level of 17-OHP is lightly elevated or normal, but **diagnostic rises after 1 hour of I.V. ACTH (0.25 mg) given.**

c. **11-hydroxylase defect:** ↑ serum level of DOC (deoxycorticosterone) and ↑ 11 deoxycortisol.

d. **3 beta-hydroxysteroid dehydrogenase defect: Definitive diagnosis by $\Delta^5\Delta^4$ steroid ratio in plasma and urine;** ↑ serum Δ^5 steroid (17 hydroxy-pregnenolone) found also in 21-hydroxylase defect.

e. Chromosome is normal for male and female.

f. In female: Injection of dye into urogenital sinus shows vagina and uterus; sonogram is helpful.

176. **Prenatal diagnosis and treatment** of ↓ 21-hydroxylase:

1st trimester: Chorionic villi biopsy (cvs), then HLA typing or DNA analysis.
2nd trimester: ↑ **17-OHP in amniotic fluid,** HLA and DNA analysis in amniotic **fluid cells.**
TREATMENT: Dexamethasone by 5th week of risky pregnancy 1.5 mg/dl in 2 or 3 divided doses. This is **not very effective.** First rimester CVS also determines sex and genotype of fetus. Only **female fetus needs treatment.**

177. Clinical presentation of **non classic** 21-hydroxylase deficiency: **Normal until puberty.** All males and some females are **asymptomatic, showing at puberty** signs of acne, hirsutism, menstrual problems and infertility. HLA-B 14, DR1 in up to 75% of patient, mutations in codon 281 are indicators for this problem.

178. **Treatment** of congenital adrenal hyperplasia:

a. **Glucocorticoid: Hydrocortisone use for the rest of patient's life.**

b. **Salt losers and ↑ renin: Add mineralocorticoid (9 alpha fluorocortisol).**

c.   Non-salt-loser and ↑ renin: Add mineralocorticoid. **Adequacy of treatment** by: Plasma level of 17-OHP, androstenedione, testosterone, and renin measure at 9 a.m., or monitor growth by osseous maturation.

d.   **Enlarged clitoris:** Surgical correction (recession rather than removal) around 6-12 months; reassure parents about child's normal sexual activity and normal menstruation in the future.

e.   **Non-salt-loser undiagnosed until child is 3-7 years of age (male):** Bone age is advanced **by 5 years,** so start treatment **with hydrocortisone** which slows growth and normalizes bone maturation; if bone age is **12 years or more** when gonadotrophin dependent tumor occurs, **hydrocortisone** will inhibit adrenal androgen, and if hypothalamus is intact, then pituitary gonadotrophin is released. This type of true precocious puberty is treated with **LHRH (luteinizing hormone releasing hormone) analog.**

f.   **Inadequate corticosteroid treatment** may cause bilateral testicular tumor due to ectopic adrenal cells in testis which might not respond to higher doses. Prolonged inadequate adrenal suppression causes adrenal tumor.

179. How to distinguish virilizing adrenocortical tumor from congenital adrenal hyperplasia in female:
Virilizing adrenocortical tumor: Initially **normal** genitalia become virilized.
Congenital adrenal hyperplasia: Virilized at birth; late onset type of virilization occurs in childhood.

180. **Virilizing adrenocortical tumor:**
In male: Symptoms **same as** non-salt-losing type of congenital adrenal hyperplasia (CAH), precocious puberty.
In female: **Virilization of normal** female. Adrenal adenoma caused intrauterine labial fusion and enlarged clitoris.
Adrenal tumor with or without Cushing syndrome and hemihypertrophy in first few years of life. Tumors also associated with **Beckwith-Wiedemann syndrome, CNS and Gu abnormalities.**
DIAGNOSIS: Serum: ↑ DHEA, ↑ DHEAS, ↑ testosterone.
Urine: ↑ 17 ketosteroid.
Sono and CT: Look for mass (carcinoma more common than adenoma).
TREATMENT: Surgical resection of mass (transperitoneal approach), follow up adrenal androgen level every month to detect recurrence. **Mitotane** (isomer of DDD) is used for **recurrence and inoperable tumor.** Neoplasm of one adrenal **inhibits ACTH** secretion which does **not** stimulate normal adrenal which gets atrophic. **Adrenal insufficiency after surgery** should be treated with **hydrocortisone.**

181. **Most common** cause of **Cushing syndrome;**
Less than 7 years: Adrenal **tumor (mostly malignant).**
More than 7 years: Adrenal **hyperplasia.**
Cushing syndrome includes **obesity, hypertension** due to ↑ cortisol level which **may or may not** depend on ACTH.
a.   ACTH-**independent** tumors (primary pigmented nodular adrenocortical disease) of **Cushing syndrome:** It is due to circulating immunoglobulin acting on ACTH receptor and stimulating steroid production. **Carney complex** includes this tumor

with cardiac and cutaneous myxomas, centrofacial lentigines, sexual precocity with testicular tumor, pituitary mass and melanotic schwannomas. It is autosomal dominant.

b. ACTH dependent tumors (cushing syndrome):

    i. **Bilateral adrenal hyperplasia:** Mostly associated with **pituitary microadenoma,** resection of it usually corrects hypercorticism.
    Nelson syndrome: Pituitary tumor becomes prominent after removal of adrenal tumor; pituitary **chromophobe** tumors causes ↑ beta-lipoprotein, ↑ beta-endorphin, ↑ ACTH.

    ii. **Ectopic ACTH causing** bilateral adrenal hyperplasia: Ectopic ACTH from islet cells carcinoma of pancreas, neuroblastoma, ganglioneuroblastoma, Wilms tumor.

    iii. Prolonged exogenous ACTH or hydrocortisone causes Cushingoid syndrome.

182. **Clinical presentation** of Cushing syndrome:

a. Infant: **Infant has symptoms** more severe than those of older children. **Moon facies** (round face, prominent cheeks and flushed appearance), **double chin,** buffalo hump, **obesity (generalized);** due to ↑ androgen (axillary and pubic hair, hypertrichosis, deep voice and, in female, large clitoris). Height is **less than 3rd** percentile **except** in case of significant virilization which causes rapid growth. High B.P., infection, **and renal stones** are common. Rarely associated with **hemihypertrophy.**

b. **Older children:** Early manifestations are **gradual obesity and growth retardation; purplish striae** on abdomen, thigh; delayed puberty, amenorrhea, high B.P., **renal stones.**

183. **Laboratory features cushing syndrome:**

CBC: ↑ Hct., ↓ lymphocyte and eosinophil.

GTT (glucose tolerance test): Diabetic despite ↑ insulin.

SMA6: ↓ K; rest are normal.

Osseous maturation: **Retarded** mostly or → or advanced in virilized tumor.

DIAGNOSIS CONFIRMED BY: 8 p.m. rise in **serum cortisol** ↑ (normal person has 8 a.m. ↑ cortisol and 50% less in 8 p.m.), so **diurnal rhythm is lost.**

Urine: ↑ free cortisol, ↑ 17 hydroxycorticosteroid.

Now differentiate between ACTH dependent or non dependent:

a. OCRH (ovine corticotrophin releasing hormone stimulation test = ACTH-dependent = ↑ ACTH and ↑ cortisol; ACTH-independent = → ACTH, → cortisol.

b. Dexamethasone stimulation test (30 to 120 µg/kg/24 hr. Q.I.D. x 2 days) = ACTH-dependent = ↓ urine free cortisol or 17 hydroxycorticosteroid (<50%), ↓ serum cortisol (<7 ug/dl).

X-ray: Osteoporosis (mostly spine), pathologic fracture; ↓ muscle, ↑ fat, absent thymic shadow due to excess cortisol.

Serum: GH ↓ (growth hormone), CT scan picks up lesion >1.5 cm (diameter).

MRI is preferred screening method: For ACTH-secreting pituitary adenoma.

184. **Treatment for cushing syndrome:**

a. **Unilateral** benign cortical adenoma: Adrenalectomy.

b. **Bilateral** benign cortical adenoma: Subtotal adrenalectomy.

c. Unilateral malignant cortical tumor: Total adrenalectomy. (Most commonly metastasis to liver and lungs).

d. Rare, bilateral malignant tumor: Bilateral adrenal removal. (Sometimes it is impossible to distinguish between benign and malignant.)

Post-operative complications of total adrenal removal: 30% of patients develop expanding pituitary mass and Nelson syndrome (melanosis, ↑↑ ACTH very high, enlarged sella turcica). To avoid this problem, the preferred treatment is now:

e. **Transsphenoidal pituitary microsurgery.**

f. **Before and after adrenal removal:**

    i. Replacement **of corticosteroid** adequately.

    ii. One gland tumor producing corticosteroid suppressing other gland (atrophy); give cortisol and corticotrophin.

g. Cyproheptadine (serotonin antagonist Block ACTH): Experimental.

185. **Postoperative complication and outcome** of Cushing syndrome: Infection, poor wound healing, collapse, pancreatitis, thrombosis. Outcome: Catch-up growth occurs but final height is less than normal.

186. Most common mineralocorticoid secreted by adrenal: Aldosterone which causes ↑ Na, ↑ Cl, ↓ K.

187. Difference between obesity and Cushing syndrome:
Obesity: ↑ urine corticosteroid suppressed by dexamethasone; **tall, obese.**
Cushing: ↑ urine corticosteroid **not** suppressed by dexamethasone; **short, obese.**

188. **Hyperaldosteronism:** Types are primary and secondary.

Primary: Rare. ↑ aldosterone, but independent of renin-angiotensin, present with ↓ B.P., ↓ K, ↓ renin-angiotensin.
Secondary: It activates ↑ renin-angiotensin, → B.P., → K.

Etiology:

a. Adenoma secreting aldosterone: Unilateral, mostly in girls between ages 3-12 years.

b. Micronodular adrenocortical hyperplasia: Bilateral, in older children, pituitary glycoprotein stimulates adrenal.

c. Glucocorticoid suppressed aldosteronism: **Response to glucocorticoid treatment,** autosomal dominant, bilateral adrenal hyperplasia.

Clinical presentations: Asymptomatic or accidental finding of **hypertension,** or with headache, dizziness; ↓ K lead to clear cell nephrosis, polyuria, polydipsia, enuresis, muscle weakness, tetany, growth failure.

If a child has **primary hyperaldosteronism,** what is the **initially** preferred investigation? **Dexamethasone suppression test (0.25 mg Q.6.H):**

a. **Marked suppression** of aldosterone and control of B.P.: Indicates patient is a **glucocorticoid responsive type.**

b. **No response:** Means adrenal adenoma (tumor). For the next step in treating adenoma, perform **CT scan** to look for tumor (perform CT scan diagnosis if more than 1.5 cm diameter). If CT scan is negative, then **catheterization in both adrenal** veins. ↑ aldosterone in **one vein means adenoma,** and ↑ aldosterone in **two veins** means hyperplasia. If venous catheterization is not successful, perform **laparotomy**

DIAGNOSIS CONFIRMED: (↑ B.P., ↓ K, ↓ renin) characteristic of the disease. Serum and urine: ↑ aldosterone. Serum: ↑ (pH, CO_2, HCO_3); ↓ (Mg, Cl); → Ca (but tetany).

TREATMENT:
a.   Glucocorticoid suppressed: Give **dexamethasone.** If no response, perform **bilateral adrenal tumor removal and then replace therapy** with steroid.
b.   Adenoma: Removal of tumor cures this.
c.   Secondary ↑ aldosterone: Treat the underlying cause.

189.   Other causes of **Aldosterone** secretion:

a.   Edematous condition with ↓ intravascular volume: Congestive cardiac failure, nephrotic, cirrhotic liver.
b.   Renal artery stenosis causing ↓ renal perfusion: ↑ renin secretion.
c.   Wilms tumor and juxtaglomerular cell tumor: Secondary ↑ aldosterone.
d.   Pseudohypoaldosteronism: Defect in aldosterone receptors, ↑ renin angiotensin activity.
e.   **Bartter syndrome:** ↓ (K,Cl), ↑ (pH, renin), → B.P., happen with ↓ **growth, defect in reabsorption of ascending limb of loop of Henle; biopsy** shows **hyperplasia of juxtaglomerular** apparatus. ↑ **PGF1 alpha** in urine cause ↑ renin in serum.

190.   Other causes of ↓ **aldosterone** secretion: **11 beta hydroxysteroid dehydrogenase activity (11 ß-OHSD),** occuring with polyuria, polydipsia, weight loss. ↓ K, ↑ B.P., **Strokes** occur. Although it **looks like** ↑ **aldosterone,** it actually ↓ aldosterone and ↓ renin, called **low renin hypertension. This enzyme converts cortisol to cortisone.** Serum cortisol is →, ↓ cortisone.
Cortisol binds with mineralocorticoid receptors, mimics hypoaldosteronism, **and is called pseudohypoaldosteronism.**

191.   Licorice causes **hypertension** because: It contains **glycyrrhetinic acid** which inhibits 11 ß-OHSD enzyme, showing conversion of **cortisol** to cortisone, ↑ **cortisone cause** ↑ **B.P.**

192.   Most common type of **catecholamine** in children: **Norepinephrine.**

193.   **First** manifestation of **feminizing adrenal tumors: Gynecomastia between 1/2 year to 7 years of age.** It secretes mostly **estrogen and then androgen;** androgen causes enlarged penis (male) and clitoris (female), advanced osseous maturation, deep voice, acne, but **normal testes.** This tumor is either **benign or malignant.**
Serum: ↑ estrogen, ↑ androgen, ↑ DHEA and DHEAS, ↓ gonadotrophin, no response to **GNRH stimulation.**
CT scan: Localize the tumor.
TREATMENT: Removal of **tumor;** gynecomastia regresses after surgery.

194.   Most common site of origin of **pheochromocytoma: Adrenal medulla.**

(Pheochromocytoma is autosomal dominant.) Other sites are sympathetic chain (mostly abdominal; thoracic, also cervical), periadrenal area, urinary bladder or ureter. Tumor more likely in **(R)** than (L) side, 20% bilateral and 30% adrenal and extra adrenal region. Patient also has **neurofibromatosis** (5% cases), which is also found in Von Hippel-Lindau disease, islet cells adenoma, and MEN types II a and II b.

195. **Hormones** secreted by pheochromocytoma: **Epinephrine and norepinephrine.**

Clinical presentations are due to epi-and norepinephrine, presentations are **hypertension (mostly sustained,** sometimes **paroxysmal, which suggests** this tumor), and **related symptoms** (vomiting, headache, palpitation, convulsion, sweating), in severe cases (precordial pain, cardiac failure, pulmonary edema, weight loss, papilledema, hemorrhage, exudate; polyuria, polydipsia suggests diabetes insipidus).

DIAGNOSIS CONFIRMED BY: ↑ **catecholamine in plasma and urine.** (In urine > 300 ug/day suggests pheochromocytoma) **detected by RIA and liquid chromatography. Gross hematuria** suggests tumors in bladder wall.

Urine: ↑ VMA (vanillylmandelic acid) (which is the metabolite of epi,-norepi-and metanephrine) which is falsely elevated by food containing vanilla.

To localize the tumor site: Best method is to give ^{131}I- **metaiodobenzyl guanidine,** which is taken by **all chromaffin tissue** of the body; others are CT scan, MRI.

196. **Treatment** for pheochromocytoma: **Surgical removal of tumor.**

Preoperative, intraoperative, and postoperative management:
Preoperative: Alpha and beta adrenergic blocker; hydration of the patient.
Operative: Laparotomy, ↑ fluid volume to avoid intraoperative or postoperative hypotension, Manipulation of tumor causes ↑ B.P. and tachycardia.
Postoperative: Maintain ↑ fluid volume for 48 hours to avoid hypotension.

197. **Biopsy** finding of pheochromocytoma: Malignancy is **rare.**

198. Family findings of pheochromocytoma: **Autosomal dominant;** check blood pressure and urinary excretion of ↑ catecholamine in family members.

199. Causes of **adrenal calcification:** Probably in **newborn, most common is hemorrhage** due to trauma or hypoxia. **Wolman syndrome has bilateral** calcification in infant (lipid disorder due to ↓ lysosomal acid lipase). Waterhouse-Friderichsen syndrome. pheochromocytoma, neuroblastoma, cortical cancer, ganglioneuroma, adrenal cyst.

200. **Wolman syndrome:** Autosomal recessive, rare **lipid (storage of cholesterylester and triglyceride) disorder** causing **extensive calcification of both adrenal** due to **deficiency** ↓ **lysosomal acid lipase,** present with ↑ liver and spleen, ↓ growth, G.I. symptom, death occurs by 4 months of age.

Prenatal diagnosis: Amniocentesis with **enzyme assay in cultured fibroblast.**

201. **Schematic diagram of hormonal changes:**

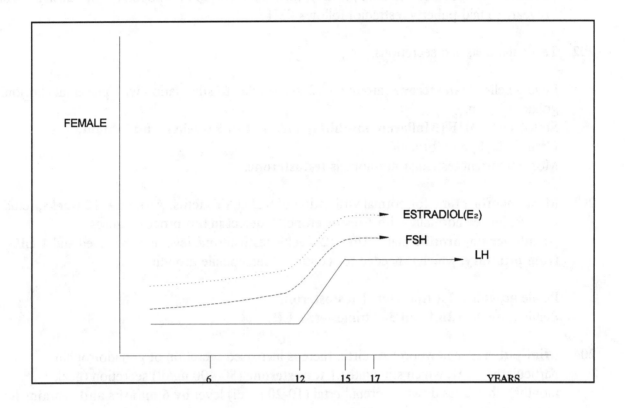

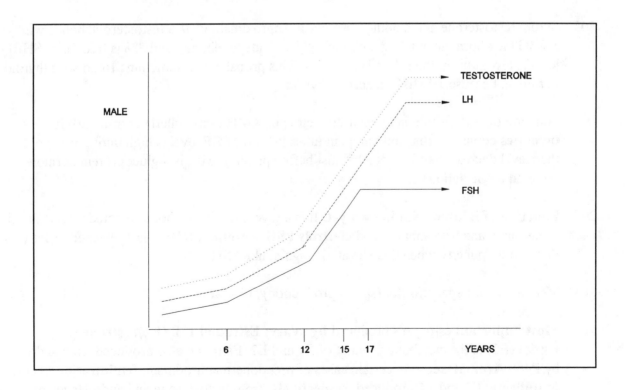

Male: ↑ FSH and LH around 6 years, sharp rise with onset of puberty, FSH increases to

mid-puberty but LH rises up to 17 years. Testosterone follows the LH.
Female: LH does **not** rise until puberty, then sharp rise to mid-puberty, FSH slowly ↑ from 6 years to mid-puberty, estradiol follows FSH.

202. Testicular cells and secretions:

     Leydig cells: **Testosterone** (around 8-12 weeks) due to stimulation with placental chorionic gonadotrophin.
     Sertoli cells: **MIF (Mullerian inhibiting factor, 4 to 6 weeks), and inhibin.**
     Germ cells: Sperm formation.
     Most important testicular hormone is **testosterone.**

203. Most important time for normal virilization of male (XY) fetus: Around **8-12 weeks,** fetus is masculinized normally with ↑ testosterone. A defect in this process causes **pseudohermaphrodite** male. After 12 weeks, testosterone level is diminished and ↑ **LH from pituitary,** which is needed for continued fetal penile growth.

     Penile growth in **1st** trimester: ↑ **testosterone.**
     Penile growth in **2nd and 3rd** trimester: ↑ **LH.**

204. **Mini-puberty** in newborn: At birth, there is increased secretion of gonadotrophin, particularly ↑ **LH,** which stimulates ↑ **testosterone** (80-400 ng/dl) secretion (peak 1-3 months), then goes down to prepubertal (10-20 ng/dl) level **by 6 months and remains low until puberty.** In newborns with testicular **atrophy or torsion,** there is ↓ **serum testosterone level and** ↑ **FSH and LH.**

205. Serum testosterone and binding hormones: Approximately 49% testosterone bonds with SHBG (sex hormone binding globulin); 49% bonds to albumin and 2% is free form. SHBG level is **low** at birth, then ↑ in 1st 10 days. This probably has something to do with thyroid hormone, because ↓ SHBG in absent thyroid.

206. Function of MIF (Mullerian inhibiting factor) or AMH (antimullerian hormone): It **involutes** cervix, uterus, and fallopian tubes in utero; MIF level is high until 2 years old, then level decreases and is detected just before puberty. MIF is a glucoprotein hormone secreted by **Sertoli cells.**

207. **Function of inhibin: Not known yet.** It is a glycoprotein hormone secreted by sertoli cells. It has alpha and beta subunit, and **controls FSH secretion.** Inhibin is ↑ elevated in 1st year, then ↓ until puberty when it is elevated ↑ again, like FSH.

208. Median age for **spermarche** (sperm production): 14 years.

209. **Most important** estrogens produced **by ovary: Estradiol 17ß (E2), estrone (E1).** Estriol (E3) is the metabolic product of E1 and E2. Estrogen also produced from androgen by **P450 Aromatase,** so in certain cases of pseudohermaphroditism, **feminization occurs at puberty.** E2 and E1 produced, **respectively,** from testosterone and androstenedione by P450 Aromatase; **E2 and E1, testosterone and androstenedione** are **interconvertible.**

210. **Hypofunction or hypogonadism** of **testes:**

Types:
a. **Primary** or hypergonadotropic hypogonadism in male: Primary defect in testes and secondary hyperfunction of pituitary due to lack of inhibition. Serum: ↑ **gonadotropin (FSH and LH),** ↓ **testosterone.**
b. **Secondary** or hypogonadotropic hypogonadism in male: Primary defect in anterior pituitary or hypothalamus and secondary hypofunction of testes. Serum: ↓ **gonadotropin (FSH and LH),** ↓ **testosterone.**

Clinical presentation, diagnosis and treatment of hypergonadotropic hypogonadism in male:

At birth: **Normal** genitalia or **very small testes and penis.**
At puberty: **Small** testes and penis (infantile) and **absent** secondary sexual character (pubic, axillary hair), fat deposits in buttock and abdomen; **long extremities** due to delayed epiphyseal closure (lower half of the body is **longer** than upper half). This is called **eunuchism.**

DIAGNOSIS:
Serum: ↓ testosterone (in all age groups), ↑↑FSH, ↑ LH (Normal person's testosterone level increases after puberty).
hCG stimulation test: Remains **low testosterone** ↓ level. (Normal person testosterone level ↑).

TREATMENT: Long-acting testosterone preparation (enanthate ester).

211. **Etiology** of primary hypogonadism:

a. Congenital anorchia: Normal external genitalia means testicular damage occurs **after 14th week** of fetal life by noxious factor.
   Serum: ↓ testosterone, ↑ FSH and LH.
   hCG stimulation test: No response to testosterone.
b. **Del Castillo syndrome** (germinal cell aplasia):**Small** testes, **small seminiferous tubules** without germ cells resulting **in azoospermia and infertility.** Normal (sexual maturation, Leydig cells).
   Serum: → testosterone, → LH, ↑ FSH, due to absence of inhibin (formed by Sertoli cell and inhibits FSH).
c. Acute orchitis due to mumps.
d. Atrophic testes due to torsion.
e. Atrophic testes due to radio and chemotherapy.
f. **Noonan syndrome:** In both **male and female, normal chromosome,** clinical presentation is like Turner syndrome (short stature, web neck), **pulmonic valvular stenosis,** characteristic facies (antimongoloid slant, hypertelorism, small chin, ptosis), 25% mentally retarded **(mostly 75% normal).**

Remember, it is associated with neurofibromatosis. It is frequently associated with undescended and small testes with either normal or diminished function, delayed puberty (2 years). Final height is **short, but within normal limits.**

212. **Chromosomal anomalies and primary hypogonadism:**

    Klinefelter syndrome: Incidence **1:1000 in the male; most common chromosomal** pattern is **47,XXY; mostly due to meiotic nondisjunction of x chromosome** at the time of prenatal gametogenesis; **extra X is contributed by mother (67%) and by father (33%).**
    Most common chromosomal abnormality in male: Klinefelter (1:1000).
    Most common chromosomal anomaly in both sexes: Down syndrome **(1:600 to :800).**
    Most common **X chromosomal** anomaly in female: **47XXX (1:1000** live births).

    First manifestation is **a behavioral or psychiatric** problem. For all boys with mental retardation or an adjustment problem in school, **rule out this syndrome; shy or aggressive behavior (e.g. fire setting behavior); tall and thin boy, delayed puberty, penis and testes remains short after puberty,** 80% has **gynecomastia. Infertility and azoospermia are present in most cases.** Higher incidence of **pulmonary disease, breast cancer, extragonadal germ cells tumor (brain and mediastinum), varicose veins.**

    DIAGNOSIS CONFIRMED BY: Chromosome.
    Serum: (**Mid-puberty** onwards) = ↓ testosterone, ↑ FSH and LH. **(In mid-puberty, testicular growth stops).**
    Testicular biopsy:
    Prepubertal: ↑ Germ cells.
    Post-pubertal: **Hyalinized seminiferous tubule, azoospermia, clumping of Leydig cells.**
    TREATMENT: Long active testosterone preparation.

213. **Klinefelter variants and primary hypogonadism: Most common type is 49, XXXXY. Mental retardation and impairment of virilization** occur with **more severity** when more than two X chromosomes are present. It is due to **sequential nondisjunction** in meiosis. It presents with severe mental retardation, mongoloid slant, large mouth, **and small** penis, scrotum and testes. Defects can **mimic Down** syndrome (single palmer crease, hypotonia, incurred terminal 5th phalanx). **Most common X-ray** finding is **radioulnar synostosis.**

214. **Etiology** of secondary hypogonadism or hypogonadotropic hypogonadism: **Most common cause is hypopituitarism.** Newborn has micropenis (< 2.5 c.m.) and ↓ GH.
    Other causes are **isolated gonadotropin deficiency. It is due to hypothalamus** rather than pituitary. It includes **Kallmann syndrome (↓ LHRH, anosmia, isolated gonadotropin deficiency.** LHRH secreting neurones arise from nasal placode, then extend into hypothalamus causing destruction of olfactory lobes); it is also associated with **X-linked type congenital adrenal hypoplasia,** polyglandular autoimmune syndrome.

215. Hypogonadotropic hypogonadism in female (secondary hypogonadism): It means **hypofunction** of **pituitary or hypothalamus** causing **hypofunction of ovary.**

    Etiology:
    a.   Hypopituitarism:
        i. Idiopathic: Hypothalamic defect, ↑ **FSH and LH with LHRH** stimulation.

    ii. Destructive: Craniopharyngioma.

  b.   Isolated gonadotropin **deficiency (deficiency of FSH** secretion in **pituitary):**

      i.   It is due to **hypothalamic defect,** so LHRH stimulation causes ↑ FSH level; **pituitary is normal.**

      ii.   Female thalassemia causes pituitary damage due to hemosiderosis.

      iii.   Kallmann syndrome (anosmia).

      iv.   Autosomal recessive disorders (Lawrence Moon-Biedl, Carpenter syndrome).

216. Diagnosis and treatment of **secondary hypogonadism:**

DIAGNOSIS:

Serum: ↓ gonadotropin (FSH, LH), ↓ gonadal steroid, **nocturnal pulsatile LH secretion** does **not** occur.

Similar picture found in **constitutional delay.** To differentiate from secondary hypogonadism, a **single dose of LHRH** will ↑ LH secretion in constitutional and **no** ↑ in hypogonadism. **Anosmia** indicates permanent gonadotropin deficiency.

TREATMENT: First rule out constitutional delay.

  a.   **Testosterone enanthate** is indicated if there is no pubertal growth by 15 years and testosterone level is less than 50 ng/dl.

  b.   **hCG** stimulates testicular growth and spermatogenesis.

  c.   **LHRH,** acts same as hCG. LHRH is more physiologic and requires 2 years of treatment to achieve ideal testicular growth and spermatogenesis.

217. **Testicular tumors** causing **pseudoprecocity:**

  a.   Leydig cell tumor.

  b.   Fragile X-syndrome.

  c.   Testicular adrenal rest.

  d.   Unilateral cryptorchidism.

218. **Characteristic microscopic** feature of Leydig cell tumor: **Reinke crystalloids** found in < 50% cases. Leydig cell tumors with **testicular growth in one testis** at around ages 5 to 9 years.

Serum: ↑ Testosterone, ↓ FSH and LH, no response to LHRH.

TREATMENT: Surgical removal.

219. **Fragile X-syndrome: Most characteristic feature is non-nodular macroorchidism in both sides** and **mental retardation.** No precocious puberty. Constriction near the end of X chromosome **Xp 27-3.** Genetic counseling and screening for the affected family are important.

220. **Testicular adrenal rest:** It **mimics Leydig** cells tumor, but Reinke crystals are **absent** (present in Leydig cells). It is bilateral and found in **congenital adrenal hyperplasia** (usually salt-losing type).

221. **Unilateral cryptorchidism and contralateral testicular** growth (25% bigger size).

222. Pathological **conditions and drugs** causing gynecomastia:

a.	Klinefelter syndrome.
b.	Peutz-Jeghers syndrome (associated with testicular sex cord tumor).
c.	Leydig cell testicular tumor.
d.	Feminizing adrenal tumor.
e.	Hypergonadotropic hypogonadism.
f.	Congenital adrenal hyperplasia (only 11 ß-hydroxylase ↓).
g.	Reifenstein syndrome.
h.	Testicular feminization syndrome.
i.	17 ketosteroid reductase deficiency.
j.	Prolactinoma (with galactorrhea).
k.	Ketoconazole (antifungal drug, inhibit testosterone synthesis).
l.	At puberty, liver cancer (fibrolamellar type).
m.	In adults: Marijuana use, digoxin use, bronchogenic carcinoma, hepatic cirrhosis, some nonsteroidal anti-inflammatory agent.

223.	**Hypofunction of ovary:**
a.	Congenital defect in development.
b.	Primary ovarian failure or hypergonadotropic hypogonadism.
c.	Secondary ovarian failure or hypogonadotropic hypogonadism.

224.	Gynecomastia in newborn due to: **Maternal hormone.** It disappears in 2 weeks. Gynecomastia in the male indicates **estrogen-androgen imbalance.** It disappears within weeks.

225.	**Physiologic pubertal gynecomastia: Mostly one** breast, but may be both with different times and degrees of enlargement, which disappears within months. Rarely present after 2 years.

Serum: All hormones are **normal.**
TREATMENT: Reassure patient and family. If breast is too big and is causing a serious emotional problem, surgery is needed, but this is rare.

226.	**Familial gynecomastia:** It is due to **increased aromatization,** i.e., peripheral **conversion from C19 steroid to estrogens** resulting in gynecomastia. Same mechanism in sporadic cases. Looks like female breast (Tanner stage 3-5) and does not reduce in size.

227.	Gynecomastia due to **exogenous estrogen: Most characteristics is the increased pigmentation of nipple and areola.** Estrogen is absorbed through skin from local application and through G.I. tract by ingestion.

228.	Most common cause of hypergonadotropic hypogonadism (primary hypogonadism): **Turner syndrome (45X0),** 1:3000 **live births.** Other causes are Noonan syndrome; gonadal dysgenesis (XX, 45X/46XY); female with (XXX,XXXX, XXXXX), ovarian defects.

229.	Presence of **goiter in Turner** syndrome indicate: **Lymphocytic thyroiditis.**

230.	Remember all the following about **Turner syndrome (important):**

a. Increased maternal age does **not** cause this syndrome (unlike Down and Klinefelter syndrome).

b. 95% of **45X0** is aborted, but mosaic form **46XX/45X is rarely** aborted, **resulting in increased survival.**

c. 45X0 contributes 5-10% of all abortuses.

d. 1.5% of all conceptions end up in 45X0.

e. Mosaic form (45XX/45X) is only 25% of all Turner syndrome cases.

f. Deletion of **short arm** of X chromosome does **not** affect ovarian function, but has Turner phenotype and short stature.

g. Deletion of **long arm** of X chromosome does cause ovarian failure (in q13-q27 band).

h. In 45X0, all oocytes disappear by 2 years of age. Finally, ovaries become **streaked, containing only connective tissues and few germ cells.** In abortus, normal gonadal ridge indicates normal process in the beginning.

231. **Recurrent G.I. bleeding in Turner** syndrome indicates: **Gastrointestinal telangiectasia.**

232. Clinical manifestation of mosaic (45X/46XX) Turner **syndrome: Most important is short stature, second is ovarian failure.** Mosaic has **less** abnormality than 45X0 Turner.

233. **Most common skeletal** anomaly in Turner syndrome; **Short 4th metatarsal and metacarpal.**

234. **Clinical manifestations** of Turner syndrome;

   At birth: Edema of dorsum of hands and feet, loose skin at the nape of neck, ↓weight, ↓ length, but normal head circumference.

   Later on manifestations:
   Growth: Short stature is most characteristic in all patients; remember they are not mentally retarded. Other features are **web neck,** epicanthic folds, high arch palate, low hairline, **wide space nipple,** small mandible, low hairline, hyperconvex nails, cubitus valgum, **delayed motor, sensory and language development. In first 3 years** of life, height growth is lower limit of **normal,** then decelerates and resulting in short stature (mean adult height 143 cm). **Delayed puberty occurs,** pigmented nevi present. **Bilateral otitis media (75%) and sensorineural hearing loss** present.
   Cardiac: Most common cardiac anomaly is nonstenotic isolated bicuspid aortic valve (33%). This is **not** a **serious** disorder, but among serious disorders (less frequent), **aortic coarctation is most common.**
   Renal: Anomalies found in 33% (pelvic kidney, horse shoe kidney, UPJ obstruction, absent one kidney, double ureter) cases.
   Ovaries:
   By 4 years: 50% has small but non streak.
   4-10 years: 90% become streak.
   Breast formation: 10-20% patient.
   Menstruation: Occasionally occur.
   Fertility: Reported in 12 patient in 45X0.

Remember, for all girls with short stature, always rule out Turner syndrome and perform chromosome analysis.

235. Most confirmatory **diagnostic procedure** of Turner: **Chromosome analysis.**

236. **Gonadotropin, level GH, thyroid hormones** and Turner syndrome; ↑ **gonadotropin (particularly ↑ FSH) at birth** until 2 years of age, when it starts declining and reaches **lowest point around 7 years,** then rises to **reach adult castrated level by 10-11** years of age.

    Remember, GH(growth hormone) has no role in this syndrome.
    Remember, antithyroid antibody detection is important. If present, then T4 and TSH level to be done.
    Remember, carbohydrate (mild) intolerance found in Turner syndrome usually improves around puberty.

237. **Treatment** for Turner syndrome;
    a. **Recombinant human growth alone or in combination with anabolic steroid** increases the height velocity.
    b. First **GH** (growth hormone), then **estrogen** therapy around 12 years of age. Daily **premarin** for 3-6 months induces puberty. **Estrogen** is cycled (day 1-23) and **provera (progestin)** (day 10-23) daily.
    c. Psychosocial support is very important.
    d. Pregnancy can be achieved by ovum donation and in vitro fertilization.

238. **Most common** chromosomal abnormality in mixed gonadal dysgenesis: 45X/46XY, 25% has dicentric Y chromosome (45X/46X, dic Y).

239. Chromosome analysis of Noonan syndrome: **Normal,** male (46XY) or female (46XX):

240. XX gonadal dysgenesis is associated with:

    Sensorineural deafness **(Perrault syndrome) XX Gonadal dysgenesis:** Patients looks **normal** phenotypically and genotypically, but **gonadal dysgenesis like Turner syndrome** is called pure gonadal (ovarian) dysgenesis. (XY dysgenesis is called Swyer syndrome. XX and XY dysgenesis is **separate** entity and **never occurrs** in the same family.)

    It **only shows up at puberty** (before that the child is normal) with delayed sexual maturation, delayed epiphyseal fusion causing **eunuchoid** stature.

    Serum: ↑ gonadotropin.
    Sonogram: Streak ovaries.
    TREATMENT: Estrogen replacement.

241. **Most common** presentation of **45X/46XY mixed** gonadal dysgenesis:
    Child: **Short stature (present in all patients).**
    Infant: **Ambiguous genitalia** is major phenotype.

Patient with **extreme** variability like Turner syndrome to male phenotype with penile urethra.

Female phenotype:
a. Streak ovary with **normal** uterus and fallopian tube (streak ovary little different from Turner syndrome: it contains mesonephric or hilar cells, and has a tubular or cord-like structure).
b. Prepubertal **enlarged clitoris,** pubertal virilization, normal mullerian structures, **intra-abdominal testis, contralateral streak gonad and fallopian tube on both sides.**
c. **Frank ambiguous genitalia, testis and vas deference in one side, streak gonad on other side, rudimentary uterus always present,** bilateral fallopian tubes.

242. Most common **gender** rearing in mixed gonadal dysgenesis: **Female:** remove the gonads (25% of the cases turn into malignanies like **gonadoblastoma),** reconstruct the vagina if needed.

243. **Prenatal** genotype diagnosis of 45X/46XY mosaicism was made. **Most likely phenotype** of this child will be: **Normal male** (out of 76 children, 72 with this diagnosis are normal males, 1 female and 3 males with hypospadias; out of 12 gonads examined, 3 were abnormal).

244. Most frequent **X chromosomal** abnormality in the **female:** 47 XXX. It is **due to maternal meiotic non-disfunction.** (In majority of cases 45X0 Turner and 50% of cases of 47XXY are defective in **paternal** sex chromosome).

Presentation of 47 XXX female:
At birth: Normal female.
Around 2 years: Delayed speech, poor coordination, behavioral immaturity.
Adolescent: Tall and gangly, behavioral disorder **or** superior academically, **normal sexual development, menarche and normal baby.**

Remember, 47 XXX predicts a phenotypically normal female in every respect except some behavioral or developmental delay.

245. **XXXX and XXXXX females: Most of them are mentally retarded and have absent or delayed sexual maturation** (e.g., one woman with XXXX syndrome gives birth to a normal child). Other features include **radioulnar synostosis,** congenital heart disease, **simian crease,** epicanthic fold.

246. Difference of Turner and Noonan syndromes:

Turner	Noonan
No mental retardation	Mental retardation often present.
Nonstenotic bicuspid aortic valve or coarctation	Pulmonary valvular stenosis.

Abnormal gonads and **abnormal** sexual maturation	Gonadal defects may be present, but **normal** sexual maturation.
Mostly 45X0	Normal chromosome.

247. Ovarian defects in either chemotherapy or radiotherapy or both in Hodgkin disease: More ovarian defects in **combined** therapy than is single treatment. Teenage girls' ovarian function **remains better or improves** more than older women's after these therapies.

248. In type 1 autoimmune polyendocrinopathy (Addison disease, hypoparathyroid, candidiasis), ovarian failure is due to: **Autoimmune disease.** It occurs mostly after 13 years, accompanied by secondary amenorrhea or delayed sexual development, **streak** ovaries with **lymphocyte infiltration, and steroid cell antibodies are present in most cases.**

249. Ovarian failure and galactosemia: Galactosemia (particularly the classic form) mostly cause ovarian damage, beginning in fetal life; ovarian damage **is mostly** due to **deficient UDP galactose** rather than to the accumulation of galactose-1- phosphate. Serum: ↑ FSH, ↑ LH at birth.

250. Ovarian failure in ataxia-telangiectasia is due to: **Unknown cause.** A few cases turn into gonadoblastoma and dysgerminoma.

251. Differentiation between **physiologic delay in puberty and isolated hypogonadotropic hypogonadism:** In isolated hypogonadotropic hypogonadism, there is ↑ **FSH and LH during sleep** which **heralds the onset of puberty.**

252. **Pseudoprecocity** due to **ovarian cyst or tumor:** Most of them **secrete estrogen** and few secrete androgen. ↑ Estrogen cause **isosexual** precocity. ↑ androgen cause **virilization.**

253. Estrogen secreting tumor of ovaries:

    Juvenile granulosa-cell tumor: It is the **most common neoplasm secreting estrogen in childhood.** It is **different** from adult similar tumor. It is associated with Ollier disease (multiple enchondromas) and Maffucci syndrome (multiple subcutaneous hemangioma). Present with **enlarged breasts and pubertal external genitalia which begin before 2 years and in 50% of cases before 10 years. No** ovulation. Pubic hair **absent** unless there is some some virilization or abdominal mass present.

    Serum: ↑↑ **estradiol** (up to 413 pg/dl; in **idiopathic** precocious puberty it is < 100 pg/dl), ↓ FSH and LH; no response to LHRH, ↑ **alpha-fetoprotein.**
    X-ray: Advance osseous maturation.
    TREATMENT: Removal of the tumor.

    Effect after tumor removal: **Immediate** vaginal bleeding after surgery. Sexual precocity reduced within few months, estrogen level becomes normal.

    Good prognosis because malignancy occurs in less than 5% of the tumors. **Sex cord tumor with annular tubules** found in Peutz-Jeghers syndrome arises from granulosa cells.

Chorionepithelioma secrete hCG which stimulates other ovary to secrete estrogen and progesterone.

254. **Stein-Leventhal syndromes or polycystic ovaries syndrome:** Most frequently present with **menstrual abnormalities and hirsutism;** obesity and bilateral polycystic ovaries also present.

Serum: ↑ FSH and LH, ↑ **response to LHRH** means ↑ FSH and LH. Free testosterone is **not** suppressed by dexamethasone (dexamethasone can suppress adrenal cause of defect). Sonogram: Polycystic ovaries.
TREATMENT: Contraceptive pills suppress ovaries, testolactone (anti-androgen and weak progestin properties) and also further inhibit the ovaries. **Obesity should be controlled** because insulin resistance disappears with obesity.

255. **Estrogen secreting** ovarian cyst:

Follicular cyst: Two types:

   a.   **Cyst formed due to stimulation of gonadotropin:**
      Serum: ↑ FSH and LH, ↑ estradiol.
      Surgical removal of the cyst or spontaneous involution brings down the FSH and LH level to normal.
   b.   **Autonomous cyst (not** dependent on gonadotropin):
      Serum: ↓ FSH and LH; ↑ estradiol, no response to LHRH stimulation.

In both the conditions, patient evidences **isosexual** precocity due to estrogen. Prepubertal girls have smaller cysts (<0.7 c.m.) and pubertal girls have larger cysts (1-6 c.m.).

DIAGNOSIS: By sonogram.
TREATMENT: It can **resolve spontaneously;** if not resolved, then aspirate or remove cyst.

256. **Gonadoblastoma:** It occurs **exclusively in dysgenetic gonads.** Occurs in **phenotypic female,** but **genotypic male** (46XY, 45X/46XY, 45X/46X fra). Virilization is found in some cases which **mimic** adrenal cortical tumor (accelerated growth, secondary sexual character, enlarged clitoris, acne). **Abdominal mass** palpable is in 50% of the cases.

Serum: ↑ **testosterone and androstenedione;** ↓ gonadotropin.
Sonogram and CT: Localize the tumor.
TREATMENT:
   a.   Unilateral tumor: Remove the tumor along with contralateral dysgenetic gonad prophylactically.
   b.   Bilateral tumor: Remove both.

257. **Androgen secreting** ovarian tumors:
   a.   Arrhenoblastoma.
   b.   Gonadoblastoma.
   c.   Juvenile granulosa cell tumor.

It is **a rare** tumor (**very rare** in prepubertal age).

258. **Factors absolutely necessary to form ovary:** 46XX chromosome. Both long and short arms of chromosome contain **gene** which is responsible for ovarian growth. **Deletion of short arm of X chromosome** results in somatic features which **mimics** Turner syndrome.

259. **Most common karyotype** in **true hermaphroditism: 46XX** (80% of cases) (**important for examination**). Other karyotypes are 46 XX/46XY mosaicism. Chimeras (chi 46XX/46XY) means Karotype was derived from more than one zygote.

260. **Hormones** responsible for **development of male genitalia:**
External genitalia: **Dehydrotestosterone** (forms penis, scrotum).
Internal genitalia: **Testosterone** (forms epididymis, seminal vesicle, vas deferens).

Dehydrotestosterone is an active metabolite of testosterone. Testosterone acts on functional **androgen receptor which is controlled by an X-linked gene.**

261. Factors responsible for **forming testes: TDF (testicular determining factor)** present **only in short arm** of Y chromosome, responsible for testicular formation. **TDF is present in SRY (sex determining region of Y).** TDF also found in **46XX male and causes male phenotype.** During meiosis Y chromosome must segregate from x chromosome, but small portion of **Y chromosome shares sequence with X chromosome.** These genes behave like autosomal gene, so they are called **pseudoautosomal genes.** TDF shows up next to pseudoautosomal gene. TDF, by **unknown** mechanism, converts **indifferent genital ridge to testes.**

262. **Hormones produced by testes:**

First hormone secreted by **Sertoli cells** of testes is **MIF** (Mullerian inhibiting factor) around **6-7 weeks** in utero. MIF inhibits mullerian duct to regress. (**Remember,** Mullerian duct forms female organs and Wolffian ducts form male organs; **M not** for **M).**

Second hormone is **testosterone** secreted by **Leydig cells of testes around 8 weeks.** hCG stimulates testosterone secretion. hCG peaks around 8-12 weeks, secreted from pituitary.

Testosterone stimulate Wolffian duct to form internal genital organs, and **dehydrotestosterone** forms external genital organs.

263. **Causes of female pseudohermaphroditism:** 46XX.

   a. **Congenital adrenal hyperplasia: Remember, this is the most common cause of this disorder. Severe** virilization in female mostly occurs in 21 and 11 hydroxylase defect, mild virilization 3 ß-hydroxy dehydrogenase defect. **Virilization more in salt-loser** than non-salt-losers type. Severe virilization causes **complete penile urethral formation, but undescended testes.**
   b. **Placental aromatase deficiency: Fetus** secretes lots of **DHEAS** which is metabolized to **androgen** which is converted to **estrogen by aromatase.** Deficiency of this enzyme causes virilization of pregnant mother and her newborn.

c. **Maternal masculinizing tumors of adrenal and ovary:** It secretes androgen which causes **maternal virilization** (hirsutism ↑ clitoris, acne, deep voice, ↓ lactation) and **fetal virilization** (↑ clitoris and labial fusion). **In case of newborn female with pseudo-hermaphroditism for unknown cause, check maternal level of testosterone and DHEAS.**

d. **Androgenic drugs** given to pregnant women: Most offending drug is progesterone, which was used for threatened abortion, but is no longer used. Testosterone and 17 methyltestosterone can cause female pseudohermaphroditism. **In case of female infant with pseudohermaphroditism** due to **unknown** cause, look for **G.U. and G.I. anomalies.**

264. **Pseudohermaphrodite and Wilms' tumor:** XY male pseudohermaphrodite has ↑ **risk of Wilms tumor, nephrosis, nephritis and renal failure.** Chromosome anomaly in Wilms' tumor is **11p⁻.** **Sporadic aniridia in male** child is associated with undescended testes, hypospadias and mental retardation.

265. **Causes of male pseudohermaphroditism:** 46XY.

a. **Testicular differentiation defect: Indifferent gonads converted into testes by** TDF (testicular determining factor) present in **short arm of Y chromosome.** Defect there will cause **female phenotype, persistent Mullerian duct and streak gonads.** Deletion of **long arm** of Y chromosome indicates a **normal** male with **azoospermia and short stature.** In other syndromes, normal Y chromosome and testes fail to differentiate.

b. **Camptomelic syndrome:** It presents with **female** phenotype **with 46XY indicating reversal of sex due to unknown cause;** uterus, fallopian tubes present and **dysgenetic** ovaries are present.

c. **Swyer syndrome of xy pure gonadal** dysgenesis: Evidenced by **female phenotype with 46XY,** but **menarche and breast development are absent. Normal** uterus, vagina and fallopian tubes. At puberty, **hypergonadotropic primary amenorrhea** appears. It is due to **defect in TDF** (receptor, gene or biologically inactive). **Gonads are streaked and can become malignant,** so **early removal** is indicated.

d. **XY gonadal agenesis syndrome:** Rare, external genitalia **slightly ambiguous,** but more **like female** (labial hypoplasia, phallus-like clitoris, labioscrotal fusion). **Absence of vagina or uterus gonadal tissues** means MIF inhibit Mullerian structures. Regression of testes **before 8 weeks of fetal life** results **in Swyer syndrome;** between **14 and 20 weeks** causes **rudimentary testis syndrome; and after 20 week is anorchia.**

266. Most common cause of true hermaphroditism: **Unknown.**

267. Male pseudohermaphroditism due to **defects in testicular hormones: 46XY.** Testosterone is **low** before puberty. To know the testicular function, **hCG stimulation test** should be done.

Five genetic defects:

a. **Leydig cell aplasia: Female** phenotype, absent uterus, shallow vagina, bilateral tests in inguinal region, **no** breasts, sparse pubic hair, ↑ LH, FSH →. It is due to **lack of**

receptor of Leydig cells.

b. **20,22 Desmolase deficiency: Lipoid adrenal hyperplasia,** fetal testes cannot synthesize testosterone, affected xy patient looks like normal female until salt loss begins.

c. **3 ß-hydroxysteroid dehydrogenase deficiency: Congenital adrenal hyperplasia** with **hypospadias** with or without bifid scrotum and cryptorchidism.

d. **17 Hydroxylase deficiency: Male with ambiguous** genitalia, hypospadias, undescended testis, **very small vagina,** ↑ B.P., ↓ K; reared as female.

e. **17-20 Desmolase deficiency:** Ambiguous genitalia, defects **in adrenal** because ACTH failed to stimulate adrenal androgen. **No mullerian** structure.

f. **17 ß-Hydroxysteroid dehydrogenase:** Completely female **until** puberty when **virilization, primary amenorrhea,** a few cases of enlarged breasts, ↑ androstenedione, Leydig cells hyperplasia, are found in **adults.** hCG stimulation test negative. **TREATMENT: Estrogen.**

g. **Uterine hernia syndrome:** Virilized male, → testosterone, ↓ MIF **with presence of Mullerian duct, normal** testicular function with spermatogenesis. **TREATMENT:** Remove Mullerian structures but keep testis, epididymis, vas deferens.

268. **Hermaphroditism (intersexuality): Mismatch of gonads and external genitalia.**

a. Male: Internal organ is **testis** and external appearance is **female.**
b. Female: Internal organ is **ovary** and external appearance is **male.**

True hermaphrodite: **Internally both testis and ovary, externally** (either male or female) with **ambiguous genitalia.**

Pseudo hermaphrodite:
a. Male: **Internally testes, 46XY (normal),** externally **female or ambiguous or partially virilized.**
b. Female: **Internally ovary, 46XX (normal),** externally **virilized genitalia.**

269. Most common **type of gonad** in true hermaphroditism: **Ovotestis.**

270. **Best way to raise** a true hermaphrodite: **As a female,** after removal of testicular tissue.

271. **Male pseudohermaphroditism (46XY) due to defect in androgen action: Testosterone synthesis is normal,** but **inherited abnormalities** in androgen action.

a. **5 alpha-reductase deficiency: Decreased dehydrotestosterone production in utero** resulting in **ambiguous external genitalia,** testosterone synthesis and action are normal. Appears with **small penis, bifid scrotum, urogenital sinus, hypospadias, normal internal** genital structures, no Mullerian structure.

b. **Testicular feminization syndrome (very important for examination):** This is the extreme example of **non-virilization.** Patient looks like a **beautiful normal female with 46XY, inguinal testes present, breasts develop** at puberty, **pubic hair absent, First manifestation is amenorrhea. Normal** level of both **testosterone and dehydrotestosterone,** but no virilization occurs **due to end organ resistance to androgens in cellular level. Vagina ends blindly, and internal organs are absent.**

> **TREATMENT:** Remove the testes and rear child as female; supplement with estrogen at puberty.

c. **Incomplete** testicular feminization: **Masculinization** (enlarged phallus, labioscrotal fusion) **at birth;** breasts, pubic and axillary hair develop **at puberty, vagina ends blindly,** uterus is **absent.** It is due to **abnormal androgen receptor or its low responsiveness.**

d. **Reifenstein syndrome:** It is due to **end-organ resistance with normal** androgen production. Present with hypospadias, small testes or undescended testes, **but normal phallus,** azoospermia and infertility. Serum: ↑ LH and FSH, ↑→ testosterone.

e. **Undetermined causes:** Most common is **45X/46XY.**

272. Diagnosis and treatment of **true hermaphroditism: Ambiguous genitals is the genetic emergency in order to know the sex of the baby,** so chromosome analysis should be done first. In the meantime do **sonogram** to look for internal organs (uterus and ovary):

a. **In virilized XX female: Uterus is present, but gonads are absent;** if there is virilization, always rule out **adrenal hyperplasia. Female hermaphrodite** should be **reared as female even with virilization.**

b. **Male pseudohermaphrodite and 46XY: Absent uterus with or without gonads. Patient should be reared as female.**

c. **5 alpha reductase deficiency with feminized infant:** Infant should be reared as **male** because **virilization normally occurs at puberty.**

d. Androgen receptor defect with feminization: To be reared as **female.** It is **easier to make female organs** than male organs.

e. **45X/46XY infant:** Reared as **female,** has short stature, uterus is present. Needs **removal of gonads. Phenotype** varies from normal male to normal female.

f. **Micropenis with XY male, suspected receptor disorder:** Treat with testosterone enanthate.

g. **Psychologic stimulation: Physician should be sensitive and** must be **expert** and experienced in this field.

h. Girls with **fetal masculinization due to congenital adrenal hyperplasia:** They **prefer male** playmates.

MISCELLANEOUS

1. Recommended fluid to drink: Cold water.

2. A phenotypically **female** child appears with **bilateral** inguinal hernia and **palpable mass** in inguinal region.

   MOST LIKELY DIAGNOSIS (important for examination): Testicular feminization syndrome.
   DIAGNOSIS CONFIRMED BY: Chromosome analysis (46XY). Initially, sonogram can be done to look for testes in inguinal canal and other internal organs. **Vaginogram shows vagina ends blindly.**

3. Tanner **stage 5 in external** genitalia, but **no breasts:** Adrenal cortical tumor. Tanner **stage 5 in breast,** but **prepubertal genitalia:** Pituitary tumor. (Prolactinoma).

4. Gynecomastia (enlarged breast) due to:

   Klinefelter syndrome.
   Cirrhosis.
   Bronchogenic carcinoma.
   Marijuana abuse.
   Ketoconazole.
   Digoxin use.

5. Wormian bones appears in the following:
   Hypopituitarism.
   Hypothyroidism.
   Down syndrome.
   Achondroplasia.
   Cleidocranial dysplasia.
   Hydrocephalus.

   [* Wormian bones are those between the two cranial bones].

6. Testicular atrophy can occur in the following:
   Cyclophosphamide therapy.
   Del Castillo syndrome.
   Klinefelter syndrome.

7. Sports and antiasthmatic medication: An asthmatic on theophylline can, before sports take proventil, alupent, or cromolyn sodium inhaler as prophylaxis to relieve theophylline induced bronchospasm. An asthmatic not taking theophylline can take it as a prophylaxis 1 hour before playing sports.

8. Different diseases and sounds produced during respiration:

Musical	Subglottic hemangioma.
Hoarseness	Laryngeal papilloma or nodule in vocal cord.
Brassy	Vascular ring, tracheitis.
Stridor, noisy	Laryngomalacia, tracheomalacia, laryngeal web.
Staccato	Chlamydia.
Metallic	Acute spasmodic laryngitis.
Croupy	Croup.
Habit cough	Disappears with sleep.

[Laryngospasm can also occur in drowning and hypocalcemic tetany.]

9. Gross hematuria occurs: * **IgA nephropathy,** acute post streptococcal glomerulonephritis.

10. Calcification found: Neuroblastoma, Pheochromocytoma. (Not in Wilms' tumor.)

11. Poisoning and its treatment:

POISONING	TREATMENT
Staph. food poison (symptoms within 1/2 hour)	Fluid only.
Salmonella food poison (Blood and pus in stool)	Fluid only.
Botulism (constipation, floppy baby)	Antitoxin, penicillin.
Mushroom, organophosphate	Atropine.
Shellfish (Mouth burning)	Emesis, lavage, enema.
Acetaminophen	Acetylcysteine (mucomist).
Alkali (caustics, lyes)	Water (orally).
Barbiturate	Dopamine, alkaline diuresis, dialysis, hemoperfusion.
Cyanide	Amylnitrite.
Phenothiazine	Diphenhydramine (benadryl).
Hydrocarbon (gasoline, carosene, naphthalene, petroleum)	Olive oil.
Methanol/ethylene glycol	Ethanol.
Iron	Desferrioxamine.
Narcotics	Naloxone.
Tricyclic antidepressant (imipramine), Anticholinergic	Physostigmine.
Carbon monoxide	Oxygen.
Mercury	BAL.
Methemoglobinemia	Methylene blue.
Salicylate	Acetazolamide, THAM solution, $NaHCO_3$.

12. IVP (intravenous pyelography) finding: Splaying of calices: Wilms' tumor.
    Ureter displaced medially and downward: neuroblastoma.

13. **CIE (Counter immuno electrophoresis)** in CSF and urine for diagnosis:
    Group B streptococci.

E. Coli.
Pneumococci.
H. influenzae type B (Not nontypable H. influenzae).
Meningococci (not Gonococci).

14. **Diabetes type 1 and management:**

Increased GL level in AM	Increase last PM dose of NPH.
Decreased GL level in AM	Decrease last PM dose of NPH.
Increased GL level in noon	Increase this AM dose of Regular insulin.
Decreased GL level in noon	Decrease this AM dose of Regular insulin.
Increased GL level in evening	Increase this AM dose of NPH.
Decreased GL level in evening	Decrease this AM dose of NPH.
Increased GL level in night	Increase this PM dose of Regular.
Decreased GL level in night	Decrease this AM dose of Regular.

15. In **hereditary spherocytosis** RBC shapes altered due to: Diminished spectin (cytoskeletal protein) which along with little actin and myosin keep the RBC shape intact.

16. **Internal genital organs** are formed by hormone: Testosterone (male). External male genital organs formed by: Dehydrotestosterone.

17. Effect of isotrenetoin (retinoic acid) in **female:** Alopecia, pseudotumor cerebri, headache, photophobia. Effect of retinoic acid in **male:** increased cholesterol.

18. Different source of **infection and different** diseases:

Chicken, pig	Salmonella (most common). Klebsiella.
Beef	Toxoplasma.
Pork	Trichinosis.
Mushroom	Acetylcholine poisoning.
Dairy products	Staphylococci.
Honey	Clostridium botulinum.

19. **Most common** cause of rectal prolapse in USA: **Cystic fibrosis.**

20. An adolescent who appears with severe throat pain and **unable to open his mouth,** refuses to eat or talk. History reveals **recent onset of acute tonsillopharyngitis.**
On exam: **Trismus or spasm** of pterygoid muscle, torticollis, high fever (105 degrees),

tonsil is enlarged and uvula is displaced to other side.

DIAGNOSIS: Peritonsillar abscess or retrotonsillar abscess.
** Most common organism is group A beta hemolytic Streptococcus.

TREATMENT: Penicillin, incision, and drainage; after 3 to 4 weeks remove the tonsils.

21. Age and appearance of sinuses:

At birth: Maxillary, anterior, and posterior ethmoidal.
3 to 5 years: Sphenoidal.
6 to 10 years: Frontal.
** In a 5 years old girl, all sinuses are present except frontal.

22. Most common sinuses involved in sinusitis: Maxillary, anterior, and posterior ethmoidal.

23. Most common organism in **acute** purulent sinusitis: Alpha hemolytic **Strep. pneumonia.**

24. Characteristics of sinusitis and site of pain/headache:

Sphenoidal: Suboccipital area.
Anterior ethmoidal: Temporal area and eyes.
Posterior ethmoidal: Trigeminal area particularly mastoid.
Maxillary: Over maxilla and teeth.

Pus in muddle meatus of nose come from maxillary, frontal, and anterior ethmoidal sinuses. Pus in superior meatus of nose come from sphenoid, and posterior ethmoid sinuses.

25. Do not breast-feed if mother has : CMV, AIDS, DIC, active T.B., postpartum psychosis, neurosis, nephritis, eclampsia, or herpetic lesion in breast.

** Hepatitis is not a contraindication of breast-feeding unless there is crack in the nipple through which contaminated blood can infect the baby.

26. Allowed breast feeding: Hepatitis, mastitis (give antibiotic and local care), inverted nipple (with difficulty).

27. Most common organism in **chronic** sinusitis: Alpha hemolytic **Strep.** pneumonia.

28. Requirement of food and food products in different ages:

Vitamin D (400 IU)	At birth.
Iron (fullterm)	At 6 weeks of age.
Iron (pre term)	After 34 weeks of gestational age.
Solid food	After 4 to 6 months.

29.   Post-nasal drip is characteristic of **chronic sinusitis.**

30.   Different kinds of milk and their characteristics:

Condensed milk	High in carbohydrates, low in fat and protein. Don't give to newborns.
Pasteurized milk	Bacteria destroyed, casein broken down.
Homogenized milk	Fat broken down and easily digested.
Evaporated milk	Softer casein and less allergenic lactalbumin.

31.   First blood gas change in acute respiratory failure: **Increase of CO_2.**

32.   A newborn was born with cyanosis and apnea at birth, but improved upon crying:

       DIAGNOSIS: Choanal atresia. It is **the most common** congenital anomaly of nose. Unilateral is less symptomatic than bilateral. Initial diagnosis is made by inability to pass catheter through nose. Final diagnosis by **CT scan.**

       TREATMENT: Oral airway; bilateral need immediate, surgical treatment, in unilateral, elective surgery is done.

33.   A child with unilateral nasal discharge due to: Foreign body.

34.   Most common cause of epistaxis: **Nose prick** which causes bleeding from Kiesselbach plexus.

35.   **Most common** organism in bronchiolitis: RSV.

36.   **Most common** organism in Croup: Parainfluenza virus.

37.   **Most common** organism in cold: Rhinovirus.

38.   **Most common** organism in pharyngitis: Virus.

39.   **Most common** bacterial pharyngitis: Group A beta hemolytic Streptococcus.

40.   A child with purulent nasal discharge, fever, pharyngitis: Pneumococci or H. flue.

41.   Adolescent abusing drugs and the role of the physician: Physician can help the child provided the patients gives detail information about type, amount, frequency of the drug used. Social service intervention is needed.

42.   Unsaturated fat is better than saturated fat, HDL better than LDL.

43.   A child with Strep. throat who received penicillin becomes **noninfectious within few**

hours.

44. A child appears with sudden onset of high fever, has **difficulty in swallowing due to throat** pain, and does not want to eat. History of **acute pharyngitis few days ago.**

    On examination: Hyperextended head, gurgling respiration, drooling with progressive difficulty in breathing, no stridor. Bulging of posterior pharyngeal wall. X-ray of neck shows retropharyngeal mass.

    DIAGNOSIS: Retropharyngeal abscess.
    Most common organism is **Staph. aureus.
    TREATMENT: Nafcillin, incision, and drainage.
    * If left untreated, the abscess rupture will cause aspiration pneumonia.

45. Most common cause of vertigo: Eustachian tube mastoid disease.

46. Most common cause of otorrhea: Otitis **externa/otitis** media with perforation.

47. Most common cause of otalgia: Otitis **externa/media.**

48. Most common organism of cellulitis or ear and external auditory canal: **Strep. pyogenes.**
    TX: Penicillin.

49. Development of ear:
    Inner ear: Develops from otocyst = reaches adult size in mid fetal life.
    External and middle ear: Develop from 1st and 2nd branchial arch, they continue to grow throughout puberty.

50. Most common cause of otitis externa: **Pseudomonas** aeruginosa, greenish discharge.
    (*Swimmer's ear due to pseudomonas infection).

    Prophylaxis: Diluted alcohol or acetic acid drops after swimming.
    TX of otitis externa: Topical preparation of neomycin, polymyxin, and corticosteroid.

51. Most common organism in furunculosis: **Staph. aureus.**

52. Cranial nerve paralysis with herpes zoster oticus **(Ramsay-Hunt syndrome).** VII cranial nerve with vesicular eruption of posterior auditory canal. A child has history of acute pain in (R) ear.

    ON EXAM: Hemorrhage or serous blebs on (R) tympanic membrane.
    DIAGNOSIS: Bullous myringitis.
    ORGANISM: Strep. pneumoniae (most common).
    TREATMENT: Antibiotic and incision of bullae (which may not reduce pain immediately).

53. Most common cause of acute otitis media: **Strep. pneumoniae.**
    (*In immunocompromised neonate: most common organism is **Pseudomonas;** next is

Staph. aureus).

54. Indication of Tympanocentesis and myringotomy:

   a. A child with history of (L) otitis media 48 hours ago, takes oral antibiotic (ceclor or augmentin), but the symptoms **persist.**
   b. **Recurrent** acute otitis media.

55. A 3 year old child with history of (R) otitis media has been on oral amoxicillin for last 48 hours, but fever still persist. No meningeal sign.

   ON EXAM: (R) otitis media.
   CAUSE: It could be due to **non-typable H. influenzae** resistant to amoxicillin.
   Tx: Augmentin or ceclor or bactrim.

56. A 5 year old girl with history of non-specific abdominal pain. No other complaint.

   ON EXAM: (R) ear effusion was found. Mother twas old that she had ear infection 6 weeks ago and was treated with antibiotic for 10 days.
   Management: No need to administer antibiotic for ear effusion because sometimes it takes 6 weeks or longer to resolve the effusion. By 2-3 months it should be normal.

57. Most common organism in chronic or persisten, otitis media with effusion: **Pseudomonas.**

58. Chronic otitis media with facial nerve paralysis:Surgery should be done immediately to relive facial nerve pressure.

59. Most common complication of otitis media: Mostly **conductive** hearing loss, may be partly **sensorineural** due to defect in round window membrane.

60. Most common organism in chronic suppurative otitis media with mastoiditis: **Gm (-)ve bacilli. Ex:** Bacillus proteus, P aeruginosa.

61. Gradenigo syndrome:

   Triad of:
   a. Otitis media with effusion.
   b. Lateral rectus muscle paralysis.
   c. Pain in lateral or retroorbital area with headache.

62. Acute otitis media with facial nerve paralysis: It means pressure on facial nerve from bony defect. **TX:** Myringotomy and I.V. antibiotics.

63. Child with history of acute or chronic otitis media develops **nystagmus, vertigo, tinnitus,** vomiting, and hearing loss.

   DX: Suppurative labyrinthitis due to bacterial invasion into the labyrinth.
   TX: I.V. antibiotic, labyrinthectomy may be necessary to prevent intracranial spread.

64. Fracture of temporal bone and complication: Most temporal bone fractures are **longitudinal** and appear with bleeding from tympanic membrane, external canal or hemotympanum; temporal bone basilar skull fracture is common in children. Transverse fracture is associated with facial palsy, and grave outcome.

65. Child with recurrent meningitis or brain abscess, always rule out: Mastoid and middle ear infection.

66. Tympanic membrane perforation:
Anterior: Due to trauma.
Center: Due to infection.

Most traumatic perforations usually heals by themselves. If they do not heal within 2 to 3 months, do surgical repair. If traumatic perforation is associated with nystagmus, vertigo, tinnitus, otorrhea, or hearing loss, then surgical intervention is an emergency.

67. X ray shows **metastatic calcification. D**iagnosis and treatment:

DX: Hypervitaminosis D.
TX: Discontinue vitamin D, decrease calcium intake; in severe cases, require aluminum hydroxide, cortisone, sodium versenate.

68. In cystic fibrosis, sodium content in sweat is **more than 60.** In burn patient, protein loss is around 4 gm%.

69. Increased anion gap found in: Chronic renal failure, diabetic ketoacidosis, lactic acidosis, large amount of penicillin, salicylate intoxication.

Cation: Na, k, Ca, Mg.
Anion: Cl, HCO_3, PO4, SO4, Protein, Organic acid.
Anion gap: $Na-(Cl + HCO_3) = 12$ (normal = 8 to 16).

70. Decreased anion gap: Nephrotic syndrome, multiple myeloma, lithium intoxication.

71. A child from 2 to 6 weeks of age appears with **projectile vomiting.**

ON EXAM: No olive mass was palpable.
LABORATORY: Na = 127, Cl = 70, K = 3.4, HCO_3 = 32.

Diagnosis and management:
DX. Pyloric stenosis. If olive mass is palpable, don't deploy sonogram, otherwise use sonogram to condirm Dx.
TX:
a. Fluid therapy.
b. Ramstead pyloromyotomy. It is better to do surgery 1 to 2 days later until fluid correction is adequate.

72. In DKA (diabetic ketoacidosis), hyperkalemia due to: **Rhabdomyolysis.**

In DKA: Every 100 mg/dl glucose increase, Na goes down by 1.6 mEq/L.

EXAMPLE: Serum glucose = 1100 mg, Na = 120 mEq, normal GL = 100 mg.
Excess glucose = 1100-100 = 1000 mg.
Every 100 mg glucose = 1.6 mEq of Na.
So 1000 mg glucose = 16 mEq of Na.
Actual Na = 120 + 16 = 136.

73. Types of fluid in DKA: Initially 0.9% saline, then add K soon because extracellular fluid level of K falls after insulin therapy. Glucose should be started in I.V. fluid when serum glucose level is 300 mg or less. Most important is hydration. Insulin can be started later unless Gl is very high.

74. Name anticonvulsant which causes rickets: Phenobarbital, dilantin.

75. Salicylate poisoning: **First respiratory alkalosis** (because salicylate causes increased sensitivity of respiratory center with CO_2); **then metabolic acidosis** (kidney starts compensating, prevents loss of Cl, but increases loss of Na, K and accumulation of acetoacetic and betahydroxybutyric acid).

    SIGN AND SYMPTOM: Hyperventilation, respiratory distress, oliguria, convulsion.
    TX: Hydration, $NaHCO_3$, peritoneal or hemodialysis.

76. In the case of a vegetarian mother who is **breast-feeding** her newborn child, what complication may arise and what management may be required?

    DIAGNOSIS: Vitamin B_{12} deficiency in mother, methylmalonic acidemia in child.
    TREATMENT: Give vitamin B_{12} to nursing mother.
    ** High fibre in carbohydrate can cause vitamin B_2 and trace mineral deficiency (zinc).

77. A child appears with severe weight loss, wrinkled skin, and constipation. What are the diagnosis and treatment? **Dx:** Marasmus (calorie insufficiency). **Tx:** Give calories.

78. A child is admitted to regular nursery with history of uncomplicated delivery and pregnancy in mother. Infant develops myoclonic seizure. History reveals that the mother took lot of vitamins to control vomiting during pregnancy. EEG shows **hypsarrhythmia.**

    What are the diagnosis and treatment:
    Dx: Vitamin **B_6 dependency seizure,** because mother took lots of vitamin B_6 during pregnancy.
    Tx: Give vitamin B_6.

79. A child appears with edema all over the body and history of diarrhea for long time. What are the diagnosis and treatment?

    Dx: Kwashiorkor (protein, calorie malnutrition).
    Tx: First non-protein diet ,then slowly increase protein and calories.
    ** Delayed bone growth, but growth hormone is increased.

80. A child between 1 and 2 years of age is brought in by its mother with a history of **swelling of wrists and ankles** for 2 weeks. Mother denies history of trauma, but child's birth weight was 4 lbs 2 oz, which is appropriate for gestational age.

    ON EXAM: Craniotabes of ping pong ball sensation, swelling of costochondral junction. X-ray shows **greenstick** fracture of long bone, epiphyseal enlargement, **cupping and fraying** of the wrist.

    What are the diagnosis and treatment? **Dx:** Rickets (vitamin D deficiency). **Tx:** Vitamin D, sunlight.
    * Craniotabes might resolve around 1 year of age, but rachitic process would continue.
    LAB: Low phosphorus, low or normal calcium, increased alk phosphate.

81. A premature newborn, born 2 weeks ago, stayed in NICU, recently appears with **swelling of the feet.** CBC shows platelet count **of 600000.**

    What are the diagnosis and treatment? **Dx:** Vitamin E deficiency. **Tx:** Vitamin E.

82. Vitamin K dependent factors are: **II, VII, IX, X.**

83. A child appears with history of polyuria, polydypsia, vomiting, and constipation. History reveals that the child received **some pills for last** few months.

    ON EXAM: High B.P., grade 2/6 systolic murmur in right upper sternal border (A.S.), retinopathy, corneal clouding. **Dx:** Hypervitaminosis. D.

84. Management of hyperactive syndrome: **Don't tell** the mother that child will **grow out of hyperactivity. To** make a diagnosis is sometimes misleading, because child **may be quiet** in the examining room in doctor's office. **Most** commonly, diagnosis made by watching the **child in classroom** and by psycho-educational testing which shows more of to reduced performance scale than verbal scale.

    MANAGEMENT:
    a.   Structure the child's environment or make a routine for the child.
    b.   Stimulant medication: methylphenidate and dextroamphetamine.

    Side effects of both medications: First one has less side effect. Difficulty in sleeping (don't give after 3 PM), abdominal pain, loss of appetite, diminished growth which gets corrected after discontinuation of medicine. Don't give to a child younger than 6 years old.

85. How to manage child with passive aggressive behavior: **Set firm limits and expectations.**

86. Most predominant form of calcium is: Ionized calcium (46%).

87. A 3-to-6 year old **boy** shows aggressive behavior. What is the outcome?
    He remains aggressive into adolescence.

88. A 3-to-6 year old **girl** shows aggressive behavior. What is the outcome?

She does not remain aggressive into adolescence.

89.   Effeminacy or cross-sex behavior in boys and how to manage it:
Two categories:
a.   First: Dresses like a girl, plays girls' roles when acting, and acts like a girl.
b.   Second: Likes female company, does not like rough games.

MANAGEMENT: Those in the first category need **early intervention during** childhood by psychiatrist and family counselor because intervention after puberty does not work. Those in the second category have fewer problem.

90.   Schizoid child and management: They are **neither out** of touch with real world, **nor** mentally retarded, but are rather immature socially and emotionally and have **delusion and hallucination.** Any stress leads them to psychotic and antisocial behavior. Later in life they mimic organically brain-damaged children or adult schizophrenics.

MANAGEMENT: Psychiatric evaluation, and long term support are necessary. Medicine may or may not be helpful.

91.   Causes of hypercalcemia: Hyperparathyroidism, vitamin D toxicity, hyperthyroidism, metastatic bone disease, milk alkali syndrome, thiazide diuretic, sarcoidosis.

William syndrome: Supra valvular aortic stenosis due to vitamin D hypersensitivity, elfin face.

92.   Normal intracellular pH and lowest level found in: pH 6.8; lowest level in mitochondria. Normal serum pH 7.35 to 7.45.

93.   Sexual abuse in the young child and the perpetrator: Perpetrator is usually **well known to the child.**

94.   Cause of hypocalcemia: Most common cause in the neonate:

Inadequate supply. Others are hypoparathyroidism, hypomagnesemia, hyperphosphatemia, acute pancreatitis.

Acidosis = ↑ Ca,   ↑K,   ↓Mg,   ↓P,   ↓Na.
Alkalosis = ↓Ca,   ↓K,   ↑Mg,   ↑P,   ↑Na.

95.   A infant under 3 months of age is brought to the E.R. with history of **excessive crying** for hours which started suddenly. **Before that, the infant was fine. ON EXAM:** Active crying, flushed face, abdomen distended ,and tense, cold feet.

What are the diagnosis and management? **Dx: Colic.** It could be due to swallowed air, high carbohydrate level, intestinal allergy ,etc. **TREATMENT:** Hold the baby upright or prone on abdomen; occasionally, sedation and temporary hospitalization in extreme condition. ** Physician should be **supportive and sympathetic.**

96.	A picture of a 6 years old girl's teeth shows damage to all upper, central, and lower peripheral teeth, but the **lower central teeth are normal.** What are the diagnosis and treatment?
	Dx: Baby-bottle syndrome.
	It means baby's teeth were damaged by proliferating bacteria in milk. This resulted in lactic acid formation which damaged the enamel. Lower central teeth are protected **by the tongue.**
	Tx: Discontinue bottle feeding, confer with dentist.

97.	Side-effects of MMR vaccine: Subacute sclerosing panencephalitis, rash, fever.

98.	Child between 2 and 5 years of age was brought to your office. Her parents were complaining that she does not want to eat properly, and they were worried about feeding. What are the diagnosis and management:

	Dx: Poor eating habits.
	It is mostly due to **excessive parenteral pressure** to feed the child.
	Tx: Don't force the child to eat. Make good meals and then enjoy mealtimes with the child.

99.	A child brought in by mother complaining of separation of skull bones.

	ON EXAM: Sign of **increased intracranial pressure,** but **normal** cranial nerves.
	LAB.: Head sonogram shows **hydrocephalus.**

	What are the diagnosis and management? **Dx: Vitamin A deficiency. Tx:** Vitamin A.
	** Also appears with night blindness, dry scaly skin, anemia. May indicate enlarged liver and spleen, or hematuria.

100.	A child appears in E.R. with history of vomiting, and lethargy. The history reveals that the child took an unknown quantity of **pills (non-prescription) a** few hours ago.

	ON EXAM.: Papilledema, bulging fontanelle, **paralysis of cranial nerves,** diplopia.
	DIAGNOSIS: Acute hypervitaminosis A (pseudotumor cerebri).
	TREATMENT: Supportive.

101.	Child lies all the time. How to approach the problem. Physician should find out first whether child understands what is he talking about. It represents a fantasy for the child.

102.	Decreased ADH secretion due to: Diabetes insipidus (central), alcohol, diphenylhydantoin, glucocorticoid.

103.	A child appears with history of pruritus, not gaining weight, bony swelling, alopecia. History reveals child has been taking some **medicine for long** time.

	ON EXAM:Increased intracranial pressure, seborrheic dermatitis, hepatosplenomegaly. **X-ray: Hyperostosis** of the middle of the shaft of long bones.
	DIAGNOSIS: Chronic hypervitaminosis A. TREATMENT: Discontinue vitamin A.

104. Most common cause of childhood nasal polyposis is **cystic fibrosis.**

105. Chronic tonsillitis and tonsillectomy: Don't do tonsillectomy in cases of chronic tonsillitis unless there is an obstruction or unless child has had more than 4 episodes of positive group A beta hemolytic Strep. infection in a year and the child is immunologically normal.

    ** **Only definite** indication is **peritonsillar and** retrotonsillar abscess.

106. Increase ADH secretion due to: Trauma, postoperative surgery, anaesthesia, meningitis, burn, prostaglandin, nicotine, nephrotic, diabetes insipidus due to end-organ resistance in collecting tubule to ADH (which may be normal), perinatal asphyxia.

107. Contraindication to MMR: Pregnant woman, child immunocompromised and/or getting immunotherapy, high fever. ** Not contraindicated when there is pregnant woman or immunocompromised household.

108. A child had tonsillectomy. What outcome do you expect? No reduction in respiratory infection, nasal allergy, or rheumatic fever. Reduction of obstruction, cervical lymphadenitis; rarely is there an improvement in nutrition.

109. If MMR is given to an adolescent girl, what advice would you give? Do not get pregnant in next 3 months, because a live virus can infect the fetus.

110. School performance in boys and girls:

    Elementary school: Girls perform better than boys except in mathematics and vocabulary and speak more fluently than boys.
    In adolescence: Boys exceed girls.
    *Learning disability occurs more in boys than girls.

111. Earliest sign of hyperactivity syndrome in toddler: **Excessive motor** activity.

112. Adopted child and foster mother: Child should be informed of the adoption **by the age of 3** years. The identity of his real parents identity should be kept **from foster** mother and child, unless real parents want to reveal themselves. Foster parents are supposed to give life-affirming atmosphere for needy child.

113. Homosexuality in boys and its management: Lack of adequate male role model or support from parents, e.g., the father criticizes him as female, or the mother overly protects him. Such boys are uncomfortable with girls.

    MANAGEMENT: Physician should **not** accuse parents, but rather suggest that family seek counseling.

114. Homosexuality in girls and its management: History of bad relations with or abandoning by mother. Some have masculine posture and attitude. Sometimes they are closer to their father than to their mother. Physician should advise the parents **neither to punish nor**

** Physician should **not** infer gender activity by looking at the posture of boys and girls.

115.   Loss of temper, its types and management:

There are two types:

a.   Temper outburst: Child **has control** and calms down after being comforted.
TREATMENT: Talk to child and comfort him.

b.   Temper tantrum: Child is **out of control** with anger. Talking to him is no help.
TREATMENT: Physical separation from parents. When child becomes quiet, don't make fun of him. Tell him that being angry is normal, but to control it is equally important.

116.   Treatment of hypercalcemia, hyperphosphatemia, hypermagnesemia:

Hypercalcemia: Steroid (causes calcuria, diminished absorption), calcitonin.
Hyperphosphatemia: Aluminum hydroxide gel.
Hypermagnesemia: No treatment is required or exchange transfusion.

117.   Child appears with hyperventilation and carpopedal spasm due to: Hypocalcemia in **respiratory alkalosis.** (Hypercalcemia in acidosis).

118.   Acidosis and alkalosis relation with K: In acidosis K goes out of the cell, so hyperkalemia. In alkalosis K goes inside the cell, so hypokalemia.

119.   How to approach a child when he has stolen something: Tell the child to return the stolen property. Don't leave anything expensive near him.
** Most children have at least one incident of stealing in their lives.

120.   First sign of hypermagnesemia in newborn: **Hyporeflexia.**

121.   A 6 to 9 year old boy was brought in by his parents with a history of **being unable to concentrate on T.V.,** having a short attention span, restlessness, engaging in purposeless movement, doing poorly in school, getting excited easily. What is the diagnosis and recommended management?

Dx: Hyperactive syndrome or **Attention deficit disorder** which usually have learning disability but not the other way around. They have minimal brain damage or cerebral dysfunction. No specific organic or biochemical defect is recognized yet.

122.   Site of brain involvement and corresponding virus:

Temporal lobe = herpes,
Entire brain = arbovirus,
Basal structure = rabies.

123.   Herpes encephalitis and its characteristics: Herpes is a DNA virus. Clinically the patient **is very sick** with a high fever and **convulsion.** In newborn a cluster of **vesicular rashes**

appear mostly in the scalp behind the ears. There is jaundice, vomiting, and lethargy.

** Newborns with a vesicular rash are assumed to have herpes until it is proved otherwise.

LAB: Increase of poly 1st, then lymph; increase of protein, but it is normal glucose.
Tx: I.V. acyclovir.

124. Types of encephalitis due to herpes: Guillain-Barre syndrome, acute cerebellar ataxia, hemiplegia, transverse myelitis.

125. Prognosis of herpes encephalitis: Poor.

126. Streptococcal infection characteristics: **Group A beta hemolytic Streptococci** is most the commonly cause of throat infection (virus is most common for throat infection). Scarlet fever caused by Strep. with characteristic scarlatiniform (sandy) rash. Impetigo appears initially with pus then crust formation (Staph. has bullous skin lesion). In newborns, **group B Strep. is the most common** infection.

   DIAGNOSIS by throat culture. **TREATMENT** with penicillin. **PROGNOSIS** is good.
   ** ASLO titer more than 166 Todd units found in pharyngitis, and rheumatic fever, but normal in Strep. pyoderma for which Anti-DNase B is best serologic test.

127. **Most common** cause of pyogenic skin infection: **Staph. aureus.**

128. Child with bacterial **endocarditis most commonly invaded by what** organism? **Strep. viridans,** which is treated with penicillin and aminoglycoside.

   Pneumococcal infection and its characteristics: In children from 6 months to 4 years, only smooth encapsulated strains are pathogenic. There is an increased chance of infection in child who lacks type-specific antibody, **sickle cell disease, asplenia.** Appears with pneumonia, otitis media, sinusitis or primary peritonitis. Most common cause of otitis media over 1 month is Strep. pneumoniae. Pneumonia has typical lobar consolidation.

   Lab: C3 deficiency. **Pneumovax** is recommended for children over 2 years of age: Sickle cell disease, asplenia, nephrotic syndrome, sickle-related hemoglobinopathy. **Prophylaxis** with medication: Penicillin.

129. Diphtheria and its characteristics: Appears with thin gray membrane over tonsil, palate, paralysis of soft palate, laryngeal diphtheria. May need tracheostomy.

   Prophylaxis: Vaccine; **Tx:** Penicillin and toxoid. Most common cause of death is myocarditis; gravis strain has poor prognosis.

130. Septic arthritis and its characteristics: More often **hematogenous than** direct,
   ** May or may **not** have fever, limping, tenderness, swelling, redness.

   Most commonly diagnosed by **arthrocentesis.** Treated with I.V. antibiotic. If patient does not improve within 48 hours, then surgical drainage is necessary.

131. Staph. aureus causes cellular death by releasing what chemical? Leukocidin.

132. **Scalded skin syndrome** caused by: Staph. aureus **group II.**

133. Protein A present in: **Staph. aureus,** but **not** in staph. epidermidis.

134. Staph. scarlet fever: Fever, and rash mimic Strep. scarlet infection, but **there is no** sore throat. It is due to **erythrogenic toxin.**

135. Most common organism in **sickle cell disease with osteomyelitis: Staph. aureus,** 2nd common is salmonella. (Heroin addict has increased vertebral osteomyelitis with Pseudomonas.)

136. **Most common** organism in **septic arthritis;**

    Newborn: Staph. aureus.
    2 mos. to 4 years:Hemophilus influenzae.
    After 4 years: Staph. aureus.

137. Meningitis and its characteristics: H. flue mostly colonizes in throat and nasopharynx. Hydrocephalus develops as a complication in newborns mostly. Most common type is communicating.

    ** Recurrent meningitis is due mostly to direct **connection between skin and meninges or fracture through paranasal sinuses.** Most common complication is **deafness.**

138. CSF findings and corresponding diseases:

Bacterial	increased poly	increased protein	decreased glucose
T.B.	increased lymph	increased protein	decreased glucose
Fungal	increased mono	increased protein	decreased glucose
Viral	increased lymph	increased protein	normal glucose
Brain abscess	1st lymph then poly	increased protein	1st normal unless abscess ruptures

139. **Most common** organism and age of patient in cases of meningitis:

    Up to 2 months: Group B Streptococcus.
    2 mos.to 12 years: Haemophilus influenzae type b.
    12 years: Strep. pneumoniae.

140. Child with meningitis with increase in head size or positive transillumination due to **subdural collection.**

141. Child with meningitis on treatment, with history of recurrence of fever: Due to **abscess formation.**

142. Most common organism in meningitis with **cystic fibrosis: Staph. aureus.** Most common organism in meningitis with **burn: Pseudomonas.**

143. **Child appears with meningitis.** History **reveals recent onset of pneumonia.** Most likely organism: **Mycoplasma pneumoniae.**

144. Diagnosis of meningitis: CSF culture, CIE (negative CIE does not exclude meningitis). Latex agglutination test is more sensitive than CIE, but more false positive.

145. **Prophylaxis** to exposure of **H. flue meningitis:** Rifampin should be given to all family members, those exposed at the day care center or nursery school, as well as to the diseased child. Doses of 20 mg/kg O.D. for 4 days.

146. Most common cause of **aseptic** meningitis: Enterovirus (coxsackie, echo. and polio). Aseptic meningitis is self-limited, culture negative. CSF shows initial poly then predominant monocyte.

147. Ideal calorie distribution in food (important):

    Protein 15%, fat 35%, carbohydrate 55%.
    Cow's milk (67 kcal/100 cc) caloric distribution:
    Protein 20%, fat 50%, carbohydrate 30%.
    Human milk (67 kcal/100 cc) caloric distribution:
    Protein 6%, fat 50%, carbohydrate 44%.

148. Evaluate a crying child: **Mother should pick up the baby.** If baby is still crying and was not fed recently, then give milk, if crying persists need for further evaluation; but it is not a good practice to hold and feed the baby all the time when crying.

149. 7-year-old boy wearing a girl's dress, is it O.K. or not; By the **age 7 child** should **know the difference between boys and girls.** They distinguish the sexes by looking at hair, dress, jewelry, sometimes breasts, rarely genitalia.

150. **Caloric contents in** each gram of: Protein and carbohydrate, 4 kcal; fatty acids (short chain, 5.3 kcal; medium chain, 8.3 kcal; long chain ,9 kcal).

151. Some characteristics of difficult children are: Low tolerance, impulsive, intense, subject to negative moods. Parents complain that their children don't listen to them, yet these children grow up to be leaders and independent thinkers.

152. Differences of fear and phobia:
    Fear: Normal.
    Phobia: Pathological.

153. When talking to a child patient, **the physician should:** Talk to the child as he would to

any other patient. Explain the problem if the patient is 3-4 years old or older. Do not laugh, or humiliate. Whispering is acceptable because it is more personal in tone.
** Never discuss the problems of one patient with another. Uncooperative children are frightened. Talk to them, try to understand them.

154. Breast-fed infant came to E.R. with profuse diarrhoea and mucous: Infectious diarrhoea.

155. When and how should a mother punish a child? Punishment should be **intense and as soon as possible after the act.** It gives **fair amount of anxiety** to child, **not so much in order to frighten** them , but rather to love them. It works best **before the child turns 6 years of age.**

156. Caloric requirement in different ages:

1st 6 months	wt x 115.
6 mos. to 1 year	wt x 105.
1 to 3 years	1300.
4 to 6 years	1700.
7 to 10 years (male)	2400.
11 to 14 years (male)	2700.
15 to 18 years **(male)**	2800.
11 to 14 years (female)	2200.
15 to 18 years (female)	2100.
Pregnancy	300 extra.
Lactation	500 extra.

157. Reasoning vs. punishment: which is better? **Reasoning is better than punishment,** but both together is better than punishment alone. Reasoning should be to the point, simple, and immediate. It works better after 7 years of age. Always encourage the child's positive behavior.

158. Sleeping arrangements of child and parents: Child should sleep in **a separate room.** If he is scared, talk to him to overcome the fear. Most of the time it works. If not, psychologic or psychiatric evaluation may be needed.

159. Child is admitted to hospital with **vague and unexplained** symptom. Its management: Psychiatric consultation.

160. Goat milk had deficiency of: **Folic acid** resulting in megaloblastic anemia; deficiency of iron, and vitamin D, as well as of sodium.

161. Child reared at home vs. child in day care: They have the same attachment to their

mothers, but the day care child is more aggressive and less co-operative.

162. A 14-year-old girl went to a **party one night, but** the next morning she could not arise from the bed and complained of **weakness (paralysis) in both lower extremities** as well as of **no vision in both eyes.**

    ON EXAM: Deep tendon reflexes are **normal,** pupillary reaction to light is **normal,** CSF is **normal.** What is your diagnosis and treatment?

    CONVERSION REACTION, because it appears **suddenly.** The girl complains of **voluntary muscle and special senses,** but exam **is normal.** It has **secondary gain.** Treatment is **psychiatric evaluation.**

    D/D: **Guillain-Barre syndrome: Ascending** paralysis, absent reflexes, increased CSF protein.
    Botulism: Descending paralysis, diplopia, dysphagia, constipation, urinary retention, normal sensory exam.

163. Nightmare types and their management:

    Two types:
    a.   Bad dreams (anxiety): REM sleep: child wakes up and **remembers** the dream. **TREATMENT:** Reassure and comfort the child.
    b.   Night terror: Non-REM stage IV, child wakes up **disoriented, confused, with increased autonomic activity** like rapid breathing, sweating, tachycardia, dilated pupil; cannot remember the dream; walks in his sleep. **TREATMENT:** Psychologic evaluation, diazepam at H.S (bedtime).

164. If a child sees both parents having sex, how should they respond? Parents should remain calm, and ask the child to leave the room.

165. A young child touches parents' genitalia, breasts, or buttock: It is **normal** for that age. They do it out of for interest and curiosity.

166. Hyperactivity and treatment: Haldol, thioridazine (both can be used in infantile autism). Psychotherapy is **not very** helpful.

167. **Rett's syndrome:** Autistic syndrome occurs only in girls of 6 to 18 months of age. Present with autistic behavior, dementia, ataxia, seizure, spasticity, dystonia, microcephaly.

    Lab: Fragile site on **Xq 27 chromosome,** abnormal EEG, cerebral atrophy; Increased ammonia and lactic acid, decreased dopamine metabolite (HVA) in CSF. Treated with anticonvulsant.

168. If young **children** do **not** want to go to school, how does one respond? They usually complain of abdominal pains or headaches. They should be made to **promptly return to school.**

If preadolescent and adolescent children do not want to go to school, however, this indicates **a serious psychopathology.** They should first undergo psychiatric evaluation and then be returned to school. **Do not force them** to go to school.

169. Complications of bronchoscopy: Hypoxia, arrythmia, laryngospasm, bronchospasm are the most common complications.

170. A child after bronchoscopy develops croup:

    Dx: Post-bronchoscopic croup.
    Tx: Oxygen, mist, racemic epinephrine and steroid PRN (when necessary).

171. Constipation and its management: Usually the infant has one or more stools in 24 hours. Explore history of constipation and do **rectal examination.** Also look for anal fissure which is very common in newborns and infants. In case of fissure, do not do rectal examination because it is painful (unless one suspects something more serious).

    MANAGEMENT:
    Newborn up to few months: 5% glucose water in between feedings.
    After 6 months: Add cereal, fruits, vegetables or prune juice.
    After 2 years: Mineral oil.
    ** Try not to use enemas or suppositories other than as temporary measures.

172. Transudate: Protein <3 gm/dl, mostly monocyte.
    Exudate: Protein >3 gm/dl, mostly polymorph.

173. Procedure of choice when making diagnosis of lung mass in infant and children: **Lung biopsy (open).**

174. When second child is born, what happens to first child? The first child develops symptoms of denial and regressive behavior like bed wetting. Managed by giving love and affection to him. Tell him the truth about the baby, hospital and birth before the second child is born.

175. OPV (oral polio virus) vaccine should not be given:
    a.   To immunocompromised child (give IPV).
    b.   In the NICU (give it to the patient just before he goes home).
    c.   To the household contact with immunocompromised child (give IPV).
    d.   To child of unimmunized parents who might get polio from the child.

176. How to handle sibling jealousy: Teach the older sibling and support the younger one.

177. **'Last name conflict;** either between both parents or between parent and adolescent: It indicates a serious problem, so refer to a psychiatrist.

178. Measles vaccine failure due to: Being given too early in life; light exposure; improper refrigeration; use of immune serum globulin at the same time.

179. Different modes of absorption of fatty acid:

     Long chain: It forms chylomicron and is absorbed through lymphatic to venous circulation. Diffusion is the principal mechanism.
     Short and medium chain: **Does not require lymphatic for absorption:** it absorbs directly into intestinal veins, then to portal vein to liver. It is better absorbed if patient has any difficulty in absorption.

180. What is the most important test for lung function? **Arterial blood gas.**

181. Principal antibody to respiratory secretion: Secretary IgA produced by plasma cell.

182. What is the most commonly involved part of lung in the aspiration of milk? Upper lobe, because of recumbent position.

183. Adolescent feelings about parents: Most adolescents accept their parents, but some don't. They wish their parent were less strict. They are more worried about the disapproval of their parents than their friends.

184. Name congenital infection which appears like autism: Rubella.

185. Metabolic disorder that causes autism: PKU.

186. Anorexia nervosa and its management: Occurs in girls in early adolescence. **Symptoms include severe weight loss (<5%),** but normal height; **fear of gaining** weight and sexual impulsiveness; **very active,** but immature and has difficult peer relationships. **Denial** is their common defense. They do well in school.

     TREATMENT: Requires hospitalization. Tell the patient that she will go home when she gains weight. If she does not eat, without threatening tell her that nasogastric feeding might be required . Psychotherapy may be required but patients do not like that.

187. Angiotensin **I forms in the kidney, II forms in the lung.**

188. Carbohydrates are stored as: Glycogen is found in liver and muscles; infant has small liver and muscle mass in comparison to adult; glycogen reserves are only 3.5% of adult values.

189. Breast-fed baby does require: **Fluoride 0.25 mg/day** supplementation.

190. Breast-fed baby **does not** require: **Iron supplementation** although iron quantity is low, but absorption is significantly high.

191. A few-weeks-old child on **breast-feeding** came to the emergency room with **active bleeding: Vitamin K deficiency,** so give vitamin K.

192. How to manage difficult adolescence: Psychiatric evaluation. A difficult child becomes a difficult adolescent and then **a difficult adult,** so **early intervention** is necessary.

193. Does perinatal asphyxia cause behavioral problems? No.

194. Maximum composition of natural fat: Triglyceride (98%).

195. Ratio of whey to casein in milk:

    Cow's milk: 18:82 (whey: casein).
    Breast milk: 60:40.

196. Treatment of cow's milk allergy: Soy formula; or goat's milk.

197. Indication for bronchoscopy: Recurrent atelectasis or pneumonia, foreign bodies, congenital malformation, hemoptysis, mass lesion.

198. The most common organism found in cases of cystic fibrosis with sinusitis : **Staph. aureus.**

199. Most common cause of osteomyelitis and septic arthritis in children: **Staph. aureus.**

200. Child came in with history of vomiting and watery diarrhea for last few hours. He had gone to his friend's house and **ate lunch 2 hours** ago.

    Most common organism that causes food poisoning: **Staph. aureus,** because onset of symptom was 2 hours ago.

201. Child appears with few hours' history of acute respiratory distress with fever. Chest X-ray shows **pneumonia with bullae formation.** Most common organism is: **Staph. aureus.** Poor prognosis. **Tx:** Nafcillin I.V.

202. To prevent Staph. infection in nursery: Strict hand-washing.

203. A 7 year old child appears with sudden onset of high fever, vomiting, abdominal pain, diarrhea.

    ON EXAM: Erythematous rash, sore throat, hypotension, oliguria, alteration in mental status.
    Most likely diagnosis is: **Toxic shock syndrome,** caused by **Staph. aureus.**
    Most commonly appears in menstruating woman using tampons.
    D/D Kawasaki disease: Occurs in children under 5 years.

204. **Meningococcal** infection and characteristics: Most commonly found in **military personal** during epidemics. Serogroup B is the most common in human being. Released endotoxins cause vasculitis and DIC.

    ** **Waterhouse-Friderichsen syndrome:** Adrenal gland bleeding with shock and sepsis due to meningococci.

    Most common site of colonization is nasopharynx, penetrating the mucosa through WBC to blood stream.

Most characteristic rash is morbilliform petechial or purpuric occuring within hours, hypotension, low platelet count, low WBC or other signs of meningitis, or acute endocarditis, myocarditis and pericarditis.

Lab: Positive culture, positive CIE in blood, urine, CSF.
COMPLICATION: Deafness, blindness, cranial nerve palsy.
Tx: Penicillin. In case of allergy give **chloramphenicol/cephalosporin.**

205. Essential amino acids are: (Nine) threonine, valine, leucine, isoleucine, lysine, tryptophane, phenylalanine, methionine, histidine.

206. Management of withdrawn child and overactive child: Withdrawn child needs an open setting. Overactive child needs a structured setting.

207. Reaction to DTP (diptheria tetanus pertussis) vaccine:
    a. Occasionally, convulsions due to pertussis part of vaccine.
    b. Crying for more than 4 hours or excessive somnolence.
    c. Swelling and tenderness at site of injection.

208. A mother asked the pediatrician as to the **best method** of to raising her child: There is **no single best method**.

209. Contraindication to DTP vaccine:
    a. Acute fever and convulsions.
    b. Previous reaction to DTP.
    c. Neurologic diseases.

210. Most important muscle of respiration: **Diaphragm.** Principal antibody to respiratory secretion: Secretary IgA produced.

211. Heterosexual interest and age:
    5% by 5 years of age.
    75% by 13 years of age.
    75% of 10 year olds, have already kissed their boy or girl friend.

212. Characteristics and examples of psychophysiologic or psychosomatic disorder: There is a gradual onset of symptoms and the **pain is real.** These disorders incline those afflicted to be **obsessive compulsive and** less sociable than others, and to look for perfection and a **higher goal in life.**
    Ex: Peptic ulcer, eczema.
    Tx: Psychotherapy and medicine.

213. Development of **secondary sexual characters first to last** male (M), female (F):
    M: Testes, penis, pubic hair, peak height velocity, axillary and facial hair.
    F: Breast, pubic hair, peak height velocity, axillary hair, menstruation.

214. Adolescent with **ascending** muscle paralysis: **Guillain-Barre syndrome.**

215. Child receiving **antibiotic develops severe diarrhoea:** Due to enterotoxin released by clostridium perfringens secondary to use of clindamycin, ampicillin.

    Mild cases: Discontinue antibiotic.
    Severe cases: Vancomycin orally.
    Dx: Pseudomembranous enterocolitis.
    * Diarrhea with **blood.**

216. Most common abdominal mass in newborn:
    Kidney: hydronephrosis.

217. Characteristics of functional heart murmur: **Vibratory, systolic; asymptomatic.**

218. Child with PPD negative, but strong clinical suspicion: Do anergy testing with panel of antigens. **Ex:** Candida, trichophyton.

219. **Most common** cause of diarrhea in children: Rotavirus (bloody stool).

220. A child travels to Mexico and develops diarrhea: E.Coli enterotoxigenic.
    Child travels to India and develops diarrhea: Giardiasis.
    Duodenal aspirate required to diagnose giardiasis.

221. Osteomyelitis and its characteristics: Usually occurs in people from 2 to 12 years of age. **Most common** organism is coagulase positive Staphylococci.

    Most common mode of spread is **hematogenous,** appearing with limping, acute fever, inability to move the site involved, tenderness, swelling, redness; increased ESR. Most common diagnostic test is Gallium scan, requiring immobilization and I.V. antibiotic for 4 weeks.

222. Essential fatty acids are: Linoleic, linolenic, arachidonic acids.

223. Juvenile delinquency: Its cause and remedy: It is due to a very rude father who does not love the child, but punishes or hits him or her very severely. This child should be punished with love and affection, but this should be done consistently.

224. Encopresis and its management: It is **normal up to the age 4 to 5 years;** unlike enuresis organic symptoms are rarely seen. It evidences a more serious emotional problem, e.g., H/O chronic constipation or psychogenic megacolon. Child cannot go to school, and parents get upset. Do not use laxative or enema. **Tx:** Be supportive and employ psychotherapy.

225. Human milk advantages: Increased secretary IgA. Increased bacterial and viral antibody, less G.I. and respiratory symptoms, increased macrophage, low pH, protects from E. coli infection.

226. A mother wants to know how much food to be given to the infant:**Do not prescribe** a definite amount. The proper amount depends on the **infant's appetite.**

227. Water content of infant: 70-75% of body weight (5% plasma, 15% interstitial fluid, 50% intracellular fluid).

228. Breast and breast-feeding:
  a.   A happy, relaxed mother feeds the baby better than a tired, worried mother.
  b.   Breast-feeding should begin as soon as possible, preferably within first two weeks of life.
  c.   Breast-feeding stimulates milk secretion.
  d.   Main cause of failure of breast-feeding is a sick infant and improper hospital practice.
  e.   Breast should be washed daily with water and kept dry.
  f.   Hold the baby in a comfortable position, alternating the breast every 5 minutes.

229. A mother asked the physician about **artificial flavors** and additives in the food which the child likes. What do you advise? **Avoid them** because they can cause allergic reaction like urticaria, respiratory difficulty, angioedema; local mouth ulceration, headache, joint pain, hyperactivity.

230. Maternal depression and child growth: Failure to thrive.

231. Increased psychiatric disorder found in: Hydrocephalus, epilepsy, brain injury, and mental retardation due to brain injury (except asphyxia at birth).

232. Growth of brain or head:
  Maximum growth (12 cm) = in 1st year (two-third of adult size).
  Less growth (2 cm) = in 2nd year (four-fifths of adult size).

233. Formula of calculating weight (in pounds):
  3 to 12 months: Age in month + 11.
  1 to 6 years: (Age in year) x 5 + 17.
  6 to 12 years: (Age in year) x 7 + 5.

  Calculation of height (in inches):
  At birth: 20 inches
  1 year: 30 inches
  2 to 12 years: (Age in year) x 5/2 + 30.

234. Around 2 years of age, **temper tantrums and breath-holding spells** are common: These actions express child's frustration and anger against social and cultural pressure. Children try to control the situation. **Loving parents can deal with this by setting necessary limits.**

235. Parents' first visit to doctor with child: Doctor should discover **parents' expectations** of their child. Usually achievement falls short of expectation.

236. 2- to-3-year-old child appears with lordosis (mild) and protuberant abdomen: It is normal for that age, so leave him alone.

237. Eye-fixation occurs in: The first day.

238. Unborn child and parents: Parents may project expectations on unborn child. They might think their child might strengthen their shaky marriage. Normally, they think the child is part of them. Pathologically, parents might try to fulfill their dreams, through the child. Sometimes they think the child will replace either someone who died recently or a child who died in a previous miscarriage.

239. When both parents have **different opinions** about rearing the child: They should compromise and rear the child as best as possible.

240. During a family planning session, a mother asked her doctor what the **interval between two children should be:** This interval should be **decided by parents only, not** by doctor.

241. When you examine a child who is **crying hard:** Give the baby back to the mother until he/she stops crying, then examine him/her.

242. **Peak height velocity (PHV)** in girls in SMR 2 at 12 years, and in boys in SMR 3 at 14 years. (SMR = sexual maturity rating).

243. Sphenoidal sinus appear around 3 years, frontal sinus at 7 years.

244. First permanent teeth is first molar which appears at 6 years, second at 14 years, third at 20 years.

245. A child between 5 and 7 years of age appears with respiratory infection 6 or 7 times a year: It may be normal for that age, so do not do extensive work up. Lymphatic tissue grows to a maximum in these years.

246. In school years a child develops: Sense of responsibilities, duties, and accomplishment. Parents sometimes get upset when the child does not achieve their goals. It is important that the child grows in his own direction, and not to be intimidated by parent desire.

247. Physical growth assessment in adolescence is most accurately measured by: **Bone age.**

248. Different electrolytes abnormalities and their management:

	Na	K	Cl	Gl	BUN	SP-GR	Diagnosis	Management
a	120	5	108	80	8	1010	Lab. error	Repeat the test
b	120	5	84	80	20	1022	↓ Na dehydration	Correct hyponatremia
c	123	4	106	700	10	1017	Pseudohyponatremia	Don't give excess sodium

d	157	4	119	70	22	1020	↑ Na dehydration	Slow correction over 48 hours
e	122	4	92	76	4	1027	↑ ADH secretion	Restrict fluid
f	151	4	118	90	25	1002	Diabetes insipidus	Increase fluid then DDAVP if necessary
g	160	4	126	88	6	1008	Salt poisoning	Remove the salt source
h	125	3.6	96	80	8	1010	Maintenance Nacl was not given	Give maintenance Nacl

Explanation of the above:
a. ↓ Na, Cl→, as cl is normal: Laboratory error.
b. ↓ Na, Cl ↓, Gl→, ↑ BUN, ↑ Sp. Gr: Hyponatremic dehydration.
c. ↓ Na, Gl ↑↑: Pseudohyponatremia.
d. ↑ Na, Cl ↑, BUN ↑, ↑ Sp.Gr: Hypernatremic dehydration.
e. ↓ Na, Cl ↓, BUN ↓, ↑ Sp. Gr: Increases ADH Secretion.
f. ↑ Na, Cl ↑, BUN ↑, ↓ Sp. Gr: Diabetes insipidus.
g. ↑ Na, Cl ↑, BUN→, → Sp. Gr: Salt poisoning (increases specific gravity and BUN in dehydration)
h. ↓ Na, cl ↓, BUN →, → Sp. Gr: Maintenance Nacl was not started in I.V. fluid.

249. **Coagulation factors:**

a. Vitamin K-dependent factors: II, VII, IX, X, Protein C, Protein S.
    Procoagulant factors (II, VII, IX, X); anticoagulant factors (protein C,S)
b   Anticoagulant factors: Protein C, Protein S, Antithrombin III, Tissue plasminogen activator (TPA).
c. Mechanism of action of protein C and protein S: Inhibits both intrinsic and extrinsic pathway.
d. Mechanism of action of antithrombin III: Inhibits both intrinsic and extrinsic pathway by inhibiting factors XII, XI, IX, X, thrombin.
e. Mechanism of action of TPA: It converts plasminogen to plasmin, which breaks the fibrin clot.
f. Factors to be tested for PT (prothrombin time): X, VII, V, II (extrinsic factors).
g. Factors to be tested for PTT (partial thromboplastin time): XII, XI, IX, VIII (intrinsic factors).
h. Factor to be tested for TT (thrombin time): I (fibrinogen).
i. **Mixing study (normal plasma is added to patient plasma, then measure PTT):**
    i.   **PTT is corrected: there is a** deficiency of PTT factors.
    ii. **PTT is not corrected: there are** inhibitors against PTT factors present.

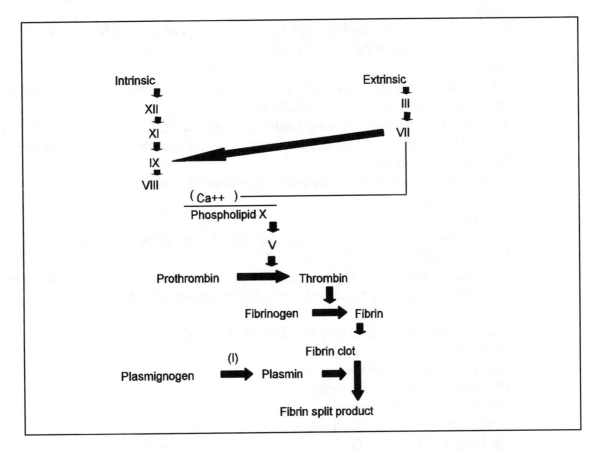

250.   Management for subconjunctival hemorrhage: Only observation.

251.   Most common infection in central line: Staph. epidermidis.
        It is the most common organism for V-P shunt infection.

252.   **Time to repair:**

        Omphalocele, gastroschisis, meningomyelocele: Surgical emergency at birth (except skin-covered **meningomyelocele).**
        Cleft lip: 1-3 months.
        Cleft palate: 12 months (starts talking at that time).
        Hypospadias: Before 18 months (time for toilet training).
        Circumcision: Not routinely recommended.

253.   Midline scalp defect posteriorly: **Trisomy 13-15 (picture of scalp will be given in the exam.)**

254.   **Different types of dysgenesis (gonads are not properly formed):**
        a.   **PURE:** (Pure gonadal problem is only undifferentiated gonads, not a chromosomal problem). Early diagnosis cannot be made, because infants look like normal females.
             i.   XY (Swyer syndrome): HY antigen present, but streak gonads did not response to it.
                   Features: External (normal female), internal (female except undifferentiated gonads), amenorrhea, no secondary sex character.
             ii.   XX: No HY antigen.

Features: External (normal female), internal (female except undifferentiated gonads), amenorrhea, no secondary sex character.

b. **Mixed:**

(Presence of both streak testes and ovaries. Chromosomal problem may be present. **Most common type 46XY,** or 45XO/46XY type.

Features: External (ambiguous genitalis with undescended testes or increased clitoris), internal (both streak ovaries and testes, other organs are either normal or abnormal male or female organs).

Early diagnosis can be made for ambiguous genitalia. Increased chances of gonadoblastoma.

c. **Partial:**

(Only in males, partial defect in testicular tissue) chromosome is normal 46XY.

Features: External (normal male).

i. Early onset (first and second trimester): Hypospadias and undescended testes.

ii. Late onset (third trimester): Anorchia or absence of testes.

255. **Abdominal pain and diagnostic procedure (important):**

a. **General:**

Allergy to food: Elimination of food.

H-S purpura: History, urinalysis.

Porphyria: Porphyria screen.

Sickle cell anemia: Electrophoresis.

Abdominal epilepsy: EEG.

b. **Genitourinary:**

UTI: Urine culture.

Congenital malformation: Ultrasonography, IVP.

Pelvic inflammatory disease: Pelvic examination.

Dysmenorrhea, endometriosis, ovarian cyst: Gynecologic consult.

c. **Gastrointestinal:**

Meckel's diverticulum: Technetium Meckel scan.

Ulcerative colitis: Rectal biopsy.

Crohn's disease: ESR, roentgenogram (barium).

Lactose intolerance: Breath hydrogen test.

Parasitic infection: Stool ova and parasite.

Intestinal tuberculosis: Tuberculin test.

Peptic ulcer: Upper G.I. series.

Pancreatitis: Amylase

Hepatitis: Liver function test.

Choledochal cyst: Ultrasonography.

Cholecystitis: Cholangiography, ultrasonography.

256. **Different tests for analyses (important):**

a. **Cognitive and Intelligence tests:**

Stanford Binet: 2 years to adult.

McCarthy scale of child ability: 2 1/2 years to 8 years.

WPPSI (Wechsler): 4-6 years.

WISC -R (Wechsler): 6 years to 16 years.

Kaufman Assessment Battery for children (KABC): 2-1/2 to 12-1/2 years.

b. **Achievement tests: (K = Kindergarden)**
Woodcock-Johnson Psycho-Educational Battery: K - 12 grade
Peabody Individual Achievement Test: School age (K - 12 grade).
Wide Range Achivement Test (WRAT): School age (K - 12 grade).
Woodcock-Reading Mastery Test: K - 12 grade
Kaufman Test of Educational Achievement (K-TEA): 1 - 12 grade

c. **Adaptive Behavior Test:** AAMD Adoptive Behavior Scale Public School Divison: 7 - 14 years.
Vineland Scales of Adaptive Behavior: Normal 0 - 19 years, Retarded of all ages.

d. **Projective tests:** Children Appreciation Test (CAT): 3 years to 8 years.
Thematic Appreciation Test (TAT): 6 years to adult.
Rorschach (Western Psychological Corporation): 3 years to adult.

e. **Other tests:** Bender Visual Motor Gestalt Test: 5 years to adult.
Berry Developmental Test of Visual Motor Integration: 2 to 16 years.
Peabody Picture Vocabulary Test - Revised: 4 to 9 years.

257. **Catch-up growth for SGA (small for gestational age):** Usually in first 6 months of life, except those who have chromosomal or viral etiology; they remain short their whole lives.

258. Most common organism in pneumonia:
First month: Group B Streptococcus.
> 1 month to 1 year: Staphylococcus.
Up to 4 years: Pneumococcus.

259. Most common organism in meningitis:
First two months: Group B Streptococcus.
> 2 months to 2 years: H. influenzae.
> 2 years: Pneumococcus.

260. Difference between hysterical and traumatic blindness:

	Hysterical	Traumatic
Pupil	Normal	Abnormal
Vision	Tunnel	No tunnel

261. **Risk factors for type I diabetes: Mumps, rubella, coxakie B4.**

262. Pertussis exposure:
a. Newborn exposed to mother with pertussis: Newborn should receive P.O. erythromycin.
b. Exposure of < 7 years of child who was immunized previously: Booster dose of DPT (unless booster dose was received in last 6 months) and oral erythromycin for 2 weeks.
c. Exposure of > 7 years old child who was immunized: Oral erythromycin for 2 weeks.
d. Exposure of person who has never been immunized: Oral erythromycin for 2 weeks after the contact has been broken. If the contact cannot be broken, then erythromycin

should continue until the cough stops in the diseased patient or if he should receive antibiotics for 7 days.

    e.   Institutional epidemics: Monovalent pertussis vaccine with oral erythromycin. Erythromycin estolate is the preferred drug because it achieves highest therapeutic level.

Effects of erythromycin in pertussis:

    a.   Eliminate B pertussis from the respiratory tract.
    b.   Reduces the spread of infection.
    c.   Reduces the symptoms of the disease.

263.   Straddle injury causes: Urethral tear and fracture of inferior pubic rami.

264.   Development of genitalia and secondary sex character in order of frequency **(first to last),** important:

Male: **Testes,** penis, pubic hair, peak height velocity, axillary hair, **facial hair.**
Female: **Breast,** pubic hair, peak height velocity, axillary hair, **menstruation.**

265.   **Hearing loss and management (important):**

Mild (30-40 db): May need hearing aid, preferential sitting in class.
Moderate (41-55 db): Hearing aid, speech therapy, preferential sitting in class.
Moderate to severe (56-70 db): Hearing aid, special class of hard of hearing.
Severe (deaf, 71-90 db): Special education for deaf, special training in speech and language.
Profound (deaf, > 90 db): Special education for deaf only.

266.   Hemoglobin electrophoresis and disease:
Hgb A1 ↑: Renal failure.
Hgb A1C ↑: Diabetes.
Hgb A2 ↑: Wilson disease.

In diabetes:
Good metabolic control (6-9%).
Fair control (9-12%).
Poor metabolic control (> 12%).

267.   Management of child whose playmate died: Reassure him and encourage him to attend funeral.

268.   Management of child in pediatric ward after another patient dies: Reassure child and explain the situation to him.

269. **Urodynamic studies and diseases:**

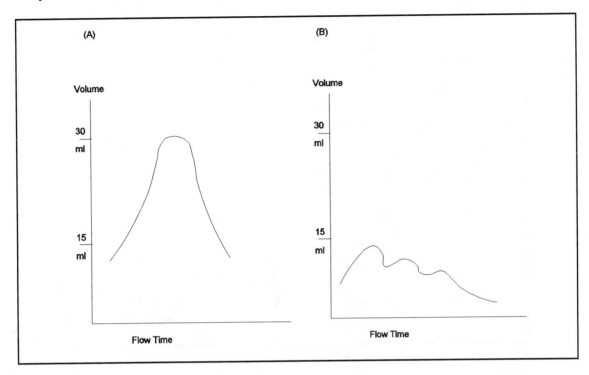

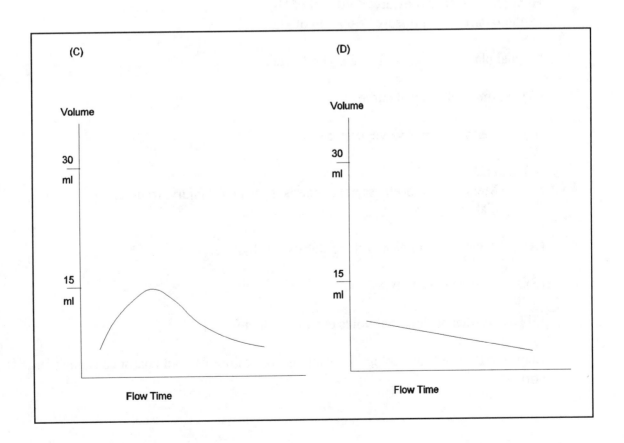

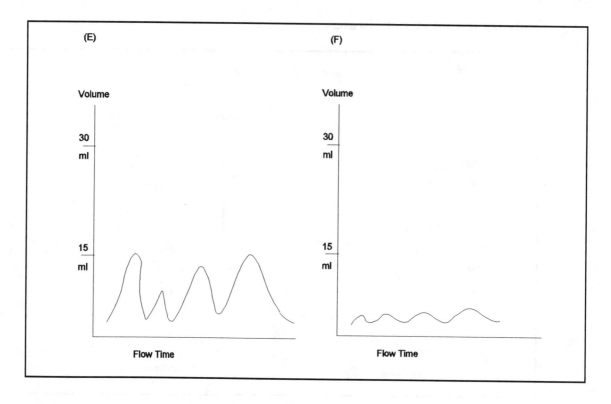

Normal voiding pressure: 20-40 mm of Hg.
Hypotonic bladder pressure: < 40 mm of Hg.
Outlet obstruction pressure: > 60 mm of Hg.

Normal bladder capacity: 10 ml/kg body weight.

(A) Normal bell-shaped curve.

(B) Posterior urethral valve, urethral stenosis.

(C) and (D)
     Meningomyelocele, sacral agenesis, spinal cord injury, traumatic paraplegia, diabetes, lues.

(E)   Abnormal straining with no detrusor activity.

(F)   Incomplete emptying.

UTI: Normal bladder, but voids early (< volume).

Enuresis: Bladder's physiologic capacity is 50% of normal, but anatomic capacity is normal.

270.　**Renogram (technetium - 99 m DTPA) and kidney diseases:**

(A)　Normal kidney.

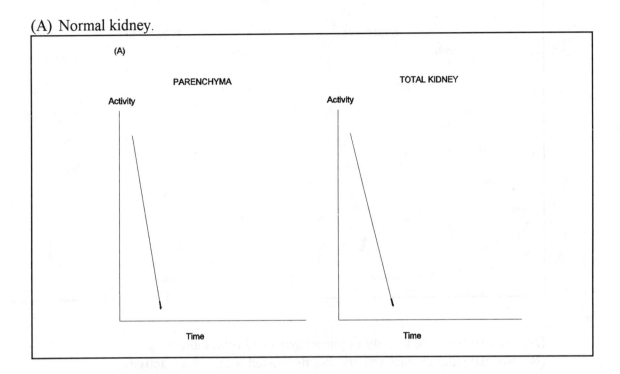

(B)　Pelvis dilated but no obstruction (reflux).

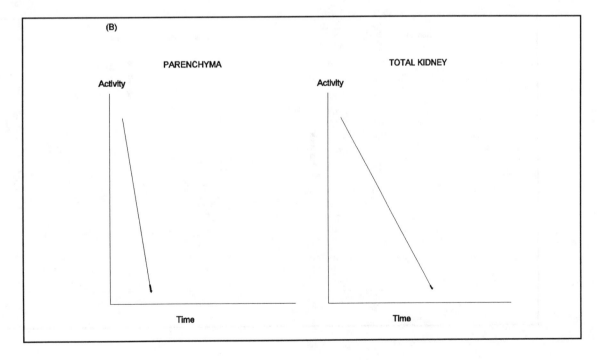

(C) Pelvis dilated and obstruction (Posterior urethral valve, UPJ obstruction).

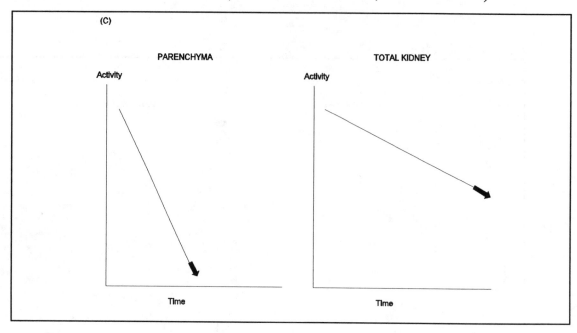

(A) Normal time and activity of parenchyma and total kidney.
(B) Normal parenchymal activity, but decreased total kidney activity.
(C) Decreased parenchymal activity and more decreased total kidney activity.

271. **Diuretics stimulated radionuclide renography in different disease states:**

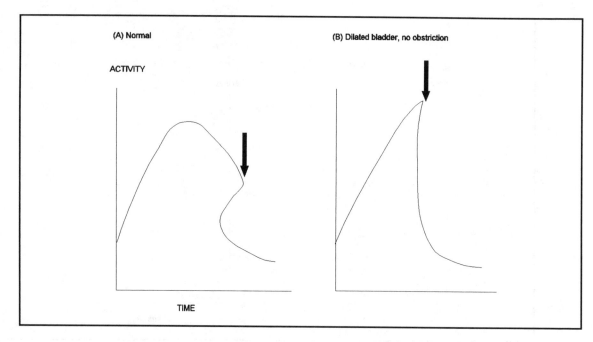

(A) Normal: Arrow (↓) means diuretics given, **voiding is enhanced** with diuretics.

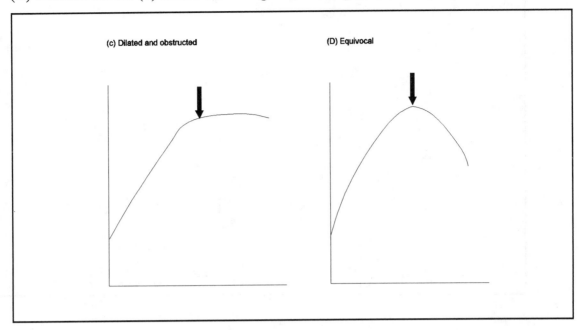

(B) Dilated bladder, but no obstruction: Arrow (↓) means diuretics given, **voiding begins** with diuretics.
(C) Dilated bladder and obstructed: Even with diuretics, **no voiding started.**
(D) Equivocal: After diuretics, voiding started, but **not normal.**

272. **Tympanometry and different disease conditions:**

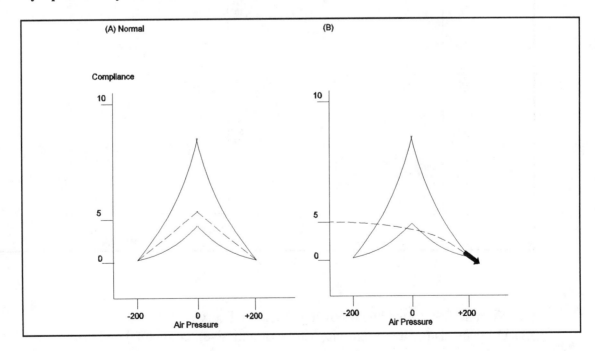

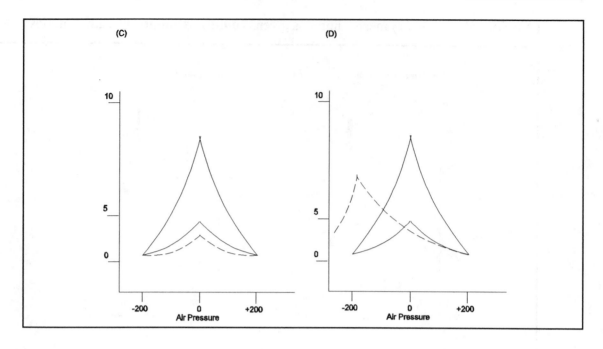

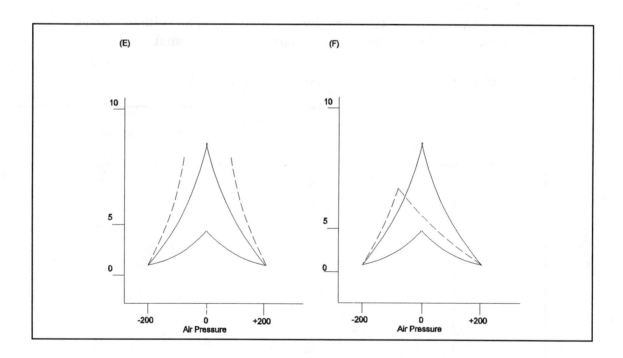

(A) Normal: See dotted line following the normal curve.
(B) Otitis media (acute or chronic; serous or adhesive), congenital middle air malformation, perforated air drum, cerumen occluding air canal, patent ventilating tube in air drum, fluid in middle ear or effusion.
(C) Otosclerosis, thickened air drum, scar ear drum, tympanosclerosis.
(D) Poor eustachian tube function, URI (upper respiratory infection).
(E) Discontinuation of ossicular chain, flaccid ear drum.

(F) Near normal.

273. **Audiometry in different diseases condition:**

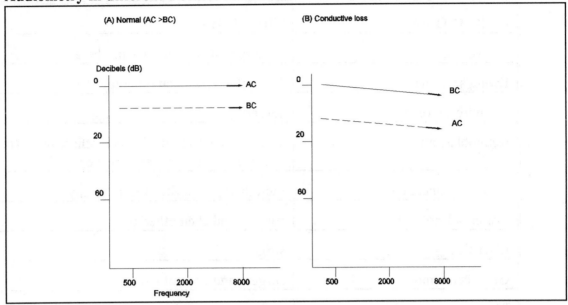

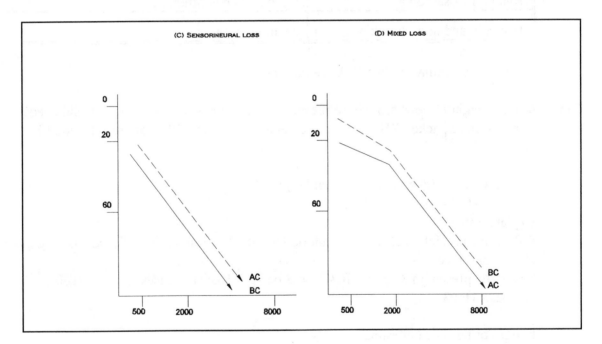

(A) Normal: No hearing loss, hearing close to 'zero' decibel, AC (air conduction)> BC (bone conduction).

(B) Conductive: Mild hearing loss, BC at least 15 db (decibel) higher than AC, usually < 20 db loss.

(C) Sensorineural: Severe hearing loss, precipitous drop of both AC and BC, usually more than 60 db.

(D) Mixed: Initially looks like conductive loss and with high frequency, sensorineural type.

274.

CARCINOMA	TREATMENT
Osteosarcoma	surgery (amputation), chemotherapy.
Ewing sarcoma	* radiotherapy, chemotherapy
Chondrosarcoma	surgery
Retinoblastoma	stage 1 (enucleation), 2 (chemotherapy), 3 (radio and chemo), 4 (radio and chemo)
Nasopharyngeal CA	radiotherapy, maybe chemotherapy
Colon (adeno) CA	surgery and chemotherapy
Liver CA	surgery
Germ cell tumor	surgery and chemotherapy
Rhabdomyosarcoma	radio and chemotherapy
Hodgkin and non-Hodgkin	chemotherapy

* Chondrosarcoma and liver CA are radioresistant.

275. 4.0 kg weight of newborn whose present hemoglobin is 5.0 mg/100 cc. Child needs transfusion of packed RBC to increase hemoglobin up to 12. **How much blood is required?**

Formula: wt. x (desired Hb - actual Hb) x 3.0 cc.
= 4 x (12 - 5) x 3 cc = 84 cc
Explanation:
P RBC means Hct of 66%, whole blood Hct of 33%, transfusion of 2 cc RBC/kg increases Hb 1 gm/100 cc
2 cc RBC present in 3 cc of P RBC, so 3 cc/kg P RBC increases Hb 1 gm/100 cc, increases Hct 3.

276. Length of newborn intestine:
S.I = 250 cm,
L.I. = 40 cm.

277. Predominant type of **sleep** in **late fetal age and newborns: REM** sleep.

Preterm infant, when it becomes fullterm by age, is **more active and alert** than fullterm who is just born.

278. **Match the following: Fetal and newborn hemoglobin.**

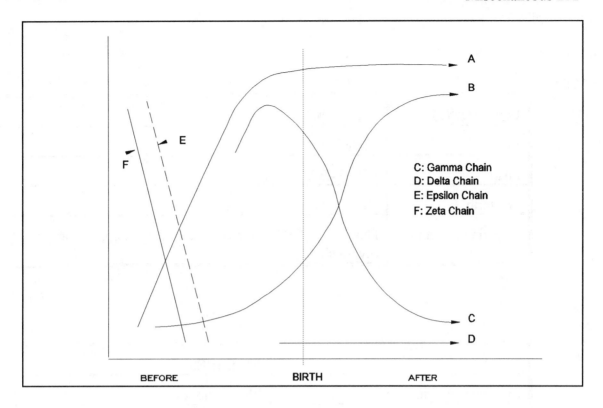

A: Alpha chain. Adult Hb `A': α2 ß2
B: Beta chain.   Fetal Hb `F': α2 Γ2 (gamma)
C: Gamma chain
D: Delta chain.
E: Epsilon chain
F: Zeta chain.

Hb 'A2': α2 δ2
Gower 1: Zeta 2, epsilon 2 (E,F)
Gower 2: Alpha 2, Epsilon 2 (A,E).

279. Behavior of infant and **Brazelton scale:**

This scale asseses in 4 dimension:

a. Motor.
b. Interactive (consolability, orientation, alertness).
c. Control of physiologic state (self-quieting, bright light attraction).
d. Response to stress (tremor, startle response).

280. Decreases RBC life span in newborn: Reduces Glutathione in RBC.

281. Mother and infant **bonding:** First one or two hours are important, let the mother hold and touch the baby.

282.

POISONING	TREATMENT
INH	Vitamin B6
Lead	EDTA; BAL (> 90)
Warfarin	Vitamin K
Digoxin (arrythmia)	Dilantin for SVT, lidocaine (ventricular ectopic beat), K (hypokalemia).

283.

RASH	DISEASES
Erythema marginatum	Rheumatic fever
Erythema chronicum migrans	Lyme disease
Erythema multiforme exudativum	Steven Johnson syndrome
Erythema multiforme Heliotrope eyelid (violaceous color)	Kawasaki disease, dermatomyositis
Erythema nodosum	Sarcoidosis, histoplasmosis, yersinia, coccidioidomycosis, birth control pill, SLE, vasculitis, regional enteritis, ulcerative colitis.

284. PPHN (persistent pulmonary hypertension) pulmonary vasoconstriction is due to: Thromboxane A 2 level is much higher in sepsis than in hypoxia.

285. Mother should not breast feed if she is taking any of the following medications:

Anticoagulants, antimicrobial (tetracycline, sulfonamide), aspirin, thiouracil, radioactive substances, antineoplastic medication.

286. Relationship of chorion to zygote:

Monochorionic is always monozygotic (two zygotes does not fuse).
Dichorionic is dizygotic in 80% of cases, monozygotic in 20% of cases.

287. Confirmation of zygocity: **DNA analysis.**

288. **Hemihypertrophy** can be found in: Wilms' tumor, adrenocortical hyperplasia/tumor,

hepatoma.

289. **Anosmia** is found in: Refsum syndrome, Kallmann syndrome.

290. **Retinitis pigmentosa** found in: Sjogren Larsen syndrome, Refsum syndrome, Abetalipoproteinemia.

291. Salt and pepper appearance of retina found in: Rubella, syphilis.

292. **GROWTH CHART IN DIFFERENT DISEASES:**

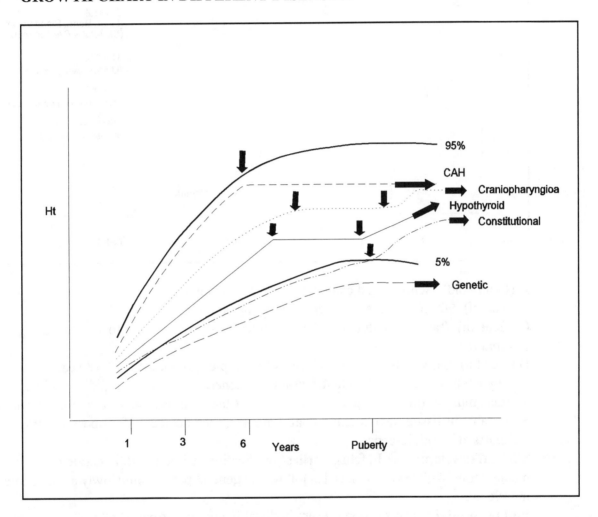

CAH (congenital adrenal hyperplasia)→ Diagnosis at 6 years. Initially tall but then no increase in Ht for 6 years.

Craniopharyngioma → Diagnosis at 9 years, surgery at puberty, then Ht. ↑.
Hypothyroid → Diagnosis at 6 years, no treatment until puberty.

Constitutional → Remains short until puberty then increases Ht, B.A < C.A.

Genetic→ Remain short for the rest of life. Both parents short. B.A. = C.A. (B.A. = bone age; C.A. = chronological age).

Postnatal development of organs and others:

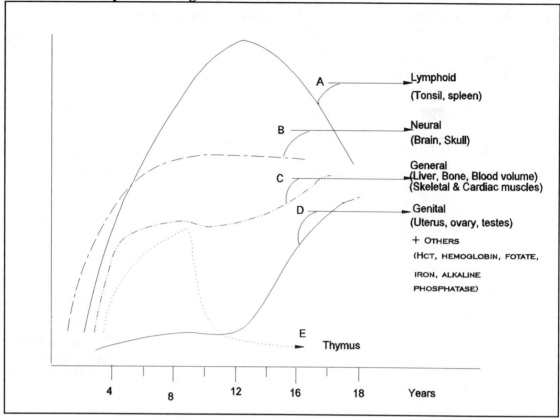

A (Lymphoid): School-aged child has more than in adult.

B (Neural): 90% of adult size is achieved by 5 years of age

C (General): Rapid growth in first 5 years, average growth from 5 to 10 years & again rapid from 10-18 years.

D (Genital): Slow growth in first 12 years then rapid growth from 12-18 years.

E (Thymus): Rapid growth in first 5 years like general & involutes rapidly in adolescence.

* Cardiac muscle: Initially larger to body size, but then follows the general growth curve.

Subcutaneous tissue (fat): Maximum at 9 months, then decreases for up to 6 years, then fat spurts at preadolescence.

Skeletal development: In fetus, **earliest** ossification at **5th** month in **clavicle** and membranous skull. Skeletal muscles follow the general pattern but slowly achieve total muscle mass.

Full term infant: Ossification present in distal femur and proximal tibia.

In adolescent girl: Fusion of humeral shaft with capitellum.

Teeth calcification: Begin at 7th month in fetal life in deciduous teeth; begins in permanent teeth just before birth.

293. COMPOSTION OF ORAL HYDRATING SOLUTION (IMPORTANT):

Fluid	Na	K	Cl	HCO$_3$	Glucose
Reformulated solution (correct answer in U.S.A.)	50	25	45	30	28
Traditional fluid	30	25	25	30	28

WHO (World Health Organization) fluid	90	20	80	30	111

294. **GROWTH CHART AND DIAGNOSIS:**

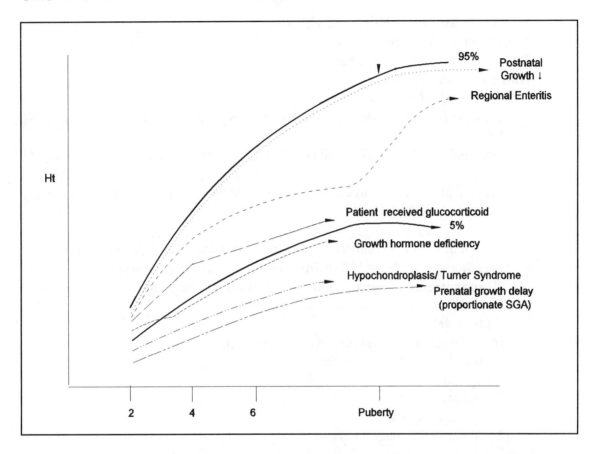

Regional Enteritis: Decreased growth rate which improves with control of the disease.
Glucocorticoid treatment: At 4 years causes growth delay but wt. ↑.
Growth hormone deficiency: Ht. and Wt. normal at birth, wt. (< 5%), Ht. steadily falls away from 5% (< 3%).
Hypochondroplasia/Turner: Ht. and Wt. both < 3%.
Proportionate SGA: Remains short for the rest of life, due to TORCH infections or genetic defects; otherwise they catch-up growth by 6 months of age.

295. Match the following acid base disorders:

DISORDERS	pH	PCO$_2$	Bicarbonate
Respiratory acidosis	↓ 7.20	↑ 60	↑ 35
Respiratory alkalosis	↑ 7.55	↓ 18	↓ 10
Metabolic alkalosis	↑ 7.55	→ 35	↑ 35
Metabolic acidosis	↓ 7.20	↓ 20	↓ 10

Compensated respiratory acidosis	→ 7.35	↑ 60	↑ 35
Compensated respiratory alkalosis	→ 7.35	↓ 18	↓ 10
Acidosis (respiratory + metabolic)	↓ 7.00	↑ 60	↓ 10
Alkalosis (respiratory + metabolic)	↑ 7.65	↓ 18	↑ 35

* ↓ CO_2 always with ↓ HCO_3 and vice versa.

*" Compensated "means pH is normal, but CO_2, HCO_3 is abnormal.

* ↓ = low, ↑ = high, → = normal.

How to remember easily:

First look at pH (low, high, normal):

a.   Low pH (acidosis): Metabolic (↓ HCO_3); respiratory (↑ CO_2); combined (↓ HCO_3, ↑ CO_2).

b.   High pH (alkalosis): Metabolic (↑ HCO_3); respiratory (↓ CO_2); combined (↑ HCO_3, ↓ CO_2).

c.   Normal pH (compensated): Respiratory acidosis (↑ CO_2, ↑ HCO_3); respiratory alkalosis (↓ CO_2, ↓ HCO_3).

296.   Calculation of fluid in hyponatremic and hypernatremic dehydration (weight 10 kg):

a.   **Hyponatremic (Na = 120 mEq/L, cold clammy, skin coma):**
     (Hyponatremia means serum Na = 130 mEq/L and less)
     Fluid = D5 water + calculated sodium.
     Sodium deficit:
     Body weight x (desired Na - Actual Na) x 0.6
     = 10 x (135 - 120) x 0.6 mEq
     = 90 mEq.
     Maintenance sodium:
     3 to 4 mEq/kg/day.
     Total correction over 24 hours.

b.   **Hypernatremic (Na = 165 mEq/L, doughy skin, irritability):**
     (Hypernatremia means serum Na = 150 mEq/L and above)
     Fluid D5 water + Nacl (25 mEq/L) + K acetate (maximum 40 mEq/L).
     Always calculate as 10% dehydration.
     Deficit = 100 ml/kg = 100 x 10 = 1000 ml.
     Maintenance for 48 hours = 1000 + 1000 = 2000 ml.
     Total = 1000 + 2000 = 3000 ml over 48 hours.
     Fluid should be corrected over 48 hours.
     Remember, serum Na level should not drop more than 10 mEq every 24 hours: rapid correction causes convulsions because water enters rapidly into cerebral cells causing cellular swelling and convulsion.

297.   **Calculation of fluid in iso natremic dehydration (weight = 10 kg):**

a.   **Isonatremic (Isonatremia means serum Na = 135-145 mEq/L):**
     5% dehydration (occurs with only tachycardia):
     Deficit = 50 ml/kg = 50 x 10 = 500 ml.
     Maintenance = 100 ml/kg = 100 x10 = 1000 ml in 24 hours.

(1st 10 kg = 100 ml/kg, 10-20 kg = 50 ml/kg, > 20 kg = 20 ml/kg).

Total = 500 + 1000 = 1500 ml over 24 hours.

Half (750 ml) over first 8 hours = repletion phase.

Next half (750 ml) over next 16 hours = recovery phase.

Fluid: D5 water + NaCl (55 mEq/L) + $NaHCO_3$

(20 mEq/L) + K acetate (20 mEq/L) or Ringer lactate (use of $NaHCO_3$ use is controversial, so use Ringer lactate).

b. **10% dehydration** (sunken eyes, dry mucous membrane, no tears, normal B.P.) =

Deficit = 100 ml/kg = 100 x 10 = 1000 ml.

Maintenance = 100 x 10 = 1000 ml.

Total = 1000 + 1000 = 2000 ml.

Emergency phase = 20 ml/kg over 1 hour = 200 ml.

Repletion phase = next 7 hours = half of remaining fluid (total 900 ml).

Recovery phase = next 16 hours = other half (900 ml) should be given.

Fluid in emergency phase = 5% albumin/Ringer lactate/0.9% NaCl/D10 W.

Fluid in recovery and repletion phase = same as 5% dehydration.

c. **15% dehydration** (same as 10% dehydration + hypotension):

Deficit = 150 ml/kg = 1500 ml.

Rest of the calculation same as 10% dehydration.

298. Different hematologic disorders and diagnosis:

DISEASES	Hgb A%	Hgb A2%	Hgb F%	Hgb S%	Hgb	MCV
Normal	95	2-4	< 1	0	N	N
Sickle cell disease	0	N	2-10 ↑	> 90 ↑↑↑	6-8 ↓↓	N
Sickle cell trait	45-55 ↓	N	N	35-45 ↑	N	N
Hgb SC disease	0	0	1 ↑	50% S, 50% C	9-10 ↓	
Thalassemia major (Beta), (cooley anemia)	< 30 ↓	N (↑ ratio A2, A)	> 70 ↑↑↑	0	< 5 ↓↓↓	45-55 ↓↓↓
Thalassemia minor (Beta)		4.5-7 ↑	1.5-6 ↑	0	9-10 ↓	55-65 ↓↓
Thalassemia (alpha)	0	N	N	0	12-14	62-75 ↓
Iron deficiency anemia	N	N	N	0	9-11 ↓	60-73 ↓
Sickle beta thalassemia	↓	↑↑	V	60-80 ↑↑		< 75 ↓

Sickle alpha thalassemia	0	N		↑↑↑	Bart ↑	↓

N = normal, V= variable, ↓ - decreased, ↑ increased.

MCV (after 1 year) = age in year + 70; Hgb (after 6 m to adult) = Around 12.

Sickle cell disease = ↑ retic (5-15%), ↓ ESR, Howell-Jolly body, spleen (initially ↑, then ↓ size).

High SC disease = huge spleen, many target cells, aseptic necrosis of femoral head and retinal damage.

Thalassemia minor = No hemolysis; poikilocyte, ovalocyte, basophilic stippling, few target cells.

Thalassemia major = Target cells, poikilocyte, huge (liver and spleen), ↓ growth.

Alpha thalassemia = Hydrops fetalis.

Both sickle thalassemia = Moderate hemolysis, mild to moderate crisis, large spleen, one parents sickle trait and other parents thalassemia trait.

299. **Treatment for encopresis:**
   a. **Primary:** Difficult; might need enema to evacuate colon initially, but avoid chronic use of enema.
   b. **Secondary:** Mineral oil and high fibre diet; sitting on toilet for 10-15 minutes after each meal; gets reward for compliance.

300. **Treatment of enuresis:**
   a. **Imipramine** is only briefly effective, and patient develops drug tolerance.
   b. Most important is to **understand the specific cause suggested by psychosocial evaluation and physical examination and try to solve that problem.**

301. **Rumination:** It is repeated regurgitation of food without nausea and G.I. problem, resulting in weight loss or not gaining weight. Found between 3 to 14 months. It may be due to psychogenic and self- stimulating factor; otherwise there is normal development, but perhaps a disturbed mother child relationship.
   Tx: Encourage proper eating habits and discourage rumination; parental counseling and family therapy.

302. **Dysthymic disorder:**
   It means intermittent depression and period of normal mood in between for days or weeks. It may be due to genetic disorder, strong family history, present with symptoms of major depression **without delusions and hallucination,** try to hide their depression, problem in school achievement and with their peers, can use drugs.
   Tx: a. Antidepressant medicine.
      b. Treat the underlying cause (means anorexia, substance abuse, chronic physical illness, personality disorder).

303. **Bipolar disorder (manic depressive):** Most common in second and third decade, but may appear before puberty. Manic features are more common than depressive features. Accompanies over-activity, insomnia, and paranoid delusion.
   Tx: a. **Lithium carbonate is the drug of choice.**
      b. Psychotherapy.

304. Etiology of attention deficit disorder: **Unknown.**

305. Homosexuality, important points to remember:
    a. If a child engages in homosexual activity, that does not mean that child has already made homosexual object choice.
    b. Physician and parents should make younger child feels safe, not guilty.
    c. Do not show anger or frustration, but rather talk to the child.
    d. If an older child is the initiator, tell him that this kind of behavior will not be tolerated in the future.
    e. Psychotherapy and legal interventions are indicated only if there is a psycological problem or physical violence.

306. **Diet for athletic activities:** Adequate calories and essential nutrients in normally balanced diet. **Special diet is not indicated.** Before and during athletic activities, water should be provided.

307. A 2-year-old child is not eating well but activities are normal. The mother is worried. What is your advice?
    It is normal in end of first year and during the second that, because of his decelerating rate of growth, the child's caloric intake is reduced. Do not force the child to eat.

308. Growth of vegetarian infant as compared to omnivorous infant: In the first two years of life, the vegetarian infant may not grow as fast as the omnivorous.

309. **Hemophilus influenzae b (Hib) vaccine:**
    a. PRP vaccine (HbOC) given at 2, 4, 6 months of age along with DPT, OPV, but in different sites of injection; 4th doses at 15 months of age.
    b. Those who did not receive first three doses should get 2 doses between 7 and 11 months and third doses at 15 months.
    c. Children between 12-15 months who did not receive any vaccine before should get 2 doses at 2 month intervals (atleast).
    d. Children older than 15 months should get a single dose of conjugated vaccine.

310. **Delayed immunization of children:**
    a. **> 2 months and < 14 months:** Same order as the normal child should receive, except Hib, which was mentioned above.
    b. **14 months to 7 years:** Give DPT, OPV, PPD in first visit if no immunization given before;
    Hib should be given as discussed,
    One month later, MMR,
    Then another month later, DPT, OPV (second dose), third dose of DPT,
    Optional OPV after 2 months of second dose and both booster after 1 year.
    If the child is **less than 4 years** and has received all the above immunization, he should get booster DPT, OPV between 5 to 7 years; but if child is more than 4 years, do not give booster dose.
    Td should be given to all children in early adolescence.

311. **Pneumococcal vaccine:** It is given in functional and anatomic asplenia after 2 years of

age. Revaccination is not necessary because of persistently good level. **Remember, it does not prevent otitis media.**

312. **Viral influenza vaccine:** It should **not** be given to normal children but is recommended for those who are at high risk for developing respiratory infection (congenital or acquired cardiac defect, cystic fibrosis, severe asthma, thalassemia, sickle cell anemia, neuromuscular disease affecting pulmonary function, BPD, immunodeficient children). **Never give small pox vaccine.**

313. **P value: It is statistically significant when < 0.01.** (That means the probability of difference between the groups due to chance is less than 1%.)

314. **Test most commonly used** for differences between proportions, i.e., comparing effect of two different medications used in two different groups: **Chi-square test.**

315. Test used for comparison of means: **Student's t-test.**

316. **Maternal-fetal conflict:** Here a pregnant woman refuses standard care that is absolutely beneficial for fetus. If the fetus is more than 26 weeks gestational age then procedure should be done according to federal court law. Pediatrician might help prenatally to initiate implementation of or support for court rules.

317. Most common organism causing peritonitis in CAPD (continuous ambulatory peritoneal dialysis):
Staph. epidermidis.
First sign of peritonitis is cloudy peritoneal dialysis i.e; neutrophil count is > 100. Other signs are pain, tenderness, guarding, rebound tenderness.
DIAGNOSIS:
Initial: Gram stain of peritoneal fluid.
Final: Positive culture of peritoneal fluid.
TREATMENT:
a.   Initial (before culture result): Intraperitoneal administration of first generation cephalosporin or vancomycin with aminoglycoside through dialysis catheter.
b.   Final: Antibiotics after sensitivity test.
c.   Fungal: I.V. Amphotericin because of poor peritoneal penetration.
d.   Removal of catheter: When there is fungal, recurrent bacterial, or complicated peritonitis.

318. Most common organism in dermal sinus tract infection:
S. epidermidis;
Other organisms are S. aureus, E. coli, Pseudomonas.

319. Functions of **immunoglobulins** in host defense:
a.   Opsonophagocytosis: IgG.
b.   Basophil and mast cell degranulation: IgE.
c.   Antibody dependent cellular cytotoxicity: IgG.
d.   Complement activation: IgG, IgM.
e.   Interfere with adherence of microorganism: IgA, IgG.

f. Neutralize toxin or virus: IgM, IgG, IgA.

320. H. influenzae meningitis and dexamethasone therapy:
It should be given **before or with** the antibiotics.
Complications of steroid use: ↑ B.P., G.I. bleeding, ↑ WBC, rebound pyrexia after the last dose.

321. Difference in blood supply of the bone in infant and children:
Infant: Epiphyseal blood vessels are connected with metaphyseal blood vessels through transphyseal vessels, so infection spread from epiphyses to metaphyses and vice versa.
Children: No connection between those blood vessels.

322. Preferred drug of choice for organisms causing osteomyelitis or septic arthritis:
a. S. aureus: Nafcillin, methicillin, oxacillin; if resistant, then vancomycin.
b. H. influenzae: Ceftriaxone, cefuroxime, or chloramphenicol.
c. Pseudomonas: Ticarcillin, timentin, gentamicin.
d. N. gonorrhoeae: Ceftriaxone, cefoxitin.
e. Fungal: Amphotericin B (intravenous, intraarticulare).

323. Most common methicillin resistant S. aureus (MRSA) strain: **Phage group II** (types 77, 83 A, 84, 85); other types are I and nontypable.
MRSA infection occurs in: Premature, burn, surgical wound, venous central line, prolonged hospitalization, from another MRSA patient.

324. Most common nosocomial infection: **S. epidermidis.**
It is one of the 11 recognized coagulase negative staphylococci (CONS). It forms slime (exo polysaccharide protective bio film) which covers the organism.
Function of slime:
a. It increases adhesion of organism with foreign body.
b. It prevents phagocytosis.
c. It inhibits penetration of antibiotic to the organism.
Treatment: Vancomycin is the drug of choice.

325. Toxic shock syndrome, S. aureus phage type and toxin:
Phage type: 29/52, noninvasive.
Toxin: Staphylococcal enterotoxin F (SEF), pyrogenic exotoxin C (PEC).

326. Most common type **of campylobacter gastroenteritis: C. jejuni.**
Most common type in septicemia is C. fetus.
Treatment for campylobacter infection:
a. Gastroenteritis: Erythromycin, tetracycline.
b. Septicemia and non enteric infection: Gentamicin.

Treatment for campylobacter pyloritis (helicobacter pylori):
Bismuth subnitrate, tetracycline, gentamicin. H. pylori is present in gastric antrum in 100% of patients with duodenal ulcer and 70% patients with gastric ulcer.
Diagnosis is confirmed by biopsy through endoscopy, rapid diagnosis by CLO test (pellet containing urea, metabolized urease produced by this organism results in change of color).

327. Hepatitis D virus (HDV), delta (δ) virus:
RNA virus. It only multiplies in the presence of hepatitis B (HBV) virus. HDV infection occurs either with HBV active infection or in chronic carrier of HBsAg. It is mostly transmitted by parenteral inoculation (drugs or blood transfusion), rarely by perinatal infection. HDV can cause fulminant hepatitis or enhance carrier state of HBsAg positive individual.

Hepatitis C virus: This is a non-A/non-B virus. It is an RNA virus which mimics both flavi and pesti virus, and is transmitted through blood, and blood products, I.V. drug, sex; results in chronic liver disease.

Hepatitis E virus: It is a non-A/non-B water borne virus which is found in developing countries, and turns into acute hepatitis.

328. **Human immunodeficiency virus (HIV) causing AIDS (acquired immunodeficiency syndrome):**
Most common is HIV-1, retrovirus, transmission mostly through cells and partly through body fluids (blood, semen, vaginal and cervical fluid, breast milk). Plasma contains 10-50 HIV particle per 1 ml and HBV (hepatitis B virus) 100 million-1 billion per 1 ml, so there is a lower risk of HIV than of HBV infection after needle stick. It is very **rarely** transmitted through saliva, tears, urine. Incubation period for perinatal infection **8 m to 3 years. Usually** becomes symptomatic by 18 months of age, but for **blood transfusion, 2 years.**

Other retroviruses are:
a. HIV-2, less common, less severe than HIV-1.
b. HTLV-1 (Human T lymphocyte virus type 1): It is transmitted through breast milk, placenta, blood, needle, syringes. **It does not cause AIDS.** Only 2-4% develop adult T cell leukemia. It is associated with tropical spastic paraparesis. It differs from HIV morphologically and genetically.
c. HTLV-2: Uncertain transmission and clinical course. It is associated with hairy cell leukemia.

Chances of infection to baby:
a. Infected mother: 20-35%. Only 8% when mother received AZT during pregnancy.
b. Previously affected child: 50-65%.

Signs and symptoms:
Failure to thrive, fever, ↑ **lymph nodes,** repeated infections, LBW (SGA). Specific features includes microcephaly, dysmorphic facial features, embryopathy, **lymphocytic interstitial** pneumonia, ↑ liver and spleen, diarrhea, cardiomyopathy, nephropathy, encephalopathy, rash, parotitis, Kaposi sarcoma.

Infections: Most common infections are pneumocystis carinii and all other types of infections.

DIAGNOSIS:
Confirmed by positive viral blood culture; DNA sequence by PCR (polymerase chain reaction), detection of IgG by ELISA method and detection of p 24 antigen. Most characteristic is reversal of T 4/T 8 ratio (normal 1.5-2.3). ↑ IgA > 1800 mg/dl at 1 year and > 2300 mg/dl at 2 years is typical of AIDS.

Prevention: Latex condom.

Treatment:

a. Most specific: AZT (azidothymidine); and treat the underlying infection.

b. Prophylaxis: Trimethoprim and sulfamethoxazole. Newborn should receive P.O. AZT 2 mg/kg/dose - Q.6.H for first 6 weeks of life.

Prognosis:

Perinatally acquired infection and infection less than one year of age have worst prognosis.

329. **Lesion of visual pathways:**

a. Optic nerve: Unilateral vision loss.

b. Optic chiasma: Bitemporal hemianopsia.

c. (R) optic tract: (L) homonymous hemianopsia.

d. (L) optic tract: (R) homonymous hemianopsia.

e. Lateral geniculate body: Homonymous hemianopsia (partial because of widely distributed fibre).

f. Optic radiation: Homonymous hemianopsia (partial).

g. Visual cortex: Homonymous hemianopsia (partial or complete).

330. Growth of brain in different stages:

a. Neuronal proliferation: 2 to 4 months in utero.

b. Neuronal migration: 3 to 5 months in utero.

c. Neuronal organization: 6 m to several years.

d. Neuronal myelination: After birth to many years postnatal.

331. **Lung maturity factors in amniotic fluid:**

Appearance of posphatidylglycerol at 35 week indicates lung maturity.

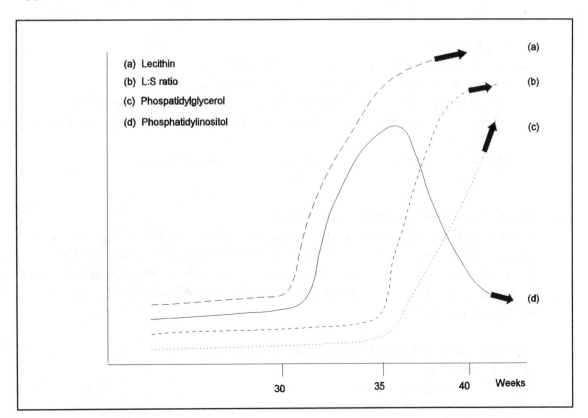

(a) Lecithin
(b) L:S ratio
(c) Phospatidylglycerol
(d) Phosphatidylinositol

332.   Most common type of anorectal anomalies:
Type III A and III B.
Different types :
Type I: Anal stenosis.
Type II: Imperforate anal membrane.
Type III A: Anal agenesis
Type III B: Rectal agenesis
Type IV: Rectal atresia.
Type I, II and III A: Low anomalies (below levator muscles).
Type III B and IV: High anomalies (above levator muscles).

Associated anomalies are:
a.   High anomalies: 50% have urinary tract and vertebral anomalies.
b.   Low anomalies: 25% have above anomalies.
* Sacral anomaly is important to predict bowel and urinary function.

High anomalies: Mostly in male, appears with rectourethral fistula (prostatic urethra); in female, it appears with fistula between rectum and posterior vaginal wall. Defect or absence of internal and defect in external anal sphincter.

Low anomalies: Intact internal and external anal sphincters. In male, anteriorly placed fistulas opening onto the skin in the midline in front of the ideal position of anus. In female, anus is ectopic (perineal, vestibular, low vaginal).
DIAGNOSIS:
a.   High lesion: Lateral X-ray in upside down position, ultrasound, CT scan, dye study for fistula.
b.   Low lesion: Repeated physical examination, dye study for fistula, ultrasound, CT scan.

TREATMENT:
a.   Anal stenosis: Dilation (digital or by instrument).
b.   Other low anomalies: Surgical correction from below.
c.   High lesion: Transverse colostomy initially, then definitive repair 6-12 m. Remember, anteriorly placed anus will **not** cause UTI, genital infection, or difficult delivery.
Prognosis: High lesion worst; Lower lesion has good prognosis.

333.   **BAER (Brainstem auditory evoke response):**
It is the electrical response generated within the auditory pathways from the VIIIth cranial nerve to diencephalon. There are 7 different waves produced from outside (VIIIth cranial nerve) to inward (thalamic radiations). Normal conduction means high altitude and reduced breathing (like tall, slim person) and abnormal conduction means low altitude and increased breathing (like short, fat person).

Different waves represent different anatomical locations:
Wave I: VIII cranial nerve.
Wave II: Cochlear nucleus.

Wave III: Superior olivary nucleus.
Wave IV: Lateral lemniscus.
Wave V: Inferior colliculus.
Wave VI: Thalamus.
Wave VII: Thalamic radiations.
Only waves I, III, and V are important to remember.

Normal:

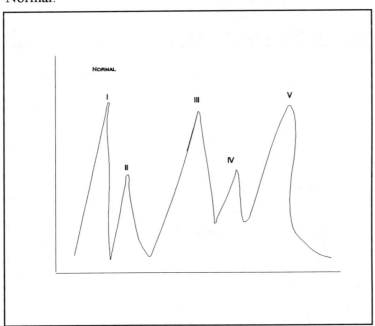

Peripheral conduction defect: Wave I and V are prolonged but distance between I to V is normal.

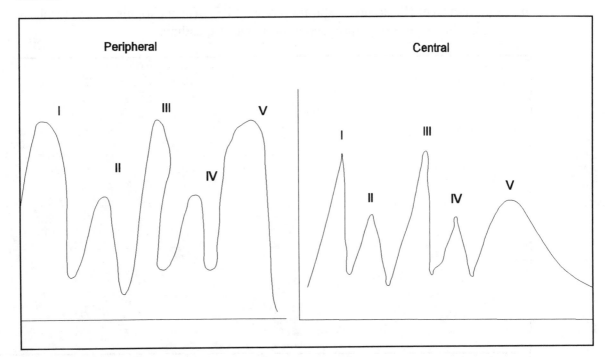

Central conduction defect: Wave V is prolonged and distance between I to V is increased.

Defects in waves in different diseases:

a. Wave I: Meningitis.

b. Wave II: Hemorrhage (intracranial).

c. Wave I and II: Viral infection (congenital).

d. Wave II and V: Hyperbilirubinemia, HIE (hypoxic ischemic encephalopathy).

334. **Flow volume curve in different lung diseases:**

a.   Normal: (Normal inspiration and expiration phases)

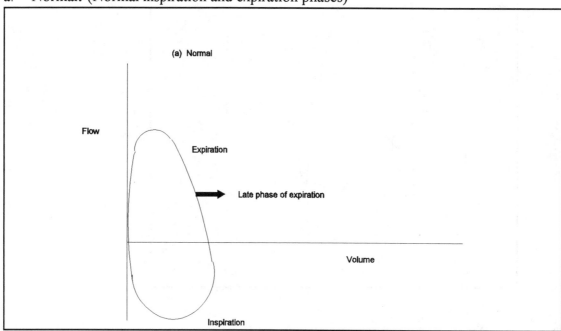

b.   **Obstructive:** (Prolonged expiration phase) BPD (bronchopulmonary dysplasia), meconium aspiration, emphysema, bronchiolitis, asthma.

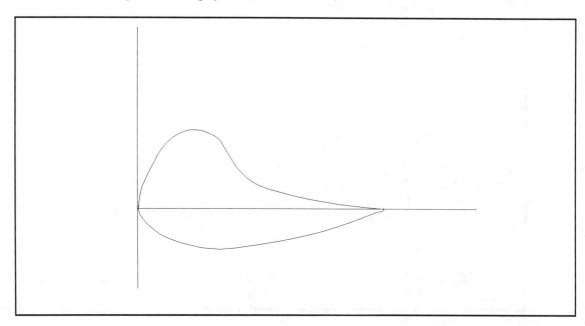

c. **Restrictive: (Reduced inspiration and expiration phases)** RDS (respiratory distress syndrome), pneumothorax, pneumonia, collapse, diaphragmatic hernia. persistent pulmonary hypertension due to collapse, pulmonary interstitial emphysema, tuberculosis.

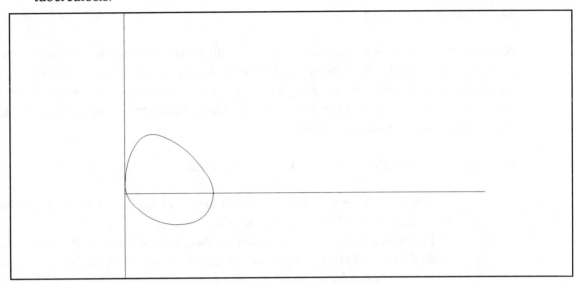

d. **Extrathoracic obstruction:** Tracheal stenosis, enlarged tonsils, epiglottitis, polyp of vocal cord and trachea.

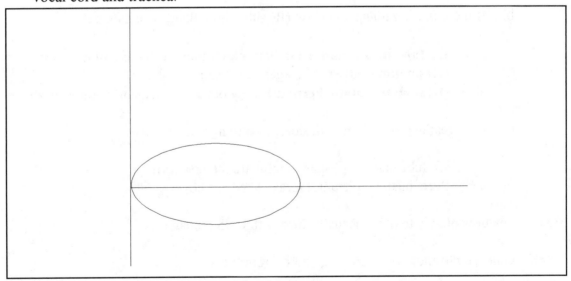

Extrathoracic tracheal obstruction is worse during inspiration than expiration. Introthoracic obstruction is worse during expiration than inspiration because during inspiration trachea is dilated by negative pleural pressure and during expiration trachea is collapsed by positive pleural pressure.

*Remember, cystic fibrosis is mixed (restrictive and obstructive) type.

335. **Lung infection test:**
   a. **Obstructive**: ↑ TLC, ↑↑ RV, ↑ FRC; ↓ ERV, ↓ VC, ↓ FEV1/FVC, ↑ RV/TLC.
   b. **Restrictive**: ↓ TLC, ↑ RV, ↓ FRC; ↓ ERV, ↓ VC, → ↑ FEV1/FVC, → ↑ RV/TLC.
   TV: Tidal volume;

RV: Residual volume.
VC: Vital capacity.
IRV: Inspiratory reserve volume.
ERV: Expiratory reserve volume;
TLC: Total lung capacity.

336. A newborn appears with respiratory distress at birth, intubated in the delivery room, still cyanotic; first thing to be checked: **Endotracheal tube position** or blocked by mucous. Check the position of the tube by laryngoscope. **Reintubate the child immediately** if there is any doubt about the position or block. Listen to the breathing sounds on each side: breathing should be equal on both sides.

    a.   If there is ↓ breath sound on (L) side, three things can happen:

        i.   **ET tube in (R) main-stem**-bronchus and (L) lung collapses: Pull out the ET tube. Clinical condition should improve.
        ii.   **(L) pneumothorax:** Here transillumination will be positive, heart sounds shifted to the (R) (but in collapsed heart sound is shifted to the same side); put a needle in chest tube on an emergency basis, then finally insert the chest tube. Patient should improve clinically.
        iii. **(L) diaphragmatic hernia:** Put NG tube. Surgical repair is needed.

    b.   If there is ↓ breathing sound on (R) side, three things can happen:

        i.   **ET tube in (L) main stem bronchus:** Pull out the ET tube.
        ii.   **(R) pneumothorax:** Management is same as above.
        iii. **(R) diaphragmatic hernia:** Rarely occurs, management same as above.

    c.   If ↓ breathing sound on both sides, two things can happen:

        i.   ET tube is in esophagus: reintubate the newborn.
        ii.   Rare, bilateral pneumothorax; same as above.

337. Features of zinc toxicity: Renal failure with CNS damage.

338. Glucose filtration, reabsorption, and excretion curve:

    a.   Maximum tubular reabsorption (TmG) = 2 mmol/minute
    b.   Maximum rate of excretion when plasma level is 16 mmol/L (PG)

ABC = Glucose filtration,
AB = Glucose reabsorption and filtration,
BC = No reabsorption, only filtration,
BEG = No reabsorption,
B = Maximum reabsorption point,
AD = No glucose excretion, all reabsorption,
DEF = All glucose excretion

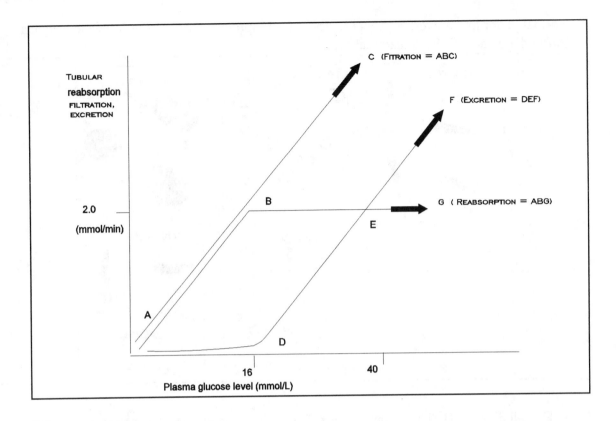

339. Peripheral blood smear and different diseases:

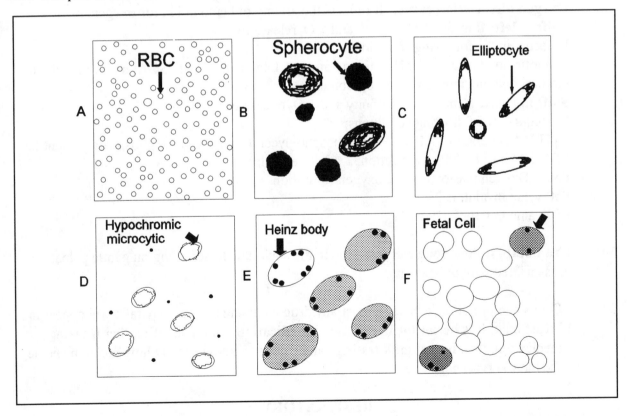

A- Normal under low power; B- Spherocytosis; C- Elliptocytosis; D- Iron-deficiency anemia
E- G6PD deficiency; F- Feto-maternal bleed

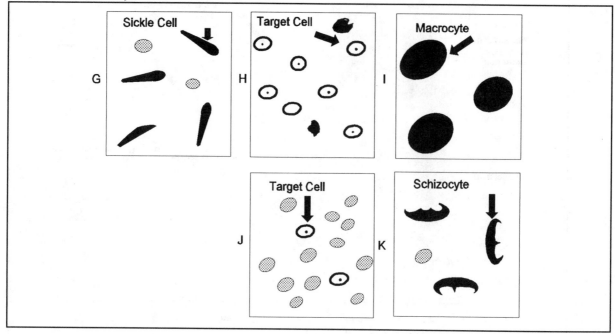

G- Sickle cell disease; H- Thalassemia major; I- Folic acid deficiency; J- Thalassemia minor; K- Hemolytic uremic syndrome

340. **Oxygen dissociation curve:** It reflects the affinity of hemoglobin for oxygen.
Shift to left: It means $\uparrow O_2$ affinity and $\downarrow O_2$ release to tissue.
It occurs in the following conditions:
Cyanotic heart disease, $\uparrow$ pH, $\downarrow$ temperature, $\uparrow$ fetal hemoglobin, SGA, infant of diabetic mother, myoglobinuria, methemoglobinemia.
Shift to right: It means $\downarrow O_2$ affinity and $\uparrow O_2$ release to tissue.
It occurs in the following conditions:
$\downarrow$ pH, $\uparrow$ temperature, $\uparrow$ 2-3 DPG (diphosphoglycerate is an organic phosphate present in RBC), $\uparrow CO_2$, $\uparrow$ ATP, $\uparrow$ ionization, $\uparrow$ adult hemoglobin.
P50 = Oxygen tension at 50% oxygen saturation.
P50 value in adult is 27.
P50 value in fetus is 19 to 21.

341. **Craniotabes:** Ping-pong ball sensation in the skull, due to softening, in gentle palpation. It is associated with prematurity.

342. Drugs and breast milk: Since almost any drug a nursing mother may take will appear in breast milk, **it is better for her to avoid medication** if possible. If mother is taking medication, then **breast milk testing** can be done to know exactly how much medicine the baby is receiving.

RESPIRATORY

1. A child appears with **a sudden onset** of cough, hoarseness, hemoptysis, dyspnea; **no**

fever.

> **ON EXAM: Croupy** cough, mild cyanosis.
> **X-ray:** Foreign body in **sagittal** plane.
> **Dx:** Foreign body in **larynx.**
> **Tx:** Removal; if child is in severe respiratory distress, **do tracheostomy first,** then **remove the foreign body.**

2. A child appears with sudden onset of cough, hoarseness, dyspnea; **no fever.**

> **ON EXAM: Audible slap, palpable thud,** and wheezing like asthma.
> **Dx:** Foreign body **trachea;** most of the time it is confirmed by **bronchoscopy.**
> **Tx:** Remove of foreign body.

3. Most common organism of acute bronchiolitis: RSV.

4. A child of a **few month appears** with URI symptom, mild fever, cough, dyspnea. **No family history** of asthma.
    ON EXAM: Prolonged expiratory phase with wheezing and retraction.
    X-ray: Hyperinflated lungs.
    CBC: Normal.
    Dx: Acute bronchiolitis.
    Tx: Supportive; cold humidified oxygen.

5. 4-year-old child appears with high fever and respiratory difficulty.

> **ON EXAM:** Rales present.
> CBC: Increase WBC.
> CXR: Pneumonia with **pleural effusion.**
> **Dx: Streptococcal pneumonia.**

6. 11-month-old child appears with acute respiratory distress with high fever and **shock-like** symptoms.

> **ON EXAM: A** few **skin lesiosn over** the body, tachypnea, rales, grunting.
> CXR: Pneumatocele, empyema, or effusion.
> CBC: Increased CBC with polymorph.
> **Dx: Staph** pneumonia.
> ** Infant with staph. pneumonia should be tested for immune deficiency and cystic fibrosis.

7. Most common cause of childhood bacterial pneumonia: **Pneumococcal** pneumonia **(lobar involvement).** ** Pneumococcal vaccine should be given to sickle cell disease patient.

8. Pneumonia with gram-negative organism:

> H. flue: Lobar pneumonia.
> Klebscilla: Lobar pneumonia with **bulging fissure.**

Pseudomonas: Serious necrotizing bronchopneumonia.
* It mostly occurs from contaminated hospital equipment or immunosuppressive therapy.

9.   A child appears with history of sudden onset of cough, choking, **which stops** when child arrives in E.R.:

ON EXAM: Wheezing on (R) side.
X-ray: Hyperinflation (R) lung and mediastinal shift to (L) side.
Dx: Foreign body (R) bronchus by bronchoscopy.
Tx: Removal by bronchoscopy.
** It means **partial** obstruction: air goes into lung during inspiration, but barely comes out in expiration.
In **complete** obstruction (R) side:
(R) lung completely collapses, then mediastinum shifts to (R) side.

10.   Kartagener syndrome (immotile cilia syndrome): Autosomal recessive, associated with **situs inversus** and **infertility in male,** defect **in ciliary motion. Appears** with **chronic** otitis media, **bronchitis,** sinusitis; wheezing, but no bronchiectasis. Usually infected with pneumococci and H. flue.

11.   Most common cause of acute laryngeal stenosis: Acute infection.

12.   Most common laryngeal tumor in childhood: Papilloma. ** Sign and symptoms: hoarseness, dyspnea.

Dx: By direct laryngoscopy.
Tx: Removal by direct laryngoscopy; cryo and laser surgery; systemic bleomycin only needed when papilloma does not respond to initial therapy.

13.   Most common pneumonia due to virus: RSV.

14.   RSV pneumonia: It is a benign condition except in infancy; usually appears with URI symptom, dyspnea, retraction.
CXR: **Diffuse infiltrate,** particularly in perihilar area.

15.   An immunocompromised child appears with fever, difficulty in breathing and coughing. History of multiple hospital admission for diarrhea and infection, but this is the first admission with respiratory problem.

CXR: Bilateral diffuse interstitial infiltrate.
Dx: Pneumocystis carinii pneumonia.
Diagnosis confirmed by discovering the organism in sputum, lung aspirate, bronchoalveolar lavage or biopsy of lungs.
Tx: Trimethoprim and sulfamethoxazole. It is also used as a prophylaxis.

16.   A child appears in E.R. with respiratory distress after feeding milk.

ON EXAM: Rales bilateral, tachypnoea, intercostal retraction noted.

X-ray: taken at 2 hours of age = negative.
Dx: Aspiration pneumonia.
* X-ray can be normal up to 6 hours of age.
Tx: Antibiotics (penicillin).
*Gastric contents have low pH, causing chemical pneumonitis.

17.   A child with history of coughing and vomiting was brought in by mother after accidental ingestion of some unknown material. A few hours later, the child develops **fever, drowsiness,** and **alteration of mental status.**

   ON EXAM: Rales bilateral.
   CXR: Early infiltrate at 3 hours of age.
   Child received antibiotics, required intubation. CXR was repeated and showed progressively increasing consolidation.

   The diagnosis: **hydrocarbon pneumonia** (e.g., gasoline, kerosene). In hydrocarbon, **gastric lavage is contraindicated** because it can go to the lungs. Routine antibiotics are not necessary, but are required when there is superimposed bacterial infection. Respiratory complications include pneumothorax, empyema, effusion, pneumatocele, but most **children survive without complication.**

18.   A child appears with persistent history of **cough** for 10 days and did not get better with different cough medications. Upon further questioning, mother stated that she was giving **cod liver oil** to increase child's weight but child swallow with difficulty.

   CXR: Showed **bilateral perihilar of increased density.** What is the diagnosis?
   Dx: Lipoid pneumonia.
   Tx: Nonspecific; don't give cod liver oil.

19.   Treatment for smoke inhalation: 100% humidified oxygen.

20.   Complication of smoke inhalation and treatment: Pulmonary edema. **Tx:** Fluid restriction and diuretics.

21.   Most common type of pulmonary hemosiderosis: Idiopathic. Other types of primary pulmonary hemosiderosis are associated with cow's milk (Heiner syndrome), with myocarditis, with glomerulonephritis (Goodpasture syndrome).

22.   A child started taking cow's milk recently, and now appears with cough, **hemoptysis,** dyspnea, wheezing, tachycardia.

   CBC: Hypochromic microcytic anemia. Low serum iron level, increase bilirubin, urobilinogen and retic count.
   CXR: May or may not have diffuse infiltrate.
   Dx: Confirm by sputum, tracheal or gastric aspirate which shows **hemosiderin in macrophage.** Sometimes open lung biopsy is required.
   Dx: Pulmonary hemosiderosis.
   Tx: Discontinue cow's milk, give corticosteroid.

23. Pulmonary alveolar proteinosis: **Rare** disease, appears with cough, dyspnea,.

     CXR: Shows infiltrate with **butterfly pattern.**
     Dx: Confirm by **biopsy.**
     Tx: Mucomist, repeated pulmonary lavage.

24. An immunocompromised child appears with acute onset of cough, mild fever and occasional wheezing.

     CXR: Showed **bilateral diffuse** infiltrate.
     CBC: Showed increased **eosinophil** count and elevation of **IgE level.**
     Dx: Pulmonary aspergillosis (fungal infection).
     Tx: Amphotericin B with 5 fluorocytosine.

25. A child appears with paroxysmal cough and dyspnea, but **no** fever. History reveals that he plays with the **dog** at home.

     ON EXAM: Hepatomegaly.
     CXR: Looks **like miliary T.B.**
     CBC: Showed very **high eosinophil count.**
     Dx: Loeffler syndrome or Eosinophilic pneumonia. It is due to Toxocara canis which is found in dogs. This patient may have **reaction to drugs** like penicillin, sulphur, aspirin.

26. Infection in burn patient: Initially the most common is Staph.aureus; after one week it is pseudomonas and klebsiella.

27. In smoke inhalation, the most important laboratory value is: Carbon monoxide level. Patient may appear with normal PaO_2 and oxygen saturation, but elevated carbon monoxide level.

28. Most common cause of **massive pulmonary atelectasis:** Postoperative patient.

29. A patient came back from operating room a few hours ago. The child started **desaturating;** examination showed diminished breathing sound on the (L) side and mediastinum shifted to the (L) side.

     Most common diagnosis: **Collapse of lung;** most common site is the **lower lobe. Bilateral collapse** needs **bronchoscopic** aspiration.

30. A fullterm newborn child was born with severe respiratory distress at birth.
     X-ray: Showed radiolucent (L) upper lobe, with shifting of mediastinum **to (R) side.**
     Dx: Congenital obstructive lobar emphysema.
     Tx: Surgical excision of the lobe.

31. Treatment for subcutaneous emphysema: No treatment necessary.

32. A child appears with tachypnea, **chest pain, cough** producing **frothy pink tinged sputum.** Medical history reveals either kidney or cardiac problem as the primary cause of

the present problem.

ON EXAM: Pale, mildly cyanotic.
CXR: **Butterfly-like** perihilar infiltrate.
Dx: Pulmonary **edema.**
Tx: Oxygen, diuretics, digoxin for cardiac failure which is non-obstructive type.
* Pulmonary edema also caused by poisoning with morphine, alcohol, barbiturate, epinephrine.
* High altitude pulmonary edema occurs within a few hours after reaching high altitude.

33.   Alpha 1 antitrypsin deficiency: It causes proteolytic destruction of pulmonary tissue resulting in **emphysema.** Normal person, pi-type MM; in this disease type ZZ. In emphysema there is growth failure, **clubbing,** increased anteroposterior diameter of the chest. **Tx** for emphysema: Nonspecific; antibiotics for infection, postural drainage of lung. History of allergy and administration of vaccine:
* Influenzae vaccine should be given every year.
* Do not give influenzae vaccine if patient is allergic to egg yolk.
* Do not give MMR vaccine if patient is allergic to neomycin.
* Do not give OPV vaccine if patient is allergic to streptomycin.

34.   An **obese** adolescent girl appears with acute onset of **substernal chest pain, radiates to the shoulder.**

ON EXAM: Pleural friction rub, rales, distant breathing sound, pain in **the calf muscle on palpation.**
CXR: Normal.
EKG: (R) ventricular hypertrophy.
Dx: Pulmonary embolism and infarction.
Tx: Heparin, oxygen.
* Pulmonary embolism occur from femoral, pelvic veins; it can occurs in sickle cell disease, cyanotic heart disease, ventriculoauricular shunt, bacterial endocarditis, severe dehydration.

35.   In a child with bronchiectasis, the most common underlying disease: Cystic fibrosis.

36.   Most common lobe involved in bronchiectasis: Right middle lobe.

37.   Most common lobe involved in hilar adenopathy: Right middle lobe.

38.   Most common lobe involved in foreign body aspiration: Right lower lobe.

39.   Middle lobe syndrome: It is due to compression of bronchus supplying middle lobe by the enlarged lymph nodes resulting in infection and bronchiectasis.

40.   A child with bronchiectasis receiving **antibiotic in aerosol form** for **long** period of time suddenly becomes very sick with high fever. Most common organism: Pseudomonas due to prolong use of aerosol therapy.

41.   A child appears with **hemoptysis** with **profuse** amount of **purulent sputum.** 10 days ago child had tonsilloadenoidectomy or went to dentist for tooth infection.

CXR: Cavity with or without fluid level.
Gram stain: Gram negative bacilli, poly.
Dx: Pulmonary abscess.

In pulmonary abscess most common organism is anaerobe treated with **penicillin.** Don't do bronchoscopy unless there is a foreign body. Don't do surgery unless you suspect of malignancy, repeated lung infection.

42.   Most common pulmonary malignancy in childhood: Metastatic lesion from Wilms' tumor. (Other metastatic lesions are osteosarcoma and hepatoblastoma).

43.   Most common cause of pleural effusion in children: Pneumococcal pneumonia.

44.   Dry pleurisy is mostly due to; Bacterial infection in lung and to tuberculosis. It involves mostly visceral pleura. Patient appears with chest pain which increases with coughing. **Friction rub appears in early stage** and **disappears later.** * Friction rub is also found in embolism.

45.   Most common organism in Empyema: Staph.aureus. It is common in infants and preschool children.

46.   Pneumothorax and features:

a.   It is common in staph. pneumonia.
b.   5% asthmatic hospitalized children can have it. It resolves spontaneously.
c.   It is found in cystic fibrosis.
d.   Spontaneous pneumothorax can occur in adolescents and young adults.
e.   Patients with collagen defect are prone to have it. e.g., Marfan syndrome, Ehlers-Danlos disease.
f.   It occurs spontaneously in newborns after first breathing.
g.   It occurs when bagging or ventilating child with high pressure or vigorous resuscitation.
h.   Asymptomatic patients do not need therapy.
i.   100% oxygen resolves pneumothorax.
j.   Tension pneumothorax needs chest tube.

47.   Most common cause of pneumomediastinum in older children and adolescents: Acute asthma.

48.   Pneumomediastinum and features:
a.   **Stabbing chest** pain which **radiates to the neck** is characteristic history.
b.   **Subcutaneous emphysema** is diagnostic, if present.
c.   Chest X-ray confirms the diagnosis.
d.   Symptomatic treatment is required.
e.   Resolves spontaneously.

49. Chylothorax and features:
    a. Most commonly found **after cardiac surgery.**
    b. Unilateral, mostly **in (L) side.**
    c. Chylothorax resolves spontaneously in 50% of infants who have it.
    d. Repeated thoracocentesis, which causes loss of calorie and protein, may be required.
    e. Should give low fat and high protein diet.

50. Asphyxiating thoracic dystrophy:
    a. Autosomal recessive.
    b. Appears with narrow thorax, short extremities.
    c. Influenzae vaccine to be given yearly to prevent infection.
    d. Progressive **renal** failure can occur.
    e. No specific therapy.

51. First restrictive then obstructive lung disease occurs in: Cystic fibrosis.

52. Cough **syncope** and features:
    a. Most commonly occurs in **asthmatics.**
    b. It is due to high intrathoracic pressure secondary to paroxysmal cough, reducing cardiac venous return, transient hypoxia to brain and syncope.
    c. No specific treatment.

53. Chromosome and cystic fibrosis: Chromosome 7 long arm.

54. Most common organism in infection with cystic fibrosis: Staph.aureus.

55. Older children with **cystic fibrosis** and X- ray sinuses: Diffuse sinusitis in all sinuses **except frontal sinus** which fails to develop. (In normal child, frontal sinus develops between **6 and 10** years of age).

56. **Prenatal diagnosis** of **cystic fibrosis: DNA analysis** of both parents to find the carrier status. DNA analysis of unborn child from **chorionic Villous sample** or **from amniotic fluid cells.** Location in **chromosome 7** middle of long arm.

57. A child shows signs of **dry hacking cough** which subsequently becomes **productive and occurs mostly in the morning or after running around. Past history of repeated admission for pneumonia. CHEST X-RAY** shows pneumonia in (R) lung **(upper lobe) and hyperinflation.**

    DX: Cystic fibrosis.
    LABORATORY: In serum **(low cl, low Na, alkaline pH).**
    DIAGNOSIS CONFIRMED BY: Sweat test **(more than 60 mEq/l of cl).**

    In **the newborn the most common** presentation of cystic fibrosis is **meconium ileus due to complete obstruction by thick sticky meconium,** develop signs and symptoms of intestinal obstruction.
    95% of males with **cystic fibrosis** have **normal** sexual function, but **are azoospermia**

(sterile) because of the defective development of Wolffian duct structure. Females with cystic fibrosis may have secondary amenorrhea probably due to pulmonary disease, **cervicitis,** blockage of cervical opening with sticky mucous, probably low fertility rate, but tolerate pregnancy well as long as pulmonary function is normal.

58.   **Newborn** with suspected cystic fibrosis and **sweat chloride test:** This test is **not** reliable in first two weeks of life. So it needs to be **repeated** after that time.

59.   **Diet** for one with cystic fibrosis: Low fat, high protein, high calorie, low roughage. Pancreatic enzyme supplement, Vitamin A,D, E, K.

60.   **Infant** with cystic fibrosis present with: **Rectal prolapse. TREATMENT:** Low roughage diet, surgery.

ADOLESCENT

1.   **Vaginal pH and age:**
First 3 weeks of life: pH 5.5 to 7.0 (acidic media resistent to bacterial growth).
3 weeks to menarche: **pH 6.5 to 7.4** (alkaline media good for bacterial growth).
After menarche: pH acidic **(less vulvovaginitis occur).**

2.   Scales type and skin disease:
Greasy scales: Seborrheic dermatitis.
Silvery scales: Psoriasis.

3.   Sex, drugs and academy recommendation: If adolescent is not sexually active, physician might suggest **'It's O.K. to say No'** to drugs and intercourse, as recommended by American Academy of Pediatrics and Ob/gyn.

4.   During gynecological examination of child, **presence of family members** is: **Helpful** for patient or physician or both in 86% cases.

5.   Most important **principle involved in pelvic exam:** To allow the **patient to be in control and command of** her body. **Patient should be** told what to expect during examination and should relax and be as comfortable as possible. For pediatric patients **frog-leg, knee-chest,** dorsal lithotomy position used are mostly. For **vulvovaginitis,** visualization of **only lower third of vagina is required.** Remember this.

6.   **Most common gynecologic problem** in childhood or adolescent: **Vulvovaginitis.** It is due to **lack of labial fat pad, lack of pubic hair,** labia minora open during squatting position, **proximity of vagina to anus, and** maybe masturbation. Thin atrophic vaginal squamous epithelium is due to low estrogen and alkaline pH which causes increased bacterial infection. Infection is **most common before pubertal age; after puberty protection** is due to increased estrogen, thick vaginal epithelium, and acidic pH (due to increased lactic and acetic acid).

7. Most common **type** of vulvovaginitis in childhood: **Nonspecific.** Non-specific vaginitis appears with **poor hygiene, brown or green discharge with bad smell and acidic vaginal** pH. **Most commonly** associated bacterial infection is **E. Coli from feces** (next is beta hemolytic Streptococcus and coagulase positive Staphylococci manually transmitted from nasopharynx). It is due to tight, rubber or plastic clothing, chemicals, soap, detergents.

   TREATMENT:
   Initial: Perineal hygiene, avoid those irritants, take sitz bath with mild soap, air- dry the vulva.
   Recurrent: Systemic amoxicillin or cephalosporin; estrogen or polysporin cream applied locally might help.

8. **Physiologic** vaginal discharge: Mostly occurs in the **6 to 12 months before** menarche, and appears with **yellow stain** in underpants. Discharge contains **Doderlein's bacilli.**
   TREATMENT: Reassurance.

9. Pathological vaginal discharge: It is due to **vulvitis,** vaginitis or both; vulvitis presents with **active vaginal** discharge, pruritus, **dysuria, local redness,** but **vaginitis** usuallyappears with **discharge only.** It is mostly due to poor hygiene, candida infection or foreign body.

10. Most common cause of **specific** vulvovaginitis in childhood: **Gardnerella vaginalis** (then candida, trichomonas). **TREATMENT:** Metronidazole.

11. **Labial adhesions:** Usually found in children younger **than 6 years** of age. They are either **asymptomatic** or show signs of recurrent UTI (20-40% cases) and local inflammation with hypoestrogenic effect of prepubertal age.

    TREATMENT:
    Asymptomatic: Reassurance (it disappears in **acidic pH** after puberty).
    Symptomatic: **Topical estrogen cream is treatment of choice;** mechanical separation advisable if it can be done easily and without trauma.

12. **Vaginal foreign body: Most common** foreign body is **wadded toilet paper.** Most common presentation is **vaginal bleeding,** second most common is smelly discharge. **DIAGNOSIS MADE:** X-ray or sonogram. **TREATMENT:** Removal.

13. **Breast diseases and management:**

    a. **Mastodynia:** Painful, engorged breast due to ovulatory menstrual cycle, found usually within 18 months of menarche. **TREATMENT:** Nonsteroidal, anti-inflammatory **analgesic** (Ibuprofen, naproxen sodium), **breast support** with bras.
    b. **Breast mass: Most common** mass is **fibroadenoma.** It is a **benign, asymptomatic mass;** in any breast tumor, **pediatrician should confer with radiologist** before conducting further investigations. Diagnosis usually confirmed **by biopsy.** Malignant tumor is rare. An important factor is the estrogen/androgen **ratio.** Androgen protects from malignancy.

c. **Macromastia or virginal hypertrophy: Massive, benign breast enlargement that** occurs mostly between the ages of 13 and 17 years. **It may be due either to an unknown** cause or to **increase estrogen sensitivity to receptors.** It appears with **discomfort and psychological problems. TREATMENT: Surgical reduction by mammoplasty is the treatment of choice** to be done in **late** adolescence to let the breast grow completely.

d. **Mastitis and abscess:** Antibiotics treatment.

e. **Trauma:** It is due to contact sports, causes **contusion, hematoma,** or fat necrosis, and resolves spontaneously. Late stage mimics malignancy, and is confirmed by biopsy.

f. **Mammary dysplasia:** It is due to hormonal imbalance, increased estrogen and decreased corpus luteum activity; appears with dysplasia in mostly the upper and outer quadrant. Diagnosis by mammography. Treated with synthetic androgen (danazol).

g. **Nipple discharge:**

h. Galactorrhea: Milk discharge, to be treated with **bromocriptine (dopamine agonist).**

i. Blood: In **duct ectasia,** or **intraductal papillomas; surgical consultation needed.**

14. Breast anomalies:

Amastia	Absence of breast (Polland syndrome and postoperative removal).
Athelia	Absence of nipple.
Polymastia	Supernumerary breast.
Polythelia	Supernumerary nipple.
Hypoplasia	Reduced size.

15. **Most common pelvic** tumor under 18 years: **Ovarian tumor. Most common ovarian tumor is teratoma. Most common presentation is abdominal pain, mass. Most characteristic X-ray finding is calcification in teratoma.**

Tumors mostly arise from **germ cells (most common is dysgerminoma).** Dysgerminoma is associated with **XY gonadal dysgenesis. Y-DNA probe helps to make the diagnosis.** Diagnosis made by **sonogram.**
TREATMENT: Surgical **removal of tumor.** Always check the **other ovary.** Specimen should be sent for **biopsy.**

16. Tumor markers are: Alpha feto protein, carcinoembryonic antigen, cancer antigen (CA) 125. They are helpful in detection of ovarian carcinoma.

17. Most common cause of **hirsutism** in adolescents: **Idiopathic.** Serum **androgen level is normal.** There may be **a decreased level of SHBG** (sex hormone binding globulin) which binds with androgen, resulting in **increased bioactive androgen.** ↑ SHBG level by estrogen and dexamethasone, ↓ SHBG level by androgen, testosterone; ↑ body weight caused ↓ SHBG level and vice versa. **Other causes of hirsutism are:**

a.   **HAIR-AN syndrome:** It is **acronym** for hirsutism, androgen excess, insulin resistance, acanthosis nigrans. **Of unknown** etiology, it may be defective in insulin receptors. Acanthosis due to ↑ androgen.

b.   Hyperprolactinemia.

c.   Polycystic ovary syndrome.

d.   21-hydroxylase deficiency in congenital adrenal hyperplasia.

e.   Ovarian hyperthecosis.

Treatment for idiopathic hirsutism and polycystic ovary syndrome. Estrogen (the predominant **oral contraceptive),** spironolactone, medroxy progesterone acetate, dexamethasone, cimetidine, GnRH agonist, cyproterone acetate.

18.   **Neonatal breast enlargement:** It is due to maternal estrogen present with a discharge called "witches milk". No treatment is required. It regresses spontaneously. Complication: Rarely causes mastitis due to Staph. infection which needs antistaphylococcal antibiotics.

19.   **Ovarian cysts (follicular):** Torsion of **ovarian cyst appears** with acute abdominal pain. It is **a surgical emergency.** Torsion of **adnexa** appears with acute, intermittent abdominal pain and radiation to ipsilateral lower extremity. **Diagnosis by sonogram.** Treatment of **unilateral torsion: Fix** the **contralateral normal ovary and adnexa.**

20.   **Ovarian autoamputation: Asymptomatic** patient, diagnosis occurs accidentally by **sonogram.** Autoamputation may be due to subclinical or antenatal ovarian **torsion** resulting in **necrosis, calcification, loss of blood supply.**

21.   Most common **cervical** neoplasm: **CIN** (cervical intraepithelial neoplasia).

22.   Most common **vaginal** carcinoma in childhood: **Sarcoma botryoides; surgery is** the treatment followed by postoperative therapy with vincristine, actinomycin-D, cyclophosphamide.

23.   Babies born to women who received DES (diethylstilbestrol) during pregnancy develop: **Adenosis** of vagina and cervix; rarely develops clear cell adenocarcinoma.

24.   **Constitutional tall stature:** Height is **more than 97%** or **more than 2 standard deviations** above the mean of the population; found in only 3% of the population. **TREATMENT:** Every patient should be treated individually. Treat the psychosocial, social and philosophical issues. **Rarely is** hormonal treatment with estrogens required.

25.   **Premature ovarian failure:**
It is **due to:**

a.   Gonadal dysgenesis.

b.   Gonadotropin-resistent ovarian syndrome.

c.   Ovarian tumors.

d.   Surgical removal or radio-or chemotherapy.
Patient appears with **secondary** amenorrhea and **hypogonadism.** Biopsy is not done routinely, but it can differentiate the following conditions:

e.   Primary ovarian failure: **No** oocytes or fewer in number.

f. Gonadotropin-resistant: Normal primordial follicles and unable to respond to gonadotropin.

g. Autoimmune: Lymphocytes and plasma cells around, but not near, the follicles.

TREATMENT: Exogenous **estrogens** and **progestin may** be added to the therapy.

26. A girl has a constitutionally **tall** stature. Which parameter decides the final adult height: **Bone age.**

27. **Estrogen treatment causes:**
a. Accelerated epiphyseal closure and reduced growth; develops secondary sexual characters and reduced acne.
b. Anxiety, neoplasm (of the genitalia, breast, or liver), thromboembolism, sterility, precipitate diabetes, gallstones, atherosclerosis.
c. Morning sickness, obesity, ↑ B.P., leukorrhea, pigmentation, night cramps.

28. Development of uterus and vagina:
Uterus: Formed from **caudal** element of mullerian duct.
Vagina: Formed from **terminal** portion of uterovaginal canal (Mullerial origin).

29. Most **frequently associated anomalies** of congenital absence of vagina (Mayer-Rokitansky-Küster-Hauser syndrome): **First renal and the skeletal anomalies** (most common **is unilateral renal agenesis).** This syndrome appears with **primary amenorrhea.**

30. Incomplete vertical fusion of vagina; This is due to **Mullerian agenesis,** together with **amenorrhea. Most commonly** associated anomaly **is renal (agenesis of one kidney)** and the skeletal.

INVESTIGATION: IVP, sonogram, bone age, chromosome.
TREATMENT: Vaginoplasty.
COMPLICATION of surgery: Squamous cell carcinoma. **Treated** with radiotherapy.

31. **Disease** and associated **mullerian anomaly:**

Mayer-Rokitansky-Küster-Hauser syndrome	Mullerian aplasia.
Kaufman-McCusick	Transverse vaginal septum.
Johnson-Blizzard, Camptobrachydactyly	Longitudinal vaginal septum.
Fraser syndrome	Incomplete mullerian fusion.
Uterine hernia syndrome	Persistent mullerian duct derivatives.

32. **Most commonly** associated **anomaly** of congenital atresia of uterine cervix: **Respiratory.** This anomaly appears with cryptomenorrhea, amenorrhea, and pelvic pain.

33. **Delayed menarche** occurs in athletes: Ballet, figure skating, gymnastics (average age of

menarche for athletes is 13.58 years; for non-athletes, 12.23 years). **Remember,** delayed menarche does **not** occur in swimmers.

Ballet: Delayed thelarche (breast) and menarche (menstruation), but pubarche and adrenarche are not affected.
Secondary amenorrhea in long distance runner is due to **decreased spontaneous luteinizing hormone pulse frequency.** Remember, secondary amenorrhea in athletes is a **diagnosis of** exclusion, so athletes should be investigated as would be nonathletes. **Most common cause of secondary amenorrhea is pregnancy,** so a test for **pregnancy and for FSH and LH levels should be done.**

34. Most common cause of death in adolescent: MVA. (motor vehicle accident). Most of such deaths (63%) occur while adolescent is the driver. Other accidents are due to sports injury and drowning.

35. Most common **underlying cause** of MVA in adolescent: **Alcohol.** Other causes are: not using a seat belt while in car a or wearing a helmet while on a motorcycle. **Most** accidents happen to **males** and between **8 pm to 4 am.** Lowering drinking age to 18 years causes a 5% increase of MVA. **Drivers educational classes bring more young drivers on the street, and this increases the likelihood of more MVA. Pediatrician** should give anticipatory guidance to adolescent and support legislation targeted to increase drinking age and mandatory use of seat belts and helmets.

36. **Athlete** and **premenstrual tension (PMT): Less PMT** due to ↓ ADH and ↑ beta endorphin.

37. **Hallmark for the depression** of young people:
    a. Persistence of depressed moods (lasting at **least 3 consecutive hours for 3 times or more in 7 days).**
    b. Absence of elation.
    c. Hopelessness and helplessness.
    d. Unable to function.

It is difficult to determine by **looking at their sad faces which adolescents are at risk** for suicide or true depression.

38. Diagnosis of **depression in adolescents:** Diagnosis can be inferred from poor school performance, frequently absence from school, alcohol or drug use, proneness to accidents. They can mask depression by alternating with euphoria, acting out behavior and sexual promiscuity. Disturbances of sleep and eating **indicate a severe problem.** It is not found in early stages, **unlike in the case of adults.** Adolescents may have **insomnia, or sleep all day, wake up during the night,** and yet are always tired. **There is strong positive family history, particularly in cases of suicide.**

39. A child **with suicidal thoughts:** Must be seen by **psychiatrist immediately.** Child might look happy at time of visit to physician, so it might be difficult to find out about present **plans for suicide. Remember,** if the child **has not** mentioned suicide, **do not** ask about it. Physician should **care for the patient in such a way that** so patient feels comfortable.

40. **Suicide: Female attempts suicide more** often than males, but **males are more successful.** Suicide is common among native Americans and Asian Americans and also in **adolescents with chronic diseases** (feelings of impotence, easily gets the medicine, feeling of loss over the death of a loved one).

41. **Breast problem** in athletes: Mastodynia, nipple irritation occurs; breast injury is uncommon. **TREATMENT:** Proper fitting bra (not too tight); adhesive strip bandage or nursing pad for nipple irritation.

42. Mentally retarded with gynecological problem: Needs **adequate** gynecological examination. **Outpatient sedation** with oral ketamine and midazolam decrease the need for examination under anaesthesia. For **any surgery,** procedure should be discussed with guardian or custodian. **An ethics advisory committee** should be consulted. For suppression of menses, depomedroxyprogesterone acetate given I.M. Q 6-12 weeks.

43. **Remember** the following **points** when patient attempts suicide:
    a. Any attempt or gesture should be considered serious.
    b. Anybody who attempted suicide before should be considered more serious because future attempts are usually more successful.
    c. Family history of suicide is significant.
    d. Suicide note should be considered serious.
    e. It is **not serious** when somebody grabs a bottle of medicine and tells everybody that he/she wants to commit suicide.

44. **Short term hospitalization** is important for patients who have attempted suicide because:
    a. It provide a secure place for the patient.
    b. It impresses the parents that problems needs to be attended to.
    c. **Most important are the psychosocial evaluation** and appropriate recommendations. (About one third of the patients follow the recommendations).
    d. Expert psychiatrist should evaluate the patient.

45. Most common **method** used for suicide in adolescents: **Ingestion of medication.** Most commonly used drug is tricyclic antidepressant (TCA). Violent methods (hanging, shooting, wrist slashing) mostly used by **males. MANAGEMENT:** Unit dose medication or bubble pack should be used.

46. Most commonly used drug by teenagers: Alcohol or marijuana (90%).

47. Substance abuse by teenagers: 66% of teenagers use illicit drug before finishing high school. 40% of them use an other drug along with marijuana. One in 18 high school seniors smoke cigarettes or drink alcohol daily.

48. **'Problem drinking'** is defined as:
    a. Drunk six times or more in the past year.
    b. Negative consequences of drinking three or more times in the past year (trouble with teachers, friends, parents).

49. Illicit drugs use and effects:

    a.   Heroin: Secondary amenorrhea due to effects on hypothalamic-pituitary-ovarian axis.

    b.   Ethanol: Body protein intake was deprived, so their is reduced muscle strength. Ethanol provides most calories.

    c.   Amphetamine: Interferes with stage 4 sleep.

50.   **Prevention** of drug use: **Teach the adolescent** not to use it and ignore peer pressure.

51.   Drug interactions and their effects:

    a.   Estrogen and alcohol: Estrogen **increases** alcohol toxication because of reduced ethanol metabolism.

    b.   Barbiturate and alcohol: Additive effect.

    c.   Metronidazole and alcohol: It causes vomiting and abdominal pain because antagonistic effect of alcohol on aldehyde.

52.   **Amotivational syndrome:** It is found in **the chronic marijuana user.** Regular use of any illicit drug incapacitates the user in the performance of regular daily tasks (at work, school, college).

53.   **Treatment** of drug abuse: **Detoxification,** then long-term medical follow-up and psychosocial support.

54.   **Abuse of opiates:** Opiates are **heroin and methadone. Heroin** is formed from **opium** and hydrolysed to **morphine** which conjugates with glucuronic acid in liver. Heroin causes **euphoria and analgesia.** It is detected in urine by chromatography **up to 48 hours** of administration.

55.   Most common cause of death in opiate (heroin) users: **Overdose syndrome. It appears** with seizure, **constricted** pupils, **respiratory depression,** cyanosis, **pulmonary edema,** stupor or coma. **Remember, death is due to pulmonary edema.**

    DIAGNOSIS confirmed by Morphine in serum. **TREATMENT:** Naloxone 0.01 mg/kg (opiate antagonist). In methadone toxicity, it may be needed for 24 hours. Supportive therapy (oxygen).

56.   Important effects of opiates (heroin) in different systems:

    a.   Respiratory: **Depression by central** inhibition. Asymptomatic patients may have pulmonary edema in X-ray, but pulmonary infection is **not** common.

    b.   CNS: **Euphoria, analgesia,** EEG-pattern-like sleep, hypothermia (by inhibiting hypothalamus), transverse myelitis; rarely Guillain-Barre syndrome, toxic amblyopia (due to quinine additive).

    c.   CVS: Vasodilatation.

    d.   Skin: **Most common is 'track'** (hypertrophic linear scar).

    e.   Muscle: Acute rhabdomyolysis with myoglobinuria after I.V. use appears with weakness, edema, tenderness.

    f.   Infection: **Most common organism is Staph. aureus;** cerebral abscess, endocarditis and HIV.

    g.   G.I.: Constipation (by inhibiting peristalsis and increaseing tone of rectal muscles).

h.   Immunologic: ↑ IgM (I.V.user), ↑ IgA (inhalation).

57.   **Earliest sign** of opiates (heroin) withdrawal: **Yawning.** Opiate withdrawal or abstinence syndrome occurs when heroin was not used for 8 hours or more, symptoms appear, up to 36 hours, with **lacrimation, dilated** pupils, **gooseflesh,** voluntary muscles cramp, diarrhea, ↑ H.R., ↑ B.P.

TREATMENT:
For detoxification: Valium.
Alternate therapy for detoxification: Methadone (it is a synthetic opiate, whose pharmacologic effect **is the same as heroins** except **there is no** euphoria. It is **not** yet considered safe for adolescents and children).

58.   Most commonly used hallucinogen: **PCP (phencyclidine).** Others are mushroom, jimsonweed, and LSD.

59.   **PCP (Phencyclidine): Mechanism of action:** Enhanced adrenergic effect by inhibiting neuronal reuptake of catecholamine.

Signs and symptoms: It is dose-related.
1-5 mg: Appears with euphoria, ataxia, nystagmus, emotional lability and distorted body image causing panic reaction.
5-15 mg: Toxic psychosis, hyperventilation, **abusive language.**
> 15 mg: Dystonia, hypotension, generalized convulsion, arrythmia.

Remember, PCP causes coma, but **does not** cause respiratory depression, **unlike** heroin, morphine. PCP can be made at home, and one of its **byproducts** causes **cramps, hematemesis, diarrhea.**

Treatment:
a.   Diazepam: If patient is agitated but not comatose.
b.   Ammonium chloride: It enhances excretion of PCP by changing urine pH acidic.
c.   Hydration: Because PCP cause sdiuresis.
d.   Keep the patient in a dark, quiet room with floor pads to prevent injury by fall.

60.   **Mushroom intoxication:** It has both cholinergic and anticholinergic effects; appears with **hallucination, euphoria (LSD-like symptoms** due to psilocybin and anticholinergic indole). TREATMENT: Induce vomiting, give activated charcoal.

61.   **Jimsonweed intoxication: CNS depression** and **anticholinergic effects** (dry skin, dry mouth, fever, dilated pupils, urinary retention), visual and auditory **hallucination.**
TREATMENT: Physostigmine (anticholinesterase). **(Physostigmine over**dose should be treated with **atropine).**

62.   **Volatile substances:**
a.   **Gasoline sniffing: Euphoria followed by violent behavior,** leads to encephalopathy.
b.   **Airplane glue: Toluene** is main ingredient, which is excreted in urine as **hippuric**

acid. Appears initially with relaxation, pleasant hallucination, person develops tolerance of and physical dependence on the drug.

Acute: Death is due to cerebral and pulmonary edema.

Chronic: Restrictive lung disease, pulmonary hypertension, peripheral neuropathy, tubular acidosis and CNS atrophy.

c. **Aerosol inhalation** (hair spray, deodorant): Arrythmia (due to epinephrine sensitization), death.

d. **Volatile nitrites (found in room deodorizer):** Euphoria, **patient appreciates music,** syncope, ↓ **B.P.,** skin flushing, followed by vasoconstriction and tachycardia.

EKG: Transient **inverted T wave and depressed ST segment. Methemoglobinemia, bronchospasm, increased intraocular pressure.**

63. Identical effects of both marijuana and alcohol: **Diminished short term memory and** coordination, causing **mental cloudiness,** prolong reaction time.

64. Hallucination in marijuana is due to: **(THC) Tetrahydrocannabinol** fraction of the resin of cannabinis sativa plant.

65. **Marijuana intoxication:** Euphoria, **diminished short term memory, loss** of judgement and time perception, **(rarely** causes distorted body image, visual hallucination **which is common in PCP), recall of frightening hallucinations** in stress or fever, ↓ temperature. ↑ H.R. (but ↑ **RR** only in experienced user). It **reduces** bronchospasms and intraocular pressure (in normal people and glaucoma patients).

66. **Important points to remember** for marijuana use:
    a. **No** physical dependence, **no** withdrawal symptoms.
    b. **No** teratogenic and carcinogenic effects **in humans.**
    c. **Increased appetite** (can be used in cancer patients with reduced appetite).
    d. **Reduced spermatogenesis and testosterone level,** may inhibit pubertal growth and development. It **is dose related:** used 4 days/week **for 6 months.**
    e. Reduce glucose tolerance if used more than 1 week.

67. Excretory product of cocaine: **Benzoyl ecgonine in urine.** Cocaine is expensive, absorbed rapidly from nasal mucosa, **metabolized in liver** and **excreted through kidney.**

68. **Cocaine intoxication:**
    Signs and symptoms: Euphoria, **decreased fatigue, increased motor activities,** ↑ H.R., ↑ B.P. ↑ temperature. **TREATMENT:** Supportive treatment and chronic medical follow up and psychosocial support.

69. **Important points to remember** for cocaine:
    a. **No** physical dependence, **no** withdrawal symptoms.
    b. **Psychological dependence afflicts** chronic user.
    c. **Increased** sexual promiscuity and greater risk of sexually transmitted disease when used in **a group** setting.
    d. Effects on fetus: **May develop** premature and LBW babies; congenital malformation (urogenital and others); developmental disorders.

70. **Effects of smoking cigarettes (chronic):**
    a. ↓ **globulin in female,** ↓ **uric acid in male.**
    b. It **enhances theophylline** metabolism by stimulating hepatic smooth endoplasmic reticulum; similar effects on endogenous hormones and some other drugs.
    c. Reduced fetal weight (dose related) by 200 gm.
    d. Chronic cough, wheezing.
    e. May cause ↓ (WBC, Hgb, Hct, MCV, creatinine, albumin), ↑ platelet aggregation.

71. **Metabolism of alcohol:**
    Absorbed from intestine and **metabolized in liver by two different pathways:**

    a. 1st pathway: Alcohol forms acetaldehyde **through alcohol dehydrogenase with** cofactor NAD, increases triglyceride causing **fatty liver** which, after necrosis and fibrosis, forms **cirrhosis.** Serum: ↑ GGTP, ↑ SGPT in **early** stages.
    b. **2nd pathway:** High serum alcohol through microsomal system with cofactor NADPH, results in reduced other drug metabolism and increased accumulation of drug (tranquilizer).
    (NADPH = Nicotinamide-adenine dinucleotide phosphate).

72. **Legal definition of alcohol** intoxication: Blood ethanol level **100 mg/dl or more.**

73. **Alcohol intoxication:**

    Signs and symptoms: Primary site of action is **CNS** occuring with euphoria, reduced short term memory, talkativeness, ↓ temperature. **Respiratory depression in high levels. Inhibits ADH** secretion results in **diuresis. Most common G.I. symptom is acute, erosive gastritis** occuring with abdominal pain, vomiting, guaiac (+)ve stool.
    DIAGNOSIS: Serum and breath analysis (level above 200 mg/dl has death risk and above 500 mg/dl has fatal outcome).

    TREATMENT:
    a. **Ventilator support:**   For respiratory depression.
    b. **Dialysis:** If blood level is above 400 mg/dl.
    c. **Chlordiazepoxide (Librium, benzodiazepine derivative):** For withdrawal or abstinence syndrome.
    [serum alcohol level drops from **400 to 0 level in 20 hours** without alcoholism].

74. **Important points to remember** in alcohol intoxication:
    a. **Physical dependence** occurs, so patient develops **withdrawal or abstinence syndrome** which begins **after 8 hours** and **lasts** up to 48 hours since last dose is taken. It appears with **insomnia, irritability, tremor, anxiety; rarely it** appears with hallucination (visual, auditory), hyperthermia, seizure those who are taking alcohol for 1 year or more.
    b. Respiratory depression is the cause of death.

75. **Sleep and growth: Complete sleep cycle** stimulates **growth by stimulating growth hormone and gonadotropin; only occurs in early puberty.** This is **not** found in anorexia nervosa. In SMR (sexual maturity rating) **3 and 4,** there is increased day time

sleep and decreased sleep latency.

76. **Important effects to remember for anabolic steroid use:**
    a. Male: Gynecomastia, atrophic testes, ↓ testosterone, ↓ gonadotropin.
    b. Female: Breast atrophy, enlarge clitoris, anovulatory menstrual abnormality, hirsutism or alopecia.
    c. CVS: ↑ LDL, ↓ HDL.
    d. **Growth:** Final height is **reduced** because of advanced epiphyseal closure, **ultimate muscle mass and strength does not improve.**
    e. **Psychological effects:** Occurs only in very high (100 times) doses, appears with **rage,** mania, depression, mood swings and alternation of sexual desire (libido).

77. Sleep **apnea-hypersomnia syndrome:** It is found in adolescence. First there is brief apnea (due to obstruction) at night resulting in his waking up several times briefly during the night, **thus** disturbing his sleep resulting in **exaggerated sleep in daytime.**

78. Most common cause of apnea in adolescence: Depression or delayed sleep phase syndrome **(delay in falling asleep,** but once sleep is started, there is no disturbance).

79. Contraceptive which helps prevent STD (sexually transmitted disease) and HIV: **Condom.**

80. **Narcolepsy syndrome** includes:
    a. During wakefulness there is REM sleep and exaggerated day time sleep.
    b. Sleep paralysis: Paralysis of voluntary muscles while falling asleep.
    c. Catalepsy: Sudden hypotonia of muscle group.
    d. Hallucinations (hypnagogic and visual), frighten.

81. Treatment for anorexia nervosa:
    a. **Recently, antidepressant medications have** been used with success.
    b. Psychotherapy (patient and family members).
    c. Nutritional therapy.
    d. Modification of behavior by therapy.

82. Important points to remember about anorexia nervosa and bulimia: (**Mostly in female, of all socioeconomic classes).**
    a. DSM-IIIR (Diagnostic and Statistical Manual of Mental Disorder) criteria for diagnosis of AN (anorexia nervosa):
        i. Tremendous fear of becoming obese.
        ii. 'They feel fat' even when they are emaciated.
        iii. **They do not** maintain body weight, but rather are 15% below than expected.
        iv. Amenorrhea for 3 consecutive months (primary or secondary).
    b. Anorexia nervosa :
        i. It is divided into , **restrictor** (restricted intake of food) and **bulimia** (binge eating followed by vomitting).
        ii. ANOREXICS are **active, good students**.
        iii. They deny their hunger, and have bizarre food habits.
    c. DSM-IIIR **distinguishes** bulimia from anorexia nervosa:
        i. It is more common than AN.

ii. Recurrent episodes of "binge" eating (i.e., eating a lot of food in two hours) then vomiting because fear of **uncontrolled** eating habit.

iii. Induced vomiting, use of laxative or severe dieting, fasting after binge eating.

iv. At least 2 binges per week for at least 3 months.

83. **Clinical presentations of anorexia nervosa (AN) and bulimia:**

a. Reduced REM, **hypothermia,** amenorrhea (due to defect in hypothalamic-pituitary-ovarian axis and ↓ **LH secretion due to hypothalamic defect)** which may **persist up to 8 years in 25% of patients despite weight gain,** constipation, esophagitis.

b. ↑ cortisol secretion, ↑ GH (growth hormone), ↓ somatomedin C.

c. ↓ T4, ↓ T3, TSH ⇁, ↑ reverse T3 (due to adaptation in low BMR due to malnutrition).

d. ↑ ADH causes peripheral edema (in some patients) **without** cardiac failure.

e. ↑ BUN, ↓ GFR (glomerular filtration rate) due to dehydration.

f. Urine: Mild protein, RBC, WBC; no bacteria.

g. CBC: ↓ WBC, ↓ RBC, rarely ↓ platelet, ↓ ESR (due to ↓ fibrinogen production from malnutrition).

h. ↑ Amylase due to bilateral parotitis, pancreatitis.

i. SMA6: ↓ K, ↓ Cl, (hypochloremic alkalosis).

j. **Very resistant to infection** (due to normal immune status and relatively good protein intake).

k. Skin: Dry, lanugo hair; **hair loss during overfeeding** state.

l. **Death: Due to electrolyte imbalance,** cardiac arrythmia or CHF (congestive heart failure) in recovery phase.

m. Heart: ↓ HR, ↓ B.P. (postural, improved with nutrition).

EKG: Low voltage, inverted T wave, ST depression, supraventricular and ventricular arrythmia.

84. Drug of choice for **syphilis (primary and secondary):** Benzathine penicillin (2.4 million units I.M.); except **in newborns,** use aqueous or procaine penicillin. Remember, benzathine penicillin does **not** cross the blood-brain barrier well.

85. **Important points to remember,** about pregnancy in **adolescent** mother:

a. Children born to adolescent mother are more prone to have **hospitalization** and **accidents** even at home.

b. Adolescent mothers have more children, are usually not married, and don't complete high school education.

c. **Most** pregnancies are **unintended,** and <50% use mostly ineffective contraceptives during 1st intercourse.

d. First medical advice is usually one year after 1st intercourse. 40% become pregnant within 2 years of 1st intercourse.

e. For successful pregnancy prevention, **motivation, information and availability of contraceptives are necessary.**

f. Pediatrician should enquire, as to why a sexually active female thinks that she is not risking becoming pregnant.

g. **Abstinence** from sexual activity is usually **not** accepted.

h. Many girls think that they are **sterile** because they have not become pregnant despite sexual activity.

i. **REMEMBER,** physician can give contraceptives to minor without telling the parents.

86. Post-coital contraception with DES (diethylstilbestrol): DES should be given within 72 hours of unprotected sex, but reluctantly, as a last resort, **because DES is teratogenic.**

87. Drug of choice for gonorrhea: **Ceftriaxone (250 mg I.M. single dose):** It is also effective in incubating syphilis. Partner should also be treated. If infection occurs in **higher pelvic organs,** give cefoxitin and doxycycline for 10 days. In **case of disseminated infection** (arthritis) give ceftriaxone for 7 days I.V.

88. Drug of choice for prophylactic treatment of syphilis in **rape** victim: **Ceftriaxone** single dose.

89. Complications of gonococcal infection (sterility, conjunctivitis) most likely due to: Associated **chlamydia** infection.

90. **Investigation of choice** to make etiologic diagnosis of salpingitis: **Laparoscopy** with tubal puncture and culture; rule out GC and chlamydia.

91. Most virulent strain of GC (gonococcus): **Piliated strains** (P+, P++ previously called T1, T2 respectively; others are non-piliated and avirulent colonies p- (previously called T3 or T4).

92. **Most of the girls have menarche** in which SMR: **SMR4 (60%)** (20% in SMR 3, 10% each in SMR 2, 5).

93. Anatomical structure and physiologic function needed for normal menstruation: Hypothalamus with higher center (pineal gland), anterior pituitary, ovary and uterus.

94. Most common cause of amenorrhea: Primary (menstruation never occurs): **imperforate hymen.** Secondary: menstruation stops for three months e.g., **pregnancy.**

Primary: ↑ FSH, ↑ LH means ovarian failure.
Secondary: ↓ FSH, ↓ LH means pituitary or hypothalamic failure.
Imperforate hymen is diagnosed by inspection. Blood filled-vagina is called **hematocolpos,** and blood filled uterus is called **hematometrium.**

95. **Diagnosis of amenorrhea:**
   a. History and complete physical examination.
   b. CBC, ESR to rule out systemic disease.
   c. Pregnancy test.
   d. Serum level: FSH, LH, prolactin, T4, T3, TSH
   e. CNS lesion: CT or MRI of head.
   f. Adrenal cause: Urine 17 ketosteroid level.
   g. Pelvic mass: Sonogram.
   h. Exploratory laparoscopy and ovarian biopsy.

96. **Treatment for amenorrhea:** It depends upon the cause of amenorrhea, so try to **correct the underlying problem.** When it is not possible to correct the cause, then **look for psychological reason** that produces **pseudo-menses.** First look for vaginal smear. If there is any **estrogen effect,** then **menstruation** can begin after **medroxyprogesterone treatment.**

    In gonadal dysgenesis: First, **give conjugated estrogen** (premarin) **followed by medroxyprogesterone.**

97. Most common cause of (DUB) dysfunctional uterine bleeding:

    Anovulatory cycle. It occurs mostly in first year postmenarche. It is due to action of estrogen on endometrium, which is not opposed by progesterone, which is secreted after ovulation. Estrogen causes continued endometrial proliferation and massive bleeding. Estrogen inhibits LH, so LH is less than FSH.

    TREATMENT: Oral 25 mg **norethynodrel (enovid)** should be given immediately. Bleeding stops with in 2 hours. Taper later doses. It corrects the **imbalance between estrogen and progesterone.**

98. An adolescent appears with **excessive first menstrual** bleeding. Always rule out:

    Coagulopathies (Von-Willebrand disease): ↑ **bleeding time,** ↓ **factor VIII level** and defect in platelet adhesiveness. **TREATMENT:** Same as DUB; in addition, **oral contraceptive during** each menstruation for the rest of her life.

99. Estrogen and factor VIII: Estrogen **increase s**factor VIII level.

100. Excessive menstrual bleeding due to thrombocytopenia management: Same as DUB; in addition, platelet transfusion may be necessary.

101. Dysmenorrhea:

    Types: Primary and secondary.
    It is found in 66% of post-menarcheal teenagers, **primary more common** than secondary.

    Secondary: Due to structural defect (cervix, uterus), foreign body (IUD, endometritis, endometriosis).
    Normal pelvic examination means primary amenorrhea.
    Primary: ↑ **prostaglandin F2α , E2** produced by myometrium, prostaglandin stimulates myometrium to contract and cause pain.

    TREATMENT:
    Primary: **Naproxen sodium** (prostaglandin synthetase inhibitor) usually for 1 day.
    (teenager with dysmenorrhea can use oral contraceptive.)
    Secondary: Correct the cause.

102. How to make diagnosis of excessive bleeding due to abortion: **B-subunit HCG**

pregnancy tests. It is positive **up to 15 days** after abortion; other pregnancy tests become negative within 5-8 days.

103. **PMS (premenstrual syndrome), treatment of choice: Gonadotropin releasing hormone agonist** (on a short term basis). Do not use vitamin B_6 and progesterone.

104. Important findings to remember in **PMS:**
    a. **Not** common in adolescents.
    b. **Not** associated with dysmenorrhea.
    c. It occurs in **late luteal phase** (second half of menstrual cycle).
    d. 33% of women of reproductive age have PMS.
    e. It appears with increased appetite **(stronger desire for sweets and salty foods),** fatigue, headache, **depression,** loss of concentration, **mood swings,** violent behavior, tenderness and fullness in breast.

105. Most common adolescent breast disorder: **Mass** (either cyst or fibroadenoma). Cyst: It varies in size with menstruation, so patient should be **reexamined in two weeks. Indication for surgical consultation: persistence** of mass or **its enlargement** in three menstrual cycles.

    First, aspirate the mass. If **no** fluid, then **perform excision biopsy** by circumareolar incision to prevent scar formation. **Most common finding** in biopsy: **Fibroadenoma** (71%).

106. **Endometriosis,** things to remember:
    a. Ectopic location of endometrial tissue, **most common site is peritoneal cavity.**
    b. Characteristics presentation is **severe pain** during menstruation.
    c. Diagnosis by **sonogram or laparoscopy.**
    TREATMENT: Oral contraceptive; in severe cases use **danazol** (antigonadotropin).

107. An adolescent appears with **several small lumps in the breast. Most likely diagnosis: Fibrocystic disease.** It can change to other diseases in the future.
    TREATMENT:
    a. Give advice and teach patient how to examine her breasts routinely.
    b. Oral contraceptives with low progesterone.

108. Contact sports and herpetic skin infection: **Wresting** can cause herpes due to contact.

109. **Tsetse syndrome: Costochondritis** of sternoclavicular junction occurs in adolescence.

110. **Male** physician examining an **adolescent female: Chaparone** should be present (because an increasing number of cases of sexual misconduct has been reported). If it is other way around (female physician examining adolescent male), chaperoning is **not** indicated.

111. Important points to remember about in **legal issues;**
    a. **Emancipated minor:** Lives away from home, married, self-supporting, or belongs to military service. They are allowed to give consent.
    b. **Mature minor role:** Many minors are very mature and are allowed to give consent

for their treatment.

c.   **Emergency situation:** In case of **life-threatening emergency,** physician can treat the patient without consent.
    In all cases, **physician should document his decisions in the chart properly.**

d.   Minors can give consent for pelvic examination and treatment of STD (sexually transmitted disease).

e.   Abortion and use of contraceptives by minors are **not** settled.

f.   Age for blood donation is 18 years **except** in Delaware (17 years).

g.   **Organ donation in minor: Both parental consent and court order are necessary.**
    First, try to find adult donor. If one not found and it is an emergency, make sure that the adolescent does not suffer physically or psychologically.

112.   **Screening tests** for normal adolescent:

a.   **Pap smear** should be done for all sexually active women regardless of age, because incidence of early neoplastic changes is 5-35/1000 examined.
    Two successive smears have 26% higher yield than one smear.

b.   Tuberculous testing.

c.   Urinalysis and urine culture during early adolescence.

d.   HIV testing for high risk patient.

e.   To find out genetic carrier state.

113.   **Androgen and Hematocrit:** It is directly proportional. SMR 1 male has Hct is 39%, whereas in **SMR 5** has **43%** (average).

114.   An adolescent, in routine physical examination, shows hypertension in **first** reading: Repeat the blood pressure test 2 to 3 times, changing the cuff size. **Most** of them has labile hypertension, 50% of them will develop hypertension in adult age. No antihypertensive is necessary in an emergency. Whether low salt diet will prevent adolescent hypertension to adult hypertension is not known.

115.   Most common testicular tumor in late adolescence and adult: **Germ cell tumor.** So, palpation of testes can diagnose early onset tumor.

116.   Most common time **for scoliosis** to occur in adolescent: **Peak height velocity** time (12 years in female and 14 years in male).

117.   **Immunization** in adolescent: **dT** at 15 years; **MMR** at 11-12 years.

NEUROLOGY

1.   Retinal hemorrhage and mode of delivery: **30 to 40% of normal full term** babies have retinal hemorrhage. It is more common in **vaginal** than cesarean section deliveries, **not** associated with birth trauma and **no** neurologic complications.
    TREATMENT: None. Problem usually **disappears** by 1-2 weeks of age.

2. Normal rate of head growth in **healthy premature:**
    0.5 cm in 1st 2 weeks.
    0.75 cm in 3rd week.
    1.0 cm in 4th week and after until 40 weeks.

3. When child achieves 20/20 (adult level) vision: 6 months of age (at birth it is 20/150).

4. **Premature baby** and its **response to light:**

    28 weeks: Blinks.
    29 weeks: Pupils react to light.
    32 weeks: Keeps its eyes closed until light is removed.
    37 weeks: Turns its head away from bright light.

5. **Nystagmus:** Involuntary rapid movement of eyes.

    Two types:
    a. Vertical: Indicates brain stem dysfunction.
    b. Horizontal: Indicates peripheral **labyrinth** abnormality or lesion in **vestibular** system or lesion in **cerebellum.**

6. **Vision test for 2-1/2 to 3-year-**old child: `E game' ,i.e., point finger in the direction of `E', because they cannot read Snellen eye chart.

7. **Ocular movement: Complete ocular movement** can be seen by 25 weeks gestational age by **doll's eye maneuver.** This maneuver is used to examine **horizontal and vertical eye movement.** "Doll's eye"refers to what is seen when the head is suddenly turned to the right and then both eyes look to the **left symmetrically.**

    Horizontal **slight** dysconjugate eye movement can be seen in premature infant, but **remember vertical dysconjugate** (skewed deviation of eyes) **movement is always abnormal.**

8. **Caloric test** to detect vestibular function: It is done for **comatose** patient. Introduce 5 cc of ice water into external auditory canal (make sure tympanic membrane is intact), then look for any **nystagmus in the opposite** direction of stimulated labyrinth. That is the **normal** response. It is absent in brain-dead patient.

9. Werdnig-Hoffmann disease and cranial nerve involvement: 12th. It innervates the tongue. Fasciculation of tongue occurs in this disease.

10. Type II Chiari malformation and cranial nerve involved: 10th (vagus). Paralysis causes **weakness of soft palate and hoarse voice** due to vocal cord paralysis.

11. Testing of 9th cranial nerve (glossopharyngeal): **Gag response** after touching **posterior pharyngeal wall.** Taste sensation of posterior third of tongue by same cranial nerve.

12. Eye muscle **paralysis** due to cranial nerves involvement and eye position:

3rd cranial nerve: Eye outward, downward; (dilated pupil, ptosis).
4th cranial nerve: Eye outward, upward.
6th cranial nerve: Eye deviated medially.

In older child, **red glass test** is used to diagnose extraocular palsy.
3rd: Oculomotor.
4th: Trochlear.
6th: Abducens nerve.

13.   **Horner syndrome** includes: Miosis, ptosis, enophthalmos, ipsilateral anhydrosis. It is either **congenital** or a lesion in **sympathetic** nervous system in brain stem, cervical spinal cord or **sympathetic plexus** near the carotid artery.

14.   Presence of **polymorph in CSF of a child: Always abnormal,** except normal newborns may have **1-2 cells** per mm^3. In children **up to 5, lymphocytes** are normal.

Normal CSF glucose: 60% of serum glucose level.
Normal CSF protein: 10-40 mg/dl (child), 120 mg/dl in neonate.
Normal CSF opening pressure: Less than 160 mm of water.
(CSF protein in newborns is reduced to **childhood range by 3 months;** in bloody tap, every 1000 RBC/mm^3 increases the protein by 1 mg/dl).
↑ CSF IgG found in: Subacute sclerosing panencephalitis; post infectious encephalomyelitis; some cases of multiple sclerosis.

15.   Most common **cause** of increased intracranial pressure: **Crying.**

16.   Normal Babinski reflex:
      a.   Adult and child: **Extension** of great toe and fanning of other toes.
      b.   Newborn: Initial **flexion** of great toe.

17.   Most common congenital anomalies of CNS: **Neural tube defects. They are** due to the failure of closure of neural tube between 3-4 weeks. **Rostral (cephalic) end closes by the 25th day and caudal end by the 27th day.**

18.   Most common type of neural tube defects: **Spina bifida occulta.** Most common site is L5 and S1.

19.   In female with meningomyelocele, what other organ is involved? Genital tract (rectovaginal fistula, vaginal septa).

20.   Most common associated anomaly in meningomyelocele: **Hydrocephalus** with type II chiari effect. So sonogram, CT, MRI should be done.

21.   Most severe form of neural tube defects (dysraphism) involving vertebral column: **Meningomyelocele;** etiology is **not known,** incidence is 1:1,000 live births.

22.   Most common site for meningomyelocele: Lumbosacral region (75% cases).

23. **Clinical presentations** of meningomyelocele: It depends on the site of location.
    a. **Low sacral:** Incontinence of bowel and bladder, anaesthesia in perineal area, intact motor function.
    b. **Midlumber: Lower** extremities flaccid paralysil; lack of pain and sensation of touch; absence of deep tendon reflexes; abnormalities of lower extremities (club feet and hip subluxation); urinary incontinence; and relaxed anal sphincter **(lower motor neurone effect).**
    c. **Lower thoracic:** More neurologic deficit than midlumber defect.
    d. **Upper thoracic and cervical: Minimal** neurologic defect and mostly does **not** cause hydrocephalus.

24. **Risk of recurrence** of meningomyelocele:

    If **previously one** child was affected: risk is **3-4%.**
    If **previously two** children were affected: risk is **10%.**
    Genetic counseling should be done as appropriate.

25. Factors (drug) causing dysraphism (neural tube defects) in pregnancy:
    a. Valproic acid (1-2% neural tube defect).
    b. Hyperthermia.
    c. Vitamin A.
    d. **Biochemical defect in basement membrane,** specifically **hyaluronate, which** causes cell division and shape of primitive neuroepithelium.

26. Factors (drugs) **preventing** neural tube defects: **Folic acid;** effects of vitamin supplementation is uncertain because of lack of randomized study.

27. **Site of meningomyelocele and hydrocephalus: Lower** the defect less the hydrocephalus (i.e., sacral defect has less hydrocephalus) **except** upper thoracic and cervical (does not cause hydrocephalus).

28. **Treatment for meningomyelocele:**
    a. **Multi-disciplinary team approach,** with surgeon, physicians, therapist, neurologist, pediatrician, advocate and coordinator of treatment program.
    b. Ruptured: Emergency surgical repair.
    c. Unruptured: Surgical repair as a non-emergency basis. (Prepare the family and finish necessary investigations.)

29. Complication of repair of meningomyelocele: **Hydrocephalus. TREATMENT:** V-P shunt (ventriculo-peritoneal shunt).

30. **Management** of genitourinary system in meningomyelocele:
    a. **Urinary incontinence: Regularly catheterize the bladder** (teach the parents and then the patient) to prevent urinary stasis and infection. Follow up with the patient regularly to rule out UTI and monitor renal function. Later on **artificial urinary sphincter placement** by surgery can make some children continent.
    b. **Rectal incontinence:** It is common. Patient **can't** go to school. **Bowel training** with suppositories and enemas in timely fashion, allows child to pass stool 1-2 times/day.

31. **Functional ambulation** in meningomyelocele:
    a. Sacral or lumber: Most of them achieve functional ambulation.
    b. Thoracic or cervical: 50% can ambulate with braces and canes.

32. Prognosis of meningomyelocele:
    a. 70% of patient shave normal intelligence.
    b. Most deaths occur before the age of 4 years.
    c. 10-15% mortality in aggressively treated patients.
    d. Seizure and learning disorder are more common than in the general population.

33. Most common type of encephalocele: **Occipital** (at or below the inion).
    Encephalocele: Etiology is the same as in meningomyelocele and anencephaly. **Most commonly** associated with **hydrocephalus** which is due to aqueductal stenosis or chiari malformation and Dandy Walker syndrome.

    Investigation: Plain X-ray. Look for bony anatomy. **Sonogram of the mass and head is the most helpful diagnostic procedure.**

34. **Crania bifidum:** Midline skull bony defect.
    Two types: Meningocele, encephalocele.
    Meningocele: Meningeal sac filled with CSF **only.**
    Encephalocele: Meningeal sac with cerebral cortex, cerebellum and part of brain stem.

35. **Hindbrain dysfunction** in hydrocephalus with Type II chiari: It appears with feeding difficulty, choking, apnea, vocal cord paralysis, stridor, lots of secretion, upper extremities spasticity. It should be treated, or it can lead to death. **TREATMENT:** Surgical decompression of medulla and cervical cord.

36. **Prognosis** of cranial meningocele, encephalocele:
    a. **Meningocele:** Good.
    b. **Encephalocele:** Microcephaly, visual defect, mental retardation, seizure.
    c. Encephalocele with hydrocephalus: Poorest.

37. **Meckel-Gruber syndrome: Autosomal recessive.** It includes occipital encephalocele, microcephaly, cleft lip or palate, abnormal genitalia, congenital nephrosis and polydactyly.

38. Antenatal diagnosis of encephalocele, meningocele:
    a. Both: ↑ alpha feto protein (when ruptured).
    b. Sonogram:
       i. Encephalocele: Increased biparietal diameter.
       ii. Meningocele: Localize the defect.

39. **Anencephaly:** Incidence 1:1000. It is due to **the failure of closure of rostral (cephalic) neuropore. It contains** only residual brainstem, and hypoplastic pituitary gland (**absence of cerebral cortex, cerebellum and pyramidal tract). Factors** causing anencephaly: Genetic, environmental, toxins, nutrition and vitamins, poverty and lower socioeconomic class.

40. Recurrence risk for anencephaly: If one child had anencephaly, risk of second child: 4%.

If two children had anencephaly, risk of third child: 10%

41. Most common abnormality associated with anencephaly: **Polyhydramnios** (50% of cases); congenital heart defect (10-20% of cases).

42. Prenatal diagnosis of anencephaly in a mother who had anencephalic baby in previous pregnancy:
    a. Amniocentesis 14-16th week and alphafetoprotein level.
    b. Sonogram between 14-16th week of gestation.

43. Most important factor which controls neuronal migration and responsible for proper placement: Radial glial fibre system.

44. **Porencephaly:** It is a **cyst or cavity** formed either due to **congenital** defect or **acquired** secondary to infarction.

    a. **Congenital or true porencephalic cyst:** Present near sylvian fissure, has **communication with ventricle,** subarachnoid space or both. It is due to **congenital developmental** defect, appears with mental retardation, spasticity, seizure, optic atrophy.
    b. **Acquired or pseudoporencephalic cyst:** It is due to **perinatal and postnatal insult** due to cerebral arterial defective or venous circulation. It is **unilateral,** does not communicate with ventricle, **no** abnormality in cellular migration, appears with focal seizure, hemiparesis in first year of life.

45. Different zones of embryonic neural tube and formation of structures: (From inside outward from central canal).
    a. Ventricular or ependymal zone: Forms glioblast (primitive CNS supportive cells) which migrate to both the outer layers and forms **astrocytes and oligodendrocyte.**
    b. Intermediate or mantle zone.
    c. Outer or marginal zone: Forms **white mater.**
    Disorders of cell migration:
    a. Lissencephaly (or agyria): Absence of cerebral convolution due to faulty neuroblast migration, smooth brain.
    b. Schizencephaly: Unilateral or bilateral cleft in cerebral hemisphere.
    c. Porencephaly: Details as before.
    All of above, diagnosis is confirmed by head CT scan.

46. Agenesis of corpus callosum is associated with: Trisomy **8 and 18.** Presentation of agenesis of corpus callosum: Either **normal** person or **with neurologic defects** (mental retardation, microcephaly, seizure, paralysis). Diagnosis confirmed by **CT scan.**

    Aicardi syndrome:
    Most characteristic finding in retina (circumscribed pits or lacunae and coloboma of optic disk), appears with **seizure in first few months (resistant to anticonvulsant),** mental retardation, hemivertebra. **Only occurs in female,** X chromosome defect.

47. Mobius syndrome and cranial nerves involved: **6th and 7th (bilateral).**

48. Microcephaly: Head circumference is 3 standard deviations less than normal population of same age and sex. Types: Primary (genetic). Secondary (non-genetic). Intrauterine noxious agents.

49. Most important **initial** evaluation of microcephaly: **Serial head circumferences measurements** (single measurement has less value) **of the patient** and family members (parents). Family history is important.

    At birth severe microcephaly: Probably means **early** intrauterine damage.
    At birth mild microcephaly: Probably means **late** intrauterine damage.
    Minimal microcephaly: When brain damage occurs **after 2 years.**

50. Investigation and treatment to be done for microcephalic child:
    a. Rule out TORCH infection.
    b. Sonogram, CT, MRI, skull X-ray.
    c. Chromosome: If associated with any other abnormal features.
    d. When no cause is found: **Maternal serum phenylalanine** level should be done. Asymptomatic mother can have **high serum phenylalanine level** in microcephalic child.

    TREATMENT: According to underlying disorder.

51. **CSF formation and control mechanism:**
    a. CSF formed by **choroid plexus in lateral ventricles.**
    b. CSF formation **stimulated by cholinergic** nerve.
    c. CSF formation **inhibited by adrenergic** nerve.

52. **CSF, its circulation and types of hydrocephalus:**
    a. Normal CSF volume is 50 cc in infant and 150 cc in adult. Every hour 20 cc of CSF are formed and absorbed.
    b. **Circulation: Lateral** ventricle through foramen of Monro into 3rd ventricle, then through aqueduct of Sylvius into 4th ventricle, then through foramen of Magendie (midline) and Luschka (lateral) into the **cisternal at** the base of brain to subarachnoid space, then circulates over the cerebrum and cerebellum, **maximally absorbed through arachnoid villi,** a very small amount absorbed through nerve sheath to paranasal sinus **lymphatic** or directly by **choroid plexus itself.**
    c. **Communicating** hydrocephalus: CSF of ventricles is **connected** with CSF of spinal canal, that is, obstruction in subarachnoid space or malfunction of arachnoid villi. Example: **Subarachnoid bleed, meningitis, leukemic infiltrate.**
    d. **Non-**communicating hydrocephalus: CSF of ventricles is **not** connected with CSF of spinal canal, that is, obstruction in any place between lateral ventricle up to foramen of Magendie and Luschka.
    Example: **aqueductal stenosis,** Arnold-chiari malformation, Dandy-Walker syndrome.

53. **Most common causes of hydrocephalus:**
    a. Obstructive (non-communicating) type: **Aqueductal stenosis. (It is the most common cause of congenital** hydrocephalus).
    b. Non-obstructive (communicating) type: **Subarachnoid hemorrhage.**

54. Clinical appearance of hydrocephalus: **Most common appearance is enlarged head.** Other findings are wide open, bulging fontanels, separation of sutures, prominent scalp veins, **'setting sun'** sign (eyes deviated downward due to impingement of enlarged suprapineal recess on tectum). Pressure effect on **corticospinal tract causes** ↑ reflexes, Babinski sign, spasticity and clonus mostly in lower extremities. **Crack pot sign (Macewen sign)** present.

    In older child: Appears with lethargy, vomiting, headache, papilledema, pyramidal tract involvement, 6th cranial nerve palsy.
    Prominent occiput: Dandy-Walker syndrome.
    Small occiput: Arnold-Chiari malformation.

55. Diagnosis and treatment of hydrocephalus: **Diagnosis confirmed by CT scan or MRI** along with **sonogram** if fontanel is open.

    TREATMENT:
    a. Communicating: Repeated lumber tap, acetazolamide, lasix; if they fail then **V-P shunt.**
    b. Non-communicating: **V-P shunt** (ventriculoperitoneal shunt).
    Treatment of choice for both types is V-P shunt.

56. Important points to remember, **regarding prognosis of hydrocephalus:**
    a. **Most child patients are pleasant,** but a few develop aggressive and delinquent behavior.
    b. **Most child patients have abnormalities in memory function,** but also **may have** ↓ I. Q. developmental delay.
    c. **Remember, prognosis does not depend on the size of cortical mantle but rather on the underlying cause.**
    d. Eye: Strabismus, visual field defect, optic atrophy, decreased vision due to increased ICP (intracranial pressure).

57. **Dandy-Walker syndrome:** 4th ventricular dilation due to **obstruction** (atresia) in the roof (foramen of Magendie and Luschka) of 4th ventricle. **Most common presentation is hydrocephalus** (90%), **prominent occiput;** long tract signs, cerebellar ataxia and delayed development are also present.

    DIAGNOSIS: Initial positive transillumination, confirmed by MRI or CT scan (Remember, CT scan is not good for **posterior fossa and spinal cord** lesion, so **MRI is the best). TREATMENT: Shunt** the cystic cavity and ventricles when hydrocephalus is present.

58. **Arnold-Chiari malformations: Most common type is type II, which is characterized by progressive hydrocephalus and meningomyelocele** due to failure of pontine flexure during embryogenesis resulting in displacement of inferior vermis, medulla and pons into cervical canal, narrowing and elongation of **4th** ventricle, kinking of brain stem. 10% of infant present with apnea, stridor and weak cry.

    Type I malformation: Not associated with hydrocephalus, symptoms appear in

adolescence, appeaar with **recurrent headache,** neck pain, spastic lower limb, urinary frequency. It is due to **displacement of cerebellar tonsils into cervical canal.**

Pathogenesis: Not known, may be due to obstruction of caudal portion of 4th ventricle during development.
DIAGNOSIS: CT scan, **MRI. TREATMENT: Surgical decompression.**

59.   **Lacunar skull (multiple areas of decreased** density in frontal, parietal bones) mostly found in: **Meningomyelocele** (important for examination). It causes hydrocephalus, increased intracranial pressure, and **thinning of skull bones.**

60.   Different types of craniosynostosis:
   a.   **Scaphocephaly: Sagittal suture (most common type).**
   b.   Occipital plagiocephaly: Lambdoid suture.
   c.   Frontal plagiocephaly: Coronal and sphenoidal suture (second most common).
   d.   Turricephaly: Coronal, sometimes sphenoidal, frontoethmoidal.
   e.   Trigonocephaly: Metopic suture.
   f.   **Acrocephaly or brachycephaly: Coronal suture.**

Remember, head **grows along the line of sutural fusion.**

   g.   **Scaphocephaly: Anteroposteriorly elongated head,** long narrow head, no hydrocephalus, **normal** child, **no** increase of intracranial pressure.
   h.   **Frontal plagiocephaly: Unilateral flattening** of forehead, elevation of orbit and eyebrow of same side.
   i.   **Occipital plagiocephaly: Unilateral occipital flattening** and bulging of frontal bone of same side.
   j.   **Turricephaly: Conical head.**
   k.   **Trigonocephaly: Triangular head.**
   l.   **Acrocephaly or brachycephaly: Round** head, **increased** intracranial pressure, exophthalmos; it is **a surgical (craniectomy) urgency.**
   m.   **Kleeblattschädel deformity:** Clover leaf skull, **prominent temporal bone only;** other bones are depressed; **hydrocephalus** is present.

61.   Most common cause of **craniosynostosis: Unknown.** (10-20% of the cases are due to genetic syndrome). It means **premature closure of cranial sutures.**

Two types: Primary (due to abnormality in skull development). Secondary (due to failure of brain growth).

Hypothesis of craniosynostosis: Development defect in base of skull causing pressure on duramater which disrupts normal sutural development.
Remember, neither osteoblast nor osteoclast is responsible for craniosynostosis.

62.   Most common **time** of presentation of craniosynostosis: **Mostly at birth,** appearing with skull deformity, bony ridge and sutural fusion. Diagnosis confirmed by: **Skull X-ray,** rarely by bone scan.

TREATMENT:
a. Primary: **Craniectomy** as soon as possible to let the brain grow.
b. Secondary: Rarely needs surgery.

63. Most commonly associated finding in **acrocephaly: Syndactyle.** (Others are cardiac, and choanal atresia).

64. **Parietal foramina:** (Important for examination). It is a congenital, well-defined defect of varying size on **each side of posterior third of sagittal suture.** It is found in normal persons. **There is no** discomfort. It may run in the family.
No treatment is required.

65. Outcome of most **uncomplicated seizure** is: **Good.**

66. **Important genetic syndrome causing craniosynostosis:**
a. **Crouzon syndrome:** Autosomal dominant; **acrocephaly or brachycephaly** due to bilateral coronal suture closure; proptosis due to underdeveloped orbit. Maxillary hypoplasia and hypertelorism are characteristic features.
b. **Apert syndrome:** Mostly sporadic; **acrocephaly; syndactyle (2nd, 3rd and 4th** fingers), mimics crouzon, **except** asymmetric face and **less** proptosis of the eyes.
c. **Carpenter syndrome:** Autosomal recessive; **clover leaf** skull; syndactyle (hands and feet); mental retardation.
d. **Pfeiffer syndrome:** Mostly sporadic; **conical head; widely spaced and prominent** eyes; short and broad (thumb and toes)
e. **Chotzen syndrome: Most commonly seen in genetic syndrome;** autosomal dominant; **ptosis eyelid; short fingers;** syndactyle (2nd and 3rd fingers); and facial asymmetry.

67. Definition of seizure (convulsion) and epilepsy:

Seizure (or convulsion): Paroxysmal involuntary disturbance of brain function which manifests as unconsciousness, abnormal motor activities, sensory and autonomic disturbance, behavioral abnormality; some seizures can appear **without** loss of consciousness.
Epilepsy: Recurrent seizure which has **no** relation to fever and cerebral **insult.**

68. Most common type of epileptic seizure in childhood: **Partial seizures (but most common is febrile seizure).**

69. A child appears with **isolated first seizure, negative** family history, EEG is **normal,** all other blood tests were **normal.** Best way to manage:
No anticonvulsant needed, but **close follow-up is absolutely necessary.**

70. **International classification of epileptic seizures:**

Partial seizures:	Generalized seizure:	Unclassified seizures.
(i) Simple partial (retained consciousness): Motor, sensory, autonomic, psychic. (ii) Complex partial (impaired consciousness): Simple partial then loss of consciousness, or consciousness impaired at the beginning. (iii) Partial seizure with secondary generalization	(i) Absence: typical, atypical. (ii) Generalized tonic-clonic. (iii) Tonic. (iv) Clonic. (v) Myotonic. (vi) Atonic. (vii) Infantile spasm.	

71. **Mechanism of seizure: Unknown.** A proposed theory holds that **recurrent seizure activity from one temporal lobe** passes through corpus callosum and stimulates the other side of temporal lobe; or **functional immaturity** of substantia nigra may cause increased seizure activity in immature brain.

    Factors that stimulate seizure: Glutamate, aspartate by neuronal stimulation on specific receptors.
    Factors that inhibit seizure: GABA (gamma amino butyric acid), **SNR** (sensitive substantia nigra pars reticulata) neurone.

72. **Partial seizures:**

    a. **Simple partial seizure (SPS): Most common symptom is motor** activity (asynchronous clonic or tonic movement in face, neck, extremities), versive seizures (conjugate eye movement with head turning) is common. **No** automatism, but some patients complain of aura (headache and chest pain). **No loss of** consciousness. EEG: Spike (or sharp wave) unilateral, bilateral, multifocal spikes.

    b. **Complex partial seizure (CPS):** It can begin with SPS with or without an aura then **loss of consciousness.** Automatism found in 50-75% of the cases (that is, **automatic behavior** like lip smacking, swallowing, picking or pulling objects, rubbing objects, walking or running). CT, MRI should be done to rule out **temporal** lobe **abnormalities** (sclerosis, hamartoma, gliosis, infarction). EEG: Sharp wave **anterior temporal** lobe and multifocal spikes.

    c. **Benign partial epilepsy with centrotemporal (BPEC)** spikes: It is common; **excellent** outcome; peaks around 10 years; normal child with normal neurologic examination. The seizure is partial, motor and sensory symptoms confined to face (numbness in tongue and gums, dysphagia, increase salivation), tonic-clonic contracture of lower face. **Seizure mostly occurs in sleep** (but CPS occurs when child is awake).
    Characteristic EEG: Repetitive spike focuses in **rolandic or centrotemporal area.**

    TREATMENT: Carbamazepine is the drug of choice for frequent seizure.

73. **Important part of counseling the** seizure patient;

   a.   Teach parents the first aid measures for handling seizures.

   b.   Child should be expected to **have normal life** without restrictions, **but he should be watched when swimming.** Gymnastic activities are **not** allowed.

   c.   Most parents and children readily adapt to the occurrence of seizures and long term treatment plan.

   d.   Most children with epilepsy will be able to control it and enjoy both normal intelligence and normal lives.

74.   **Diagnosis** for epilepsy:

DIAGNOSIS:

   a.   **Uncomplicated** epilepsy: **By EEG.** (Remember, normal EEG does **not** rule out seizure, interictal EEG can be negative for up to 40% of patients).

   b.   **Complicated, uncontrolled epilepsy: By prolonged EEG monitoring with simultaneous closed circuit video, recording** is the method of choice. It is extremely helpful in the classification of seizures, in determining their location, and frequency, and in ruling out pseudoseizures.

   c.   **Initial work up should include serum SMA6, calcium, magnesium. (Remember,** do spinal tap only when infection is suspected, and do CT and MRI only when mass or any other intracranial lesion is suspected.)

75.   **Seizures and treatment of choice:**

Infantile spasm	ACTH (adrenocorticotropic hormone). Prednisone is equally effective.
Intractable seizure, not responsive to anticonvulsant	Surgery.
Recalcitrant seizure	Ketogenic diet.
Neonatal	Phenobarbital.
Partial seizure, generalized tonic-clonic.	Carbamazepine.
Absence, myoclonic seizure	Sodium valproate.

76.   Most common cause of **recurrent** seizures in a seizure patient **on anticonvulsant therapy: Noncompliance.** Diagnosis by history and **confirmed by serum sub therapeutic level.**

77.   **How to make diagnosis of Absence seizure: Hyperventilation** for 3-4 minutes produces absence seizure.

78.   **Generalized seizures:**

   a.   **Absence seizures** (petit mal): **No aura, no** postictal state, appears with **sudden cessation of speech or motor activity with blank facial expression, no** loss of consciousness. EEG: Typical 3/sec spike and generalized wave discharge.

b. **Generalized tonic-clonic (grand-mal):** Aura present, **loss** of consciousness, eyes rolling back, tonic-clonic convulsion of whole body, loss of sphincter control, tongue biting, then postictal state. It is **common** in childhood.
Idiopathic seizure: When **no** cause is found, a generalized tonic-clonic seizure is called an idiopathic seizure. **Factors that stimulate this seizure:** Theophylline, methylphenidate, psychotropic medicine; fever, fatigue, stress, infection.

c. **Myoclonic epilepsies of childhood: Repetitive seizures** with muscle contractions (symmetric), **loss of** muscle tone ,and history of **falling. Lennox-Gastaut syndrome:** It is **combined myoclonic and tonic** seizure. **Interictal EEG shows spikes.**

d. **Infantile spasm:** Occurs between 4 to 8 months of age, appears with brief, symmetric contraction of neck, trunk, and extremities. Three types are flexor, extensor, and mixed; **Mixed type is the most common** (flexor type causes flexion, and extensor type causes extension). **Characteristics of EEG: Hypsarrhythmia.**

Classified in two groups: Symptomatic (most common) and cryptogenic.
Symptomatic: History of **pre-peri-and postnatal insult** (HIE, PVL, infection, trauma). 80-90% **of patients are mentally retarded. Poor** prognosis. Cryptogenic: **No** history of insult. **The child is normal** and **bears no** risk.

79. Side effects of anticonvulsant medications:
    a. **Carbamazepine: ↓ WBC (leukopenia),** hepatic damage, idiosyncratic drug reaction. **Erythromycin should not be given simultaneously with this drug** because they compete for metabolism in liver. **Its plasma level is reduced by** phenobarbital, phenytoin, and valproate. When sodium valproate is added to this drug, **toxicity develops even with normal serum levels,** because active metabolite is **carbamazepine 10,11 epoxide which produces toxicity.** Serum half life is **8-20 hours. Monitor CBC, and serum drug level routinely.**

    b. **Phenobarbital and primidone:** 25% of children develop **behavioral** changes, **includig reduced attention span and cognitive** performance. Valproate **inhibits** the metabolism of phenobarbital **resulting in ↑ phenobarbital level and toxicity, even with therapeutic doses. Monitor serum level, but not the CBC.**

    c. **Phenytoin: Steven-Johnson syndrome:** lymphadenopathy, gum hyperplasia, megaloblastic anemia, polyneuropathy, lupus-like disease, rickets. Suspension is **not** recommended because it cannot be mixed well and ↑ serum Na level erratically. **Not a popular drug.**

    d. **Sodium valproate: Rarely** causes behavioral changes. G.I. symptoms, loss of hair, tremor, **hyperphagia. Two rare, but serious, effects are Reye-like syndrome, irreversible hepatic damage. (Reye-like syndrome** includes lethargy, ↑ NH4, ↓ serum carnitine level).
    Treatment is to discontinue the medication. Symptom disappear in a few days.
    2 year-old child: Develops idiosyncratic hepatotoxic syndrome (abdominal pain, retching, weight loss).
    TREATMENT: Reduce doses or discontinue.

    e. **ACTH: ↑** glucose, ↑ B.P., **transient brain shrinkage,** G.I. symptoms.

    f. **Ketogenic diet:** Restricted CHO and protein, but **includes plenty of fat,** so it tastes bad to children.

80.   A child appears with isolated first seizure **with abnormal EEG or recurrent** seizures. Best way to manage: Anticonvulsant therapy and follow up.

81.   **Drug of choice** for status epilepticus:
   a. **Diazepam or lorazepam (I.V.) immediately** (side effects of diazepam is respiratory depression, hypotension, short duration of action). With lorazepam those effects are less and the duration of action is longer.
   b. If seizure is controlled or persists after diazepam/lorazepam: Second drug to use is **phenytoin** (Some centers use **phenobarbital.**)
   c. If seizure **still persists** use: **Diazepam drip,** I.V. paraldehyde, lidocaine or general anaesthesia.
       (Rectal or I.M. paraldehyde causes tissue sloughing, so do **not** use those means unless they are absolutely necessary. **Diazepam drip is better** than paraldehyde.)
   d. If seizure is still **not** controlled, then produce: **Phenobarbital coma.**

82.   Most common cause of neonatal seizure: **HIE** (Hypoxic ischemic encephalopathy).

83.   Most common type of **seizure in drug withdrawal neonate: Myoclonic.**

84.   **Pertinent things to remember for febrile seizures:**
   a. **Between 9 months to 5 years of age,** strong family history indicates genetic condition.
   b. **From studies of animals:** Arginine-vasopressin may be an important factor in the pathogenesis of febrile seizure.
   c. **Spontaneous remission** occurs; **epilepsy rarely** develops.
   d. **Most common** seizure disorder in childhood is febrile seizure.
   e. **Tonic-clonic convulsion** when core temperature is 39 degrees or more. Maximum duration of seizure is 10 minutes (>15 minutes duration indicates an organic cause).
   f. If there is any suspicion of **meningitis, do spinal tap** and look for other causes of infection.
   g. EEG is usually not necessary **except in atypical febrile seizure** (>15 minutes duration repeated convulsions for hours/days, focal seizures) or there is a **risk of developing epilepsy** (onset before 9 months, strong family history, atypical febrile seizures, abnormal neurologic finding, delayed development). **EEG should be done** in atypical febrile seizure and where there is a risk of developing epilepsy.
   h. Incidence of epilepsy is **9%** with risk factors and **1%** without it.
   i. **Management:**
       i.   **Simple** febrile seizure: Antipyretics and reassurance.
       ii. If any bacterial infection is present: Antibiotics.
       iii. **Acute prolonged febrile seizure:** Drug of choice is diazepam or lorazepam per rectal **(only in acute condition).**
       Remember, do **not** use anticonvulsant for simple febrile seizures. Phenobarbital does not prevent the recurrence of febrile seizure.

85.   Most important **initial** management of status epilepticus: **Maintain the airway** (Ambu bag, intubation).

86.   **Most common type** of Neonatal seizure and other types:

a. Most common is **Subtle type** (chewing, lip smacking, blinking, nystagmus, apnea, bicycling, pedaling, color change).

b. Focal clonic seizure: Rhythmic focal clonic movement of muscles (found in **metabolic, focal, brain lesion, infection, subarachnoid hemorrhage).**

c. Multi-focal clonic type: Multiple focal clonic movement of muscles of extremities. (Moves from one limb to another, and is found in **hypoxic ischemic encephalopathy).**

d. Tonic seizure: Tonic posture of extremities and trunk (found in **intraventricular hemorrhage).**

e. Myoclonic: Focal or generalized jerky movement of (mostly distal) muscles. (Found in **drug withdrawal.)**

EEG classification of neonatal seizures:

f. Clinical seizure with **consistent** EEG changes (focal clonic and tonic, some myoclonic; responds to anticonvulsant).

g. Clinical seizure with **inconsistent** EEG changes (generalized tonic, subtle, some myoclonic; mostly non-epileptogenic; may not require or respond to anticonvulsant).

h. No clinical seizures with **positive EEG** changes (focal clonic or tonic seizure **with** anticonvulsant; comatose condition **without** anticonvulsant).

87. Prognosis for status epilepticus: Improves significantly due to modern ICU care. Mortality occurs in 5% of cases.

88. **Pyridoxine dependent seizure:** Autosomal recessive. This seizure can appear **in utero or shortly after birth** with generalized tonic-clonic movement. It does **not** respond to anticonvulsant. **Pyridoxine** is necessary to synthesize **glutamic acid decarboxylase** which in turn is necessary to synthesis **GABA,** which prevents convulsion.

    TREATMENT: I.V. pyridoxine 100-200 mg. (Seizure stops immediately and EEG normalizes within few hours), life long supplementation with oral pyridoxine 10 mg/day is necessary. Untreated patient will suffer persistent convulsions and mental retardation.

89. Most common cause of status epilepticus: Febrile seizure for 30 minutes (particularly in children under 3 years of age).

    Status epilepticus: Convulsions lasting more than 30 minutes or series of convulsions for 30 minutes without return of consciousness.
    Area of brain damage by status epilepticus: Hippocampus, cerebellum, amygdaloid body, thalamus, middle cortical areas.
    Earliest histological change: **Cellular ischemia** (then neuronophagia, cell damage, proliferation of microglia, increased reactive astrocyte).
    Acute pathological change: **Venous congestion,** few petechial bleed, edema.

90. A child with **benign paroxysmal vertigo (BPV)** is likely to develop **in the future: Motion sickness and migraine (which develops several years later).**

    BPV: Always develops in **toddler only,** appears with **sudden attack** of **ataxia, begins to**

fall while walking, refuses to walk, vomiting (no lethargy), **nystagmus, vertigo** which lasts from **seconds to minutes** either **daily, weekly or monthly.**
DIAGNOSIS: By ice water calorie testing, **abnormal vestibular function.**
TREATMENT: **Dimenhydrinate.**

91. Treatment for protracted **night terror:**
    a. Diazepam or imipramine.
    b. Underlying emotional disorder should be treated.

92. **Breath holding spell:** Two types: Cyanotic and pallid.
    a. **Cyanotic: Most common type.** It is provoked by upsetting the infant, appears with **apnea, cyanosis, unconsciousness** with or without generalized convulsion, opisthotonos, bradycardia. It can recur frequently, but it is stereotyped. Mostly occurs in 2 year olds (6 months-5 years). EEG: **Normal.** TREATMENT: Support and reassure the parents.
    b. **Pallid:** Less common. It is provoked by pain (trauma), appears with **stopped breathing, unconsciousness, paleness, hypotonia, tonic convulsion, bradycardia.** TREATMENT: Same as cyanotic type; in **refractory cases,** when **bradycardia persists then only use atropine which blocks the vagal effect.** Atropine causes high fever in hot weather.

93. **Syncope:** Two types are simple syncope and cough syncope.
    a. **Simple:** Mostly in children over 10 years of age. It is due to **diminished cerebral circulation** due to hypotension (normally, autoregulation maintains cerebral circulation even with hypotension). Ischemia of cerebral cortex withdraws the **inhibitory** influence on reticular activating system (RAS), so excessive discharge from RAS causes **brief tonic contraction of muscles of face and extremities in 50% of patients.** Patient may appear with **upward deviation of eyes which mimics epilepsy.** EEG: No seizure, but **there is transient slow** activity. **TREATMENT:** None.
    b. **Cough:** Mostly found in **asthmatics.** It is due to **increased intrapleural pressure** (due to cough) which inhibits venous return to (R) side of heart, so there is a **diminished (L) ventricular output, diminished cerebral circulation, hypoxia, unconsciousness.** It begins **shortly after sleep.** Child wakes up with coughing, and redness, fright, sweating, unconsciousness, hypotonia, and vertical upward eye movement. **Episodes last for few seconds. Recovers within a few seconds, but** doesn't remember anything about the attack **except** the coughing. **TREATMENT: Prevention of bronchoconstriction in asthmatic.**

94. **Treatment** for familial paroxysmal choreoathetosis: **Clonazepam is sometimes effective.** It is rare autosomal dominant disorder. Appears with sudden onset of **choreoathetosis** precipitated by movement (like walking after waking up), and lasts for few seconds. It is **not** a seizure.

95. Shuddering (or shivering) attack: Child is 4 months to 7 years old: Attack occurs with sudden flexion of head, trunk and shivering as if somebody poured ice cold water on the body.

96. Narcolepsy and catalepsy:
Narcolepsy: Paroxysmal attack of irrepressible sleep. Mostly occurs after adolescence.
Catalepsy: Narcolepsy with muscle hypotonia. EEG: **REM sleep. TREATMENT:**
Schedule naps, **amphetamines,** methylphenidate, tricyclic antidepressant.

97. Difference between true seizures and pseudo seizures:

True	Pseudo
Any age	Between 10-18 years.
History of epilepsy may or may not present	May have history of epilepsy.
Cyanosis present, abnormal pupil	No cyanosis, normal pupil.
Loss of sphincter control	No loss of sphincter control.
Tongue bite present	No tongue bite.
No moaning or crying	Moaning or crying during seizure.
No neurotic personality	Neurotic personality present.
Diagnosis confirm positive EEG	**EEG is normal.**
Respond to anticonvulsant	No response.
↑ prolactin level after seizure	No increase in prolactin level.

98. **Most important causes of headaches in children: Migraine (most common).**
Increased intracranial pressure and stress. (Less common causes are refractive error, strabismus, teeth malocclusion, sinusitis.)

99. Most common etiology of migraine: **Unknown; may be due to vasomotor instability.**
There is an increased level of circulating serotonin, and substance P, a polypeptide (vasodilator) which acts on both intracranial and extracranial blood vessels.

100. Most common type of migraine: **Common migraine** (90% of sufferers have positive family history).
Other types are: Classic migraine, migraine variants, and complicated migraine.
Characteristics of migraine: At least three of the following symptoms will be present: throbbing headache, unilateral side, abdominal pain, nausea or vomiting, associated with visual, motor, sensory aura; relief after sleep; positive family history.

Diagnosis and treatment for migraine: Diagnosis of migraine: by history and physical examination.
TREATMENT:
a. **Behavioral:** Biofeedback and self-hypnosis exercise.
b. Prevention: Avoid stress and anxiety, avoid certain food (nuts, chocolate, cold drinks, hot dogs, Chinese food containing monosodium glutamate), avoid sunlight, loud noise, drugs (alcohol, oral contraceptive).
c. Medical: Mild cases: Acetaminophen. Severe cases: Ergotamine. For vomiting:

Dimenhydrinate. Prophylaxis: Propranolol (more then 2-4 attacks monthly) for one year.

101. Difference between organic and psychogenic (stress) headaches:

Organic	Psychogenic (stress or tension)
Any age group	Common **after puberty.**
Most common in **early morning and relieved after vomiting**	Most common in **school days** or examination days, infrequently in morning.
Nausea, vomiting due to increased intracranial pressure	No nausea, no vomiting, normal intracranial pressure.
Constant pain, **gradual** onset	Hurting or aching **pain (intermittent)** and acute onset.
Mostly **frontal and occipital** region (or diffuse)	**Mostly frontal;** or vertex or occipital region.
Diagnosis **by CT, MRI**	**Diagnosis by exclusion** after history and physical examination.
Treatment: According to cause.	**TREATMENT: Reassurance, acetaminophen** or other analgesic. Severe cases: Brief hospitalization and observation. Some patients respond to biofeedback and self-hypnosis exercises.

102. Most common cause of neurocutaneous syndrome: **Unknown.** (Mostly familial, may be due to defect in differentiation of primitive ectoderm.)

103. **Most common type** of neurofibromatosis: **(90%) NF-1** (gene location on chromosome 17); NF.2.

104. Mode of inheritance in neurofibromatosis or Von Recklinghausen disease: **Autosomal dominant.** It is due to **abnormality in neural crest differentiation and migration** during early part of embryogenesis (probably related to nerve or glial cells growth factor).

105. **Most common presentation** of neurofibromatosis: **Cafe-au-lait spots** present in 100% cases.

106. Diagnosis of NF.1 is made if two if the following features are present:
   a. Cafe-au-lait spots:
      i. Prepubertal patient
         At least 5 spots over 5mm in diameter.
      ii. Postpubertal patient: At least 6 spots over 15 mm in diameter.
   b. Lisch nodules (two or more): Hamartoma in iris is diagnosed by slit lamp

examination. It is absent in NF.2.

   c. Two or more neurofibromas or one plexiform neurofibroma.

   d. Optic glioma (benign tumor, 80% of patients have normal vision; asymptomatic).

   e. Axillary or inguinal freckling (hyperpigmented areas).

   f. Bony defect: Most common is kyphoscoliosis (40% patient).

   g. First degree relative with NF.1.

107. Complications of NF-1:

   a. Neurologic complication:

      i.   Speech and learning delay, and attention deficit disorder due to abnormal signal by MRI in globus pallidus, thalamus, internal capsule. (Not picked up CT scan).

      ii.   Macrocephaly with normal ventricle (**rarely** hydrocephalus).

      iii. Hemiparesis and intellectual deficit due to occlusion of cerebral vessels.

   b. **Psychologic disturbances.**

   c. **Malignant changes:**

Neurofibrosarcoma, schwannoma; ↑ incidence of pheochromocytoma, leukemia, Wilms tumor, rhabdomyosarcoma.

108. Most characteristic features of **NF-2: Bilateral acoustic neuromas;** (NF-2 gene located in chromosome 22).

109. Diagnosis of NF-2 is made when one of the following is present:

   a. **Bilateral** 8th cranial nerves acoustic neuromas diagnosed by CT or MRI.

   b. A family history of NF-2 in parent, sibling or child and either **unilateral** 8th cranial nerve tumor or **any two** of these = neurofibroma, glioma, meningioma, schwannoma or juvenile subcapsular (posterior) lenticular cataract.

110. Clinical presentation of NF-2: Hearing loss, unsteady gait, facial weakness, posterior subcapsular cataract (50% cases), CNS tumors (schwann cell, glial cell and meningioma like NF-1).

111. Treatment of neurofibromatosis:

   a. No specific treatment.

   b. Asymptomatic patient:

Reexamination every year.

112. What is the chance a **mother with neurofibromatosis** of giving the disease to her baby? **50% (important for examination). No** prenatal diagnosis is available. If child has the disease, then **both parents should be examined very carefully.**

113. Characteristic **brain lesion** of tuberous sclerosis: **Tubers,** present specifically in **subependymal** region, become **calcified and project into ventricle** (candle dripping appearance). **Tuberous sclerosis: Autosomal dominant;** gene located on chromosome 9.

114. An infant appears with **infantile spasm;** EEG shows **hypsarrhythmia.** Most likely diagnosis: **Tuberous sclerosis.** Characteristic other features are:

   a. **Ash leaf** (90% cases, hypopigmented skin lesion).

b. Periventricular tubers (around 3 years of age).

c. Generalized seizure (myoclonic type in later age).

d. Mental retardation (may have normal intelligence).

e. Sebaceous gland hyperplasia.

f. **Shagreen patch** (rough, raised lesion in lumbosacral region).

g. Subungual or periungual **fibroma.**

h. **Heart**   Rhabdomyoma (50% of cases).

i. Retina: Mulberry tumors or phakoma.

j. **Kidney: Hamartoma or polycystic disease (in most patients).**

115. Diagnosis and treatment of tuberous sclerosis: Diagnosis **confirmed by CT scan or MRI in most cases.** Always look for skin and retinal lesion.

    TREATMENT: According to the presentation.
    a. Seizure: Anticonvulsant.
    b. Hydrocephalus (due to tubers blocking foramen of Monroe): V-P shunt.

116. A child appears with **unilateral facial nevus (port wine stain),** seizure, intracranial calcification, hemiparesis mental retardation. Most likely diagnosis: **Sturge-Weber syndrome.** It is due to **abnormal development of primordial vascular bed** during early part of cerebral vascularization. **Remember: not** all patients with facial nevus have Sturge-Weber syndrome. Focal tonic-clonic **seizures** occur mostly in first year of life on the **contralateral** side of the lesion, but **glaucoma or buphthalmos** occurs on **same** side. **Mental retardation occurs after 1 year (50% of cases)** due to **persistent seizure.** Cerebral atrophy is due to hypoxia and use of multiple anticonvulsant.

    DIAGNOSIS:
    Skull X-ray: **Rail-road track sign** due to **calcification** in occipitoparietal region.
    CT scan: Unilateral **cortical atrophy** and same-sided **ventricular dilatation.**
    TREATMENT:
    a. **Seizure:** Anticonvulsant. If **no** response and to prevent mental retardation, **lobectomy or hemispherectomy is indicated.**
    b. Treat for glaucoma.
    c. Port wine stain: Flash-lamp pulsed laser treatment.
    d. Developmental delay: Special program for education.

117. Most common cause of **death in Von Hippel-Lindau disease: Renal cancer.**

    Von-Hippel-Lindau disease: Autosomal dominant. **Most common neurologic finding is cerebellar hemangioblastoma** (present early in life with increased intracranial pressure). Retinal angiomata also present.
    Diagnosis by CT scan: Cystic lesion with vascular mural nodule.
    TREATMENT: Surgical removal of tumor.

118. **Eye finding** in linear nevus syndrome: **Homonymous hemianopia.** This syndrome usually appears with facial nevus, mental retardation, generalized myoclonic or focal seizure.

119. **Preferred method of investigation** for posterior fossa mass (cerebellum, vermis and other structures): **MRI. It is also the preferred method for investigating any spinal mass.**

120. Agenesis of cerebellar vermis: Autosomal recessive. Appears in **infancy** with **generalized hypotonia, diminished deep tendon reflexes, characteristic respiration (alternate hyperpnea and apnea),** ataxia, mental retardation.

121. **Acute cerebellar ataxia** secondary to **viral** (varicella, coxsackie or echovirus) infection mostly due to: **Autoimmune disease.** It is a **self-limited** disease. Prognosis is very good.

122. Acute labyrinthitis is associated with: **Otitis media,** vertigo, abnormal labyrinth function by ice water calorie testing.

123. Toxic causes of ataxia: **Alcohol, dilantin** (>30 µg/ml serum level), thallium.

124. Most common type of **tumors** occur in **ataxia telangiectasia are lymphoreticular tumors** (lymphoma, leukemia, Hodgkin disease), and brain tumors.

125. Most common type of **degenerative ataxia: Ataxia-telangiectasia, autosomal recessive. Ataxia appears** around 2 years of age and telangiectasia is found in mid childhood.

      Serum: ↓ (IgA, IgG2, IgG4, IgE), ↑ alpha fetoprotein.
      Secretary: ↓ IgA
      Chromosome: 14 chromosome breakage.
      Death: Due to infection or tumor spread.

126. Most common cause of death in Friedreich ataxia: **Hypertrophic cardiomyopathy and congestive cardiac failure.**

      Friedreich ataxia: Ataxia appears between 3-10 years, **mostly involving the lower limb. Romberg test is positive; planter response is extensor; absence of achilles reflex. Most common characteristics are explosiveness; dysarthric speech; nystagmus (which is present in most children,** with this condition); normal intelligence; and loss of vibration and position sense due to degeneration in posterior column, per cavus.
      Roussy-Levy disease: As in Friedreich ataxia, there is atrophy of lower limb muscles.
      Ramsay-Hunt syndrome: As in Friedreich ataxia, there is myoclonic epilepsy.

127. Most common **acquired chorea in childhood: Sydenham chorea.**

128. **Sole neurologic manifestation** of rheumatic fever: **Sydenham chorea.**

129. **Three** major features of Sydenham chorea: Chorea, hypotonia, emotionally labile.

      Other features are: Symmetric **chorea** is prominent in face, trunk, and distal limbs. **It is increased by stress and disappears with sleep.** Mood swings (uncontrolled crying). **Typical features: Milkmaid's grip** (relaxing and tightening of fingers in handshake), **darting tongue** (unable to protrude tongue for more than few seconds).

TREATMENT: Phenothiazine, haloperidol; penicillin prophylaxis is necessary because these patients are susceptible to rheumatic carditis (particularly mitral valve).

130. **Most common cause** of **dystonia or athetosis** (slow intermittent twisting motion which causes turning and posturing of trunk and limbs). **Perinatal asphyxia.** Other causes are dystonia musculorum deformans, Wilson disease, drugs, Hallervorden-Spatz disease.

131. Preferred method of treatment for **drug**-related dystonia: **I.V. diphenhydramine.** Drugs causing dystonia (athetosis): Phenytoin, phenothiazine, carbamazepine.

132. **Kaiser-Fleischer ring** (due to copper deposition in Descemet membrane) found in: **Wilson disease.** It is autosomal recessive. Appears with **acute hepatic failure** (<10 years of age), **progressive dystonia** (>10 years of age) due to basal ganglia degeneration, **wing-beating tremor.**

   CT or MRI: Cerebral atrophy, dilated ventricle, lesion in thalamus and basal ganglia.
   Initial screening test: ↓ Ceruloplasmin level.
   Diagnosis confirmed by liver biopsy.
   Treatment: Penicillamine (ß, ß-dimethylcysteine), vitamin B6 (penicillamine is an antimetabolite of B6). If cannot tolerate penicillamine, use trimethylene tetramine dihydrochloride.

133. Treatment for **extreme form** of DMD (dystonia musculorum deformans) when medical treatment (trihexyphenidyl, carbamazepine, levodopa, diazepam, bromocriptine) fails: **Cryothalamectomy.** DMD has **unknown** cause. (It may be due to abnormalities of catecholamine metabolism in the CNS). Occurs in childhood, **appears with extended and outward rotation of lower limbs,** then progresses to all four extremities, trunk, and axial musculature.

134. Most common cause of Cerebral Palsy(C.P.): **Unknown.** (Only <10% of patients had perinatal asphyxia.)
   C.P.: Nonprogressive motor disorder mostly involving the extremities. C.P. may be associated with delayed development, mental retardation, epilepsy, visual speech, hearing, cognitive and behavioral abnormalities (motor handicap is the **least** problem).

135. Most common **type of tics** in children: **Transient tics.** Other types are: Chronic tic, **Gilles de la Tourette syndrome.**

136. Differences between tremor and seizure:

Tremor	Seizure
No eye movement	Abnormal eye movement.
Increases with stimulus	No change with stimulus.
Jitteriness	Clonic movement.
Stopped by flexion of limb	Does not stop.

137. Most **severe** form of C.P. : **Spastic quadriplegia. (Most common type is spastic diplegia.)**

138. Type of C.P. that occurs in bilirubin encephalopathy: **Athetoid C.P.** It is now very rare.

139. In **spastic diplegia,** the most common neuropathologic finding is: **PVL** (periventricular leukomalacia), which is due to perinatal asphyxia. PVL damages the fibres of internal capsule supplying the legs.

140. Common manifestation of HIV (human immune deficiency virus) in CNS: **Encephalopathy. Primary features of AIDS encephalopathy:** Brain growth stops, development is delayed and neurologic signs manifest.

141. Diagnosis and treatment for C.P.: Diagnosis by history, physical; baseline CT scan; EEG. **Treatment:** Multidisciplinary approach from different sub-specialties.
    a. Severe spastic diplegia: Rhizotomy might help.
    b. For spasticity: Dantrolene sodium, benzodiazepine, baclofen.
    c. Severe athetosis: Levodopa.
    d. Dystonia: Carbamazepine, trihexyphenidyl.

142. What is the **laboratory characteristic** of Leigh disease (subacute necrotizing encephalomyelopathy)? ↑ **serum lactate level.**
    Leigh disease: It is due to deficiency of **pyruvate dehydrogenase** complex (i and iv of respiratory chain). Autosomal recessive. Appears with difficulty in feeding and swallowing, vomiting, failure to thrive, seizure, hypotonia, ataxia, nystagmus, and delayed motor and language development. Most patients die within 6 months. CT scan: symmetric low attenuation in basal ganglia.

143. Zellweger syndrome (cerebrohepatorenal syndrome): **Autosomal recessive.** Appears with **frontal bossing,** large anterior fontanel, **hypotonia,** excessive skin folds in neck, **areflexia, generalized seizure, developmental delay, hearing** loss, eye findings (cataract, nystagmus, optic atrophy), ↑ liver and prolonged jaundice. Most of patients die within 1 year.

144. Encephalomyopathies:
    a. Mitochondrial defect: Reye syndrome, Leigh disease.
    b. Peroxisomal defect: Zellweger syndrome.

    MELAS (mitochondrial myopathy, encephalopathy, lactic acidosis and stroke): Manifestations **begin after** few years. Appears with **short stature, seizure** (focal or generalized), **acute hemiparesis,** hemianopia, dementia and cortical blindness. CT: Basal ganglia calcification, lucent areas. No treatment available.
    MERRF (myoclonic epilepsy, ragged-red fires): Manifestations **begin after few years.** Appears with myoclonic epilepsy, progressive ataxia, dysarthria, nystagmus, **rarely** optic atrophia and pes cavus, progressive intellectual deterioration; short stature and positive family history like MELAS. **Degeneration** of neurones in dentate nuclei and cerebellar white mater.

Kearns-Sayre syndrome: It includes ophthalmoplegia, retinal degeneration and ataxia. Short stature and perceptive deafness (> 50% cases). **Rarely** is there a positive family history and seizure.

MELAS, MERRF, KEARNS-SAYRE SYNDROME: Muscle mitochondrial study shows reduced activities of complex 1 (NADH-CoQ reductase) and or complex IV (cytochrome oxidase) **defect in mitochondrial DNA.**

145. Most common clinical manifestation of **burn encephalopathy: Seizure.** Burn encephalopathy is due to **multiple factors** like carbon monoxide, smoke, laryngeo spasm, bacterial infection, cortical venous thrombosis, electrolyte imbalance, cerebral edema, emotional stress, and drug reactions.

146. **Hypertensive encephalopathy** is most commonly associated with: **Renal diseases.** This **encephalopathy** appears with severe headache, seizure, blurred vision, hemiparesis, transient cortical blindness. **Treatment:** Antihypertensive, anticonvulsant.

147. Encephalopathy due to radiation: Two types: Acute and late onset.
   Acute: It is due to excessive radiation which causes cerebral edema and hemorrhage secondary to ↑ permeability to cerebral blood vessels, present with focal seizure or hemiparesis. **It commonly occurs.**

   Treatment: Steroids. Late onset: Rare, of unknown cause, appears same as above **except** no bleeding. CT shows **atrophic** brain, calcification. Found in leukemia after therapy.

148. In basilar skull fracture, the most characteristic sign is: Battle sign (bruise over mastoid).

149. **Intubation** is necessary in which Glasgow coma scale: **Seven or less.**

150. The outcome of intracranial pressure (ICP) and cerebral perfusion pressure (CPP):

   If ICP < 15 mm Hg and CPP > 50 mm Hg: Better outcome.
   If ICP > 50mm Hg and CPP < 40 mm Hg: Poor prognosis.

151. **Factors which reduce ICP** (intracranial CO_2 pressure):
   a. Mechanical hyperventilation (Pa CO_2 < 30 mm Hg).
   b. Diuretics: Mannitol, lasix.
   c. Sedation: Phenobarbital, morphine, diazepam.
   d. Paralysis: Pavulon (pancuronium).
   Remember, ↓ CCP (cerebral perfusion pressure), along with ↓ systemic pressure, give colloid to ↑ systemic pressure.

152. Prognosis or outcome of coma patient:
   a. Is **not** influence by pentobarbital coma or steroid.
   b. It depends on **underlying causes** of coma (diabetic coma has better outcome than Reye syndrome).
   c. **Poor outcome** when EEG shows **burst** suppression, alpha-like activity, very low voltage, electrocerebral silence.

    d. **Somatosensory evoke potential is the most sensitive and reliable method of predicting neurologic outcome.**

    e. Modifies Glasgow score, eye movement, pupillary reaction to light, seizure, motor activities.

153. Evaluation of **brain stem function** by: **Ice water caloric test.** It should **not** be done on perforated ear drum.

154. Most common organism causing infection in basilar skull fracture: **Streptococcus pneumoniae. (Meningitis,** which is due to communication between nasopharynx, middle ear with the brain). Remember, the use of prophylactic antibiotic is controversial and not used in the first seven days of CSF rhinorrhea.

155. Principles of treatment of comatose patient:

    a. 1st is to maintain **airway.**

    b. 2nd is to maintain normal cardiovascular status.

    c. 3rd is to correct fluid and electrolyte abnormalities.

    d. Use anticonvulsant for seizures.

    e. **Goal of treatment is to find the cause.**

156. Criteria for brain death:

    a. **Patient condition:** Comatose, apneic, normotensive, normothermic, no voluntary movement and no vocalization. Apnea is **confirmed** when patient is unable to breath after 15 minutes, or until the PCO_2 reaches 60. Patient should be on mechanical ventilator with positive airway pressure on 100% O_2. Apnea testing should be **done only when brain death is definite.**

    b. Every brain stem function is absent. Pupils are dilated fixed midline. There is an **absence** of auriculo ocular (response to loud noise); absence of vestibulo-ocular (no response to ice water caloric test); no lateral eye movement with turning head (doll's eye test); no corneal reflex; and all other reflexes (gag, sucking, cough) are absent.

    c. EEG: Electrocerebral silence.

    d. Flaccidity and no spontaneous movement **except** withdrawal of spinal cord reflexes and myoclonus.

    e. Longer period of observation in newborns (premature and fullterm) is required because the cause of asphyxia or coma is unknown.

    f. Nuclear brain scan: Absence of brain circulation. Remember, EEG and brain scan are not definitive tests. **Diagnosis of brain death should therefore be made** on the basis of the above mentioned criteria, physical examination, and observation.

157. Most common type of skull fracture: **Linear and non-**depressed fracture. A rarely occuring complication of this fracture is **leptomeningeal cyst** (protrusion of leptomeninges and accumulation of CSF through the fracture).

158. Different sites of **fracture** and **manifestations:**

Fracture	Manifestations.
Temporal bone	Bloody discharge from middle ear (hematotympanum).

Basilar skull	**Raccoon's eye sign** (bilateral ecchymosis and swelling of upper eyelids, which means anterior fossa basilar fracture), **6th to 7th cranial nerves palsy, CSF otorrhea, rhinorrhea present.** **Battle sign:** Ecchymosis over mastoid area.
Sphenoid bone	3,4,6 cranial nerve palsy.

159. Treatment for **depressed skull fracture:** Surgery is indicated when there is:
    a. Neurologic deficit.
    b. Compound wound.
    c. Depression more than 3-5 mm in depth.
    Surgery:**Debridement of bony fragments pressing on cerebrum.**

160. A child appears with head trauma. **Immediate management should be** directed to: **Cardiovascular and respiratory system for adequate** oxygenation to prevent further tissue damage.

161. Important points to remember for head injury skull fracture:
    a. **X-ray: All children younger than 5 years** should have X-rays done and provide history of head trauma to rule out fracture (because of unreliable history and examination findings). If there is any signs and symptoms **present** then X-ray is indicated but **diagnosis confirmed by CT scan or MRI. After 5 years, routine X-ray is no longer needed.**
    b. Skull fracture does not always indicate underlying brain injury (33% of skull fractures have normal neurologic examination; 50% of deaths due to brain injury have no skull fracture).
    c. **Subdural** hematoma more often occurs **without** than with fracture.
    d. **Epidural** hematoma associated **equally** with or without fracture.
    e. **Importance of seat belt or car seat:** When head is **fixed, much more powerful** forces are needed to cause the kind of injuries when head is **not fixed.** (Head is more or less fixed with seat belt of car seat.)
    f. 5-10% of physical and mental retardation is due to head injuries.
    g. Most common cause of serious head injuries due to motor vehicle (automobile) accident.
    h. Male to female ratio 2:1.

162. Difference between subdural and epidural hematoma:

Subdural	Epidural
Blood between duramater and cerebral mantle.	Blood outside the duramater.
Bleeding from **cortical veins.**	Bleeding from **middle meningeal artery** and rarely from veins.
Found in shaken baby syndrome, trauma.	Not found in shaken baby syndrome, but there is trauma.

No lucid interval.	Lucid interval (minute to days) present (1st unconscious then looks good, then get worse).
Appears with focal or generalized seizure and/or poor feeding, irritability, lethargy, vomiting, fever.	When hematoma is pressing on temporal lobe, there is a progressive loss of consciousness and focal seizure.
Examination: 50% of patients have retinal or subhyaloid hemorrhage; tense anterior fontanel or increased head circumference.	Examination: Ipsilateral 3rd cranial nerve palsy, contralateral hemiparesis, skull fracture in 50% of cases.
Diagnosis confirmed by: **CT** or MRI.	Diagnosis confirmed by: **CT** or MRI.
Treatment: Subdural tap which may be repeated.	Treatment: Surgical removal of hematoma.

163.   Preferred method treatment for post-traumatic seizure: **Phenytoin (does not alter mental status). Early post-traumatic seizure** usually occurs **within the first two days** after trauma due to **cerebral edema, petechial or hemorrhagic lesion, or penetrating wound.** If patient develops a brief seizure within a few minutes or hours after the trauma, it is due to **mechanical or neurochemical changes in the CNS.** It does **not** require anticonvulsant, because the seizure does not recur.

164.   **Concussion:** It is a **brief, reversible and transient loss** of consciousness with areflexia and amnesia about the events surrounding the trauma. It is probably due to a temporary reduction of cerebral blood flow and oxygen consumption, the stretching of nerve fibres within the white mater, and transient paralysis of nerve fibres and alternation in neurotransmitter release. **Patient appears with** hypotonia, areflexia, transient apnea, pupillary dilation, transient cortical blindness (due to edema around calcarine fissure); **confusion,** vomiting and lethargy during the recovery phase. **Excellent outcome. Treatment:** None required.

165.   Most common cause of death in first few days after accident: **Cerebral edema. Diagnosis:**   Papilledema by examination; **CT scan or MRI. Management:**
    a.   Monitor ICP (intracranial pressure).
    b.   Elevate head at a 30 degrees angle.
    c.   Restrict fluids because of ↑ ADH secretion.
    d.   Hyperventilation to keep the PCO_2 at 25-30, adequate oxygenation (↓ PCO_2 is cerebral vasoconstrictor).
    e.   Medicine:
        i.   Mannitol and lasix (diuretic action).
        ii.   Dexamethasone (reduces cerebral edema).
        iii.   Glucocorticoid (stabilizes blood brain barrier; action begins after 24 hours).
        iv.   Cooling by ice pack or cooling blanket (temperature: 32-33 degrees) for 2-3 days. (Reduces cerebral edema).

166.   Indicator of severity of trauma in concussion: **Duration of amnesia** (retrograde and post-

traumatic).

167. Indication for **admission to hospital for observation** in concussion:
    a. Skull fracture with focal neurologic sign.
    b. Seizure.
    c. **Worsening** of level of consciousness, persistent lethargy and vomiting.
    d. History of trauma is uncertain.

168. Most common cause of death in Tay-Sachs disease: **Bronchopneumonia.** (Patients usually die before reaching 4 years of age.)

169. A child appears with **hyperactivity, short attention** span, disturbances in sleep, bad temperament; there is history of minor head trauma. **Most likely diagnosis: Post-traumatic syndrome. Treatment:** Self-limited disease, so all that nedded are reassurance and carrier detection.

170. Prenatal diagnosis and carrier detection of Tay-Sachs disease (TSD). **(Important for examination):**
    a. Prenatal diagnosis by: CVS (chorionic villous sampling) in first trimester.
    b. Carrier detection in asymptomatic parents: Serum or leukocyte **hexosaminidase A** determination.

171. Tay-Sachs disease (TSD): Most common type of GM2 gangliosidosis. Autosomal recessive. **Hexosaminidase A deficiency.** Clinical manifestations **begin after 6 months** of age (except **startled response means hyperacusis** after birth) with developmental delay. Around one year of age, child appears with **macrocephaly** (excessive GM_2 ganglioside deposit in brain), is unable to sit, stand, or talk, shows spasticity (after hypotonia), blindness, deafness, convulsion. Cherry-red spot in retina is the most characteristic finding. Treatment: None.

172. Most important sources of information about neurodegenerative disorders of childhood: Detailed history and physical examination. **History: Regression** of developmental milestones.

    Physical examination to determine **white or gray** mater involvement:
    a. White: Early onset of upper motor neurone lesion.
    b. Gray: Convulsion, visual defect, intellectual deficit.

173. Complication of cerebral aneurysm and arterio venous malformation: **Rupture.**

174. Cherry-red spot (lipid surrounding the retinal ganglion cells) found in:
    a. Tay-Sachs disease.
    b. Niemann-Pick disease.
    c. Sandhoff disease.

175. Neurodegenerative disorder, its mode of inheritance and biochemical defect: All are **autosomal recessive** except adrenoleukodystrophy, which is XLR (X-linked recessive).
    a. **Sphingolipidosis (all of them are diagnosed by leukocyte and skin fibroblast):**

    i.   GM1 gangliosidosis: ß galactosidase.
    ii.   GM2 gangliosidosis: Hexosaminidase A (Tay-Sachs), A and B (Sandhoff).
    iii. Krabbe disease: Galactocerebrosidase.
    iv. Metachromatic leukodystrophy: Arylsulfatase A.
  b. Sialidosis: Neuraminidase (diagnose by skin fibroblast).
  c. Adrenoleukodystrophy: Very long chain of fatty acid oxidation (diagnose by plasma, skin fibroblast).
  d. Neuronal ceroid lipofuscinoses: Unknown enzyme (diagnose by electron microscopic findings in skin biopsy).

176.   A child appears with **congestive cardiac failure**, progressive hydrocephalus. Most likely diagnosis?
Arteriovenous malformation of vein of Galen. (Hydrocephalus due to obstruction of CSF pathway) Remember, intracranial bruit can be heard on auscultation in arteriorenous malformation. Diagnosis **confirmed** by **angiography;** second choice is CT with contrast.
Treatment: Surgical resection.

177.   Most important is **study to diagnose MS** (multiple sclerosis): **MRI** detection.
Multiple sclerosis:
Pathology: Demyelination and plaque formation.
Etiology: Unknown. May due to genetic, immunologic or infectious factors.
Presentations: Most frequent finding is unilateral weakness or ataxia; diplopia and visual loss are due to optic neuritis.
Treatment: Surgical resection.

178.   Most common site of **cerebral aneurysm:** At **carotid bifurcation** or on the **anterior and posterior cerebral arteries (not** in circle of Willis).
Diagnosis confirmed by: **Angiography. Treatment:** Surgical resection.

179.   Cerebral aneurysm is associated with: Type III collagen vascular disease (sometimes).

180.   Most common organism in brain abscess: **Staph. aureus** (other organisms are microaerophilic Streptococci, aerobe, anaerobe, fungi, parasite).

181.   Most common **solid** tumor in childhood: **Brain tumor.** Brain tumor is second most common form of **malignancy** in childhood. (First if leukemia).

182.   Diagnosis and treatment of brain **abscess:**
Diagnosis by: CT scan (abscess cavity), brain scan (area of enhancement due to disrupted blood-brain barrier).
Treatment: Surgical drainage and antibiotics for 6 weeks. First give broad spectrum antibiotics (penicillin and chloramphenicol), then choose antibiotics according to culture and sensitivity.

183.   Most important investigation for **stroke: Head CT or MRI.** (History and physical examination are very important; brain scan is helpful in focal encephalitis, cerebritis, cerebral abscess, infarction of brain).

184. Most common **site and type** of brain tumor in childhood:
Site: **Infratentorial (posterior fossa).**
Type: **Glial cell tumor.** (First **is cerebellar astrocytoma;** second is medulloblastoma; third is brain stem glioma then ependymoma), all are **posterior fossa tumor.**

185. Immunologic diseases causing brain tumor: Ataxia telangiectasia and AIDS are the most common causes of lymphoma.

186. Most common **supratentorial** tumor in childhood: **Craniopharyngioma (characteristic is calcification).**

187. Clinical manifestations of **brain tumors.** It depends on site, type, and rate of growth. **There are both focal neurologic sign and increased intracranial pressure** (vomiting, papilledema, diplopia), ataxia.

188. **Cerebellar astrocytoma: Most common tumor.** Appears with hydrocephalus and increased intracranial pressure due to obstruction of aqueduct of Sylvius or fourth ventricle.

   Histology: Protoplasmic and fibrillary astrocytes appears in radial fashion interspersed with Rosenthal fibres.
   Treatment of choice: Surgical resection; second choice is radiation for high grade astrocytoma or postoperative tumor progression.
   Prognosis: No other tumor has as good a prognosis.

189. **Medulloblastoma:** Second most common is the posterior fossa tumor, **of unknown site of origin.** Metastasises to **extracranial site. Histologically: Pseudorosettes** formation of deeply staining nuclei with scant cytoplasm.
   Treatment:
   a. Very young patient: Surgery and chemotherapy (vincristine, lomustine, prednisone).
   b. Older patient: Surgery and radiation. (* Younger patients don't tolerate radiation.)

190. **Craniopharyngioma:** Most common supratentorial tumor in childhood. Most common characteristic is **calcification** (90% of cases). First clinical manifestation may be the **short stature.** Examination reveals **bitemporal visual** defect and hydrocephalus with increased intracranial pressure (vomiting, papilledema).
   Diagnosis:
   X-ray skull: Calcification.
   CT scan or MRI: Mass.
   Preferred method of treatment: Surgical removal (subfrontal craniotomy).

191. **Brain stem glioma:** Most common cranial nerve is **abducens (diplopia)** and facial (facial weakness). **Personality changes** are characteristic of brain stem gliomas (lethargy, irritability and aggressive behavior). Preferred method of treatment: **Radiotherapy.**

192. **Ependymomas:** They arise from inside the fourth ventricle and appear with hydrocephalus and increased intracranial pressure (vomiting, diplopia). Preferred method of treatment: **Surgical resection and radiation.**

193. **Best diagnostic** study for all brain and spinal cord tumors (important for examination): **MRI.** Definitive diagnosis by **biopsy.**

194. **Diencephalic syndrome** is due to which brain tumor? **Optic nerve glioma** when involving optic chiasma and hypothalamus. This syndrome appears with **visual defect, emaciation** (no subcutaneous fat), but **normal linear growth, hyper alertness,** euphoria. When hypothalamus is involved, there is obesity, excessive appetite, **diabetes insipidus,** and hypogonadism. Treatment for optic nerve glioma:
    a. **Resection of tumor** to prevent further spread, but can cause blindness.
    b. Hypothalamic and chiasma involvement:
       i. **Younger** patient: Actinomycin D and vincristine chemotherapy and later on radiotherapy.
       ii. Older patient: Radiotherapy (>3 years).

195. Hypervitaminosis A and vitamin A deficiency cause: Pseudotumor cerebri (important for examination).

196. **Parinaud syndrome:** This syndrome is produced by **tumor of pineal** gland causing **pressure on quadrigeminal plate,** appears with **paralysis of upward conjugate movement of the eyes and poorly reactive pupil. Diagnosis confirmed** by: Biopsy (different pineal gland tumors are sensitive to different treatments).

    Treatment:
    a. Teratoma: Surgical removal.
    b. Germinoma: Radiotherapy.
    c. Pinealomas: Chemotherapy.

197. Complications of cranial radiotherapy:
    a. Changed in cognitive behavior.
    b. Reduced verbal performance.
    c. Reduced academic achievement.
    d. Reduced perceptive motor function.

198. **Pseudotumor cerebri (no focal sign):** It **mimics** brain tumor and appears with **increased intracranial pressure,** but shows normal CSF cell counts and protein; ventricular size and anatomy are normal. **Most frequent** symptoms are **headache, diplopia (due to 6th cranial nerve paralysis),** sometimes vomiting.
    Most consistent examination finding is **papilledema with enlarged blind spot;** separation of sutures, cracked pot or resonant sound (Macewen sign). **Treatment:** Self-limited; treat the underlying cause.

199. Most significant **complication** of pseudotumor cerebri: **Optic atrophy and blindness.**

200. Most common **intramedullary spinal cord tumor: Low grade astrocytoma.** (Second is ependymoma).

201. Most common presentations of **spinal cord tumor: Gait disturbances and back pain. Cervical** spinal cord tumor: Lower motor neurone lesion (flaccidity, hyporeflexia) in

upper extremities and upper motor neurone lesion (spasticity, hyperreflexia) in lower extremities. Decreased chest wall movement and weak cough. In **lower** extremities there is loss of sensation of pain, temperature and touch. **Brown-Sequard syndrome due to extramedullary tumor:** Ipsilateral spasticity, ataxia, weakness and contralateral loss of pain and temperature. **Diagnostic study of choice: MRI.** X-ray shows: Widening of interpedicular distance in 40% of patients

Treatment:
a. **Surgical resection** is preferref treatment.
b. Neuroblastoma **metastasize** to extradural spinal space.
Radiation therapy prevents laminectomy.

202. Spinal cord **trauma** mostly due to:
a. MVA.
b. Breech delivery in newborns.
c. Down syndrome: Vertebral anomaly.

203. Most common site for **fracture-dislocation** of spinal cord: C_5-C_6. It produces flaccid quadriparesis, loss of sphincter tone and sensory level to upper sternum.

204. Presentation of severe spinal cord injury: **Spinal shock** which includes loss of sensation, areflexia and flaccidity for four weeks. Reflex **flexor** movement develops then **extensor** movement develops with **hyperreflexia,** spasticity, and autonomic bladder.

205. Conus medullaris syndrome: It is due to fracture at T_{12}-L_1, accompanying loss of sphincter (bladder and rectal) control, flaccid paralysis, diminished sensation in the legs.

206. Central spinal cord lesion: It is due to **hemorrhage and contusion; upper** extremities are more involved than lower; appears with lower motor neurone signs in lower extremities; dysfunction of urinary bladder; sensory loss below the lesion.

207. Diagnosis and treatment of spinal cord injury: **Diagnosis confirmed by MRI.** Initially X-ray spine: It is positive only 50% of cases of severe spinal injury.
Treatment:
a. **First, immobilize and stabilize spine** by cervical collar or sand bag.
b. Maintain airway (oxygen, ambu bag, intubation and mechanical ventilation).
c. Correct shock by intravenous volume expanders.
d. Fracture, dislocation: Traction and immobilization, if the vertebral fusion is unstable.
e. Hemorrhage (epidural, intraspinal), progressive neurologic worsening: Laminectomy, inspection of cord.
f. Supportive measures for urinary and rectal incontinence, skin care, nutrition.

208. Most common **radiologic finding** in tethered cord: **Spina bifida. Tethered cord:** It is due to persistence of **thickened** rope-like filum terminale which connect the conus medullaris at or below L_2 level. (**Normally,** filum terminale becomes fibre-like structure and has conus medullaris ends at L_1.) It appears with **cutaneous** (dimple, lipoma) **defect** over the lesion, **asymmetrical foot growth and muscle wasting.** Diastematomyelia is the associated finding. **Diagnosis confirmed by MRI. Treatment: Surgical resection of**

filum terminale.

209. Most common **site** for diastematomyelia: **L₁- L₃.** It means **division of spinal cord into two,** by bony or fibrocartilaginous septum arising from posterior vertebral body extending backward. It is associated with vertebral anomalies and overlying skin defect (hemangioma). Most commonly present with unilateral foot abnormalities (talipes equinovarus, gastrocnemius atrophy, reduced pain and thermal sensation). Diagnosis **confirmed by MRI.** Treatment: Surgical resection of septum.

210. Most common site of **arterio venous malformation (AVM)** in spinal cord: **Thoracic region.**
     `Steal' phenomenon: It is found in AVM when blood shunts through abnormal **veins and bypasses the spinal cord.** It causes either **transient or progressive loss** of neurologic function. Patient appears to have difficulty walking, low back pain, dysfunction of bladder and rectum, **hyporeflexia** and Babinski reflex present. Diagnosis **confirmed by selective spinal angiography. Treatment:** Surgical excision.

211. A child appears with **rapidly progressive scoliosis and trophic ulcers** in hands and feet. Most likely diagnosis?

     Syringomyelia. It means **there is a cystic cavity** within the spinal cord. Two types:
     a. Communicating (with CSF),
     b. Non-communicating.
     (It is called syringobulbia when it is in medulla.) Pathogenesis: Not known;

     Communicating type is associated with **Chiari type 1** malformation and non-communicating type is susceptible to tumors, trauma, arachnoiditis and vascular accidents. It involves different spinal tracts and produces symptoms:
     a. **Lateral spinothalamic tract:** Upper extremity. (There is the loss of pain and temperature, but touch is intact. This is called **dissociation.)**
     b. **Corticospinal tract:** Upper limb (muscle wasting, absent reflex) and upper motor neurone lesion in lower extremities.

212. Diagnosis and treatment of syringomyelia: **Diagnosis confirmed by MRI. Treatment: Surgery.** When associated with type 1 chiari: Decompression of foramen magnum and upper cervical vertebra.

213. **CPK or CK** (creatinine phosphokinase): It is **not** a universal screening test for neuromuscular disease, because it is normal in many diseases. It is **elevated** in **Duchenne muscular dystrophy.**

214. **NCV** (nerve conduction velocity): It is electrophysiologic measurement of both motor and sensory nerve condition. It measures **only the fastest** conducting nerve in nerve fibres. Neuropathies are diagnosed by **decreased conduction,** which is found when 80% of the total nerve fibres are affected.

215. A child appears with history of **viral** infection; now experiences **abrupt** onset of progressive **weakness; flaccidity** in lower extremities; urinary incontinence; **and pain in**

lower back and abdomen. **Initial** examination reveals loss of **pain; light touch; temperature sensation,** but joint position and vibration sense are intact; hyporeflexia.

Later on patient develops **spasticity and upper motor neurone signs in lower extremities.** CSF: Increased lymphocytes, increased or normal protein. **Most likely diagnosis: Transverse myelitis (important for examination).** It is characterized **initially** by hypotonia and hyporeflexia and **finally** by hypertonia and hyperreflexia. **Diagnosis confirmed by MRI.**
Treatment:
a. Self-limited disease. Complete cure occurs over weeks or months in 60% of the cases.
b. Bladder care (intermittent catheterization).
c. Physiotherapy.
Remember, steroids do **not** work.

216. EMG (electromyography): It is **least** useful in pediatrics because of uncooperativeness of patients. It can diagnose myotonia.

217. A child develops **malignant hyperthermia after anaesthesia** is given for surgery. Examination reveals hypotonia, and wasted proximal muscles (face and neck) with weakness.
Most likely diagnosis: Central core disease.
Serum CPK: Normal, **except** it is elevated in crises like malignant hyperthermia.

218. **Most definite** diagnosis of study in neuromuscular disorder: **Muscle biopsy. Open biopsy** better than needle biopsy. Specimens are **most** commonly obtained from **vastus lateralis (quadriceps femoris)** under local anaesthesia in outpatient (**avoid** deltoid muscles because they contain 80% type 1 fibre, making it **difficult** to recognize different **fibre distribution patterns).** Study under EM (electron microscope) of a frozen section specimen.

219. Nerve biopsy: Most common site of biopsy is **sural nerve.**

220. Most common mode of inheritance of myotubular myopathy: **X-linked recessive (Xq28;** in Duchenne and Baker it is Xp21). **Myotubular myopathy:** It is due to **maturational arrest** of fetal muscles around 8-15 weeks. It appears with **decreased fetal movement** in utero. At birth, there is **thin** muscle mass; **hypotonia;** ineffective respiration and the need for ventilator support; poor sucking and swallowing; so **gavage feed is needed.** (**No** cardiomyopathy, **no** CNS malformation, **no** characteristic facies).
Diagnosis confirmed by: Biopsy; (CPK, EMG, NCV, EKG. All are normal). Prognosis: 75% die within a month's time.

221. CMFTD (congenital muscle fibre type disproportion): It is due to an embryologic defect of fibre-type growth and differentiation. It is a **non-progressive benign** disorder present **at birth with hypotonia, hyporeflexia, delayed motor (walking)** development in infancy, **dolichocephalic head, facial weakness,** high arch palate. **Diagnosis confirmed by: Biopsy;** (CPK, EMG, NCV, EKG. All are normal). **Treatment:** Physiotherapy.

222. **Nemaline rod disease** (Autosomal dominant/recessive). It is due to **rod-shaped** inclusion

structure within muscle fibres. It **mimics** CMFTD, but here patient has **a serious disease,** which appears in infant or children with **hypotonia, thin muscle mass** (proximal and distal), **weak respiratory and bulbar** muscles, dolichocephalic, high arch or cleft palate. Usually a survivor sufferes from gastrostomy and is confined to wheelchair. (**No** cardiomyopathy.) **Diagnosis confirmed by: Biopsy** (CPK is normal).

223. Common complication of benign congenital hypotonia: Recurrent joint dislocation (mainly shoulder). Benign congenital hypotonia: Benign condition (not diseased) with non-progressive **hypotonia which persists until adult life.** Physical examination is **normal.** Biopsy and other laboratory studies are **normal. Diagnosis by exclusion. Treatment:** None. **Prevention: Avoid gymnastics,** because any excessive mobility of the spine can cause a stretch injury, compression, or vascular injury to spinal cord.

224. Detection of carrier state of Duchenne muscular dystrophy. Mother is carrier in X-linked recessive disease, but 30% are **fresh mutations** (i.e., mother is not carrier). Lyon hypothesis can explain when **some females** are affected (one X chromosome becomes inactive and gene-deleted chromosome becomes active), particularly with Turner syndrome. In **asymptomatic carrier:** CPK is elevated in 80% of cases. In 20% it is normal. Muscle biopsy will identify carrier state in 10% (out of 20% of normal CPK). **New definitive molecular DNA analysis:** Isolation and cloning of Duchenne gene and **specific deficiency of dystrophin (encoded protein)** will help in prenatal diagnosis, carrier state, disease state and future therapy.

225. Most common **hereditary** neuromuscular disease (very important): **Duchenne muscular dystrophy, X linked recessive (Xp21 locus). First sign** of manifestation may be **poor head control,** but the disease usually does **not** manifest **until person is 2 years** old. Apears with **lordotic posture (to compensate for gluteal weakness) and Gowers' sign by 3 years of age, and Trendelenburg gait (or waddling gait) by** 5-6 years of age. Most of them can walk by 12 years of age. **Proximal muscles are weak,** but distal muscles functions are preserved. **Pseudohypertrophy of calf muscles and wasting of thigh muscles are typical disease presentations. Remember, extraocular muscles function are normal. There is no** anal or bladder incontinence until late stage. There is, however, weakness in respiratory and pharyngeal muscles.

    Progressive scoliosis: contracture mostly found in ankle, knee, hip, elbow. Next to calf muscle, tongue hypertrophy (no fasciculation) is the second most common finding, forearm hypertrophy is the third most common finding. Cardiomyopathy and lowered I.Q is common. (**No muscle pain, no muscle spasm and no** cancer.) Death **is mostly due** to respiratory failure in sleep around 18 years of age. **Diagnosis confirmed by: Muscle biopsy** (vastus lateralis, gastrocnemius). Serum: **Very high CPK level** (from birth to death). EMG: Nonspecific myopathy. CXR and EKG: Should be done. DNA probe: Most specific method of future diagnosis.

226. **Protein deficiency in Duchenne muscular dystrophy: Dystrophin.**

227. Mode of inheritance of myotonic muscular dystrophy: **Autosomal dominant.** If mother has the disease, then **there is a 50% chance** that baby will also.

228. Treatment for Duchenne muscular dystrophy:
   a. No specific treatment.
   b. Myoblast transfer: New experimental treatment.
   c. Cardiac failure: Digoxin.
   d. Pulmonary infection: Antibiotics and prevention.
   e. Nutritional support: Supplement with **calcium and fluoride.** (Do **not** give vitamins.)
   f. Do **not** give steroids (they worsens the condition).
   g. Physiotherapy: It delays, but can't prevent, contracture.

229. Diagnosis and treatment of myotonic dystrophy:
   a. In typical cases: **Clinical diagnosis** is enough; biopsy not necessary.
   b. Suspected, atypical, or severe neonatal form: **Biopsy confirms** the diagnosis. (EMG: Characteristic myotonic EMG appears **after** 2 years of age. CPK: Normal or slightly elevated).
   Treatment: No specific treatment.
   a. Physiotherapy and orthopedic consultation for contracture.
   b. Treat the cardiac, G.I., eye, and endocrine problem.
   c. For myotonia: Phenytoin, carbamazepine, quinidine, procainamide. These drugs increase depolarization threshold of muscle membrane resulting in improved myotonic condition and muscle function. Anticonvulsant should be given in same doses like seizure.
   d. If **only** weakness (**no** myotonia): Do **not** use above medications.

230. Clinical manifestations of myotonic muscular dystrophy:
   At birth: Mostly normal or hypotonia of facial weakness. Facial features are inverted: **'V'** shaped upper lip, thin cheeks, narrow head, high arch palate. **Initial** wasting of **distal** muscles and eventually **proximal** muscles wasting as well. Wasted thenar and hypothenar muscles, **atrophic tongue, winging of scapula.** Gower sign is present (**normal** reflexes).
   Myotonia: It is absent **until patient reaches 3 years** of age. It is a **slow relaxation of muscles after contraction** (patient is **unable** to open the hand quickly after making fist). It can be demonstrated in affected mother of a child with hypotonia to make the diagnosis. (**No** muscle pain present.) Speech difficulty, swallowing difficulty causing aspiration, sometimes extraocular muscular weakness are present.
   Smooth muscle weakness: Weak uterine contraction causes **ineffective labor;** weak peristolsis causes **constipation.**
   Cardiac: Block with arrythmia (**no cardiomyopathy** unlike most other muscular dystrophies).
   Endocrine: Hypothyroid, hypoadrenalism, diabetes mellitus, delayed puberty, testicular atrophy, frontal baldness (in male).
   Eye: Cataract, abnormal visual evoke potential.
   Development: Mild mental retardation (50% of cases), (**no** epilepsy).
   Serum: ↓ IgG.

231. **Severe neonatal form of** myotonic dystrophy: Rare. Appears with multiple joint contracture (extremities, spine), hypotonia, weakness. Patient requires ventilator support, gavage or gastrostomy feed. Constipation and abdominal distension are due to smooth muscle weakness. 75% of patients die within their first year of life.

232. **Facioscapulohumeral (FSH) muscular dystrophy** (Landouzy-Dejerine disease): Autosomal dominant. Appears with weakness of facial and shoulder girdle muscles (winging of scapula). Muscles of hip girdles and thighs become atrophic (Gowers sign and Trendelberg gait are present). Lumber lordosis, kyphoscoliosis, foot drop are also present. Asymmetry of weakness appears unlike that of any other muscular dystrophy. **Diagnosis confirmed by: Muscle biopsy. Treatment:**
    a. Foot drop and scoliosis: Orthopedic treatment.
    b. **No** physiotherapy because it does not help.

233. Congenital muscular dystrophy: **Autosomal recessive.** Characteristic presentation is **arthrogryposis at birth,** hypotonia, hyporeflexia, **thin muscle** mass in trunk and limbs. **Diagnosis confirmed by:** Muscle biopsy.

234. Myopathies and other conditions:
    a. Hypothyroidism and steroid myopathies: Proximal muscles.
    b. Hyperthyroidism: Muscles wasting.
    c. Hypokalemia, carnitine deficiency: Proximal muscles.

235. Treatment for **carnitine deficiency** (muscle and systemic): **L-carnitine.**

236. Type II Glycogenesis (Pompe's disease) (important): **Autosomal recessive. Deficiency of acid maltase.** Appears in these forms:
    a. Infantile: **Myopathy, cardiomegaly, hepatomegaly, hypotonia, weakness.**
    b. Late childhood: Milder forms of myopathy and others are absent. **Diagnosis confirmed by**: Quantitative assay of **acid maltase in liver or muscle biopsy.**

237. Most serious complication of dermatomyositis: **Calcinosis (dermal and subdermal).**

238. Neonatal myasthenia gravis (transient and congenital):

Transient	Congenital
Mother is **affected,** but there is **no** correlation between maternal duration and the severity of the diseases on baby's condition.	Mother is normal.
Full recovery in 5-47 days.	**Persistent** problem.
Future pregnancies **are affected.**	Does **not** affect future pregnancies.
Fatigue, poor feeding, respiratory distress (but **normal** eye muscles).	Same as transient type; in addition, **extraocular muscular weakness is present.**
Diagnosis: In newborns **(Neostigmine, atropine test). In older children (Edrophonium chloride).** Improves clinical condition. **EMG confirms** the diagnosis.	**Diagnosis:** Same as transient type.

Treatment: P.O. Neostigmine or pyridostiginine **(cholinesterase inhibitor).** Discontinue medications after few days or sometimes weeks.	Treatment: P.O. **Neostigmine or pyridostigmine, steroid, thymectomy. Try to discontinue medication after improvement. May require long term therapy.**
Maternal antibody (Anti-Ach) crosses the placenta, blocks the Ach receptors, and produces symptoms.	**No maternal** antibody present.
Prognosis: Good.	**Prognosis:** Varies. Some improve within months or years, but in others symptoms persist into adult life. Immunosuppression, removal of thymus, and hypothyroid treatment may cure the patient.

239. Myasthenia Gravis, clear picture: In normal person, acetylcholine (Ach) is released from nerve ending, Ach acts on **postsynaptic receptor** and causes **cholinergic** effect. Ach is broken down by **cholinesterase enzyme. In myasthenia gravis,** there is **a reduced number** of receptors available (due to receptor blockade by anti-Ach antibody), or reduced receptor function. This results in **decreased cholinergic** action producing weakness or hypotonia. **To make diagnosis, cholinesterase inhibitor** is used: it prevents the breakdown of Ach, thus potentiating the Ach action and reducing the symptoms. It is also used for **treatment.**

240. **Dermatomyositis:** It includes:
    a. Symmetric proximal muscle weakness.
    b. Serum CPK is high.
    c. Multifocal EMG changes.
    d. Muscle biopsy (vacuole, ischemia, degeneration and regeneration of muscles with lymphocyte infiltration).
    Diagnosis confirmed by: Muscle biopsy.
    Treatment: Prednisone, salicylate, physical therapy.

241. Defect in myasthenia gravis and its clinical manifestation: It is due to **postsynaptic neuromuscular blockade.** There is the result either of a **decreased response or decreased numbers of cholinergic receptors (due to circulating receptor binding acetylcholine antibodies).** It is an **autoimmune** disease.
    Its appearance: **Earliest and most constant** findings are **ptosis and extraocular muscular** weakness. Older children have diplopia, but **normal** pupillary reaction. **Feeding difficulties and facial weakness** are the important findings. **Rapid muscle fatigue is the diseases's unique characteristic. If untreated, it progressively gets worse, involving the respiratory muscles and leading to possible aspiration. (Remember, familial myasthenia gravis is non-progressive.)**

242. Myasthenia gravis could be due to:
    a. Hypothyroidism (usually Hashimoto's thyroiditis).

b.   Collagen vascular diseases. Thyroid function test should therefore **always** be done for this patient.

243.   Antibiotics which **enhance** myasthenia: Kanamycin, streptomycin. (Avoid these medications.)

244.   Agents causing **neuromuscular blockade and mimic myasthenia.**
   a.   Organophosphate.
   b.   Tick paralysis (**neurotoxin inhibits the release** of Ach from axonal ending).
   c.   Botulism (cranial nerves involved, **Guanidine** treatment is effective for extraocular and limb muscles, but not for respiratory muscles).
All of the above conditions are diagnosed by **EMG** along with identification of toxins and ticks in different conditions.

245.   **Spinal muscle atrophy (SMA): Autosomal recessive.** Etiology: **Unknown.** There are many theories. Classification of SMA according to time and severity of onset:
   a.   SMA type 1: (**Werdnig-Hoffman disease:** severe infantile form).
   b.   SMA type 2:   (Late infantile form).
   c.   SMA type 3:   (Kugelberg-Welander disease).
   d.   Variant of SMA: (Fazio-Londe disease: Bulbar palsy due to motor neurone degeneration of brain stem.)
Clinical presentations are:
(**Severe**) **SMA type 1: Tongue fasciculation,** hypotonia, weakness, poor suck and swallow, atrophic muscles, areflexia, (no involvement of sphincter and extraocular muscles, child looks very alert), sometimes respiratory distress at birth, 66% die **within 2 years.**
(**Moderate**) **SMA type 2: No symptoms in early infancy.** Later develops scoliosis, nasal speech, and progressive weakness. May survive in **school years** and use a wheelchair.
(Mild) SMA type 3: Normal in infancy. Later develops proximal muscular (shoulder-girdle) weakness. Live into **adulthood.**
All types present with: Muscles **fasciculation and brightness.**
Diagnosis confirmed by: Muscle biopsy (or EMG). In type 1, diagnosis is usually made **clinically.** NCV is normal. Chromosome location is 5.
Treatment: Nonspecific. Only supportive measures (orthopedic, physiotherapy, uses computer keyboard better than pencil).

246.   In peroneal muscle atrophy (Charcot-Marie-Tooth disease, HMSN type 1), diagnosis is confirmed by: **NCV (nerve conduction velocity) is reduced.** It is **autosomal dominant. It is the most common genetically determined neuropathy.** It appears with **tibial and peroneal** nerve involvement resulting in clumsiness, falling easily, wasted anterior compartment muscles (stork-like), tingling, enlarged thickened palpable nerves.(No pain, no cranial nerve involvement, normal I.Q.; other organs are normal.)
Treatment:
   a.   Stabilization of ankle.
   b.   Leg should be protected from trauma.
Detection: Asymptomatic parents should be tested for NCV.

247.   Argyll-Robertson pupil (no reaction to light but accommodation) found in: HMSN type III

(Defense Sottas disease).

248. Treatment for Refsum's disease: **Avoid green vegetables, nuts, and coffee.** Refsum's disease: It is due to **block in alpha oxidation,** which converts phytanic acid to prostanoic acid. ↑ phytanic acid (found in green vegetables, nuts, coffee) in CSF, blood, brain. Appears between 4-7 years with ataxia, retinitis pigmentosa, and perceptive hearing loss. NCV is delayed.

249. **Familial dysautonomia (Riley-Day syndrome): Autosomal recessive.**

    It is due to reduced unmyelinated nerve fibres which carry sensations of pain, temperature and taste. Appears with **aspiration pneumonia due to poor sucking and swallowing,** breath-holding spells and syncope, ↑ sweating, and blotchy skin erythema. **Insensitivity to pain causes more trauma** (corneal ulceration, tongue bite) and **non cerebellar ataxia.**

    Autonomic crisis (after 3 years): **Cyclic vomiting** lasts for 1-3 days with retching, ↓ B.P., sweating, skin blotching; sometimes hematemesis.
    Diagnosis made by:
    a. **2.5% methacholine drop into one conjunctival sac:** Miosis of pupil in this disease. (**No** action in normal person. Other eye acts as control.)
    b. I.V. norepinephrine infusion: Increased pressure response.
    Treatment: Symptomatic and supportive measures for respiratory, G.I., eye, bony problem. Death: Due to chronic respiratory failure or aspiration in childhood.

250. **Most effective treatment** for Guillain-Barre syndrome: **Plasmapheresis (both in acute and chronic condition).** Other treatment includes: Respiratory care, prevention of decubitus ulcer and infection. Some **chronic** cases respond to methylprednisolone.

251. Diagnosis of Guillain-Barre syndrome: CSF (↑ protein, **normal** cell and glucose) and clinical manifestations (ascending paralysis, areflexia).

252. **Miller-Fisher syndrome:** It is found in Guillain-barre syndrome, appearing with **acute ophthalmoplegia, areflexia, ataxia.**

253. Acute Guillain-Barre syndrome and its associations: It is **post-infectious polyneuropathy** causing demyelination of mostly motor and some sensory nerves. Associated with mycoplasma pneumoniae, and campylobacter infection of the respiratory system.

254. **Etiology** of Bell's palsy (unilateral facial palsy): Post-infectious, allergic or immune demyelinating facial neuritis.

255. Treatment for Bell's palsy:
    a. Do **not** give steroids. Surgery is **not** effective.
    b. Methylcellular eye drop to protect cornea.

256. Prognosis for Bell's palsy: Excellent.

257. Congenital **absence** of depressor angularis oris muscle: It causes **facial asymmetry,**

particularly when infant cries. No difficulty in feeding. Normal eyes. (**Facial nerve palsy:** Facial asymmetry all the time, difficulty in feeding, unable to close eyelids).

258. Most common **cause** of hearing impairment **in childhood: Genetic** (Trisomy 13-15, 18, 21; Waardenburg syndrome).

259. **Non genetic-congenital** causes of **sensorineural** hearing loss:
   a. Ototoxic medication (streptomycin, quinine, thalidomide).
   b. Infection (rubella, CMV).
   c. Radiation.
   d. PPHN (persistent pulmonary hypertension).
   All of the above factors cause 50% of hearing loss in newborns. CMV causes deafness in both symptomatic and asymptomatic patients.

260. **Auditory Brain stem response (ABR):** Remember, it does **not** assess hearing, but rather measures **auditory neuronal electric response** that is usually correlated to behavioral hearing. Normal ABR means **auditory structures up to the midbrain** are responsive. Abnormal ABR does not always mean the absence of hearing. Use:
   a. It is used for screening the hearing of **newborns hearing screening to** detect the ability of peripheral auditory and system to transmit information to VIII cranial nerve and brain stem.
   b. To detect the CNS pathology.

MUSCULOSKELETAL

1. Most common congenital foot deformity: **Metatarsus adductus.** It is due to intrauterine position. Forefoot can be brought to midline neutral position. It **resolves spontaneously in 90% of cases,** but 10% might need cast. (Metatarsus varus: **Fixed** deformity, it is due to medial subluxation of tarsometatarsal joints, adduction and inversion of metatarsal bone. Foot can't be brought to midline position).

2. **Syndactyle:** Most common **between second and third toes; between long and ring fingers.**

3. **Otitic hydrocephalus:** It is a complication of acute otitis media. It appears with **increased intracranial pressure** (headache, vomiting, diplopia, papilledema, 6th cranial nerve paralysis, draining ear) with **normal ventricle and CSF.** Etiology: Unknown. **Investigation:** First do **CT scan** to rule out brain herniation. **Complication: Optic atrophy. Treatment:** Antibiotics, repeated lumber tap, acetazolamide, furosemide, lumboperitoneal shunt.

4. **Polydactyly:** Autosomal dominant. Most common site for extra digit is **ulnar side (little finger side).**

5. Different rotational problems:

a. **Out-toeing in infancy: Normal, more lateral** than medial hip rotation, resolves spontaneously by 2 years when child starts walking.

b. **In-turned feet in the 1st year (Pigeon-toed):** Metatarsus varus/adduction due to intrauterine position.

c. **In-toeing feet in 2nd year:** It is due to medial **tibial** torsion. Resolves spontaneously with observation.

d. **In-toeing in early childhood:** It is due to medial **femoral** torsion. It resolves spontaneously with observation.

e. **In-toeing or out-toeing in late childhood and adolescence:** Rare. It is due to failure of rotational problem. Needs **surgical** correction around 8-10 years of age.

6. Most common cause of CDH (congenital dislocation of hip): **Mechanical cause due to positional problem.**

7. Most common ultrasound finding in CDH (congenital dislocation of hip). **Normal** hip joint and structure (60% cases).

8. Most **definitive method to diagnose** CDH (congenital dislocation of hip): **Ultrasound.**

9. **Preferred method of treatment** in CDH (congenital dislocation of hip): **Pavlik harness (splint);** if this fails, then traction. If traction fails, open or closed reduction.

10. **Complication** of CDH: Aseptic necrosis of femoral head.

11. Most common cause of **limping** (due to hip problem) between **3-6 years** of age: **Toxic synovitis (irritable hip).** It is preceded by URI symptoms. Appears with **limping. May have pain** in the hip, anteromedial side of thigh and knee, restriction of abduction and medial rotation of hip joints. Joint fluids are **normal and sterile.** Sonogram shows joint **effusion.** Radionuclide **scan** shows normal or increased uptake. Septic arthritis: **Pus in** joint cavity, fever, ↑ ESR, ↑ uptake in bone scan. Osteomyelitis: Same as septic arthritis **except** there is pus in the joint.

Treatment for toxic synovitis:
a. Bed rest at home; resolves within 7-10 days.
b. Nonsteroidal anti-inflammatory drug only.

12. **Legg-calve-perthes disease:** It is juvenile **idiopathic avascular** necrosis of femoral head with **unknown** etiology. **Four** stages of the disease formation:
a. Synovitic stage (1st): Joint stiffness, effusion.
b. Necrotic stage (2nd): Bone necrosis.
c. Fragmentation stage (3rd): New bones **replace** the dead bones.
d. Reconstitution stage (4th): Restoration of normal structure.
Sign and symptoms: Gradual onset of **limping, stiffness, pain aggravated by movement and relieved by rest.**
DIAGNOSIS:
a. **1st few weeks: Bone scan (↓ uptake); MRI.**
b. **After few weeks: X-ray hip joint; Bone scan (↑ uptake).**
TREATMENT:

   a. **1st step** to give **rest** to reduce synovitis.
   b. **2nd step** is containment (keep head inside the acetabulum): **Surgery** is preferred (because return to normal activity in 4-6 months) to abduction bracing.

13. Most common clinical type of lordosis is: **Benign juvenile form.** Lordosis is the accentuation of normal lumbar curve. Appears with **prominent buttock** in prepubertal child (no pain, normal movement of spine). **DIAGNOSIS CONFIRMED** by **lateral x-ray spinal column. TREATMENT:** Observation.

14. **Slipped capital femoral epiphysis (SCFE): It** is a **stress** fracture **separating femoral head from neck.** SCFE occurs **during maximum** pubertal growth **before** epiphyseal closure. **Boys and blacks** are more affected than girls and whites.

   Clinical presentations:
   a. **Chronic** (most common): **Groin pain referred** to medial side of thigh and knee, limping, **local tenderness in hip joint which is laterally rotated,** restricted internal rotation, atrophy and shortening of limb.
   b. Acute or chronic SCFE.
   c. Acute SCFE.
   d. Pre-slip or minimal slip.
   Diagnosis confirmed by X-ray hip: Medial displacement of epiphysis.
   TREATMENT: Surgery (emergency, pinning or external fixation). **PROBLEMS:** Chondrolysis of femoral head and acetabulum; stiff joints, avascular necrosis, postoperative pain and fracture.

15. **Congenital** scoliosis: In utero, malposture does **not** produce scoliosis. It is due to **anomalous vertebral segmentation** (hemivertebrae) which causes scoliosis with postnatal growth. Most (80%) of the congenital scoliosis progressively worsens. It is associated with G.U., cardiac anomalies and other syndromes (VATER, Goldenhar, Klippel-Feil syndromes).
   TREATMENT:
   a. **Long flexible curve:** Nonoperative (spinal orthosis: Milwaukee brace).
   b. **Short rigid curve:** Surgical correction.

16. Scoliosis (congenital or idiopathic) progresses **rapidly** during: **Growth spurt and in adolescence.**

17. **Idiopathic scoliosis:** Most common type of **idiopathic** scoliosis is **adolescent type.** Etiology: Unknown. Signs and symptoms of scoliosis are **subtle. Most commonly done** screening test is `the forward bend test'. Remember, there is **no** pain in scoliosis. **DIAGNOSIS CONFIRMED** by **X-ray spine and vertebrae. TREATMENT:** Should begin on time before severe progression.
   a. Observation: Curve < 20 degrees in preadolescent and < 30 degrees in mature person.
   b. Orthotic (Milwaukee brace) therapy: Curve > 25-30 degrees in immature patient and < 40 degrees.
   c. Surgery internal fixation (Harrington rod or C-D instrumentation) and arthrodesis (posterior spinal fusion): Curve > 50 degrees and progressively increases as disease progresses.

Untreated patient: Reduced pulmonary function, cor pulmonale, degenerative arthritis, impingement on nerves (**no** spinal cord compression).

Congenital kyphosis (kyphosis is enhancement of normal dorsal curve): $T_{10}-L_2$, either appears in infancy or when child started walking. It is due to **failure of vertebral formation. X-ray confirms the diagnosis. Do MRI** to rule **out** cord compression. **Extra vertebral anomalies are present,** e.g., paraplegia in severe cases. TREATMENT: **Surgical therapy is the only effective treatment** (arthrodesis, local spinal fusion).

18. **Idiopathic Kyphosis:** Found in adolescent. Etiology: Unknown. Occurs with pain, localized tenderness, fatigue, (**unusual** neurologic complication). X-ray confirms the diagnosis.
    TREATMENT:
    a.   **Milwaukee brace** in skeletal immature patient.
    b.   **Rarely** needs surgery.

19. Most common **site for spondylolisthesis:** At L_5 there is a fracture in **pars reticularis,** a part of the posterior vertebral arch. It is a fracture of L_5 **mostly due to stress,** less likely from trauma. Appears with upright posture, lumber lordosis, back pain, stiffness. X-ray confirms the diagnosis.
    TREATMENT:
    a.   Asymptomatic patient (slippage < 50 degrees): Observation.
    b.   Symptomatic patient: Brace.
    c.   If slip > 50 degrees, severe pain, neurologic sign and brace ineffective: Surgery.

20. Most common organism for diskitis: **Staph. aureus** (others are viral or unidentified causes). **Diskitis:** Common site is the upper lumber, lower thoracic. It is a benign, self-limited condition, occuring with mild fever, back pain, and refusal to sit, walk or stand; ↑ ESR. **DIAGNOSIS** confirmed by MRI. **TREATMENT:** Rest, immobilization, nonsteroidal anti-inflammatory drug, antibiotics.

21. Atlantoaxial joint instability found in: **Down syndrome.** This joint instability causes **cord compression,** paresthesia of upper limbs, neck pain, in severe cases quadriplegia. Open mouth AP view to visualize rotary displacement. CT scan for bones and MRI for cord compression.
    TREATMENT:
    a.   Unstable joint: Posterior fixation of upper cervical spine.
    b.   Subluxation: Reduction, cast, brace, immobilization.

22. Most common type of persistent torticollis: **Infantile congenital muscular torticollis.** Other types are: Trauma, inflammation, neurologic and other causes. Treatment for congenital type: Mostly **resolves spontaneously.** Operation needed if it persists for more than 2 years. The effect of passive exercise is doubtful. Treatment for drug induced dystonic spasmodic torticollis: Diphenhydramine (benadryl).

23. Most common elbow fracture: **Supracondylar.** It can cause Volkmann ischemia or contracture due to neurovascular injury which can cause paralysis and contracture of forearm muscles.

24. Absence of part of the limb in newborn found in: Intrauterine early **chicken pox** infection (1st trimester).

25. **Compartment syndrome (important):** It is found in **forearm, lower part of leg trauma** resulting in ischemic injury distal to site of swelling due to tight fascial compartment. Appears with increased pain, swelling and distal ischemia.

   TREATMENT: Remove all the pressure (dressing, bandage). If no improvement, then **fasciotomy should be done.**

26. Most common **type** of Salter Harris epiphyseal fracture: **Type II** (easily reducible, growth is **normal).**

   Type I: **No** reduction necessary, **normal** growth.
   Type III: Needs **reduction, normal** growth, intra-articular shearing force causing injury.
   Type IV: Need **internal fixation.** May cause **growth arrest.**
   Type V: **Need cast, arrest of growth.**

27. **Classification** of Salter-Harris fracture:

   a. Type I: Epiphysis separated from metaphyses. Germinal cells are (growth) intact. There is normal growth. X-ray may be **negative** but tenderness over growth plate may be the only sign.
   b. Type II: Same as type I and small piece of metaphysis breaks and stays with epiphyses. There is normal growth. This is the most common type.
   c. Type III: Separation along the growth plate with variable distance. There is normal growth.
   d. Type IV: Fracture extends from joint through growth plate into metaphysis. Growth arrest is possible.
   e. Type V: Crush injury causing death of germinal cells (growth plate). There is growth arrest.

28. Treatment for clavicular fracture: **Sling to provide rest to arm.**

29. **Nursemaid's elbow (subluxation of radial head):** It occurs in < 4 years old child when elbow is **pulled suddenly** with **longitudinal traction (elbow extended** and forearm pronated). Usually there is **clicky noise, normal** flexion and extension, **limited supination.** X-ray is normal.

   TREATMENT: Gentle supination with arm in 90 degrees flexion.

30. **Overuse injuries:** It occurs in second decade in immature athletes with **very high ambitions** resulting **in overuse** injuries. Repeated traumatic events cause irritation, inflammation, and microfractures. Diagnosis made by **history of high risk** attitude and **point tenderness.**

31. Treatment for **stress** fractures: Rest, **cast** for complete fracture, physiotherapy. **Stress fracture:** It is due chronic repetitive muscular action on a bony insertion site or repetitive

trauma to that side (example standing causes first metacarpal sesamoid fracture; marching cause metatarsal shaft fracture).

32. Fracture of cervical spine and different sports: C_1, C_2 : Diving, surfing, water skiing, trampolines. C_3 -C_7:   Football.
    Injuries in different sports:
    a. **Wrestling:** Skin (herpes and other infection), brachial plexus pinching or stretching called (**'stingers' and `burners'),** shoulder subluxation, knee injury, hand injury.
    b. **Hockey:** Specific injury (ankle sprains, hip adductor injury, shoulder injury).
    c. **Gymnastics:** Common problem is **overuse and traumatic injury** to (ankle, wrist, spine). Most common injury with floor exercise.
    d. **Football: Most injuries are minor, 'stingers and burners' as in** wrestling, injury to knee, shoulder, ankle, **myositis** ossificans, turf toe (forceful dorsiflexion of 1st metatarsophalangeal joint).
    e. **Ballet: Delayed menarche and eating disorder, medial snapping hip syndrome** (due to iliopsoas tendon passing over anterior hip capsule), injury to feet, ankle, leg, knee, hip, spine.
    f. **Baseball: Most common injury is to shoulder and elbow,** particularly among pitchers.
    g. **Swimming: Most common is shoulder injury** (swimmer's shoulder: Tendinitis of supraspinatus or biceps).
    h. **Running: Mostly overuse injury** to lower extremity. Iliotibial band syndrome (bursitis, tendinitis, mechanical friction of band, i.e., extension of tensor fasciae latae and lateral femoral condyle), **compartment syndrome.**
    i. **Soccer:** Injury to hip (iliac crest contusion: **hip pointer),** knee (ligaments, menisci).
    j. **Skiing:** Injury to **thumb (salter type III),** ankle, tibial spinal fracture.
    k. **Tennis:** Tendinitis (shoulder, elbow), injury to (ankle, abdomen). **Treatment for pain in all injuries:** Rest, nonsteroidal anti-inflammatory agent.

33. **Marfan syndrome: Autosomal dominant.** May be due to defect in collagen or defective dermal microfibril. **Clinical manifestations:** Tall, slim, hypotonia, lax ligaments, **increase** in lower portion of body greater than in upper portion, narrow maxilla, dental crowding. Defective gene at **chromosome 15.** Eye: Most common **is ectopia lentis;** severe myopia, blue sclera, iris tumor. Skeletal: Long, thin arms and legs; **diminished upper-lower segment ratio;** funnel chest or pigeon breast. CNS: **Dural ectasia;** learning disability, hyperactivity.
    TREATMENT:
    a. **Beta blocker:** To prevent aortic dilatation.
    b. Multiple subspecialty (orthopedic, cardiac, ophthalmology) approach.
    c. Physiotherapy: To improve neuromuscular tone.
    d. Prophylactic antibiotics: To avoid endocarditis. * Genetic counseling is important for the patient and family.

34. Chondrodysplasia punctata (Conradi-Hunermann syndrome): X-ray: Stippled calcification of epiphyses and growth plate.

35. Most common osteoporotic syndrome of childhood: **Osteogenesis imperfecta.** It causes skeletal deformities and fractures.

Osteogenesis imperfecta (OI):

a.   **Type I: Most common type of OI. Autosomal dominant. Appears with blue sclera, osteoporosis, multiple fractures** (from minimal trauma and rarely at birth), hearing loss after first decade, **dentinogenesis imperfecta (yellow broken teeth),** kyphoscoliosis (20% cases), **spontaneously improved** as puberty like type IV. **Culture of skin fibroblast shows diminished type 1 collagen.**

b.   **Type II: Lethal** disease. Autosomal recessive. 50% **of cases lead to stillbirth. The rest die** from respiratory difficulty due to defective thoracic cage, **LBW, soft skull, multiple** fractures. Defect in **alpha 1 (I) chains of type I collagen,** which is the main collagen.

c.   **Type III:** Autosomal recessive. Appears in newborn with blue sclera, multiple fractures (normal birth weight and length). Cardiorespiratory failure before childhood causes death.

d.   Type IV: Autosomal dominant. A mild disease (less fracture, less hearing loss, fewer dental problems), blue sclera at birth improves with age. As in **type I, there is spontaneous improvement at puberty.**

TREATMENT:

a.   Type II: **No** treatment is effective against this serious disease.

b.   Type I, III, IV: Firm mattress or pillow to prevent fracture, aggressive orthopedic management (splinting). **Don't give** calcium, vitamin C, fluoride, calcitonin, or magnesium oxide.

Prenatal diagnosis: Not available for all types, but type II is diagnosed by sonogram, X-ray, biochemical study.

36.   Treatment for **Caffey disease (infantile cortical hyperostosis): Corticosteroid.** It appears within first three months of life with **fever,** severe **soft tissue swelling** over the face and jaws, **progressive cortical thickening of** both long and flat bones, **exacerbations and remissions** with **spontaneous regression** after few years. Alkaline phosphatase slightly increased.

37.   **Defects in skeletal growth (short stature or dysplasia):**

Achondroplasia	Thanatotropic dysplasia	Hypochondroplasia
Autosomal dominant, 50% new mutation, etiology is unknown.	Sporadic, **most lethal congenital skeletal dysplasia.**	**Autosomal dominant.**
May be associated with hydrocephalus due to foramen magnum obstruction.	Familial: Clover leaf skull with hydrocephalus.	**No** hydrocephalus.
Large head circumference.	Large head.	**Normal** head.
No respiratory distress.	Respiratory difficulty, **narrow** chest.	**Normal** respiratory status.

Dental malocclusion, otitis media and conductive hearing loss.		
At birth: Rhizomelic limb shortening, large head, short stature, hypotonia which resolves later on, depressed nasal bridge.	**At birth: Shorter** than achondroplasia, large head, short limb, depressed nasal bridge.	**At birth: Normal; manifest later** with short stature, stocky, muscular built, normal head.
Xray: Reduce interpedicular distance L_1- L_5 (characteristic).	Xray: Inverted 'U' shaped and flattened lumber vertebrae (characteristic).	Xray: Same as achondroplasia, but mild variety.

38. Most common **cardiac lesion** in Marfan syndrome: **Aortic insufficiency** due to aortic root dilation. (MVP also occurs with equal frequency).

39. Most common cause of **death in Marfan syndrome: Progressive MVP** (mitral valve prolapse). It causes arrythmia, endocarditis, thromboembolism, and heart failure. **(Idiopathic MVP = non progressive).**

40. **Arthrogryposis: Sporadic,** appears **in utero** (breech, oligohydramnios, reduced fetal movements) and **at birth (fixed deformed flexed knee,** wrist, elbow and other joints, **dislocated hip,** club feet), less mental retardation, **thickened skin. TREATMENT:**
    a. Physiotherapy: Passive joint movement.
    b. Orthopedic: Splint, cast or surgery.

RICKETS, TETANY

1. **Mode of inheritance** of familial hypophosphatemia (vitamin D-resistant rickets, **X-linked hypophosphatemia): X-lined dominant That is,** the mother of the affected child has either bowing, short stature or **only fasting** hypophosphatemia.

2. Vitamin D-**dependent** rickets (Pseudovitamin D deficiency, hypocalcemic vitamin D resistant rickets): **Autosomal recessive. It is due to deficiency of enzyme 25 (OH) D-1 alpha hydroxylase,** which is required for the formation of 1,25 $(OH)_2$ D. The level of 1,25 $(OH)_2$ D (vitamin D_3) will be **low** in serum. Usually appears with rickets **around 3-6 months of** age in an infant who is **already taking vitamin D (400-600 IU/day** also develops **dental enamel hypoplasia, secondary** hyper parathyroidism, glucosuria, aminoaciduria, and renal tubular acidosis). Serum: ↓ Ca, ↓ P, ↑ alkaline phosphatase. ↑ **PTH,** ↓ 1,25 $(OH)_2$D.

   TREATMENT: Large dose of vitamin D_2, or **small** dose of vitamin D_3 (1-2 µG/day). **Above mentioned** clinical condition is called **type I vitamin D dependent rickets.** What is type II?

Type II: Some of the above mentioned patients **will not** respond to large doses of vitamin D_2 or small doses of vitamin D_3. This is due to **defect in end organ (skin, bone) receptors of** $1, 25 (OH)_2$ D in cytoplasm or nucleus: these **receptors are producing abnormal genes.** Patient appears with **short stature and alopecia totalis.** It is common in children of **marriages,** between first cousins, so type II **represents hereditary resistance to 1, 25 $(OH)_2$ D. TREATMENT: Large dose** (15-30 µg/day) of $1,25 (OH)_2$ D will improve rickets, but **not** the alopecia.

3. **Hypophosphatemic bone disease:** Autosomal dominant. Appears with ↓ P in serum, ↑ P excretion in urine, but normal X-ray, normal height, → $1, 25 (OH)2$ D in serum. **TREATMENT: Oral phosphate with 1, 25 $(OH)_2$ D.**

4. **Familial hypophosphatemia:** Defect in **proximal tubular reabsorption of phosphate and conversion of 25 (OH) D to 1, 25 $(OH)_2$ D. Clinical presentations: Bowing** of lower limb when starting to walk, **waddling gait, short stature, intraglobular dentin** (characteristic teeth **pulp** deformity, normal enamel; enamel defect found in calcium deficient rickets, but periapical infection found in both rickets). X-ray: Widening, fraying, and cupping of metaphysis; coarse trabecular bone. Serum: ↓ Ca, ↓ P, ↑ alkaline phosphatase. → **PTH,** ↓ $1, 25 (OH)_2$ D. Urine: ↑ P excretion despite ↓ P in serum.

   TREATMENT: Oral phosphate with vitamin D (dihydrotachysterol or D_3).

5. **Etiology of hepatic** rickets and discussion: **Reduced absorption of Vitamin D in intestine** due to lack of bile salt secretion by liver. (It is **not** due to impairment of 25-hydroxylation in liver.) It can be due to extrahepatic biliary atresia, neonatal hepatitis, or TPN (total parenteral nutrition). **Serum:** ↓ **Ca,** ↓ **25, (OH) D,** ↑ alkaline phosphatase. **X-ray:** Positive for rickets (cupping, fraying, widening of metaphysis). **TREATMENT:** 4000-10,000 IU of **vitamin D_2** (100-250 µG) or 50 µG of **25 (OH) D** or 0.2 µG/kg of **1, 25 $(OH)_2$ D** along with oral **calcium.**

6. **Primary chondrodystrophy (metaphyseal dysplasia):** Patient will have short stature for the rest of his life. Appears also with bow legs and waddling gait. Serum: **All normal** (Ca, P, alkaline phosphatase, Vitamin D metabolite).

7. **Etiology of rickets due to anticonvulsant therapy** and discussion: **Anticonvulsant increases hepatic enzyme (cytochrome P-450 hydroxylase) activities,** resulting **in increased** conversion of 25 (OH) D to 1, 25 $(OH)_2$ D. As many patients do not take enough dairy products (source of calcium) or exposure to sun, relatively **normal** serum level of 1, 25 $(OH)_2$ D is comparatively low in relation to degree of ↓ Ca, ↓ P, ↑ PTH in serum. **TREATMENT: Vitamin D_2** (500-1000 IU/day). Remember, all anticonvulsants can cause rickets, particularly phenobarbital and phenytoin.

8. **Etiology of oncogenous** rickets (primary hypophosphatemic rickets associated with tumor) and discussion: Tumor releases **unidentified substance** which **increases phosphaturia and inhibits the conversion of 25 (OH) D to 1, 25 $(OH)_2$ D.** It is found in **neurofibromatosis, epidermal nevus, and linear nevus syndrome. TREATMENT:**
   a. **Removal of the tumor cures the rickets.**
   b. If malignant or cannot be removed, **give 1, 25 $(OH)_2$ D with oral phosphate.**

9. **Etiology** of rickets due to **renal tubular acidosis (RTA)** and discussion: It is due to **phosphaturic hypophosphatemia.** RTA appears as hyperchloremic metabolic acidosis with loss of bicarbonate, calcium, K, phosphate in urine. **Proximal or type II:** It can cause **full-blown rickets.** Distal or type I: **Only bone demineralization without** overt rickets. Both types appear with **bone pain, diminished growth, osteopenia (rarely** fracture).
    TREATMENT:
    a. Distal type: Sodium bicarbonate.
    b. Proximal type: Sodium bicarbonate with oral phosphate. To prevent oral phosphate that causes secondary hyperparathyroidism, give **vitamin D.**

10. **Hypophosphatasia:** Autosomal recessive. It is **defined as low serum alkaline phosphatase activity.** It is classified into two types:
    a. **Congenital lethal** hypophosphatasia **(severe** infantile form): **Deficient** alkaline phosphatase activity **only in liver, bone and kidney** (normal in intestine and placenta). Appears with **moth-eaten** appearance of end of long bones **(resulting in severe shortening)** and **severe deficiency of ossification, Wormian bones (intersutural bones),** nephrocalcinosis due to hypercalcemia, diminished calcification of skull bones, premature loss of teeth.
    b. **Hypophosphatasia tarda (milder** childhood or late adolescence form): Appears with **bowing** of leg, slight **shortening of height,** bone pain, fracture, mild bony defect, and tooth loss. In both the conditions: Serum: ↑ inorganic pyrophosphate and pyridoxal 5-phosphate. Urine: ↑ phosphoethanolamine (it is metabolized by alkaline phosphatase).
    TREATMENT: No satisfactory treatment, but **infusion of plasma rich alkaline phosphatase helps in healing bones. Pseudohypophosphatasia:** Patient appears exactly as in hypophosphatasia, but **there is normal** alkaline phosphatase activity. It may be due to mutant alkaline phosphate isoenzyme.

11. Most common **cardiac defect in William syndrome** (idiopathic hypercalcemia): **Supravalvular aortic stenosis.**

12. **Idiopathic hypercalcemia:** Three different forms:
    a. **William syndrome (elfin facies syndrome):** Facial features consist of prominent maxilla, hypoplastic mandible, cupid's bow curve in upper lip, caries with peg-shaped teeth; **failure to thrive due to poor feeding, mild mental retardation and** unusual `cocktail party patter' behavior is characteristic. **Hypercalcemia is an infrequent finding.**
        Serum: **Normal vitamin D metabolite (most cases),** (few have ↑ vitamin D metabolite even with normal intake of baby and mother).
        TREATMENT: **Social support and special school** for the mentally retarded.
    b. Mild idiopathic hypercalcemia: Transient, **normal** looking child, normal vitamin D metabolism, but sometimes nephrocalcinosis is due to hypercalcuria.
    c. Familial hypocalcuric hypercalcemia: Autosomal dominant, **asymptomatic patient** (neonate may manifest **severe parathyroid hyperplasia),** most patients have **mild** parathyroid hyperplasia **despite ↑ serum Ca** (> 18 mg/dl) due to inappropriate response of parathyroid gland. Parents has ↑ serum Ca (12-15 mg/dl). Normal vitamin D metabolism. Serum: **Mg level is elevated.**
        TREATMENT:

      i.   Only in cases of serious hyperparathyroidism: Emergency parathyroid **removal.**

      ii.   All other cases: No treatment is required.

13.   a.   **Hyperphosphatasia (Juvenile Paget disease):** Autosomal recessive. It is due to **elevation of bone isoenzyme of alkaline phosphatase in serum. Appears** around 2-3 years of age with **painful bony deformity with growth failure,** sometimes fracture, large skull with **wide diploic space.** Serum: → Ca, → P, ↑ alkaline phosphatase, ↑ acid phosphatase. Urine: ↑ leucine amino acid peptidase. **TREATMENT: Calcitonin** (reduces rapid bone turnover).

      b.   **Transient** hyperphosphatasia: Unknown, **benign, asymptomatic** patient, ↑ bone and liver isoenzyme, begins from 2 months to 2 years of age and resolves within 6 months of its occurence.

      c.   **Familial** hyperphosphatasia:**Autosomal dominant,** benign, asymptomatic, ↑ serum alkaline phosphatase.

14.   **Earliest sign** of renal osteodystrophy: **Growth failure** (occurs before skeletal changes).

15.   **Earliest indication of bone disease** (osteitis fibrosa) in renal osteodystrophy: ↑ **PTH level in serum.**

16.   **Earliest bony changes** (osteitis fibrosa) in renal osteodystrophy: **Subperiosteal erosion of middle and distal phalanx.**

17.   Most common cause of Fanconi syndrome and its features: **Idiopathic.** (Other causes are inborn errors of metabolism, heavy metals, certain drugs like tetracycline, gentamicin.) **Fanconi syndrome:** Clinical characteristics are **growth failure** and **rickets due to hypophosphatemia with phosphaturia.** Vomiting, dehydration, polyuria, polydypsia, constipation. Urine: Loss of (amino acid, glucose, phosphate, bicarbonate, uric acid, protein, Na, K). Serum: ↓ (P, K, protein, pH), ↑ **Cl (hyperchloremic metabolic acidosis),** → Glucose. **DIAGNOSIS: No** definite test. **TREATMENT:**

      a.   Secondary Fanconi syndrome: **Treat underlying cause.**

      b.   Rickets: Large dose of **vitamin D.**

      c.   Primary Fanconi syndrome: **Mineral and electrolyte; correct dehydration.**

      d.   Metabolic acidosis: Large dose of **alkali** (sodium bicarbonate, polycitra, Shohl solution). Sodium bicarbonate and Shohl solution have 1mEq of base = 1 ml. but polycitra has 2 mEq of base = 1 ml.

18.   Prenatal diagnosis of cystinosis (Fanconi syndrome with cystinosis): **Increased cystine in amniotic fluid.**

19.   **Cystinosis:**

Etiology: **Unknown.** Autosomal recessive. It is due to **abnormal accumulation of cystine in lysosome and failure of lysosomal release of cystine. No** enzyme defect: remember, Fanconi syndrome is **not** due to effect of cystine on tubules. Cystine **is deposited in R.E. (reticulo-endothelial) system** (liver, spleen, lymph nodes, bone marrow), but not in brain and muscle. **Renal deposition causes 'swan neck'** (atrophy, shortening of proximal tubule), **renal failure** due to glomerular sclerosis and interstitial fibrosis.

Clinical presentation:

a. **Infantile or nephropathic form: Blond hair and fair complexion** (defect in melanin synthesis), photophobia (cystine deposit in conjunctivae and cornea), **Fanconi syndrome (3-12 months), growth retardation, hypothyroidism, severe renal disease.**

b. Adolescent or intermediate form: **Mild renal** defect in second decade.

c. Adult type: Benign, normal kidney.

Laboratory: Same as Fanconi syndrome + cystine deposit.

DIAGNOSIS:

a. Asymptomatic patient: ↑ **cystine content in leukocyte or fibroblast.**

b. Slit lamp examination: Shows cystine in cornea.

TREATMENT:

a. **Same as Fanconi syndrome.**

b. **Cysteamine** (sulfhydryl binder): It reduces intracellular cystine. It can **reduce Fanconi** syndrome, but can't reverse it.

c. Renal failure (end stage): Hemodialysis and transplant. (Hemodialysis does **not** reduce tissue cystine level.)

Effects of renal transplant in cystinosis:

a. **Renal function of patient: Improves** like any other chronic kidney disease needing a transplant, so **increases survival chances of patient.**

b. **Progressive photophobia** and retinopathy: Cysteamine eye drop.

c. Extrarenal presentations: Swallowing difficulty, myopathy, pancreatic insufficiency (endocrine, exocrine), CNS (seizure, cerebral atrophy).

20. Difference between **cystinuria and cystinosis:**

Cystinuria: Inborn errors of transport of cystine (amino acid); no cystine deposition; no Fanconi syndrome.

Cystinosis: Already discussed.

Lowe syndrome (oculo cerebro renal dystrophy): X-linked recessive, etiology: **Unknown.** May be due to abnormality in collagen (splitting of glomerular basement membrane).

Presentation:

a. Initial: Eye (cataract, glaucoma, buphthalmos), mental retardation.

b. Later on: Fanconi syndrome (may resolve spontaneously or lead to chronic renal failure).

TREATMENT: Same as Fanconi syndrome.

21. **Renal osteodystrophy: Pathogenesis:** In the early phase of the disease, there is ↓ GFR, normal phosphate (intake in food) suppresses vitamin D_3 formation in kidney, ↓ vitamin D_3 cause ↓ Ca and P absorption, resulting in ↑ PTH secretion which keeps serum Ca→ and P ↓ or → (due to phosphaturia); when GFR ↓ to 25-30% of normal, then phosphaturia by PTH does not occurs, so **compensatory hyperparathyroidism occurs to keep Ca →.**

Bone biopsy: Osteomalacia and **osteitis fibrosa (not** rickets) (degree of ↑ PTH correlates with osteitis fibrosa, but not with osteomalacia.) **Clinical presentations: Osteodystrophy is directly proportional** to the degree and duration of renal failure. Appears with **growth**

failure (first sign), metabolic acidosis, protein calorie malnutrition, anemia. In advanced disease condition, it appears with **bone pain and deformity,** weak muscles, slipped epiphyses, metastatic calcification, **itching.** Genu varum, dental anomalies present.

Tetany is rare (despite ↓ serum Ca) because acidosis and hyperparathyroidism protect the condition. Serum:↓ Ca (mild), ↑ P, ↑ alkaline phosphatase, ↑ PTH.

TREATMENT:
a. **Restrict dietary phosphorus and increase dietary calcium.**
b. **Vitamin D$_3$.**
c. High P in serum: **Phosphate binder** (avoid aluminum-hydroxide because it causes toxicity).
d. Hemodialysis or peritoneal dialysis (↓ or ↑ bone disease).
e. **Calcium carbonate.**
f. **Hyperparathyroidism: Needs** autotransplantation.

22. **Important findings to remember for tetany:**
Definition: Hyperexcitability of CNS and peripheral nervous system due to ionic alternation.
a. Tetany is caused by ↓ (H^+, Ca^{2+}, Mg^{2+}).
b. Alkalosis (↓ H^+) causes tetany with → (Ca^{2+}, Mg^{2+}).
c. ↓ K^+ prevent and ↑ K^+ precipitate ↓ Ca^+ tetany.
d. K^+ has no effect on ↓ Mg^{2+} tetany.
e. Ionized calcium is **40-50% (4.0-5.2 mg/dl)** of total calcium. Tetany mostly develops when Ca^{2+} (ionized) < 2.5 mg/dl (equivalent to total Ca 5 mg/dl).
f. In hypoalbuminemia (nephrotic syndrome), total Ca is low (<7 mg/dl), but **ionized Ca^{2+} is normal,** so no tetany.
g. Ionized magnesium is 75% of total Mg (1.6-2.6 mg/dl), < 1.0 mg/dl may cause tetany.
h. Tetany manifests with carpopedal (wrist and ankle) spasm, laryngospasm.
i. **Latent** tetany: **Only** manifests after stimulation, ischemia. **Trousseau sign** (tourniquet application causes ischemia and tetany), **chvostek sign** (stimulation of facial nerve causes twitching of upper lip, entire mouth, orbicularis oris muscles).
j. ↓ Ca 2^+ causes prolong QT interval in EKG.

23. Most common cause of **early (first 36 hours) hypocalcemia in** newborns **(important):** **Transient hypoparathyroidism** (it is the most common dysfunction of parathyroid gland). **TREATMENT: Calcium gluconate.** (Remember, when ↓ Ca is associated with ↓ Mg, then **MgSO4** should be added to the therapy.)

24. Treatment for **alkalotic tetany** due to **hyperventilation (important): Blow air into a bag or balloon** to increase PCO_2. Remember, **the most common cause of hyperventilation is psychogenic. Relation of alkalosis and tetany:**
a. **Both** respiratory alkalosis (hyperventilation) and metabolic alkalosis (sodium bicarbonate) cause tetany.
b. Remember, metabolic alkalosis (hypochloremic) due to pyloric obstruction does **not** cause tetany.
c. Alkalotic tetany in renal patient is **protected by concurrent metabolic acidosis. Correction of acidosis** results in tetany and convulsion.

25. Most common cause of **late (mostly occurs in first 5-10 days,** and as late as 6 weeks) hypocalcemia of newborn **(important): High phosphate milk (cow milk).**
TREATMENT: Discontinue that milk.

26. **Early** hypocalcemia usually occurs in: Premature, LBW, IUGR, IDM (diabetic), babies and those delivered after prolonged labor.

27. How high phosphate milk in neonates causes hypocalcemia: High P milk cause ↑ serum P level (by increasing tubular reabsorption and ↓ GFR) resulting in ↓ serum Ca level. In newborns, response of parathyroid gland to hypocalcemia is **inadequate,** resulting in progressive hypocalcemia and tetany.

28. Treatment of choice for **hypocalcemia (tetany) in DiGeorge syndrome** (aplasia of both thymus and parathyroid gland): Dihydrotachysterol or highly active vitamin D metabolite (1, 25 dihydroxy vitamin D 3). Remember, simple calcium therapy **does not** work.

29. A newborn nursed **exclusively on breast milk** may develop (important):
    a. Vitamin D deficiency: Needs vitamin D supplement.
    b. Fluoride deficiency:
    Needs fluoride (0.25 mg/dl). Remember, nutritional vitamin D deficiency is **very rare.**

30. Preferred method of treatment for **hypocalcemia (tetany) in vitamin D deficiency:** Concentrated vitamin D supplement (initially, I.V. calcium is given).

31. Etiology of transient hypomagnesemia (↓ Mg): **Unknown.** It occurs due to ↓ **Mg absorption from** intestine and kidney. **Intestinal loss** in inflammatory bowel disease and resection of bowel. **Renal loss** found in Bartter syndrome (↓ Mg. ↓ K, tetany due to tubular defect), aminoglycoside, cis-platinum. Remember, ↓ Mg is usually associated with ↓ Ca, ↓ Mg stimulates parathyroid secretion like ↓ Ca.
TREATMENT: Magnesium sulfate (I.V. or I.M.), magnesium chloride/gluconate (oral).

32. **Most common cause** of failure to thrive:
Psychosocial (emotional deprivation, neglect or abuse like withholding food from children). Other causes are organic (malabsorption, infection and systemic diseases), chromosomal disorder, malignancy, immunodeficiency (e.g., AIDS).

33. Treatment for failure to thrive (FTT) due to psychosocial cause:
    a. **Temporary hospital admission in order to remove baby from that negative environment.**
    b. FTT due to any other causes: Treat the underlying cause.

INJURY

1. Most common **cause of death between 1-14** years old: **Accident** (second is malignancy). Most common accident is MVA (motor vehicle accident). MVA is most common cause of

death between **1-25 years. Pedestrian being hit by motor vehicle** occurs most commonly **between 3-7 years. Boys** have more accident than girls.

2.	Bicycle accident: Most common cause is **bicycle product-related injury.** Most common site of injury is **craniofacial (67% of** cases).

3.	Home related injury: Mostly between **2-3 years old.** Most common injury is **falling downstairs** or hit with low furniture. **Severity of injury in fall depends on the surface impacted** rather than number of stairs. Walker **is** very risky (1 out of 3) and only **delays walking** rather than helps.

4.	School related injury:
	a.	Older children are only mildly injured in **physical education activities.**
	b.	Playground injuries mostly occur in **the head and neck, and are often product related.**
	c.	Interscholastic sports injuries: Most common for **boys is football,** and for **girls, basketball.**
	d.	More injuries occur **during practice** than during competition.
	e.	50% hockey players suffer significant **facial trauma.**

5.	**Farm related injury:** It is due to **increased use of farm equipment and lack of supervision of children.** Occurs mostly during planting and harvesting time when parents are busy.

6.	'Accident-prone **period'** rather than `accident prone **child':** The latter** term should be replaced by "**accident prone period"** which refers to **age, developmental level, and social stress.** "Accident **prone** child" describes **personality**.

7.	Most common EMS calls for children are due to: **Trauma (54%).** Most frequent medical conditions are seizure, respiratory problems, and poison ingestion.

8.	Most common cause of **poor** success rate for pediatric prehospital CPR: Due to **specific cause of pediatric cardiopulmonary failure, (e.g., SIDS, drowning) not due** to poor resuscitation. **Most common cause of prehospital pediatric cardiopulmonary arrest is SIDS.** Second most common is drowning. Third is unknown.

9.	Prehospital primary survey in **order of ABCD:**
	A:	Airway.
	B:	Breathing.
	C:	Circulation.
	D:	Disability (modified Glasgow coma scale).

10.	Prevention of **pedestrian** MVA: Clothing reflector, walking facing traffic, begin walking instruction at 2 years of age.

11.	**Prevention of MVA (motor vehicle accident) and age:**
	a.	Up to 30 lbs (up to 2 years): Infant safety seat or convertible safety seat.
	b.	30-60 lbs (2-8 years): Booster seat or safety lock.

    c.   8-16 years: Seat belts (lap and shoulder).

    d.   Above 16 years: Seat belts, ↑ drinking age, SADD (Students Against Drunk Driving) program.

    e.   Person driving: Active (reduce driving speed, use seat belt); Passive (air bag, automatic seat belt).

Remember, drivers education **enhances MVA** because it **increases the number of teenage drivers.**

12.   To prevent **bicycle and motorcycle** injuries: **Wear helmet,** ride with traffic, don't use headphone, and wear reflective clothing .

13.   **To prevent Drowning:**

    a.   Up to 5 years: Water safety education; children always should be attended to; certified life preserver as floating device.

    b.   15-21 years: Tamper-proof pool cover should be installed. Hyperventilation is dangerous before diving.

14.   To prevent **firearms** injuries: Don't keep gun at home with children. Always lock it away. Adults should be held responsible for such injuries.

15.   To prevent **falls:**

    a.   Up to 4 years: Non-accordion stairway gate, carpet in stairway, shopping cart seat belt.

    b.   1-10 years: Playground surface and equipment should be modified.

    c.   11-21 years: Avoid trampolines in gymnastics.

16.   To prevent **poisoning:** Poison prevention education. Keep medicine locked, and safety caps on bottles.

17.   To prevent **burns:**

Up to 5 years: Routine fire inspections. Fire escape should be accessible. Teach child to be careful with hot water and materials.

18.   To prevent **sports** injuries: Proper conditions and equipment, strict rules, rehabilitation.

19.   Social factors causing accidental injury:

    a.   Maternal: Single, unemployed, uneducated, pregnant, abusing drugs or alcohol.

    b.   Family matters: Death of friend or family member, birth of a sibling, move to a new house, change of job, marriage of parent.

20.   Most commonly used **screening test** for head injury patient: MGCS (modified Glasgow coma scale).

21.   **Different drugs and effects:**

| Nitroprusside | Cyanide toxicity. |

Isoproterenol	Tachycardia, ↓ myocardial O_2 demand, subendocardial ischemia, arrythmia.
Dopamine	Selective renal vasodilator in low doses, also vasodilate splanchnic vessels.
Dobutamine	Increase myocardial contractility, so use in cardiac failure.
Epinephrine	Tachycardia, severe vasoconstriction in higher doses, use in cardiac arrest.

22. CVP (central venous pressure) **does not:**
   a. Correlate with LVEDP (left ventricular end diastolic pressure).
   b. Reflect true mixed venous gases (pulmonary artery).

23. **Modified Glasgow coma scale (MGCS):**
   a. **Best verbal response:**

Score	> 5 years	2-5 years	0-23 months
5	Oriented and converses.	Appropriate words and phrases.	Smiles, coos.
4	Disoriented and converses.	Inappropriate words.	Cries, consolable.
3	Inappropriate words.	Persistent cries/screams.	Inappropriate cries or screams persistently.
2	Sounds not understandable.	Grunts.	Grunts restless, agitated.
1	No response.	No response.	No response.

   b. **Best motor response:**

Score	>1 year	<1 year.
6	Obeys.	Spontaneous.
5	Localizes pain.	Localizes pain.
4	Flexion withdrawal.	Flexion withdrawal.
3	Decorticate rigidity.	Decerebrate rigidity.
2	Decerebrate rigidity.	Decerebrate rigidity.
1	No response.	No response.

   c. **Eyes opening:**

Score	> 1 year	< 1 year.
4	Spontaneously.	Spontaneously.
3	To verbal command.	To loud voice.
2	To painful stimuli.	To painful stimuli.
1	No response.	No response.

Intubation is required when MGCS scale is 8 or less.

24. Most common cause of **pediatric trauma mortality: CNS injury (60%).**

25. Most common type of trauma in pediatric age group: **Blunt trauma.**

26. Child appears with **abdominal trauma (tenderness,** superficial bruise, distension). What is preferred investigative method?
    a. Stable child: Abdominal CT with contrast (include lower chest).
    b. Unstable child: Peritoneal lavage.

27. **Outcome** of major trauma in pediatrics:
    a. Excellent (> 95% have **no or minimal** residual damage).
    b. Comatose patient (more than 24 hours): > 50% have reasonable recovery.

28. Things to be looked for in any severe trauma patient: **First ABCD** (airway, breathing, circulation, disability), then HEENT examination (head, ear, eyes, nose, throat). Examine the body cavities, and bones. Do rectal examination. Put Foley catheter into bladder. Laboratory studies: CBC, amylase, LFT, urinalysis.

29. Decorticate and decerebrate posture **(important):**
    a. Decorticate: Flexion of upper extremities and extension of lower extremities (Indicating cerebral **irritation).**
    b. Decerebrate: Extension of both upper and lower extremities. (It indicates more serious problem like **herniation.)**

30. MOFS (multiple organ failure syndrome): Severe progressive worsening of body function is due either to sepsis or to pan-systemic involvement. ARDS (adult respiratory distress syndrome) is the pulmonary part of MOFS. ARDS is due to damage of alveoli and capillaries resulting in abnormal collection of fluid, protein, and electrolytes into the alveoli resulting in diminished ventilation-perfusion ratio and hypoxia. ARDS pathologically mimics infantile RDS.

31. Circulatory collapse/shock:

Types of shock	Management
Cardiogenic (heart failure).	Dopamine, dobutamine, epinephrine.

Obstructive (vascular obstruction).	Remove the obstruction; **never give digoxin.**
Hypovolemic (reduced blood volume).	Colloid (10 cc/kg) or crystalloid (20 cc/kg). Blood loss should be replaced.
Distributive (poor perfusion in sepsis).	Antibiotics, cardiovascular support.

32. Mortality in ARDS (60%) is due mostly to: Dysfunction of other organs (except lungs: only a few deaths are due to lungs).

33. Most important ABG change in status asthmaticus: ↑ CO_2 (> 55 in respiratory failure).

34. **Treatment for status asthmaticus that is unresponsive to initial therapy:**
    a. Give oxygen to correct hypoxia.
    b. Fluid to correct dehydration.
    c. To relief bronchospasm: Beta 2 sympathomimetics, theophylline.
    d. Corticosteroid; atropine (inhalation).
    e. Treat the infection, if any.
    f. **Rarely** requires ventilator. Setting is different from conventional ventilation. Use **very low ventilator rate with prolonged expiration** because of delayed emptying of the lungs.

35. Treatment of choice for metabolic collapse (acidosis):
    a. **Slow infusion of sodium bicarbonate** (1-2 mEq/kg).
    b. Always look for, and then treat, the underlying cause.
    (example: if hypoxia is the cause, then give oxygen.)

DROWNING

1. Most common cause of death in **drowning:** Suffocation due to **respiratory obstruction** causing hypoxia (aspiration of water may or may not occur).
   Near drowning: Successful resuscitation. Patient may survive or die later on (near drowning with delayed death). **Most (92%) recover completely.**

2. Most common cause of drowning: **Accidental.** Most common < 25 years, especially between **1-4 years.** Common in **non-white** male.

3. Age group and different sites of drowning:
   10-12 months: Bathtub (unsupervised).
   1-3 years: Swimming pool (unsupervised, no fence around the pool).
   Management (prevention):
   a. Swimming pool should be covered with fence with self-latching gate.
   b. Children always should be supervised during bathing and swimming.

4. **Blood volume** in drowning and aspiration: **Increase of blood volume** with aspiration, so

during resuscitation excessive fluid causes more damage, and ↑ **third spacing.**
Remember, in **first 15 minutes there** is **no** electrolyte abnormality if resuscitation was successful.

5. **Drowning:** It causes hypoxic damage to all body organs. **Severity** of drowning of depends on:
    a. Duration of submersion.
    b. Aspiration into lungs (occurs in 80-90% of cases).
    c. Individual response.
    Duration which causes irreversible brain damage is unknown; probably > 3-5 minutes. In **cold** water because of hypothermia patient tolerated hypoxia better. Full recovery is rare if hypoxia > 20 minutes but **resuscitation should always be attempted.** In **hot** water (hot tubs, jacuzzi) drowning, **irreversible CNS damage occurs < 3-5 minutes.**

6. Difference between sea water and fresh water pulmonary aspiration **(important):**
    a. **Sea water (hypertonic, 3% saline):** It **draws water within** the alveoli, resulting in hypoxia.
    b. **Fresh water (hypotonic):** It **reduces surface tension** of alveoli causing **collapse** and hypoxia.
    In both types: Intrapulmonary shunting, ↓ lung compliance, ↑ airway resistance, abnormal ventilation perfusion, ↑ ratio between dead space and tidal volume.

7. **Step by step effects** after drowning:
    1st: Panic, anxiety, breath-holding.
    2nd: Swallowing water, unconsciousness.
    3rd: Involuntary respiration.
    4th: Apnea (due to medullary depression).
    5th: Cardiac irregularities, bradycardia, pulselessness.
    6th: Cardiac arrest.
    Most important organs that respond to this situation are **CNS and heart.**

8. **Drowning in ice cold water** and hyperventilation:
    a. **Large amount aspiration:** Ice cold water rapidly enter the circulation through alveoli and cause **massive intravascular hemolysis with ↑ k** resulting **in cardiac arrest** or **ventricular fibrillation.**
    b. **Small amount of aspiration:** Mild hemolysis, hematuria and perhaps renal failure.

9. **ABG** changes in aspiration with drowning:
    a. Oxygen: Hypoxia persists for **few days in severe** aspiration.
    b. CO_2: CO_2 **rapidly ↑ after** aspiration and **rapidly ↓ after ventilation, even with severe aspiration,** so exhalation of CO_2 is **not** a problem.

10. **Definitive autopsy findings in** lung after drowning: Presence of **diatoms, algae, flagellates** in the lungs **confirm death by drowning** (forensic medicine).
    (Autopsy findings in brain: Edema, perivascular hemorrhage in early death, cystic degeneration of basal ganglia or midbrain in late death.)

11. Clinical presentation in drowning: Hypothermic child may look clinically dead, but that does not mean biological death (vigorous resuscitation is therefore indicated).
Lung: Pulmonary edema, secondary infection.
Heart: Myocardial failure.
CNS: Hypoxia, ischemia (**rare** cerebral edema).
Clinical condition depends on **water temperature** (discussed before).

12. **Treatment** for drowning: **All patients should be resuscitated. Follow ABCD rule.**
    a. **Airway** and breathing: Maintain normal ventilation by any means (like mouth-to-mouth, oxygen, CPAP, intubation).
    b. **Circulation:** CPR, dopamine, plasma.
    c. **Metabolic acidosis:** Sodium bicarbonate.
    d. **Nasogastric tube to decompress the stomach (important).**
    e. **Bronchospasm:** Nebulized isoproterenol; aminophylline or epinephrine.
    f. **For ↑ ICP (intracranial pressure):** Hyperventilation, diuretics, mannitol, phenobarbital.
    g. After circulation is established: **Diuretics.**
    h. Don't use **prophylactic corticosteroid and antibiotics.**

13. **Most serious complication** in drowning and near drowning: **Neurologic damage** (0-21%) (mortality about 20%).
    a. When patient **appears comatose** in the hospital: After resuscitation, **50% have normal outcome.**
    b. When patient is **awake** or **unconscious at the scene,** but **awake in hospital: No** serious neurologic damage.

BURN

1. **Criteria for hospital admission** in burn:
    a. Burn > **10%** of body surface.
    b. Burn in **face, hands, feet, genitalia.**

2. **Classification of burn** (4 degrees):
    a. **1st degree: Only epithelium** damaged; pain and redness. Complete recovery.
    b. **2nd degree: Epithelium and part of corium damaged** but dermal appendages which cause **reepithelialization are intact.**
    c. **3rd degree: Full thickness dermis damage,** only growth from skin margin. **Skin graft needed.**
    d. **4th degree:** Damaged tissues underneath (subcutaneous, fascia, muscle, bone). **Grafting and flap needed.**
       i. Mild: < 10% burned.
       ii. Moderate: 10-30% burned.
       iii. Severe: > 30% burned.

3. Temperature and **protein denaturation** that occurs in burn: **More than 45 degrees C (113 degrees F).** (Human skin tolerates up to **44 degrees C** or 111 degrees F.)

4. **Etiology of burn** in different age group:
   a. First 3 years: **Scald** is the most important type of burn injury. It is **mild.**
   b. Older children: Burn from **combustible material.** It is **severe.**

5. **Cardiac function** and burn:
   a. Within seconds of burn: ↓ Cardiac output (due to excessive reflex response and reduced venous return).
   b. Later on: ↓ myocardial contractility (due to **plasma factor).**

6. **Renal function** and burn:
   a. **Within minutes** of severe burn: ↓ plasma flow to kidney, ↓ GFR, **oliguria,** abnormal tubular function;
   b. **First 12-24 hours:** ↑ ADH and ↑ aldosterone (↑ Na reabsorption and ↑ K excretion) resulting **in water retention.**

7. **Emergency management** of severe burns:
   a. First maintain the airway.
   b. **Inspect** wound, assess cardiorespiratory status, evaluate of any other injury.
   c. Fluid: Ringer lactate/saline/plasma 20 cc/kg/hour for 1-2 hours.
   d. NG tube and bladder catheter (to measure urinary output).
   e. Measure surface area by measuring weight and length.
   f. Wound care: Clean, debride and apply antibiotics locally.
   g. Analgesia: Morphine, valium.
   h. Infection (Beta hemolytic Strep.): Benzathine penicillin.
   i. Tetanus prophylaxis: Toxoid (active); TIG (tetanus immunoglobulin, passive) for those who received no or only one toxoid injection before).

8. **Rehabilitation and burn: Rehabilitation is extremely important** because burns causes physical and psychological trauma. The goal is to **return the child to a normal life** as early as possible.

9. **Fluid therapy in first 24 hours of recovering burn (important):**
   Goal of therapy: To keep the normal fluid volume and electrolyte balance without edema formation.
   Fluid of choice to be mixed: Add **12.5 gm of human** serum albumin (50 cc of 25% solution) to **950 cc of Ringer lactate in 5% dextrose.**
   (**Mixture contains** = Na 132 mEq/L, Cl 109 mEq/L, lactate 28 mEq/L, K 4 mEq/L, glucose 47.5 g/L, albumin 12.5 g/L).
   Calculation of fluid (first 24 hours): 2000 ml/m2 of body surface/24 hours + 5000 ml/m2 of **burned** surface/24 hours. Half of this should be given in the first 8 hours, the rest half in next 16 hours.
   Example: 3 year-old child with body surface area 0.66 m^2, has 3rd degree burn on 30% of his body surface.
   (2000 x 0.66 = 1320 cc/24 hour) + (5000 x 0.66 x 0.3 = 990 cc/24 hour).
   Total amount = 1320 + 990 = 2310 cc/24 hours.
   Half (1155 cc) will be given during first 8 hours = 144 cc/hour for 8 hours.
   Remaining half (1155 cc) will be given in next 16 hours = 72 cc/hour for 16 hours.

Remember, first emergency phase of fluid (20 cc/kg) for 1-2 hours should be given (Ringer lactate/saline/plasma). This fluid is **separate** from fluid given during first 24 hours.

Fluid of choice for < 1 year age (more likely to develop hypernatremia, so less Na is required):

930 cc of 5% dextrose in 0.3% Nacl solution with 20 cc of $NaHCO_3$ (1 mEq/1 cc), 50 cc of 25% human albumin (mixture contains Na 77 mEq/L, Cl 57 mEq/L, bicarbonate 20 mEq/L, glucose 46.5 g/l, albumin 12.5 mg/l).

Don't add K in first 24 hours, because multiple tissue breakdown causes ↑ serum K and poor renal function.

10. Fluid therapy **after 24 hours:** It is 3/4th's of the first day's requirement.
    Fluid: Na 50 mEq/L (< 1 year 35-40 mEq/l); **add K 30-40 mEq/L** if normal renal function.
    Formula: 1500 ml/m² body surface/24 hour + 3750 ml/m² burned surface/24 hour.
    Start **oral feeding slowly on second day and reduce I.V. fluid accordingly.**
    Weight gain (edema) reaches a maximum in **3 days,** then patient starts to lose weight untill **the 13-14th postburn day** and then returns to `preburn' weight.

11. **Calorie requirements** for burn patient:
    25 Kcal/kg + 40 Kcal/% burned body surface/24 hours.
    Example: 10 kg weight child with 30% burn:
    (25 x 10 + 40 x 30) Kcal/24 hours = 1450 Kcal/24 hours.

    In children:
    Maintenance: 1800 Kcal/m² body surface/day.
    For burn: 2200 Kcal/m² burned surface/day.

12. Most common complication **causing death** in burn patient: **Pulmonary lesion (80%).**
    (most common: edema, tracheobronchitis, bronchopneumonia, alveolar capillary block syndrome.) Other complications of burns:
    a. Cardiac dysfunction.
    b. Oliguria (due to ↑ ADH and ↓ GFR).
    c. Renal failure (transient or persist, treated with peritoneal or hemodialysis).
    d. Sepsis (most common organism is staph. aureus and pseudomonas).

TRANSPLANT

1. In transplant, one recognizes donor's foreign alloantigen by: **MHC** (major histocompatibility complex) which **initiates graft rejection by T lymphocytes.** MHC is called **HLA** (human leukocyte antigen) which is present in **short arm of chromosome 6.**
   Class I HLA: HLA-A, HLA-B, HLA-C.
   Class II HLA: HLA-DP, HLA-DQ, HLA-DR.
   Class I present in all nucleated cells.
   Class II present in a few cells (macrophage, monocyte, dendritic cells, **B-lymphocyte).**

2. **Strongest** transplantation antigen: **HLA-DR.**

3.   **How allograft rejection occurs: MHC** presents the **foreign antigen to donor's T lymphocyte,** then **CD** 4 (helper cells) initiates the rejection and **releases cytokines (interferon, interleukin), CD8** (suppressor cells) **thus amplifying** the process of rejection.

4.   GVHD (Graft-versus-host disease) type:
     a.   Acute GVHD: Usually **occurs 7-14 days** after transplant (not after 100 days). It has a **grade of 1 to 4 depending on** severity of infection.
     b.   Chronic GVHD: Usually occurs **after 100** days of bone marrow transplant.
     Treatment for both: **Prednisone, cyclosporin, anti thymocyte globulin.**

5.   Principles of action of immunosuppressive drugs: It **prevents and treats** allograft rejection and GVHD.

6.   **Mechanism of action** of immunosuppressive drugs:
     a.   **Corticosteroid (prednisone):**
          i.   **Prevents T lymphocyte proliferation** by blocking **directly** the genes of (IL) interleukin 1 and 6, **indirectly** blocking IL-2 which depends on IL 1 and 6.
          ii.   **Anti-inflammatory** response by producing **lipocortin** which inhibits **phospholipase A2,** finally **reducing synthesis of prostaglandin** (which causes inflammation).
          iii. It destroys some activated lymphocytes and inhibits the migration of monocytes to site of inflammation.
     b.   **Azathioprine** and 6 MP (6-mercaptopurine): It inhibits **T cell** activation and **monocyte migration. It cannot reverse allograft rejection.**
     c.   **Cyclosporine:** It specifically **inhibits** IL 2 mRNA and **IL 2 synthesis** by CD 4 (helper) cells. **T cell activation is inhibited due to absence of IL 2.** (It may inhibit IL 1, 3 and gamma interferon production.) It **prevents tissue rejection.**
     d.   **FK 506:** It is produced by fungus. **The action is the same as cyclosporine,** but chemically different.
     e.   **Anti-thymocyte globulin: T cell depletion.**
     f.   **OK T 3:**
          i.   It eliminates T lymphocyte through R.E. cells of liver and spleen.
          ii.   It inhibits T cell activation by binding with lymphocytes.
          iii. It reverses the graft rejection.

7.   **Side effects of immunosuppressive drugs:**
     a.   **Corticosteroid (Prednisone):**
          i.   **Immediate effect:** Serious **opportunistic** infections (bacteria, virus, fungus).
          ii.   **Late effect: Growth retardation,** hypertension, cataract, cushingoid feature, G.I. bleeding, **hyperglycemia,** osteoporosis, aseptic necrosis femoral head, pituitary adrenal axis suppression.
     b.   **Azathioprine and 6-MP: Myelosuppressive effect (↓ WBC),** secondary infection, anemia (megaloblastic), hepatitis, pancreatitis, malignancy (lymphoma and squamous cell cancer).
     c.   **Cyclosporine:** It is a very important drug because it does not suppress bone marrow, or create anti-inflammatory action.
          Metabolism: In liver by cytochrome P 450.

Side effects: **Nephrotoxicity (biopsy** is needed to distinguish between **cyclosporin toxicity and rejection in renal transplant).**

Management of nephrotoxicity: Reduce the dose or change to azathioprine.

Acute toxicity ($\uparrow$ creatinine in serum, $\uparrow$ B.P., oliguria, fluid retention), **chronic** toxicity (fibrosis, atrophy).

Others are: Neurotoxicity, hepatotoxicity, endocrine disorder (gynecomastia, $\downarrow$ testosterone, $\uparrow$ prolactin), **hypertrichosis, gingival hyperplasia.**

    d.   **FK 506:** $\downarrow$ **Cholesterol,** nephrotoxicity, neurotoxicity.

    e.   **Anti-thymocyte globulin: First doses flu-like symptom** due to lymphocytosis and cytokine release. **Later** develops **serum sickness** (anaphylaxis).

    f.   **OKT 3:** It produces **OKT 3 antibody and reduces drug effectiveness. First dose produces** (fever, chill, wheezing, dyspnea, vomiting, diarrhea) by cytokine and this reaction is reduced by methyprednisone.

8.   **Complications** of bone marrow transplant:
    a.   Oppotunistic infection.
    b.   Acute and chronic GVHD, graft rejection.
    c.   **Recurrent malignancy** and induced **secondary cancer** (EBV positive non-Hodgkin B lymphoma, leukemia).

9.   **Indications** for bone marrow transplant:
    a.   Bone marrow failure (*aplastic anemia).
    b.   Immune deficiency syndrome.
    c.   Malignancy. (In ALL, **transplant is done in second remission. First** is chemotherapy.)

10.   **Types of bone marrow used:**
    a.   Autologous: Patients' own stored marrow.
    b.   Syngeneic: Identical twin.
    c.   Allogenic: Sibling or unrelated donor.
    Most frequently used is **allogenic type.**

11.   **Most troublesome complication of autologous** marrow graft: **Recurrent malignancy** (either at original site of tumor or in marrow).

12.   Difference between bone marrow transplant and solid organ transplant: Donor marrow contains **viable lymphocytes** which react with **host antigens** to cause acute and chronic GVHD (graft versus host disease). It is **absent** in solid organ transplant.

13.   **Renal transplant:**
Indication: ESRD (end stage renal disease) is due to **reflux nephropathy,** dysplastic kidney, **obstructive** renal disease, acquired chronic glomerulonephritis.
Contraindication: Active systemic infection, I.V. drug abuse, systemic malignancy and irreversible brain or other organ damage. Remember, in allograft the **risk of recurrence** of primary renal disease is not a contraindication.
Match: HLA and ABO tissue match.
Surgery: Recipient's native kidney **should be kept inside except** in intractable nephrotic syndrome, **cancer, severe** $\uparrow$ **B.P.,** or refractory infection.

Complications of surgery:
a. Child receives **adult** kidney: Severe loss of fluid and electrolytes (Ca, Mg, Na, HCO_3). **Replacement therapy needed.**
b. **Oliguria:** Colloid or crystalloid and diuretics.
c. **Rejection:** Immunosuppressive therapy (mentioned before).

Prognosis:
a. Up to 70% of chances of surviving 5 years with anti-rejection therapy.
b. **Living donor kidney better** than cadaveric.
c. **Poor** prognosis if it is done **< 2 years** of age and better outcome after 10-15 years.
d. Survival 85-90% (not allograft); better quality of life.

14. **Most common method used** for removing residual cancer cells (in autologous transplant): **Use monoclonal antibodies directed against cancer cells.**

15. **Most common cause** of liver transplant in pediatrics: **Biliary atresia.** (Other causes are fulminant hepatitis, alpha 1 antitrypsin deficiency, intrahepatic cholestasis, inborn error of metabolism).

16. **Contraindications** to liver transplant: **(Remember,** chronic hepatitis B is **not** a contraindication for liver transplant).
a. Extrahepatic cancer (primary or metastatic).
b. Irreversible **non-hepatic** infection.
c. Alternative therapy is available.
d. Damage of extrahepatic organs and serious disease.
e. Pulmonary severe A-V shunting with hypoxia.

17. Matching of organ in liver transplant: Not HLA, but `ABO' matching.

18. **Complications after liver transplant: ↑ B.P., abdominal hemorrhage,** opportunistic infection, convulsion, encephalopathy, vanishing bile duct syndrome (due to ischemia), secondary lymphoma.

19. **Prognosis** for liver transplant: **Usually excellent** (if operative and postoperative complications have been resolved).

20. **Post operative** immunosuppressive therapy in **liver, lung, cardiac and kidney transplant:**
Begin: Cyclosporin, methylprednisolone, azathioprine therapy, **rejection occurs in 75% patient.**
Then use: Methylprednisolone, OKT 3.

21. Most common indication of **cardiac transplant: Hypoplastic (L) heart syndrome.**
Cardiac transplant:
a. **Contraindications:** Uncontrolled systemic infection, cancer, active peptic ulcer disease, poorly controlled diabetes.
b. Tissue match: Not HLA but **ABO.**
c. **Rejection:** Immunosuppressive therapy (same as liver, renal, lung).
d. Prognosis: 60-70% chance of 5 year survival.

22. Lung transplant:
    Indication: Chronic pulmonary disease (cystic fibrosis).

23. Heart-lung transplant:
    Indication: Chronic pulmonary disease with cor-pulmonale, Eisenmenger syndrome.

24. **Pancreatic** transplant:
    Indication: Diabetes with severe retinal or renal disease.

25. **Age group** most susceptible to serious complications of anaesthesia:
    a. Less than 6 months of age.
    b. Less than 36 weeks gestational age in newborn.
    Both age groups: Develops periodic breathing, apnea, bradycardia, cardiac arrest.

26. **Preoperative or preanesthetic preparation should include: Correct dehydration and acidosis, correct anemia and blood volume, reduce fever.**

27. **Intraoperative monitoring:**
    a. All vital signs should be normal (monitor and auscultation).
    b. Oxygenation should be adequate (pulse oximeter, ABG).
    c. Fluid should be appropriate (do **not** overload with fluid).

28. **Postoperative** or postanesthetic follow up and complications:
    Complications: Excitement, pain, vomiting, fever; subglottic edema between 6 months to 6 years if there was a history of croup. **TREATMENT:** According to complications.

PAIN

1. **Pain management** in children:
   a. **No children should suffer from pain.**
   b. Medication use: Bupivacaine with morphine or fentanyl.
   c. Chronic terminal patient: Antidepressant and analgesic.
   d. Other therapy: Relaxation and hypnosis.

2. **Right conceptions of pain** in preterm, fullterm and children:
   a. Preterm and fullterm have normal pain sensation and memory.
   b. Neurosensory pathway for pain sensation is intact.
   c. Early fetal age: Peripheral nerves connecting to CNS through dorsal root of spinal cord is present.
   d. Pain fibers in spinal tract are **myelinated** by mid-and late gestational age.
   e. Synaptic pain transmission to neocortex is myelinated by late gestational age.
   f. Substance P (nociceptive transmitters) and endogenous opioids (pain modulator substance) functions are normal and **concentrations increased in perinatal period.**
   g. Nociceptive informations are transmitted peripherally by **unmyelinated C fibers in**

neonate (like adult).

h. Nerve impulse transmission through **A-delta fibers** is delayed unless myelination is completed after birth.

i. Lack of inhibitory control in newborn results in **hyperalgesic response** to afferent stimuli until myelination is completed postnatally.

j. Increased **autonomic response** to painful procedure without anesthesia in newborn. (↑ B.P., ↑ heart rate, Palmer sweating, ↑ ICP, ↑ catecholamines, ↑ corticosteroid, ↑ growth hormone, ↑ glucagon, ↓ insulin, ↑ glucose. These responses are reduced by **inhalation of anaesthesia or fentanyl anaesthesia.**)

3. **Side effects** of meperidine as analgesic: **Seizure.** It is due to its long-acting metabolite **normeperidine.**

4. **Postoperative** management of pain:
   a. **Severe pain.**
      i. **Morphine and fentanyl** can be used without problems in children 3 months and older.
      ii. If it is used in children youner than 3 months, monitor **for apnea** for 24 hours after the last dose.
      iii. PCA (patient controlled analgesia) in older children:
      This computerized pump device is very good because opioid analgesia is controlled by the patient in a timely fashion.
   b. **Mild to moderate pain:** Non-opioid analgesic. There is an upper limit to its effect on pain. Beyond that, higher doses cause toxicity.

5. **These are misconceptions about children and pain (important):**
   a. Biological immaturity causes decreased pain perception.
   b. Higher tolerance to pain.
   c. Little or no memory of painful experience.
   d. Worse side effects of analgesic.
   e. Higher risk of addiction to narcotics.
   All of the above are **wrong conceptions of adults to children.**

6. Single most **important factor** to help children cope with pain **during procedure (important): Presence of parents. By "procedure" is meant:** burn dressing; intrathecal chemotherapy; bone marrow aspiration; lumber puncture.)
   Here **cognitive behavioral techniques and hypnosis are very helpful in pain therapy.**
   All these procedures can be done effectively **without** sedatives and analgesics.
   Skin suturing: Pain can be reduced by **adding a small amount of sodium bicarbonate** with the anaesthetic solution used for local anaesthesia.

7. **Side effect of midazolam (benzodiazepine), alfentanil or fentanyl as analgesics: Hypoventilation and airway obstruction.**

PHARMACOLOGIC CALCULATIONS

1.   Most important organ for drug metabolism: **Liver.**

2.   **Volume of distribution of drug (VD): It** means **total amount** of drug present in the body in relation to its serum concentration.

   Example: A newborn received loading doses of **phenobarbital** for convulsions. Phenobarb initial level was 40; **after 96 hours** level drop **20;** then maintenance (5 mg/kg) started immediately and the repeat level was **30.**

   Formula: Volume of distribution (VD) $= \dfrac{\text{Dose (mg/kg)}}{\text{Plasma level (CP)}}$

$$= \frac{5.0 \text{ mg/kg}}{(30-20)\text{mg/L}}$$

$$= 5/10 = 0.50 \text{ L/kg}.$$

   * If one plasma level is given, then use that level only.

3.   **Half life of drug (T 1/2):**

   $T\ 1/2 = \dfrac{0.693 \times VD}{Cl \text{ (clearance)}}$

   It is a **time** when drug serum level **drops by half (50%).** In order to calculate from formula, VD and Cl values **will be provided in the question.**

   Example: **(In newborn)** phenobarbital level initially = 40,
                 After 96 hours = 20, i.e.,
                 phenobarbital half life = 96 hours.

4.   **Clearance (CL):** It is the amount of **drug removed per unit of time from the body.**

   Formula: $CL = \dfrac{0.693 \times VD}{T\ 1/2}$

   In order to calculate CL; VD and T 1/2 values will be provided.

5.   **Steady state of drug:**

   $CSS \text{ (steady state)} = \dfrac{Rinf \text{ (rate of infusion)}}{Cl \text{ (clearance)}}$

   It is **5 times** half life.

   Example: Dopamine half life is 2 minutes, so steady state will occur in 10 minutes. **"Steady state"** tissues are in equilibrium (amount of **drug infused is equal to amount of drug eliminated).**

INVESTIGATIONS OF CHOICE

1. Preferred investigative procedure for mediastinum and lung disease:

   MRI: Mediastinum.
   CT: Lungs.

2. **Preferred investigative procedure after first UTI** in infant and young children:
   VCUG (voiding cystourethrogram).

   a. If reflux is present, then do **excretory urography** (IVP).
   b. If **no** reflux present, then do **ultrasonography.**
   c. **After first infection** in late childhood, **only ultrasonography is good enough.**

3. **Preferred investigative procedure for congenital dysplasia of hip: Ultrasonography.**

4. Preferred investigative procedure for **recent** head trauma: **CT scan** . It is simple, and shows acute hemorrhage and bony abnormalities better than does MRI.

5. **Preferred investigative procedure for tumor, demyelinating disease and for distinguishing white from gray matter: MRI.**

6. Preferred investigative procedure for **abdominal trauma, retroperitoneal tumors** (Wilms', neuroblastoma), **lymphoma with retroperitoneal lymphadenopathy, testicular tumor: CT scan.**

7. Preferred investigative procedure for **tumorous destruction of cortical bones: CT scan.** But MRI is better for surrounding soft tissue and bone marrow examination.

8. Preferred investigative procedure for **soft tissue neck, face, thyroid, cervical adenitis:** Ultrasonography.

9. Preferred investigative procedure (in newborn) for **intraventricular hemorrhage, meningomyelocele for ventricular dilation, dysmorphic facial features** (rule out intracranial pathology), **large head (rule out ventricular dilation): Ultrasonography (through anterior fontanel).**

10. Preferred investigative procedure for **pyloric stenosis,** gall stone, renal stone, renal and perirenal **mass, congenital anomalies** of **kidney, ureter, bladder: Ultrasonography.** It also helps to diagnose appendicitis, and intussusception.

11. Preferred investigative procedure for **prenatal diagnosis** (growth and development, malformations): **Ultrasonography.** Under sonography guidance amniocentesis, PUBS (periumbilical blood sampling), CVS (chronic villous sampling) is done.

12. Preferred investigative procedure for **malrotation:** Upper G.I. series.

13. Preferred investigative procedure for **intussusception: Barium enema** (but **air enema** is becoming popular in many centers).

14. Preferred investigative procedure for **pelvic mass (ovary, uterus): Ultrasonography.**

15. Preferred investigative procedure for **testicular mass or swelling: Testicular scan.**

16. Preferred investigative procedure for **obstructive and restrictive lung disease: Ventilation-perfusion scan.**

17. To distinguish biliary atresia from neonatal hepatitis: **Hepatobiliary scan.**

18. **MRI** is an **excellent** procedure for the following:
    CNS: White and gray mater, CSF, tumor, fat, marrow, muscles, ligament, tendon, solid abdominal organs. (CT scan is preferred for renal mass.) (MRI is not sensitive for calcium and cortical bones.)

GENETICS

1. **Gene:** It is a **functional unit of DNA** from which RNA is copied (transcribed). In any genetic disease, **gene can be identified** through examination of DNA from any cells from the patient.

2. **Gene therapy (somatic cell genetic correction):** DNA containing functional gene should be introduced into the cells and these cells must be replaced in the individual from which they are taken.

3. **Single mutant gene:**
   Each single mutant gene presents one of the four patterns of Mendelian inheritance:
   Autosomal recessive.
   Autosomal dominant.
   X-linked recessive.
   X-linked dominant.

4. **Recessive** gene and **dominant** gene:
   Recessive gene: When mutant gene **does not** affect heterozygous person.
   Dominant gene: When mutant gene **does** affect heterozygous person.
   Homozygous: Same mutant gene at both **homologous** loci in a person.
   Autosomal recessive gene: Manifests clinically in **homozygous** state.

5. Rate of recurrence in multifactorial inheritance: **2-10%** among all **first degree** relatives (parent, sibling, offspring).
   If one sibling had cleft lip and palate: Risk of recurrence is **4% in next sibling.**

If one **parent** had cleft lip and palate: Risk of first child will be **affected is 4%.**

6. **Pyloric stenosis (important):**
    a. **If mother had pyloric stenosis** in childhood: Then baby will be affected **25% of the time.**
    b. **If father** had pyloric stenosis in childhood: Then baby will be affected **4% of the time.**

7. Malformation and same identical twin:
    Chances of having same malformation in **identical twin: < 100%.** It is much higher than in the case of non-identical twin.

8. Risk of recurrence of **cleft lip and palate:**
    a. One affected child: 4%.
    b. Two affected children: 9%.

9. Risk of recurrence of **congenital intestinal aganglionosis:**
    a. Large segment involved: Higher recurrence.
    b. Small segment involved: Lower recurrence.

10. Diseases caused by deletion of mitochondrial DNA: Kearns-Sayre syndrome (mitochondrial myopathy), Leber hereditary optic neuropathy.

11. Risk of recurrence for **trisomy 21 (Down syndrome):** 1%.

12. **Fragile X chromosome** is associated with (important): Mental retardation.

13. **Incidence:**
    a. Incidence of chromosomal abnormality in newborn: 1:150.
    b. Incidence of Down syndrome: 1:800.
    c. Most common chromosomal abnormality is **(balanced structural** rearrangement): 1:520.
    d. Most common chromosomal abnormality in male **(Klinefelter):** 1:1000.
    e. Most common chromosomal abnormality in female (poly-x anomalies): 1:1000.

14. In karyotype abnormality, chances of **having aborted fetus is: 90%** (only 10% for live birth). (Chromosomal abnormalities are associated with 50% of cases or primary amenorrhea; 20% cases of mental retardation; and 10% cases of male infertility).

15. Trisomy 18 (important points to remember):
    a. Incidence of 1:8000 births; **born full term, but LBW (low birth weight); cardiac defects (VSD most common) almost always present which might cause early death** (usually within 3 months).
    b. **Clinical features are: Hypertonia and mental retardation, FT, LBW,** (more in female), **prominent occiput, small chin, low set ears, horseshoe kidney,** hernia (inguinal or umbilical), cryptorchidism, **rockerbottom feet, single umbilical artery,** cleft (lip or palate), **hypoplastic nails, flexion deformity of finger,** simian crease; heart **(VSD, PDA), short-sternum, diaphragmatic** hernia.

In picture: Prominent occiput, rocker bottom feet, hypertonic posture.

16.   Definition of chromosomal abnormalities:
Haploid: 23 chromosomes.
Diploid: Normal 46 chromosomes.
Euploid: Multiplications of haploid (46, 69, 92).
Polypoid: Euploid, but more than 46 chromosomes (69,92).

Aneuploid: Cells **deviated** from euploid (Trisomy is most common).
Trisomy: 3 homologous chromosomes instead of 2. Trisomy is the **most common type of aneuploidy.** Example: Down syndrome, trisomy 21, trisomy (18, 13).
Monosomy: 1 chromosome short of normal 2.
Triploidy: 69 chromosomes (3 haploid sets).
Nondisjunction: Failure to separate during meiosis or mitosis, the latter form mosaicism.
Mosaicism: More than one population of cells, but **different chromosome number** in same person. Example: Turner mosaic = 45x/46xy.
Robertsonian translocation (or centric fusion): Chromosomal breakage close to centromere in acrocentric chromosome. Example: Down syndrome from centric fusion of 14, 21.
p represents: Short arm of chromosome (18 p = short arm of chromosome 18).
q represents: Long arm of chromosome (18 q = long arm of chromosome 18).

(+) and (-) sign: Addition and deletion of chromosome respectively.

17.   Risk of recurrence in subsequent pregnancy after the first baby is born with **Trisomy 21** (Down syndrome) **(important):** 1%.

18.   **Down syndrome:** 95% due to trisomy, 5% translocation.
    a.   **Trisomy 21 (important points to remember).**
        i.   **Most frequent human chromosomal abnormality.**
        ii.   > 50% are spontaneously aborted in early pregnancy.
        iii.   **Increased maternal age** causes nondisjunction (by unknown cause) resulting in trisomy. (Paternal cause of nondisjunction occurs in 10-20% cases). **Very friendly child.**
        iv.   Clinical **features: Hypotonic** child with **mental retardation,** malformed ears, **oblique palpebral fissures** with epicanthic folds, Brushfield spots in iris (speckled), **endocardial cushion defect (most common), simian crease with short broad hands,** ↑ **gap between 1st and 2nd toes, furrowed tongue, duodenal atresia** and imperforate anus, Hirschsprung disease, small acetabular and iliac angle, small penis and cryptorchidism.
        In picture, note oblique eyes, protruding tongue, hypertelorism, malformed ears.
    b.   **Translocation:**
        i.   **Most common type due to centric fusion of chromosome 21 and 14** t(14q 21 q); another is 21 with 13 and 15 chromosome.
        ii.   5% of cases are inherited from **carrier parents** when chromosome 21 or 22 involved.
        iii.   100% chance Down syndrome occuring if carrier has **t(21q 21q).**

    iv.   If carrier has **t(21q 22q)** then offspring can be normal, a carrier, or abnormal.

    v.   Down syndrome patients with **apparently normal karyotypes are very** likely to have mosaic with low frequencies of trisomic cells.

    vi.   Clinical features same as Trisomy 21.

19.   Leukemia and chromosome abnormalities:
    a.   Down syndrome: ALL (acute lymphoblastic leukemia).
    b.   Philadelphia chromosome (chromosome 22): Chronic myelogenous leukemia.

20.   Superoxide dismutase (SODs) cellular level and trisomy 21: SODs level is 1.5 times of normal in trisomy 21.

21.   **Increased maternal age causes (important): All** Trisomies and nondysjunction.

22.   **Trisomy 13 (important points to remember):**
Clinical features are: Midline scalp defects, cleft lip, cleft palate, microcephaly, small eyes. Remember apnea and seizure (characteristic). Mental retardation, **persistent fetal hemoglobin and nuclear projection in neutrophil, heart (mostly VSD; PDA), polycystic kidney,** cryptorchidism, bicornuate uterus, polydactyl, omphalocele, single umbilical artery.
In picture: Midline defects, cleft lip and palate, hypotelorism.

23.   Trisomy 9 features: **Fish mouth, abnormal cranial sutures,** microcephaly, forehead prominent with deep-set eyes, dislocated hip and knee (congenital), mental retardation.

24.   Trisomy 8 features: **Plump nose with broad base, strabismus, short stature,** LBW, patellar dysplasia, restricted joint movement.

25.   **5p-syndrome (deletion** of short arm of chromosome 5): **Cat-like cry.** (Important for examination).

26.   **11 p- syndrome: Aniridia, Wilms' tumor,** gonadoblastoma, ambiguous genitalia.

27.   **9 q- syndrome** (deletion of long arm of chromosome 9): **Trigonocephaly,** long fingers.

28.   4 p- syndrome: Delayed ossification, eye (coloboma, ptosis).

29.   **13 q- syndrome: Retinoblastoma,** coloboma, ptosis, hip dysplasia.

30.   18 p- syndrome: As in Turner, large floppy ears, short stature.

31.   18 q- syndrome: Hypotonia, seizure, **carp mouth,** small genitalia, narrow ear canal.

32.   21 q- syndrome: Hypertonia, **pyloric stenosis,** downward palpebral fissures.

33.   22 q- syndrome: Hypotonia, **bifid uvula,** ptosis.

34.   **Turner syndrome (important points to remember):**

   a. **Most common chromosomal defect in all abortuses examined.**

   b. 95% of 45X0 are spontaneously aborted.

   c. 55% of all Turner syndrome are **45X0 (most common).**

   d. Incidence of 1:3000 in females, only well documented monosomy in human.

   e. **Chromosomal analysis is mandatory** in any suspected causes of Turner syndrome.

   f. **Fertility: Most 45X0 are not fertile. Few cases** of fertility have been reported. But in **mosaic form (45x/46xx) fertility,** menses and secondary sexual character were reported.

   g. **Most common mosaic form 45x/46xx.**

   h. **Gonadal dysgenesis** (can turn into malignancy, so should be removed) found in another mosaic form 45x/46xy.

   i. **Remember this well; increased maternal age has no relation to this syndrome (but autosomal trisomies and Klinefelter syndrome increase with advanced maternal age).**

   j. **No mental retardation (please note).**

   k. Paternal x or y is absent in 75% of cases of testable Turner syndrome.

   l. **Clinical features are: Short stature, primary amenorrhea, gonadal dysgenesis and streak gonads. No** mental retardation, but a few cases of **spatial perception problem were** reported.

35.   **47, XYY male:** Antisocial behavior, problems in school, tall stature.

36.   46, XX with phenotypic male: Internal and external genitalia like male. Diagnosed at puberty (like Klinefelter) for delayed puberty and sterility.

37.   **Different chromosomal abnormalities in Turner syndrome** (important for exam):

   a. 45,X.

   b. 45, X/46, XX; 45, X/47, XXX.

   c. 45, X/46, XY.

   d. 46, X, i (Xq).

   e. 46, X, del (Xq).

   f. del(Xp), r(X).

38.   **Klinefelter syndrome (47, XXY):**

   a. Incidence of 1:1000 **(male). Most common chromosomal abnormality in the male,** very rarely aborted.

   b. **It is associated with advanced maternal age.**

   c. **Clinical presentations are:** Usually not diagnosed until puberty. Then this evidence appears: **infertility, small testes, azoospermia,** small patterns on digits with low ridge count. Persons with this syndrome **usually have normal life.**

39.   46, XY with phenotypic female:

It is due to:

   a. XY pure gonadal dysgenesis (Swyer syndrome).

   b. End organ resistance to androgen (Testicular feminization syndrome).

   c. Testes are unresponsive to LH and hCG (Leydig cell aplasia).

   d. Defect in testosterone synthesis.

40. **Fragile X syndrome (very important):**
    a. Most common site of fragility is long arm of X chromosome (band q 27-28).
    b. **Mental retardation** may or may not associated with **macro orchidism (large testes in male).**
    c. **In any male with mental retardation, always look for testicular and chromosomal abnormality.**
    d. It probably represents about 30% of all X-linked male mental retardation and 10% of retardation (mild) in females.

41. 47, XXX female: Looks like **a normal** female, has **normal** gonadal function, **is fertile,** diagnosis is made by chance.

42. Most common chromosomal abnormality in all spontaneous abortuses **(important):** **Trisomy (aneuploidy). Trisomy 16 is the most common among all trisomies** (trisomy 13 **is less** likely to be aborted unlike other trisomies). Polyploidy (particularly triploidy) is common in abortuses. Birth control pills have no effect on polyploidy or other aberrations.

43. A women who had **two or more spontaneous abortions.** Investigation to be done: **Chromosome analysis for balanced translocation** (which is found in 5-10% cases). In balanced translocation, parents looks normal.

44. Collagen defect in Ehlers-Danlos syndrome:
    a. Type IV: Lack of type III collagen.
    b. Type VI: Lack of hydroxylysine in collagen.
    c. Type VII: Unable to convert procollagen to collagen.

45. **Congenital malformations (important points to remember):**
    a. Major malformations: Structural defects which result in serious medical, surgical or cosmetic problems.
    b. Minor malformation: No serious outcome.
    c. Major is 2% and minor is 4% of all births.
    d. **Most common cause of major malformations is genetic (51%).** (Next is unknown: 43%).
    e. **Chromosome analysis should be done in multiple major malformations.**

46. Mode of inheritance and defects:
    a. Duchenne muscular dystrophy: X- linked recessive.
    b. Becker muscular dystrophy: Same as above (milder form).
    c. Infantile polycystic kidney: Autosomal dominant.
    d. Unilateral multicystic kidney: Nonhereditary.
    e. **Cleft lip and palate:** Multifactorial.
    f. **Cleft lip and palate with lip pits:** Autosomal dominant.

47. Hemifacial microsomia is due to: Around 6th to 7th week of gestational age, there is a failure of **switching of vascular supply from stapedial artery to external carotid artery.**

48. Synostosis of long bones is due to: **Failure of death of cells** between the long bones.

49. Probable causes of congenital malformations:
    a. Collagen defect (Ehlers-Danlos syndrome).
    b. Cellular shape defect (neural cells defect).
    c. Circulation defect (hemifacial microsomia).
    d. Cellular death defect (synostosis of long bones).

50. Metabolic disease with malformation: **Glutaric aciduria type II** is associated with some malformations, **particularly GU (genitourinary) anomaly (G for G).**

51. **First step** in genetic counseling: **Make sure that the diagnosis is correct.**

52. **Parental reaction** in genetic counseling:
    a. Denial, depression, anger (usually), but each family behaves differently.
    b. To avoid parental difficulty in understanding different genetic terms, it is better to show them **both normal and abnormal pictures and then compare and contrast them.**
    c. Sometimes parents think that **nobody** in the family has the problem, so it can't be hereditary. It is an absolutely wrong idea, because **healthy parents can have a baby with hereditary defects.** This point should be made clear to the parents.

53. **Detection of carrier** by DNA analysis in the following diseases:
    a. **Hemophilia A, Duchenne muscular dystrophy** (both x-linked recessive).
    b. Hemoglobin S and C, thalassemia.
    c. Alpha 1 antitrypsin deficiency.
    d. Tay-Sachs disease.

54. When a child has either **an excess or deficiency** of chromosomal material (translocation), look for: **Balanced translocation** in both parents (because then patient is normal).

55. **Most common cause** for prenatal diagnosis: **Advanced maternal age (over 35 years).** Incidence of any chromosomal anomaly over 35 years: 1%.
    Because of routine prenatal diagnosis of women over 35 years of age, now 80% of Down syndrome babies are born to women **under 35 years,** because they don't go for prenatal diagnosis. In 20% of cases, the extra chromosome in **Trisomy 21 is from the father.**

56. **Prenatal diagnosis (important):**
    a. **Amniocentesis:** Done in **15th or 16th week** of gestational age under ultrasound guidance. Fetal tissues placed in culture, then **chromosome, DNA analysis and enzyme assay can be done.** Fetal loss is 0.5%.
    b. **CVS (chronic villous sampling):** Done in 9th to 11th **week** of gestational age. Fetal tissues should be analyzed as mentioned above. **Fetal loss is about same as amniocentesis** and **additional 1% chance of mosaicism** for which amniocentesis should be done. Reported ↑ incidence **of limb anomalies.**

57. Alpha felo protein (AFP) is **synthesized by:** Fetal liver, G.I. tract, yolk sac.
    In amniotic fluid, AFP is highest between 14-18 weeks, then level falls progressively.
    So, ultrasonography should be done to estimate gestational age before amniocentesis.

58. ↑ **alpha feto protein level** in the following conditions: **Anencephaly, meningomyelocele, omphalocele (not hereditary), Meckel syndrome** (autosomal recessive: it consists of encephalocele, polycystic kidney, genital and eye abnormalities, cleft lip and palate, polydactyl), **congenital nephrosis (autosomal recessive),** twin gestation, fetal demise, intestinal atresia, spontaneous abortion, Rh sensitization, contaminated with fetal blood, growth retardation.

59. **Most common indication** to measure alpha felo protein in a pregnant woman (important): History of child with neural tube defects (anencephaly, meningomyelocele, encephalocele; but **not** omphalocele which is non hereditary defect).

60. ↓ **alpha feto protein level** in the following conditions: **Trisomy 21 and 18** (found in 20% cases).

61. **PUBS (Percutaneous umbilical cord blood sampling):** Done around 20 weeks of gestational age for chromosome study after detection of fetal anomalies by ultrasound. Fetal blood also used for other studies.

62. Outcome of most congenital deformities: 90% of cases resolve spontaneously.

63. Most common type of deformities of newborns: **Musculoskeletal** (it is due to intrauterine molding).

64. **Teratogenicity in newborn when mother is involved with:**

Parvovirus	**Hydrops fetalis,** hemolytic anemia, still-birth.
Varicella	**Hypoplastic limb,** skin scar.
Diabetes mellitus	**Sacral agenesis, asymmetric septal hypertrophy (heart).**
Cigarettes, marijuana	**Decrease birth weight.**
Lupus	**Congenital heart block.**
Alcohol	**IUGR, mental retardation.**
PKU (phenylketonuria)	**Microcephaly,** mental retardation.
Isotretinoin	**Truncus arteriosus,** CNS malformation, absent thymus.
Diethylstilbestrol	Female (vaginal cancer, adenosis), male (G.U. anomaly).
Thalidomide	**Phocomelia.**
Warfarin	**Hypoplastic nose, stippled epiphyses.**
Cocaine	**Abruptio placenta,** prematurity.
Carbamazepine	**Craniofacial defect.**
Valproic acid	**Spina bifida.**

Tetracycline	Hypoplastic enamel.
Phenytoin	Hypoplastic nail, heart defect.
Mercury	Microcephaly.
Iodine, propylthiouracil	Fetal hypothyroidism, goitre.
Aminopterin/amethopterin	Craniosynostosis, hydrocephalus.
Angiotensin converting enzyme	Hypoplastic skull, dysplastic kidney.
Rubella	Cataract, PDA.
Toxoplasmosis	Hydrocephalus, microcephaly, diffuse calcification.
CMV	Periventricular calcification, microcephaly.

65. Radiation to mother and fetus:
    a. Diagnostic or therapeutic radiation usually will **not** cause fetal malformation.
    b. Radiation should **not exceed** 500 millirads for the entire pregnancy period.
    c. Abortion is indicated when exposure exceeds 10000 mrad.

66. **Amniotic band disruption sequence:** It is a fibrous band of amnion (extending from placenta up to chorion) causing fetal craniofacial and limb defect. This fibrous band either prevents the normal development or damages the already formed structures.

67. VATER association and VACTER anomalies:
    V: Vertebral defect.
    A: Anal atresia.
    TE: Tracheo esophageal fistula with esophageal atresia.
    R: Radial hypoplasia, renal abnormality.
    (VACTER same as VATER. Also, C is cardiac defect is VSD). Single umbilical artery and genital anomalies are also associated with these defects.

68. In PKU, enzyme **deficiencies** are:
    a. Phenylalanine hydroxylase.
    b. Tetrahydrobiopterin cofactor.
    Resulting in accumulation of phenylalanine in body fluids.

69. **Diseases and chromosome:**

Cystic Fibrosis	Chromosome	7
Prader Willi Syndrome	Chromosome	15
Insulin Dependent Diabetes	Chromosome	6
Wilms' Tumor	Chromosome	11 p-

Retinoblastoma	Chromosome	13 q-
Thalassemia (ß,√,δ)	Chromosome	11
Thalassemia (α)	Chromosome	16

70. **Autosomal recessive:**

Ataxia telangiectasia	**Kartagener syndrome.**
Alpha 1 antitrypsin deficiency	Macular corneal dystrophy.
Albinism (tyrosinase + and -)	Farber disease.
Adrenogenital syndrome	Wolman disease.
Hemoglobinopathies	**Chediak-Higashi disease.**
(SS, SC, Sß, ß thalassemia)	Schwachman syndrome.
Tay-Sachs disease	Fanconi anemia.
Hurler syndrome	Pendred syndrome.
Phenylketonuria	Metachromatic leukodystrophy.
Wilson disease	**Galactosemia.**

Autosomal dominant:

Nail-patella syndrome	**Tuberous sclerosis.**
Hereditary angioedema	**Retinoblastoma.**
Hereditary spherocytosis	**Polycystic kidney.**
Alport syndrome	**Aniridia.**
Waardenburg syndrome	Huntington chorea.
Peutz-Jeghers syndrome	Apert syndrome.
Gardner syndrome	**Achondroplasia.**
Neurofibromatosis	Thanatophoric dwarfism.
Marfan syndrome	Hyperlipoproteinemia type II.
Dentinogenesis imperfecta	Facioscapulohumeral muscular dystrophy.

X-linked recessive:

Color blindness	Ocular albinism.
Retinitis pigmentosa	Nephrogenic diabetes insipidus.
Hemophilia (A,B)	**Glucose 6 phosphate dehydrogenase deficiency.**
Gout	**Duchenne muscular dystrophy.**
Lesch-nyhan syndrome	**Chronic granulomatous disease.**
Menkes (kinky hair) syndrome	**Hunter syndrome.**
Wiskott-Aldrich syndrome	Ichthyosis.
Testicular feminization syndrome	Bruton agammaglobulinemia.
Familial congenital hypoparathyroidism.	Fabry disease.

X-linked dominant:

Vitamin D resistant rickets	**Pseudohypoparathyroidism.**
Telecanthus hypospadias syndrome	↓ TBG (thyroid binding globulin).
Incontinentia pigmenti	↑ TBG (thyroid binding globulin).

71. Mode of transmission of the disease:

a. **Autosomal recessive:** Affected individual (homozygous) should receive one mutant gene from each parents (heterozygous). Here, only homozygous state has the disease and heterozygous is the carrier. When both parents are heterozygous then offspring can have four different conditions. The offspring can get normal allele from both parents and become normal, or a normal allele from the father and a mutant allele from the mother and become unaffected but heterozygous or a normal allele form the mother and a mutant allele from the father and become unaffected but heterozygous or the mutant allele from both parents and has the disease (homozygous). So, the chances are 1 in 4 is homozygous, 1 in 2 is heterozygous for mutant gene and thus 2 in 3 heterozygous, if child is unaffected.

The children of the diseased (homozygous) person are all carrier (heterozygous) when the spouse is not affected. The children could be affected (homozygous) when the spouse is carrier (heterozygous) which is rare.

Only one generation of the family will have the disease. That means **one child or his sibling** (brother or sister) has the disease. Child, parents, offspring, cousin, nephew, niece, uncle, **or aunt will not have the disease.** In description of family tree, when **anybody other than** the child 's own brother or sister is affected, it is **not** autosomal recessive. **Diseased (25%), carrier (50%), normal (25%); male and female equally affected. Most common type.**

Example:

Cystis fibrosis or any Autosomal recessive: Let us assume that person A has autosomal recessive disease, his **sibling is B** married to an unrelated spouse C, wants to know the chances that his children will get the disease. The B has 2/3 chances of being heterozygous.

P = Frequency of normal allele

q^2 = Frequency of CF phenotype

p + q = 1

$(p+q)^2 = 1$

q^2 = 1 in 2000 (let us assume the frequency of CF gene in the general population).

$$\therefore q = \sqrt{\left(\frac{1}{2000}\right)} = \frac{1}{45}$$

$$p = 1 - q = 1 - \frac{1}{45} = \frac{44}{45}$$

The proportion of carriers (frequency of heterozygote) is 2 pq

$$= 2 X \frac{44}{45} X \frac{1}{45} = \frac{1}{22} = 5\% (approximately \;\;)$$

So, C has 1/22 chances of being heterozygous (carrier).

Both B and C will be heterozygous = 2/3 X 1/22 = 1/33 (3%)

The probability of first child will be affected

= 1/4 X 1/33 = 1/132 = < 1% (1/4 = autosomal recessive)

The person A has a sister D married to an unrelated spouse. They want to know about the risk of her first child being affected: The same as above i.e.; < 1%

The risk of birth defect in a newborn of unrelated parents, is 2-3 %

The risk of birth defect, in a newborn of related (first cousin) parents, is 4-6% (double).

b. **Autosomal dominant:** Each individual who **inherits the gene will have the disease.** Affected individual will inherit the gene from his/her **affected one parent** except in fresh mutation which is very rare. Other parent is normal. This affected individual (e.g., he) is heterozygous. He will probably marry a girl who is not affected. His children will inherit normal allele from his wife and either the normal or mutant (abnormal) allele from him, so **his children will each have 1:1 chance** of having the mutant gene and the disease.

(Rarely, if **both parents** carry the gene, i.e., heterozygous, then their children can inherit either normal or mutant (abnormal)allele from each parent and become homozygous. So, the chances of children become normal 1 in 4 , heterozygous 2 in 4 or homozygous 1 in 4; so 3 out of 4 being affected.)

Generation after generation is affected. That means mother or father or uncle or aunt or brother or sister or nephew or niece or cousin is **affected.** More than one generation is affected. **Diseased (50%), normal (50%), no carrier. Male and female equally affected. Second most** common type.

c. **X-linked recessive:** Each son of a carrier female has a 50% (1/2) chance of having the disease and each daughter has 50% (1/2) chance of being carrier. All daughters of the affected male are carriers of the mutant gene but all sons are normal. Carrier daughter may have affected sons. In each pregnancy the female carrier has a 25% chance of having affected son, 25% chance of carrier daughter and 50% chance of normal children (son and daughter).

Only male is affected and **female is the carrier.** More than one generation is affected. Child's brother, male cousin, nephew, or grandfather **has the disease,** but sister, niece, female cousin, uncle, aunt, father, mother **are not affected.** If female is affected, exclude X-linked recessive.
Diseased (25%), carrier (25%), normal (50%). In each pregnancy of a carrier, 50% of male children are affected and 50% of female children are carriers.

Example: X-linked recessive (e.g., hemophiliac A):

i. A consultand's female whose mother is a carrier and father is normal, but maternal grandfather had the disease and grandmother was normal. The risk that she is a carrier is 1/2 (50%) and the risk of having an affected son is 1/2 (carrier) x 1/4 (x-linked recessive transmission risk) = 1/8.

ii. A consultand's female whose sister become a carrier from her mother and rest of the conditions are same as above. The risk of her become the carrier and her son being affected are the same as above.

iii. A consultand's female whose mother is not a carrier and father is normal, but maternal uncle had the disease and grandmother was the carrier but grandfather was normal. The risk that she is a carrier is 1/33 (3%) and risk of having an affected son is 1/33 x 1/4 = 1/132 = < 1%.

iv. A consultand's male whose brother has the disease, one sister is the carrier and other sister is not the carrier. The chances that he is a carrier zero because male cannot be the carrier and the chances of having an affected son is zero if the mother is not a carrier.

v. A consultand's female whose is a carrier, the chances of having an affected child already been discussed.

d. **X-linked dominant: Generation after generation. More than one generation is affected.** Child's father or mother, brother and or sister, nephew and or niece, uncle and/or aunt **has the disease. All daughters of the affected father will be affected, but none of his sons. If mother is affected, both the sons and daughters** will be affected, and it will then be difficult to differentiate this from auto-dominant.

Diseased (50%), normal (50%), no carrier; equal male and female, but male is seriously affected.

How to solve this problem when history is given:

(1)   See if more than one generation has been affected: **Exclude** auto. recessive.

(2)   See if a female has the disease: You **exclude** X-linked recessive.

(3)   See if mother and father are **not** affected: Diagnosis **autosomal or X-linked recessive.**

(4)   If mother or father is affected: Diagnosis **autosomal or X- linked dominant.**

(5)   See if the father and all his daughters are affected but none of his sons: X-linked dominant.

(6)   See if the father and half of his daughters and half of his sons are affected: Autosomal dominant.

(7)   See if the mother and half of her daughters and half of her sons are affected: Either autosomal or X-linked dominant. In X-linked dominant sons are affected more seriously.

72.   **Increased alpha feto protein: Incorrect gestational age, multiple** pregnancy, meningomyelocele (ruptured), omphalocele, spina bifida, anencephaly, **congenital nephrosis,** threatened abortion, feto maternal bleeding, acardia, **Turner syndrome,** cystic hygroma, renal agenesis, polycystic kidney, epidermolysis bullosa, lesion of placenta and umbilical cord, hereditary persistence (Autosomal dominant trait).

Decreased alpha feto protein: Wrong gestational age, trisomy 21, 18, IUGR (intrauterine growth retardation).

Alpha feto protein produced by: Liver, G.I. tract, **yolk sac.**

73.   **Down syndrome present with:** ↑ HCG, ↓ alpha feto protein (33%), ↑ nuchal fat.

METABOLIC DISEASES

1.   **Most common lipid** responsible for atherosclerotic heart disease: **LDL-Cholesterol.** Cholesterol does **not** present in free state, when it binds with **LDL** (low density lipoprotein), it forms **LDL-Cholesterol** in type II hyperlipidemia.

2.   Which form of lipid **protect** the heart from atherosclerosis: **HDL (High density lipoprotein) bind with cholesterol protect** the heart.

3.   **Hyperlipidemia** and **features:**

Types are: I, IIA, IIB, III, IV, V. **Types** manifest in **children** are: **I, IIA, IIB.** Out of these three types, **type IIA is most important.**

Type I
Present with **abdominal pain, pancreatitis, xanthoma,** lipid deposit in retina. **No heart lesion.**
Plasma: chylomicron present, cholesterol normal or elevated, **triglyceride level very high.**
Biochemical: **Decreased lipoprotein lipase.**
Electrophoresis: Heavy band at origin.
Treatment: Low fat diet.

Type IIA
Present with normal or **severe coronary artery, disease,** xanthoma, tendinitis.
Plasma: Increased LDL, normal VLDL, elevated cholesterol, normal triglyceride.
Biochemical: Decrease non hepatic LDL cell receptor.
Electrophoresis: Increased B band density.
Treatment: Low fat diet, drugs (colestipol, probucol, nicotinic acid).

Type IIB
Sign and symptoms same as type IIA.
Plasma: **Increased** (LDL, VLDL, cholesterol triglyceride).
Biochemical: not known.
Electrophoresis: Increased B and pre B band density.
Treatment: Same as IIA, **loose weight** if obese.

4. **Inborn errors of metabolism and abnormal odor:**

Phenylketonuria	**Mousy or musty.**
Tyrosinemia	**Cabbage like, rancid, fishy.**
Methionine malabsorption	**Cabbage.**
Maple syrup urine disease	**Maple syrup.**
Isovaleric acidemia	**Sweaty feet.**
Beta methylcrotonylglycinurea	**Tomcat fish.**
Trimethylaminuria	Rotting fish.
Hawkinsinuria	Swimming pool.
Oasthouse urine disease	Hop-like.
Glutaric acidemia type II	Sweaty feet.

5. Usual presentation and approach to metabolic diseases:
Presentation: Vomiting, lethargy, poor feeding, convulsion, coma.
Approach:
a. First rule out systemic infection : No infection.

b. Serum ammonia level:
   i. If high level then obtain.
      Blood pH, CO_2: → Normal: Urea cycle defects.
      → Acidosis: Organic acidemias.
   ii. If normal level then obtain.
      Blood pH, CO_2: → Normal: Aminoacidopathies or galactosemia.
      → Acidosis: Organic acidemia.

6. **Clinical manifestations** of **classic PKU (most common type): Normal at birth and remains asymptomatic for first few months. Appears** with **severe mental retardation, vomiting, blond hair, blue eyes, fair skin;** sometimes seborrheic or eczematous skin lesion which improves with aging, but older children with PKU have purposeless movement, rocking, athetosis present.

   Musty or mousy odor due to phenylacetic acid, ↑ tone, ↑ reflexes, seizure, EEG abnormalities, microcephaly, growth retardation.

7. **Diagnosis of** classic PKU:
   a. **Initial** newborn screening test of Guthrie. Blood should be drawn **after 72 hours and after protein feeding.**
   b. Following criteria to **confirm the diagnosis:**
      i. Serum phenylalanine level over 20 mg/dl.
      ii. Normal serum tyrosine level.
      iii. ↑ urinary excretion of metabolites (phenylpyruvic acid and o-hydroxyphenylacetic acid).
      iv. Normal level of cofactor tetrahydrobiopterin.

8. **Treatment** for classic PKU **(should begin soon after birth):**
   a. **Lofenalac** (low phenylalanine) diet to keep the serum level between 3-15 mg/dl.
      Overtreatment: Cause phenylalanine deficiency **(lethargy, rashes, diarrhea,** anemia anorexia, and death).
      Undertreatment: Phenylketonuria.
   b. **Tyrosine: Adequate** intake.

9. For a **pregnant mother with PKU,** when should low phenylalanine diet begin **(important)? Before conception.** Try to keep the phenylalanine level less than 10 mg/dl throughout pregnancy.

10. A pregnant mother with PKU did not take low phenyl alanine diet. What is effect on fetus:
    a. ↑ risk of spontaneous abortion.
    b. Mental retardation.
    c. Congenital cardiac defect.

11. Hyperphenylalaninemia as a result of deficiency of cofactor tetrahydrobiopterin (BH4):
    It is a cofactor for tyrosine and tryptophan hydroxylases, which is required for biosynthesis of neurotransmitters (dopamine and serotonin). This patient **deteriorates even with normal serum phenylalanine level.** BH4 is synthesized from guanosine triphosphate and oxidized to BH2 (quininoid dihydrobiopterin). BH2 is reduced to BH4

by enzyme dihydropteridine reductase.

Clinical presentations: Same as classic PKU. Normal until 3 months of age, then comes down with hypertonia, poor head control, **myoclonic seizure,** dysphagia.

Diagnosis of BH4 deficiency in hyperphenylalaninemia:

a.   **Urinary** measurement of neoptrin (oxidative product of dihydropterin triphosphate) and biopterin (oxidative product of dihydro and tetrahydrobiopterin):

    i.   6-pyruvoyltetrahydropterin synthase deficiency:

       ↑ neoptrin and ↓ biopterin (in urine).

    ii.   GTP cyclohydrolase deficiency:

       ↓ neoptrin and ↓ biopterin (in urine).

    iii.   Dihydropteridine reductase deficiency:

       → neoptrin and ↑ biopterin (in urine).

b.   **BH4 loading test:** Loading dose (oral or I.V.) normalizes serum phenylalanine level within 4-6 hours in patient with BH4 deficiency. This test should be performed when patient is receiving normal amount of phenylalanine in the diet.

c.   **Enzyme assay:**

    i.   Dihydropteridine reductase: Measured in liver, WBC, RBC, cultured fibroblast.

    ii.   6-Pyruvoyltetrahydropterin synthase: Measured in liver and kidney, RBC.

    iii.   GTP cyclohydrolase: Measured in liver and phytohemagglutinin-stimulated lymphocytes.

12.   **Treatment** for BH4 deficiency in hyperalaninemia:

a.   **Low phenylalanine diet:** It does not prevent neurologic damage. This diet should be combined with the therapies in (b) and (c) for at least 2 years. High phenylalanine inhibits neurotransmitter synthesis.

b.   **Neurotransmitter precursors** (L-dopa and 5 hydroxy tryptophan): They prevent neurologic damage. Remember, every patient with PKU and hyperphenylalaninemia **should be tested for BH4 deficiency,** because if treatment is delayed **beyond 6 months, there is irreversible neurologic damage.**

c.   **BH4 replacement in high doses (20-40 mg/kg/day): High** doses easily cross blood-brain barrier and prevent neurologic damage.

13.   **Benign hyperphenylalaninemia: Asymptomatic** patient with **serum level of less than 20 mg/dl; no** urinary excretion of phenylpyruvic acid; **deficiency of phenylalanine hydroxylase enzyme** (1-35% of normal) activity.

Diagnosis made by serum: Phenylalanine and BH4 level.

TREATMENT:

a.   Asymptomatic, diagnosed after serum testing routinely: No treatment is required.

b.   No PKU, normal tyrosine, serum phenylalanine (10-20 mg/dl): Simple reduction of dietary protein. If this fails, then put patient on low phenylalanine diet.

All infants who were not treated will need close follow up for phenylalanine level and development.

14. **Prenatal diagnosis and carrier for PKU (Autosomal recessive): By specific genetic probe after CVS (chronic villous biopsy).**

15. **Transient hyperphenylalaninemia:**

   a. It is found in newborns with **transient tyrosinemia.** When tyrosine oxidation matures both levels (tyrosine and phenylalanine) **become normal.**
   b. It is also produced by delayed or absent of maturation of phenylalanine transaminase when patient received milk with high protein.

16. **Pathway of phenylalanine metabolism:**

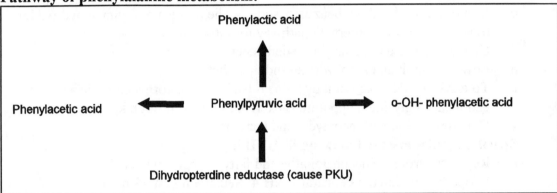

17. **Richner-Hanhart syndrome (Tyrosinemia II, oculocutaneous Type):**
   Signs and symptoms: Keratoconjunctivitis palmoplantars.
   Diagnosis: ↓ Tyrosine aminotransferase in hepatic mitochondria.
   Treatment: Diet restriction of phenylalanine and tyrosine.

18. **Neonatal tyrosinemia:**
   Types: Acute, chronic and hypermethionemia.
   Signs and symptoms: Acute hepatic disease with or without renal tubular dysfunction **(ascites, bleeding disorder, coma,** vomiting, diarrhea, lethargy).
   Diagnosis: Plasma (↑ tyrosine or ↑ methionine or both or may be ↑ phenylalanine); ↓ WBC, ↓ platelet count.
   Enzyme: ↓ parahydroxyl phenylpyruvic oxidase.
   Treatment: Diet low in (phenylalanine, tyrosine, methionine), carbohydrate as glucose (for hypoglycemia).

19. **Nonketotic hyperglycinemia:**
   Signs and symptoms: Seriously ill child in first few days of life (most die in first 2 weeks) appear with ↓ reflex, ↓ tone, apnea, seizure (myoclonic, generalized), coma. Those who survive in first 2 weeks appear with waxing and waning (muscle spasm, then relaxation), ↓ motor and mental development.
   Diagnosis: ↑ Glycine in CSF (plasma and urine are nonspecific).
   Enzyme: Defect in glycine cleavage system.
   Treatment: **No effective treatment.** Strychnine and diazepam might work in mild form.

20. **Hyperammoniemia (↑ NH4), urea cycle disorder:**

Signs and symptoms: Progressive illness, tachypnea, seizures (generalized or focal), waxing and waning of consciousness, coma, death, pulmonary hemorrhage without pulmonary disease.

Diagnosis:

a. Plasma: ↑ **NH4,** ↓ **BUN.**

b. Diagnosis confirmed by liver enzyme assay.

Treatment:

a. **Preferred method of choice: Hemodialysis** is most effective, but not readily available, so **peritoneal dialysis is the most practical treatment.**

b. Exchange transfusion: Is not that effective. It is done when dialysis is not available and in newborn with jaundice.

c. Combination of sodium benzoate, sodium phenylacetate, arginine hydrochloride together helps clear alternate pathway for nitrogen excretion .

d. Give arginine except in arginase deficiency.

e. Low protein, high carbohydrate, and lipid diet.

f. To enhance NH4 excretion by kidney: Na benzoate forms hippuric acid with endogenous glycine. Hippurate is excreted rapidly through kidney.

g. Gut sterilization with neomycin and lactulose.

Specific entities are the following in ↑ NH4:

a. Reye's syndrome: Encephalopathy and fatty changes in liver.

b. Idiopathic self limited neonatal ↑ NH 4: Seizure in first 48 hours.

c. Carbamyl phosphate synthetase deficiency: Defect in transport of ornithine into mitochondria.

d. Ornithine carbamyl transferase deficiency (X-linked dominant): Plasma (↑ glutamine, ↑ alanine), diagnosis by enzyme assay in liver.

e. Arginase deficiency: Strong family history, asymptomatic, diagnosis by enzyme assay, diet low in arginine.

f. Arginosuccinic aciduria: ↓ arginosuccinic lyase, neonate with friable hair, diagnosis by enzyme assay.

g. ↓ N acetylglutamate synthetase: Treatment with carbamyl glutamate, supplemental arginine, low protein diet.

21. **Alcaptonuria:**

Signs: **Darkening of diaper** on standing.

Diagnosis: Confirmed by measurement of homogentisic acid in urine.

Enzyme: Disorder of oxidation of homogentisic acid.

Treatment: Diet low in (phenylalanine and Tyrosine) have little justification to prevent melanin-like by-product deposition in joint cartilage.

22. **Homocystinuria (type 1, classic homocystinuria)**

Signs and symptoms:

a. Neonatal: Asymptomatic.

b. Symptoms which develop later are: Ectopic (**downward** dislocated) lens (2 to 3 years), features like Marfan syndrome (posterior lens dislocation), intelligence deficit, thrombotic episodes in arteries, malar flush, livido reticularis.

Prenatal diagnosis: Enzyme assay of cultured amniotic cells or chorionic villi.

Diagnosis: Homocysteine in urine (in blood not reliable).

Enzyme: ↓ cystathione synthetase activity.

Treatment: Pyridoxine (large dose), a cofactor of enzyme mentioned above, and folic acid. If no response, then prescribe diet low in methionine and high in cystine.

23. **MSUD (maple syrup urine disease, defect in organic acid):**
Signs and symptoms: **Normal at birth.** Profound illness within one week. Appears with shallow, rapid breathing, diminished consciousness, alternate ($\downarrow$ tone and $\uparrow$ tone), **odor of maple syrup (burnt sugar),** tonic seizures. **Death results from respiratory failure.**
Diagnosis: $\uparrow$ **Plasma (leucine, isoleucine, valine), $\downarrow$ alanine.**
Enzyme: Defective decarboxylation of leucine, isoleucine and valine.
Treatment:
   a. **Life long dietary restriction of leucine, isoleucine, valine, and monitor plasma level periodically.**
   b. Neonate in acute condition or crisis before diet: **Peritoneal dialysis** is the preferred treatment.
   c. Some response to thiamine.

24. **Propionic acidemia:**
Signs and symptoms: Appears in neonatal period with lethargy, tachypnea, poorly fed, worsened by protein diet, no seizure, coma.
Prenatal diagnosis: Enzyme activity in cultured amniotic cells and uncultured chorionic villi.
Diagnosis:
   a. Definitive: By enzyme assay in WBC or cultured fibroblast.
   b. $\uparrow$ Plasma (NH4 and glycine) is virtually diagnostic; $\downarrow$ WBC, $\downarrow$ platelet.
Enzyme: Propionyl CoA carboxylase deficiency.
Treatment:
   a. **P.O. Biotin and I.M. vitamin B_{12} (megadose).**
   b. **Sterilize the gut promptly with neomycin.**
   c. Correct dehydration, acidosis, low protein and high carbohydrate diet.
   d. Administration of L-carnitine (deficiency of carnitine) improves fatty acid oxidation and correct sacidosis.
   e. $\uparrow$ NH 4: Treat for $\uparrow$ NH 4 (peritoneal and hemodialysis).
   f. Long term therapy with low protein (natural) and L-carnitine.

25. **CLA (congenital lactic acidosis, disorder of organic acid metabolism):**
Signs and symptoms: **Mostly acidotic at birth,** $\downarrow$ tone, **optic atrophy,** seizures (myoclonic, generalized), **tetany** (due to calcium lactate complex in plasma), physically normal at birth, but becomes **obese rapidly.**
Diagnosis: $\uparrow$ **plasma (pyruvate and alanine),** $\uparrow$ anion gap, $\uparrow$ lactate in plasma.
Treatment:
   a. **Megavitamin therapy (Biotin, thiamine, lipoic acid, steroid), but most patients do not improve.**
   b. Metabolic acidosis: $NaHCO_3$.

26. **Isovaleric acidemia (sweaty feet syndrome; organic acid disorder):**

Signs and symptoms: **Odor of sweaty feet. Patient normal at birth,** but become **tachypneic** in neonatal period. **Seizures, CNS depression and serious infections.**

Diagnosis: Urine ↑ (isovaleric acid and its metabolites).

Diagnosis confirmed: Enzyme assay of skin fibroblast.

Prenatal diagnosis: By measuring isovaleryl glycine in amniotic fluid.

Enzyme: Defect in leucine catabolism.

Treatment:

a.   Correct hydration and metabolic acidosis.

b.   **Glycine and carnitine** enhance urinary excretion of isovaleric acid.

c.   **Peritoneal dialysis for ↑ NH 4.**

d.   **Long term diet (↑ calorie, ↓ protein) and oral glycine and carnitine supplement.**

27.   **Glutaric acidemia type II** (organic acid defect):

Signs and symptoms: **Sweaty feet.** All die in neonatal period.

Mode of transmission: X-linked in neonatal. Later onset is autosomal recessive.

Remember, most of the enzyme defects in any metabolic disorders are autosomal recessive.

Enzyme: Molecular defect in electron transport system that connects several dehydrogenases with **coenzyme Q.**

28.   **Neonatal diabetes mellitus:**

Signs and symptoms: Starts from 4th to 44th day of life. Appears with weight loss, dehydration due to polyuria.

Diagnosis: ↑ **plasma glucose (245 to 2300 mg/dl),** → insulin, ↓ **pH (metabolic), but no ketonuria.**

Etiology: **Unknown,** no problem in pancreas. It is found in postmature, LBW. Higher incidence with family history of diabetes.

Treatment:

a.   **Fluid, electrolytes** to correct dehydration.

b.   **Regular insulin;** (monitor serum glucose level) twice a day, keep plasma glucose > 130 mg/dl. Remember, **the presence of glucose in urine is O.K. Don't try to make aglycosuria.**

c.   **Diet: Liberal amount of protein and carbohydrates.**

Prognosis:

a.   **Most of them are transient** . They required treatment for approximately 65 days.

b.   Some develop permanent diabetes mellitus.

c.   Few develop diabetes mellitus.

29.   **Galactosemia:**

Signs and symptoms: At birth normal or LBW. Within first few days of life, **appears with fulminant** clinical pictures **(hepatosplenomegaly, jaundice,** vomiting, diarrhea, **renal tubular acidosis, cataract,** anemia).

Preliminary diagnosis: Presence of **reducing substance in urine.**

Diagnosis : In **RBC enzyme ↓ (galactose 1-phosphate uridyl transferase activity).**

Remember, galactose 1 phosphate level will be ↑. Never do galactose tolerance test.

Treatment:

a.   **Remove galactose from milk** (give nutramigen, prosobee).

b.   **Try to keep galactose 1 phosphate level < 4 mg/gm of hemoglobin** (normal is < 1 mg/gm of hemoglobin).

These are very important points to remember:

a.   **Elimination of galactose from the diet does not invalidate the enzyme assay, irrespective of duration of elimination.**

b.   Organ damages (liver, kidney, eye cataract) are **reversible** with the diet.

c.   The earlier the onset of therapy, the better the intellectual outcome.

d.   Behavioral and learning disorders has been noted in both the treated and untreated groups.

e.   Cataract due to ↑ galactitol.

f.   Liver and kidney dysfunction due to ↑ galactose 1 phosphate.

30.   **Galactokinase deficiency** (disorder of galactose metabolism):

Signs and symptoms: Newborn appears with **cataract and pseudotumor** cerebri (cataract resolves with restriction of diet). Normal kidney and liver.

Diagnosis: In **RBC, ↓ galactokinase activity.**

Enzyme: Galactokinase normally converts galactose to galactose 1 phosphate.

Treatment: Life-long dietary restriction of galactose (give nutramigen, prosobee).

Remember, galactitol causes lens swelling.

31.   **Hereditary fructose intolerance:**

Signs and symptoms: **Normal at birth. Intolerance** appears after fructose intake with **postprandial seizures,** ↑ liver size, **obstructive jaundice,** bleeding, **renal tubular acidosis,** vomiting, sometimes diarrhea. **Striking aversion to sweets.**

Diagnosis:

a.   Liver biopsy and enzyme assay ↓ **1-phosphofructaldolase.**

b.   If diagnosis of this intolerance is suspected, then discontinue fructose from diet in neonate so that definitive diagnosis can be done one or two years later.

Treatment: **Give glucose** (don't give fructose or sucrose, even avoid medicines that contain fructose or sucrose).

Prognosis: Excellent.

32.   **Pompe disease (type II glycogenosis):**

Signs and symptoms: Normal at birth. Symptoms manifest in first few months with cardiomegaly, hepatomegaly, hypotonia, ↓ reflex, **normal CNS. Death results from respiratory failure.**

Diagnosis: Lysosomal storage of glycogen in RBC, liver and skeletal muscle and enzyme study after biopsy.

Prenatal diagnosis: Demonstration of **abnormal lysosomes in uncultured amniotic cells and enzyme assay in cultured amniotic cells.**

Treatment: Don't give glycogen, only supportive.

Enzyme: ↓ alpha-glucosidase.

EKG: ↓ PR, ↑ QRS, **(L) axis deviation.**

EMG: Myotonic discharge.

NCV: Slowed (NCV = Nerve conduction velocity).

33.   **Glycogenosis type I (type I a and I b):**

Signs and symptoms: Normal at birth. Appears later with ↑ liver, **hypoglycemic seizures, tachypnea** due to lactic acidosis. **Depressed infant wakes up only for feeding.** Type Ib same as type Ia, but there is **more neutropenia in type Ib.**

Diagnosis:

a. Definitive (type Ia): **Skin fibroblast culture** showing ↓ glucose 6 phosphatase.
b. Definitive type Ib: **Transport defect** for glucose 6 phosphate at microsomal membrane.
c. Glucagon stimulation test: No response means **no ↑ glucose,** but ↑ of lactate in type I.
d. Plasma: ↓ glucose, ↑ lactate.

Prenatal diagnosis: Not possible because this enzyme is absent in skin fibroblast and in WBC.

Treatment:
a. Goal is to prevent hypoglycemia: Frequent feeding Q 2.H and continuous feeding at night with **glucose and its polymers** in order to reduce glycogen store.
b. Acidosis (metabolic): $NaHCO_3$.
c. ↑ uric acid: Allopurinol.
d. ↑ lipid and xanthomatosis: MCT oil.

Enzymes:
a. Type Ia: ↓ glucose 6 phosphatase.
b. Type Ib: **Failure of translocator** that permits glucose 6 phosphate into microsomes where enzymes are localized.

34. **Defects in peroxisomal functions:**
    a. **Zellweger's syndrome** (cerebrohepatorenal syndrome);
       Signs and symptoms: **Genital abnormalities, ↓ tone, seizures, nystagmus, failure to thrive,** wide anterior fontanel, micrognathia, high forehead. Death usually within 1 year.
       Diagnosis: Confirmed by ↓ plasmalogen in RBC and cultured fibroblast.
       Prenatal diagnosis: ↓ **plasmalogen level** in amniotic cell and chorionic villi.
       Treatment: None.
       Autopsy:
       i. Liver: Fibrosis, iron storage.
       ii. Kidney: Small in size, multiple small cyst.
       iii. Brain: Polymicrogyria, pachygyria, ↑ water content.
       Defect: **Functional disorder of peroxisome.**
       Two others disorders of peroxisomes are:
       i. Neonatal adrenoleukodystrophy.
       ii. Infantile Refsum's disease.
    b. Neonatal adrenoleukodystrophy:

       Signs and symptoms: **CNS** (↓ tone, nystagmus, developmental delay), **no** dysmorphism, **normal** liver and kidney.
       Diagnosis: Same as above in (a). Treatment: None.
    c. Infantile Refsum's disease:
       Signs and symptoms: **Retinitis pigmentosa,** sensorineural deafness, developmental delay, ↑ liver.
       Diagnosis: Same as in (a), ↑ phytanic acid.
       Treatment: **Restriction of phytanic acid in the diet.**
       Defect: Accumulation of phytanic acid.

35. **Congenital lipodystrophy:**
    Signs and symptoms: **Long and thin newborn;** hepatomegaly develops later. In pediatric

age group, appears with **insulin resistent diabetes mellitus,** acanthosis nigricans, ↑ liver, advanced bone age.

Diagnosis: **Plasma (↑ insulin, ↓glucose), ↑ chylomicron.**

Treatment: Low fat diet.

Defect: ↓ **activity of insulin on adipose tissue,** ↓ fat storage.

36. **Wolman disease (neutral lipidosis):**

    Signs and symptoms: **Failure to thrive since birth, ↑↑ liver and spleen;** vomiting and diarrhea.

    Prenatal diagnosis: Enzyme assay in cultured chorionic villi or amniocyte.

    Diagnosis: **Confirmed by ↓ enzyme assay in WBC** or **cultured skin fibroblast.**

    Pathognomonic sign: Calcified adrenal gland.

    Treatment: None, except steroid for adrenal failure.

    Enzyme: ↓ **acid lipase activities.**

    Prognosis: Poor,;death likely within 6 months.

37. **Farber's disease:**

    Signs and symptoms: Appears **in first week of life with painful swelling of multiple joints, hoarseness, strider, nodules in skin and subcutaneous tissue,** cherry rod spot in retina.

    Diagnosis: Enzyme ceramidase activity in skin fibroblast or WBC.

    Prenatal diagnosis: Presence of ceramidase levels in cultured chorionic villi or amniocyte.

    Treatment: Nonspecific; anti-inflammatory drugs.

38. **Gaucher's disease (lysosomal dysfunction);**

    a. **Malignant infantile form:**

       Signs and symptoms: Appear within first 2 years of life with ↑ liver and spleen, ascites, ↓tone, **cough and respiratory difficulty, vegetative state of CNS, no** cherry red spot (↓ beta glucosidase).

       Diagnosis: **Enzyme assay (↓ beta glucosidase) in WBC and skin fibroblast.**

       Enzyme: ↓ Beta glucosidase activity.

       Prenatal diagnosis: It is possible with enzyme assay in amniotic cells or chorionic villi.

    b. **Chronic juvenile form: First clinical manifestation is enlarged spleen.** Neurologic damage appears later in life.

       Diagnosis: Same as above.

       Treatment: Splenectomy causes remission for few years; glucocerebrosidase and marrow transplant are under investigation.

39. **Most common complication of meconium ileus with cystic fibrosis: Intestinal perforation with meconium peritonitis.**

40. **Tay Sachs disease (ganglioside storage disease):**

    Signs and symptoms:

    a. **Infantile form:** Appear after 3 months and before 8 months with **hyperacusis, CNS** (↓ tone, seizures **large head without hydrocephalus** spasticity). Cherry red spot appears after neonatal period.

    b. **Late onset or juvenile form:** Appears with ataxia, and choreoathetetosis. **There is** no cherry red spot. Atrophic brain with ↑ ventricle (MRI, CT).

Diagnosis: Confirmed by **absence of enzymes in WBC, cultured skin fibroblast, and plasma.**

Prenatal diagnosis: Enzyme activity in amniotic cells or chorionic villi.

Enzyme: ↓ activity of beta hexosaminidase A, so ↑ accumulation of GM2 ganglioside in all tissues. In CNS, **gray mater involved (early** involvement causes shrunken brain with dilated ventricle, **late** involvement causes enlarged brain with small ventricle).

Treatment: None.

41. **Niemann Pick disease (lysosomal dysfunction):**
    a. **Type A:**
       Signs and symptoms: Appear after neonatal period, with ↑ liver and jaundice, **cherry red spot in retina,** CNS deterioration after neonatal period.
       Diagnosis: **Confirmed by enzyme assay (↓ sphingomyelinase),** activity in **skin fibroblast, marrow culture, WBC.**
       Treatment: Nonspecific.
    b. Type B: Same as type 'A', except no **CNS involvement. Normal life span expected.**

42. **Generalized gangliosidosis (mucolipidosis type I).**
    Signs and symptoms: Of Hurler syndrome, **Hurler facies,** ↑ liver and spleen, skeletal defects, **tense ascites, growth and mental retardation,** macular cherry red spot. Death occurs in the first 2 years due to pulmonary complications.
    Prenatal diagnosis: Enzyme assay in cultured amnionic cells.
    Diagnosis: **Confirmed by enzyme (↓ neuraminidase activity)on skin fibroblast and WBC.**
    Treatment: Nonspecific.
    Enzyme: ↓ **neuraminidase activity.**

43. **Tyrosinemia:**
    a. **Type I: Tyrosinosis, Hereditary tyrosinemia, Hepatorenal tyrosinemia:**
       Enzyme: ↓ Fumarylacetoacetate hydrolyse. (Autosomal recessive.) Organs involved:Liver, kidney, CNS.
       Signs and symptoms:
       i. **Acute** (within first 6 months): **Cabbage -ike odor,** ↑ liver and spleen, ↓ glucose, jaundice, failure to thrive, vomiting, ↑ bleeding (melena, hematuria, ecchymosis).
       ii. **Chronic (after 1 year): Vitamin D resistant rickets, Fanconi** syndrome (renal tubular dysfunction), cirrhosis, growth and developmental delay.
       Diagnosis:
       Serum and urine: Presence of succinylacetoacetate, succinylacetone.
       Confirmed: **Enzyme assay** in liver biopsy or fibroblast culture.
       Treatment: Diet low in tyrosine, phenylalanine, methionine. If no response, then liver transplant.
       Prenatal diagnosis:
       i. **Amniotic** fluid: Measure succinylacetone level.
       ii. CVS: Enzyme assay.
    b. Type II (Richner-Hanhart syndrome, oculocutaneous tyrosinemia):
       Enzyme: ↓ cytosolic fraction of hepatic tyrosine amino transferase.
       Organs involved: CNS, eye, skin.

Signs and symptoms: Mental retardation, herpetiform corneal ulcer (due to tyrosine deposit), hyperkeratosis (palm and sole).

Diagnosis: ↑ tyrosine in serum and urine, **confirmed by enzyme assay.**

Treatment: Diet low in tyrosine and phenylalanine.

NEONATOLOGY

1. **Constipation in newborn:**
   a. Constipation is **not present at birth,** but appears around first month of life, indicating **congenital aganglionic megacolon, cretinism, anal stenosis.**
   b. > 90% of fullterms pass stool within 24 hours; the rest pass in 36 hours.
   Treatment:
   a. Functional: 5% glucose water.
   b. Treat the underlying cause.

2. Treatment for meconium plug syndrome: **Gastrografin enema. (Use in diluted form,** or it can cause dehydration due to rapid loss of fluid with enema. It can be removed by **mucomyst or isotonic saline enema also.)**
   After removal of meconium plug, infant should be observed for congenital aganglionic megacolon. It is associated with cystic fibrosis.
   Clinical presentation of meconium plug syndrome: Intestinal obstruction (vomiting, abdominal distension), **sometimes passes inspissated meconium stool 1-2 times.**

   Abd X-ray: Dilated proximal intestine and bubbly appearance (meconium infiltrated with gas).
   Associated findings are: Intestinal atresia and stenosis, volvulus.

3. **Pneumopericardium: Asymptomatic** or **appears with** sudden shock with tachycardia, muffled heart sound, diminished peripheral pulses.
   Diagnosis: Confirmed by chest X-ray. (Air around the heart)
   Treatment:
   a. Asymptomatic: No treatment.
   b. Symptomatic: Pericardial tube placement.

4. Treatment for **chlamydia or ureaplasma pneumonia** in BPD patient: **Erythromycin.**

5. Most common cause of lung cyst: **Acquired. (Either from alveolar rupture by over-inflation or infection by Staphylococci.** Congenital cyst is rare).
   Lung cyst: Mostly asymptomatic. If symptomatic then tachypnea and cyst infection appear.
   Diagnosis by: Chest X-ray.
   Treatment:
   a. Asymptomatic: No treatment (spontaneously resolves).
   b. **Severe respiratory distress: Surgical removal,** but before that, do CT scan.

6. **Pulmonary hemorrhage:**
   a. **Bleeding mostly from alveoli** (in 66% of cases); the rest are interstitial.
   b. **Most common clinical presentation is bleeding from endotracheal tube.**
   c. Diagnosis by chest X-ray: Butterfly opacity of perihilar area.
   d. **Treatment:** Blood, high PEEP (positive end expiratory pressure, epinephrine aerosols).

7. **Tension pneumothorax:** It is less common, and is due to **accumulation of air in pleural space** resulting in intrapleural pressure that exceeds atmospheric pressure. It cause ipsilateral lung collapse, shifting of mediastinum (superior vena cava compression venous engorgement of cerebral veins resulting in IVH or intracerebral bleeding).

8. **Pneumothorax Clinical manifestations:**
   a. **Asymptomatic:** Diminished breath sound on affected side. May or may not have mild tachypnea.
   b. **Symptomatic:** Usually there is a sudden onset of cyanosis, tachypnea, respiratory distress, irritability, apnea, asymmetric chest (bulging on affected side), ↓ breath sound and hyperresonance on affected side. Heart sound is deviated to opposite side. Only 10% of cases have bilateral pneumothorax, 90% unilateral.

   Diagnosis:
   a. Initial: Positive transillumination.
   b. Final: Confirmed by chest X-ray (showing air collection in pleural space, collapsed lung, mediastinal shift to opposite side).

   Treatment:
   a. Asymptomatic patient: Only close observation.
   b. Symptomatic: Emergency needle aspiration then placement of chest tube. (100% O_2 can absorb pneumothorax rapidly by reducing nitrogen tension in blood).

9. **Pneumomediastinum:**
   a. Most pathognomonic sign of pneumomediastinum in newborn: **Subcutaneous emphysema.**
   b. Most common presentation is **asymptomatic.** (If symptomatic, then it appears with tachypnea, engorged neck veins, hypotension, subcutaneous emphysema.)
   c. 25% of cases of pneumothorax have pneumomediastinum.
   d. Diagnosis confirmed by chest X-ray.
   e. Spontaneously resolves, require only supportive treatment.

10. **Most common cause of pneumothorax:** Over-inflation causing alveolar rupture.

11. **Most common presentation** of pneumothorax: **Asymptomatic** (occurs in 1-2% of all live births). (Pneumothorax is more common in **term and post term** than preterm, **male** more than female. **Less common** is symptomatic type).

12. **Mechanism of pneumothorax:**
    Alveolar rupture → air leak into interstitial space → interstitial emphysema or travel along peribronchial and perivascular connective tissue sheath to the root of the lung → causing pneumomediastinum, pneumothorax, subcutaneous emphysema.

13. **Most important factor** causing pneumothorax in a patient on mechanical ventilator: **High PIP** (positive inspiratory pressure). Next is PEEP (positive end expiratory pressure).

14. **Complications of ECMO: Most common complication is intracerebral bleeding** due to heparinization. Other complications are **inability to keep PCO_2 normal** (usually CO_2 is very low), thromboembolism, stroke, seizures, ↓ platelet and ↓ WBC, atelectasis, cholestatic jaundice, hemolysis, edema and ↑ B.P.

15. Most commonly used bypass in ECMO: **Veno-arterial** (internal jugular vein with carotid artery). Other is veno-venous (internal jugular vein with femoral vein).

16. **A-a gradient (alveolar-arterial oxygen gradient);**
    a. **Simplified equation:**
       $(A-a) DO_2 = (PATM - PH2O) - (PaO_{2+} PaCO_2)$.
    b. Mostly used equation:
       i. $(A-a) DO_2 = PAO_2 - PaO_2$.
       ii. $PAO_2 = PiO_2 - PACO_2/R + PaCO_2 \times FiO_2 (I-R)/R$.
    PATM = Atmospheric pressure, PH2O = Partial pressure of H2O vapor,
    PAO_2 = alveolar oxygen tension, PaO_2 = arterial oxygen tension,
    $PACO_2$ = alveolar CO_2 tension, $PaCO_2$ = arterial CO_2 tension.
    $PiO_2 = FiO_2 (PATM - PH2O)$.
    R = Respiratory exchange ratio.
    In 100% oxygen, $FiO_2 = 1$, $PACO_2$ and $PaCO_2$ is equal, R = 1, so simplified formula can be used.
    A-a gradient more than 620 for 12 hours = 100% mortality.
    A-a gradient more than 600 for 12 hours = 94% mortality.

17. Prognosis of PPHN with ECMO therapy:
    a. PPHN: 85-90% survive. Out of that, 70-75% appear normal at 1 year of age.
    b. PPHN: With diaphragmatic hernia, there usually is a poor prognosis (due to pulmonary hypoplasia) if **PCO_2 is over 40 in pre-and postoperative on mechanical ventilator.**

18. **Indications for ECMO in PPHN:**
    a. 5-10% of **PPHN** (unresponsive to ventilator management) patients with **$AaDO_2$ greater than 620 for 8-12 hours and oxygenation index (OI) is more than 40%.**
    b. **Hypoxic patient of diaphragmatic hernia,** especially when **ventilation index** (rate x mean airway pressure) **exceeds 1000 and PCO_2 exceeds 40 mm Hg.**
    c. Selected patient of HMD, meconium aspiration, group B Strep. infection.
       Oxygenation index (OI): (mean airway pressure x FiO_2 x 100) ÷ Postductal PaO_2.

19. **Contraindications ot ECMO:**
    a. **Absolute contraindications:**
       i. Presence of intracranial hemorrhage.
       ii. **Patient at risk for IVH** (weight < 2000 gm, < 35 week gestational age).
       iii. Congenital and or neurological abnormalities with poor outcome.
    b. **Relative contraindications:**

    i.   Congenital heart disease.

    ii.   Ventilator therapy > 7 days.

20.   **PPHN (persistent pulmonary hypertension) or PFC (persistent fetal circulation):**
Age group: Usually term and post term.
Etiology: Asphyxia, meconium aspiration, group B strep. infection, pulmonary hypoplasia (due to diaphragmatic hernia and other causes), HMD, hypoglycemia, polycythemia.
Normal physiology at birth: After first breathing, pulmonary alveoli expand, pulmonary capillaries dilate, pulmonary pressure drops, (R) ventricular pressure drops, systemic pressure and aortic pressure **increase, shunting (R) to (L) through PDA and foramen ovale stops, normal physiologic condition is established.**
Factors causing pulmonary vasodilatation at birth: Gas filled alveoli, ↑ PaO_2, ↑ pH, release of vasoactive substances.

Factors causing increased pulmonary vascular constriction (resistance):
a.   **Maladaptation:** Pulmonary vessels did not dilate even with high oxygen and other changes mentioned above.
b.   **Smooth muscle proliferation in pulmonary arteriole and increased muscle thickness: Due to hypoxia.**
c.   **Dysplastic capillaries, hypoplastic lungs:** In diaphragmatic hernia, Potter syndrome.
d.   **Obstructive:** Polycythemia and increased blood viscosity.

21.   **PPHN (signs and symptoms, diagnosis, treatment):**
Signs and symptoms: Sick-looking child with severe cyanosis, respiratory distress, tachypnea, mitral and tricuspid regurgitation (due to ischemic papillary muscle dysfunction and is usually present within first 12 hours of life.
Shunting: Two level (foramen ovale, ductus arteriosus).
Diagnosis:
a.   **Initial hyperoxia test (100% oxygen): PaO_2 < 100 = PPHN (like cyanotic** heart disease), but sometimes improves oxygenation with bag and mask and hyperventilation (**unlike cyanotic** heart disease).
b.   **Preductal (right arm) and post ductal (umbilical artery) PaO_2 gradient: If > 20 mm Hg** = suggests PPHN shunting through ductus, but remember there should be **no** difference if shunting through foramen ovale.
c.   Diagnosis confirmed by echocardiogram with color doppler flow study demonstrate shunting.
Treatment:
a.   Always treat the underlying causes (↓ **glucose, infection, ↑ Hct).**
b.   **One approach is normal ventilation without pancuronium paralysis:** To keep PaO_2 50-70 mm Hg, PCO_2 50-55 mm Hg; **Tolazoline** (nonselective, alpha adrenergic antagonist; it **causes vasodilation of all the blood vessels of the body except in kidney where it causes vasoconstriction)** and **dopamine** to counteract tolazoline's inducing of hypotension.
c.   Second **approach is hyperventilation (mostly with pancuronium paralysis):** To keep PCO_2 20-25 mm Hg, pH 7.50-7.60, PaO_2 90-100 mm Hg. (Recent development: low PCO_2 has no effect on pulmonary vasodilation, which is caused by alkaline pH and high oxygen). Sometimes $NaHCO_3$ infusion can be given to cause pulmonary

vasodilation if PCO_2 is normal. To achieve the goal, often ↑ PIP, ↑ RR, is required and use pavulon to paralyse the muscles.

   d.   ECMO (extracorporeal membrane oxygenation).

22.   **Complication of pavulon:** Edema.

23.   **Meconium aspiration:**
Age group: Term or post term.
Etiology: Usually fetal distress and hypoxia in utero or at birth.
Signs and Symptoms: At birth, appears with respiratory distress, tachypnea, cyanosis, retraction in severely aspirated patient. Chest is overdistended.
Diagnosis: Confirmed by chest X-ray; Patchy infiltrate, increased anteroposterior diameter, coarse streaks in the both lung fields.

Prevention:
   a.   Monitor for fetal distress and prompt initiation of delivery to avoid hypoxia in fetus (by obgyn. physician).
   b.   DeLee suction of oropharynx after the head is delivered (by obgyn. physician).
Treatment:
   a.   Thin meconium, no asphyxia: May need minimal suction.
   b.   Thick meconium, asphyxiated newborn: Endotracheal intubation and suction attached directly to the tube.
   c.   Mild aspiration and mild cyanosis: Oxygen by oxyhood usually correct hypoxia.
   d.   Moderate to severe aspiration, severe cyanosis: Mechanical ventilation (use higher rate, higher oxygen, **lower** PIP and PEEP to avoid pneumothorax, pneumomediastinum). **The goal is to ventilate the infant properly.**
Prognosis: Depends upon the **degree of CNS injury due to asphyxia. Lung problem usually resolves** but tachypnea may persist up to several weeks. **Very rarely** is there coughing, wheezing, and hyperinflated chest remain for 5-10 years.
Ball-valve mechanism: Meconium blocks the airway. In inspiration, air goes inside the alveoli, but in **expiration the airway collapses,** resulting in air trapping in the alveoli, distension of alveoli ,and air leaks.

24.   **Complications of hyperventilation in PPHN:** ↓ cardiac output and cerebral blood flow, barotrauma, pneumothorax, ↓ fluid requirement, hyperinflation of lungs.

25.   **Prognosis for HMD patient:**
   a.   65% survive in < 1000 gm.
   b.   **95%** sick infants survive > 2,500 gm.
   c.   **85-90%** of all patient of HMD on mechanical ventilator become normal.
   d.   **80%** have **normal** neurologic outcome in < 1500 gm.

26.   **TTNB (transient tachypnea of newborn) or RDS type II:** It is due to **slow absorption of fetal lung fluid** resulting in ↓ pulmonary compliance, ↓ tidal volume, and ↑ dead space.
Signs and symptoms: Tachypnea, expiratory grunting, **rarely** retraction and cyanosis (resolved by oxygen).
It is found in both **term and preterm vaginal delivery and cesarean section delivery. Diagnosis made by exclusion.**

Chest X-ray: Fluid line in fissures, ↑ pulmonary vascular marking, hyper aeration, flat diaphragm, rarely pleural fluid.
Treatment: Supportive.

27. Most common cause of **aspiration of amniotic fluid with or without meconium in utero:** Fetal distress (due to hypoxia for prolonged labor or difficult deliveries) causing vigorous respiratory movements in utero resulting in aspiration. Pneumonia is the complication. Diagnosis confirmed by X-ray.
Treatment: Respiratory support, antibiotics.

28. **Complications of BPD: Growth retardation,** transient psychomotor delay, parental stress, nephrolithiasis (due to diuretics and TPN), osteopenia, subglottic stenosis.

29. **PDA (patent ductus arteriosus);**
Factors that keep the duct open:
↓ O_2, ↓ pH, ↑ pulmonary artery pressure,
↓ B.P. (systemic), ↑ PGE, prematurity. (When HMD resolves, pulmonary pressure drop, ↑ (L) to (R) shunt, pulmonary edema, (L) ventricular volume overload).
Signs and symptoms of PDA:
a. Unexplained **apnea** in a patient recovering from HMD.
b. ↑ CO_2, ↓ PaO_2.
c. Wide pulse pressure, bounding peripheral pulse, active precordium, systolic or to and fro murmur.
d. CXR: ↑ heart size, ↑ pulmonary circulation.
e. ↑ liver size.
Diagnosis confirmed by Echocardiogram.
Treatment:
a. **Fluid restriction and diuretics.**
b. If they fail then give **indomethacin** (inhibit prostaglandin secretion).
c. If that fails, then perform **surgical closure.**
Contraindications of indomethacin:
↓ platelet (< 50,000/mm^3), ↑ creatinine (> 1.8 mg/dl), bleeding disorder, ↑ BUN (> 20 mg/dl).

30. Most common cause of **anemia in HMD: Frequent withdrawal of blood samples.**
Remember, oxygen dependent infants should have hematocrit close to **40.**
Major cause of death in BPD: (R) heart failure and viral necrotizing bronchiolitis.

31. **Infants at risk** for BPD are the following:
a. Severe RDS with prolonged mechanical ventilation and oxygen therapy.
b. **Other factors are:** PIE (pulmonary interstitial emphysema), prematurity, PDA, high PIP (positive inspiratory pressure), increased airway resistance in first week of life, **pulmonary infection with Ureaplasma urealyticum, male sex,** ↓ CO_2 at 48 hours with possibly a family history of asthma.

32. **BPD (bronchopulmonary dysplasia);**
Acceptable ABG (arterial blood gas) in BPD patient is pH > 7.30, PCO_2 50-70 mm Hg, PaO_2 55-60 mm Hg with oxygen saturation 90-95%.

Blue spell in BPD: It may be due to **airway obstruction** in BPD (mucous, edema, bronchospasm and collapse of acquired tracheomalacia) or may be due to **acute cor pulmonale** or **myocardial ischemia.**
Treatment:

a. Bronchodilators (aerosolized beta 2 adrenergic drug or theophylline).
b. Diuretics and fluid restriction.
c. Treat infection with U.urealyticum, respiratory syncytial virus.
d. High calorie nutrition for growth.
e. CPAP for tracheomalacia.
f. Dexamethasone (it helps to wean patient off mechanical ventilator).
g. Older patient may respond to vasodilator therapy to ↓ pulmonary artery pressure.

33. **Prevention of umbilical artery thrombus formation: Heparin flush or continuous infusion (1-10 u/ml), or using smooth-tipped catheter with hole only at the end.**

34. **Complication of umbilical vein catheterization:** Liver cirrhosis from portal vein thrombosis (other complications may be same as in umbilical artery).

35. **Oxygen toxicity in prematurity:**
Lung: BPD.
Eye: ROP.

36. **BPD (bronchopulmonary dysplasia):** It is a **radiological diagnosis.**
Stage II is complete opacification obscuring the cardiac border. Probably indicates pulmonary edema.
Stage III is multiple cystic changes mostly around perihilar region.
Stage IV is multiple cystic areas all over the lung with hyperlucency.
Pathological diagnosis: Stage I is same as HMD.
Stage II is a **period of** regeneration and proliferation of bronchial epithelium, necrosis and repair of alveolar epithelium.
Stage III is **period of** transition to chronic disease, extensive repair with membrane phagocytosis and epithelial regeneration, interstitial fibrosis and bronchiolar metaplasia.
Stage IV is chronic disease, obliterative bronchiolitis with interstitial fibrosis and squamous cell metaplasia.
Most surviving neonate with chronic radiological changes usually recovers by 6-12 months.

37. **Antibiotics of choice for early onset neonatal sepsis: Ampicillin and gentamicin.**

38. **Ventilator management of RDS or HMD:**
Goal is to keep pH between 7.35-7.45 (up to 7.25 is acceptable), PaO_2 55-70, PCO_2 35-55.
a. First **try oxyhood:** If PaO_2 cannot be maintained above 50, even with 70% oxyhood, then try CPAP.
b. **CPAP** (6-10 cm of H_2O pressure) by nasal prongs: If PaO_2 cannot be maintained above 50, even with 100% oxygen, then try mechanical ventilator.
c. **Conventional ventilator setting:**

Ventilator rate 10-60 breaths/min,

PIP = 16-18 cm H2O,

PEEP = 4-6 cm H_2O,

Inspiratory time = 0.4-0.6 second.

High frequency jet ventilator rate 150-600/min.

High frequency oscillatory ventilator rate 300-1800/min.

Try to keep the above mentioned goal.

d. **Surfactant therapy (bovine or synthetic).**

e. **Respiratory acidosis (↑ CO_2, ↓ pH):** ↑ ventilator rate.

f. **Respiratory alkalosis (↓ CO_2, ↑ pH):** ↓ ventilator rate.

g. **Metabolic acidosis (→ CO_2, ↓ pH):** First to correct then underlying cause then give $NaHCO_3$.

h. **Both metabolic and respiratory acidosis (↑ CO_2, ↓ pH, ↓ HCO_3):** Remember, **first correct respiratory acidosis** (by ↑ ventilator rate), **then correct metabolic acidosis (by $NaHCO_3$).**

i. **Weaning off from mechanical ventilator: The first two parameters that should be reduced is (a) PIP,** because it causes maximum barotrauma and **(b) oxygen because it causes ROP (retinopathy of prematurity) and BPD (bronchopulmonary dysplasia).**

39. **Most serious complication of tracheal intubation: Asphyxia due to obstruction of the tube.** (Other complications are cardiac arrest due to vagal stimulation. Long term complication is subglottic stenosis)

40. Most common complication of umbilical artery catheterization: **Clot formation** in and about the catheter in 95% of cases shown by aortography (but autopsy shows 1-23%). Other complications are infection (most common organism is staph. epidermidis), embolism, thrombus, spasm, perforation.

41. Management of **blanching of leg** due to umbilical artery catheterization: **Removal of catheter:** If blanching persists, then **warm up the other leg.This** causes reflex vasodilatation of affected leg through splanchnic nerve plexus. Try to put catheter in other umbilical artery. (Spasm of radial artery or thrombosis can be managed in the same way as umbilical artery.)
Arterial spasm can be relieved by local infusion of tolazoline 1-2 mg over 5 minutes. Catheter should be removed immediately if there is no free flow of blood.

42. **High frequency oscillatory ventilator (HFOV):**
Advantage: Helps in CO_2 elimination, ↓ MAP (mean airway pressure), occasionally improves oxygenation in a patient not responding to conventional ventilator (example = RDS, pulmonary interstitial emphysema, meconium aspiration, multiple pneumothoraces).
Disadvantage: Increased air leak, ↑ IVH, ↑ PVL, ↑ air trapping.

43. **High frequency jet ventilator (HFJV):**
Advantage: Same as HFOV.
Disadvantage: Necrotizing tracheal damage (especially with hypotension and poor humidification), ↑ air trapping.

44. **Complications of ET (endotracheal) tube: Plugging,** extubation, subglottic granuloma, and stenosis.

45. **Complications of mechanical ventilations in RDS:**
    a. **Short term:** Pneumothorax, PIE (pulmonary interstitial emphysema), ↓ cardiac output.
    b. **Long term:** Chronic lung changes (BPD).

46. Most of the HMD/RDS are: **Self-limited, and improve by third day of life.**

47. **Corticosteroid and RDS/HMD:** It can be given to a woman who do **not** have toxemia, diabetes or renal disease; her **amniocentesis shows pulmonary immaturity of fetus and she is likely to deliver after 48 hours and before 72 hours.** One or two doses of betamethasone can be given I.M.

48. **Surfactant administration and RDS/HMD:** If surfactant is given immediately after birth or within 24 hours of age, **it will definitely improve pulmonary function (but it may not reduce either the mortality from RDS or the incidence of BPD).**

49. **Excessive fluid and RDS/HMD:** Excessive fluid increases the incidence of PDA, particularly in first few days of life, resulting in (L) to (R) shunt from aorta to pulmonary artery, and ↑ pulmonary edema which causes worsening of RDS.

50. Most common cause of neonatal death: **Hyaline membrane disease and its complication.**

51. **A few** important points about lung surfactant:
    a. It is present in high concentration in fetal lung by the 20th week of gestational age, but does **not** appear in alveoli.
    b. It appears in amniotic fluid from the 28th to the 32nd week.
    c. Mature level of surfactant is achieved **after 35 weeks** when phosphatidylglycerol appears in amniotic fluid.
    d. It is synthesized by type II cells.
    e. Surfactant production is reduced by the following: Hypoxia, pulmonary ischemia, ↓ B.P., cold, hypovolemia, high O_2 and high ventilator pressure.
    f. Surfactant deficiency in lung results in failure to achieve FRC (functional residual capacity) resulting atelectasis.

52. Most common cause of ALTE (acute-life threatening events): **Apnea of infancy.** Apnea of infancy occurs **mostly in fullterm infants in first 6 months of life,** showing **isolated apnea of 5 to 15 seconds with or without periodic breathing,** no bradycardia, no color change and it resolves spontaneously. Some infants have apnea longer than 20 seconds, or shorter when associated with bradycardia or color change. Both resolve spontaneously.

    ALTE: Some infants with apnea of infancy, usually after discharge from the hospital, develop acute life-threatening events which require vigorous resuscitation or positive pressure ventilation. **50% of ALTE are due to apnea of infancy.** Other causes are gastroesophageal reflux, convulsions, infection, heart disease, breath holding spell, pharyngeal incoordination, central hypoventilation syndrome, CNS anomaly, accidental or incidental maternal smothering.

Infants with ALTE have higher incidence of periodic breathing and apnea than normal population. They also have **slow brainstem conduction, reduced CNS sensitivity to CO_2, reduced arousal response to hypoxia and hypoventilation** but all these effects are the either result of ALTE or present before ALTE.
Later on significant number of patients of ALTE die suddenly.

53. **HMD (hyaline membrane disease) or RDS:**
     Clinical presentation: Premature babies appear immediately after birth with respiratory distress, cyanosis, tachypnea, grunting, retraction (intercostal).
     Diagnosis confirmed by chest X-ray.
     Differential diagnosis: **Remember, group B Strep infection cannot be distinguished from RDS. Total anomalous pulmonary venous return (TAPVR) also mimic RDS.**

54. **Clinical presentations and treatment in apnea: Clinical presentations:** Idiopathic apnea of prematurity varies **inversely with gestational** age. Apnea is **rare in first** 24 hours: if mostly occurs from the 2nd to the 7th **day of life.** If apnea develops suddenly on the 2nd day in a previously well child,there is a serious illness. **95% of cases bradycardia are associated with apnea.** In premature infant, apnea of more than 10-15 secs is serious.

     Treatment:
     a. Infant should be on an apnea monitor.
     b. **Mild apnea:** Gentle cutaneous stimulation.
     c. **Recurrent and prolonged apnea:**
        i. Bag and mask ventilation with oxygen.
        ii. Theophylline: It decreases diaphragmatic muscle fatigue, ↑ CO_2 sensitivity to CNS.
        iii. Anemia: Transfusion of packed RBC.
     d. **Obstructive or mixed apnea:** CPAP, 3-5 cm H2O pressure (nasal continuous positive airway pressure). CPAP splints the upper airway and prevents collapse.
     e. **Apnea due to other causes:** Treat the underlying cause, but maintain oxygenation and airway stability.

55. **Relation of apnea with SIDS** (sudden infant death syndrome): **Apnea does not predict future SIDS.** Apnea usually resolves by 36 weeks of gestational age and has a good outcome.

56. **Most common type** of apnea in premature infants (important):
     Mixed type (50%), i.e., combination of both obstructive (10%) and central type (40%).
     Obstructive type: It is due to upper airway obstruction due to pharyngeal instability, flexion of neck ,or nasal blockage, pharyngeal collapse due to negative pharyngeal pressure during inspiration, or incoordination of the tongue and other upper airway muscles.
     Central type: It is due to immaturity of the reticular activating system in respiratory

center resulting in diminished response to ↑ CO_2 and paradoxic response to hypoxia.

57. Apnea and its relation to sleep state:
Apnea: It is the cessation of breathing for 20 seconds or more (longer apnea), or < 20 seconds with bradycardia and color change. Short apneas (10 seconds) are rarely associated with bradycardia.
Apnea and sleep: Most apneas occur **during active sleep with rapid eye movement (REM).** Newborns and premature infants sleep 80% of the time (adults, 30%). Out of that, **> 50% is active sleep in premature infant.** During active sleep, there is low voltage electrocortical state, ↓ muscle tone, ↓ arousal from sleep, ↓ respiratory drive, irregular breathing, inspiratory chest wall distortion, absence of upper airway adductor activities.

58. Lung fluid is absorbed after birth **mostly by: Pulmonary circulation;** rest is absorbed by lymphatics, expelled from trachea (30 cc), or swallowed into stomach. Removal of fluid is impaired by C- section or by sedation.

59. **Management of respiratory difficulty or failure:**
    a. **First, establish ventilation,** irrespective of the causes of this problem, and correct hypoxia.
    b. Second, **establish good peripheral circulation.**
    c. If problem is due to narcotics (morphine, demerol), give **narcan**.
    d. Cardiac stimulation: Cardiac massage, epinephrine.
    e. Metabolic acidosis due to hypoxia: $NaHCO_3$ should be given after ventilation was established and hypoxia was corrected.
    f. Hypothermia should be corrected.
    g. Duct-dependent cardiac lesion: PGE1 infusion.
    h. RDS: Mechanical ventilator, surfactant.
    i. Pneumothorax (tension): Needle aspiration, chest tube.
    j. Sepsis: Antibiotics.
    k. Hypotension without hypovolemia: Dopamine.
    l. Chronic cardiac failure: Dobutamine.
    m. Erythroblastosis fetalis with anemia: Exchange transfusion with half volume (40 cc/kg) with packed RBC.
    n. Erythroblastosis fetalis with polycythemia (due to cyanotic heart disease): Partial exchange transfusion with 5% albumin.

60. **Periodic breathing:** In first months of life, both in FT and preterm develop periodic breathing during sleep i.e., **apneic pauses of 5-10 secs** followed by bursts of **rapid breathing 50-60/minute for 10-15 seconds.** Preterm infants usually have periodic breathing until the 36th week gestational age. **Periodic breathing is normal and does not require any therapy.**

61. Diagnosis of choice for respiratory distress: **Chest X-ray.**

62. **Stages of HIE and prognosis:**
    Three stages 1 to 3 (better to worse):
    a. **Stage I: Hyper alert patient,** normal (muscle tone, posture, EEG), ↑ **reflexes and**

strong Moro reflex, dilated pupil. **Good** prognosis.

b. **Stage II: Lethargic, diminished** muscle tone, ↑ reflexes, but weak Moro reflex, **flexed** posture, **constricted pupils, seizures occur** and EEG shows low voltage. **Variable** prognosis.

c. **Stage III: Stuporous or comatose, flaccid** muscle tone, **decerebrate posture and seizures, absent** (reflexes and Moro reflex), EEG shows **burst suppression to isoelectric** pattern. **Poor prognosis and death.**

63. **Most common and serious** emergencies in newborns at birth:
    Respiratory difficulty and failure is due to the following:
    a. **Central:** Depressed respiratory center either from hypoxia, drugs (narcotics), IVH, or anomaly.
    b. **Peripheral:** Lung immaturity, meconium aspiration, pneumonia, pneumothorax, lung hypoplasia. It is diagnosed by chest X-ray.
    c. **Mechanical:** Choanal atresia causing obstruction, Pierre-Robin syndrome causing a problem due to posterior displacement of the tongue, diaphragmatic hernia.
    d. **Cardiac:** Cyanotic heart disease with failure.
    e. **Sepsis:** Bacterial infections.

64. **First breathing, stimulus, and pressure:**
    Stimulus for first breathing:
    ↓ O_2, ↑ CO_2, ↓ pH, ↓ temperature, ↑ tactile stimulation.
    Pressure generates in first breathing:
    10-50 cm water pressure. It is the maximum for any time in life. Normal newborns and adult breathe with 4 cm water pressure. Spontaneous pneumothorax occurs due to high pressure. 20-30 cc of air stays in the lung to form FRC in first breathing.

65. Most common site of bone injury in newborn at birth: **Clavicle.**
    It is due to traumatic delivery. Appears with immobilization of ipsilateral upper limb. Examination reveals crepitation and bony irregularities. (In **greenstick** fracture, there is no movement limitation, but Moro reflex is present.)

    Diagnosis: Confirmed by X-ray.
    Treatment: Immobilization of arm and shoulder.
    Prognosis: Excellent: heals within week by callous formation.

66. Treatment for fracture humerus: Immobilization of arm (for 2-4 weeks) strapped in the chest by triangular splint and Velpeau bandage. Fracture humerus is rare. Excellent prognosis.

67. Most common nose injury in newborn at birth: **Dislocation of cartilaginous** portion of septum. Appears with nose irregularity. **Treatment:** Surgical repair.

68. Most common cause of facial nerve palsy in newborn: **Pressure effect of facial nerve** due to forceps or difficult delivery. Present with unilateral facial paralysis with eyes open. Most commonly associated with 6th cranial nerve palsy. Prognosis for facial nerve edema is better than severity of nerve injury.

69. **Hypoxic ischemic encephalopathy (HIE):** HIE is one of the important causes of permanent damage to CNS resulting in mental retardation, sometimes cerebral palsy, or death.

    Etiology:
    a. **Fetal hypoxia** in utero due to the following:
        i. Maternal hypoxia due to hypoventilation due to anaesthesia, cardiac failure, or carbon monoxide poisoning.
        ii. Maternal hypotension due to anaesthesia or pressure on vena cava or aorta.
        iii. Early placental separation.
        iv. Placenta insufficiency.
        v. Excessive uterine contraction due to oxytocin.
    b. **Neonatal hypoxia** after birth due to the following:
        i. Anemia due to hemorrhage or hemolytic diseases.
        ii. Respiratory failure due to narcotics, injury, or cerebral defect.
        iii. Shock due to IVH, adrenal hemorrhage, sepsis, or severe blood loss.
        iv. Cyanotic heart disease.
        v. Severe meconium aspiration (it can cause fetal hypoxia as well).

    Effects of hypoxia in newborns (important):
    a. **Fullterm:** Cortical neuronal necrosis and subsequent cortical atrophy, parasagittal ischemic injury, focal seizure, and hemiplegia are more common in fullterm than in preterm.
    b. **Preterm:** PVL and subsequent spastic diplegia, IVH, status marmoratus of basal ganglia.

    Diagnosis confirmed by CT or MRI.

    Clinical manifestations:
    a. **Fetus: IUGR and increased vascular resistance are usually the first indication of fetal hypoxia.** Appearance of **variable or late deceleration** with **loss of beat-to-beat variability, and scalp pH < 7.20** indicates severe fetal distress. At this point early delivery is indicated.
    b. **Newborn:** Developed meconium-stained amniotic fluid, respiratory distress, bradycardia, cyanosis, initial hypotonia, then hypertonia, lethargy, unresponsive to resuscitation. During the next 24 hours, patient develops seizure, cerebral edema, ↓ Ca, ↓ glucose, persistent pulmonary hypertension, G.I. perforation, acute tubular necrosis.

70. **Phrenic nerve injury causing diaphragmatic paralysis:** It may be associated with brachial plexus injury. Appears with difficulty in breathing, irregular respiration, cyanosis, ↓ breathing sound in paralysed side.

    Diagnosis confirmed by ultrasonography or fluoroscopy.
    Treatment: Nonspecific; placed on affected side; give oxygen if cyanotic; rarely surgical plication of diaphragm.
    Complication: Pulmonary infections.
    Prognosis: Usually recovers in 1-3 months.

71. **Factors causing IVH** (intraventricular hemorrhage): **Most important factor is fluctuation of cerebral blood flow in premature infant. Example: Asphyxia, vigorous**

suctioning.
Reperfusion injury to the damaged vessels; increased venous pressure due to increased intrathoracic pressure like pneumothorax; hypo-and hypertension; hypertonic solution like rapid I.V. push of sodium bicarbonate and vitamin E, RDS.

72.   Most common site of spinal cord injury in difficult delivery: C_7 and T_1.
Injury to spinal cord, that occurs in breech and difficult shoulder deliveries, resulting in hemorrhage, edema or complete separation of spinal cord.
Presentations: Motor paralysis below the site of injury. Severe cases appear with respiratory difficulty, and shock. Initially appears with areflexia, flaccidity. A few weeks or months later they appear with hyperreflexia, flexion rigidity.

Brachial nerve palsy:
   a.   **Erb-Duchenne paralysis:** Injury at C_5, C_6, **appears** with **adduction, internal rotation** of the arm with pronation of forearm, **absent Moro** on that side, some sensory loss in outer side of arm, **normal hand grasp.** Better prognosis than with Klumpke paralysis. Actually depends on severity of injury.
   b.   **Klumpke paralysis:** Injury at C_7, C_8 and T_1; appears **paralyzed hand, absent** hand grasp; ipsilateral ptosis and miosis if sympathetic fibers of T_1 are involved.
Diagnosis confirmed by MRI.
Treatment:
   a.   **Immobilization with brace or splint,** keep arm 90 degree abducted, external rotation of shoulder, supination of forearm, neutral position of wrist. Immobilization should be intermittent throughout 24 hours.
   b.   **Entire arm paralysis:** Same as above and also **gentle massage and range-of-motion exercises** begin within 7-10 days. If no improvement by 3-6 months, then neuroplasty, neurolysis, end-to-end anastomosis, and nerve graft should be done.

73.   **PVL (periventricular leukomalacia):** It is the **necrosis of periventricular white matter due to anoxic ischemic injury. Most common site of PVL is external angle of lateral ventricle. 75% of cases occur in preterm, 25% in term infants.** Other important factors are endotoxin and lack of autoregulation of cerebral blood flow. PVL may, or may not, be present with IVH.
Most common clinical presentation is spastic diplegia syndrome.

74.   **Watershed infarction:** It is found in **fullterm** infant; appears with **cortical infarction** at the junction of anterior, middle and posterior cerebral arteries **due to ischemic injury.** It is usually **absent in premature** due to presence of **meningeal anastomosis** among those three arteries which is **characteristically found in fetal life.**

75.   **Visceral injury in newborn:**
   a.   Liver: Most common injury next to CNS is breech presentation causing pressure on liver resulting in rupture and subcapsular hematoma. Appears with abdominal distension, tachypnea, tachycardia, shock.
         Diagnosis: By ultrasonography.
         Treatment: Surgical repair.
   b.   Spleen: Rupture of spleen may, or may not, be associated with liver rupture. Presentation, diagnosis and treatment is the same as for liver.

c.   Adrenal: Due to breech delivery or anoxia, stress, or infection. Appears with shock, cyanosis and later **calcification.**

Diagnosis: By ultrasonography.

Treatment: Steroid for adrenal failure.

76.   **IVH (intraventricular hemorrhage):**

Clinical presentations: Most commonly found in severely premature **(500-750 gm)** infants, most commonly found within first **3 days of life. Most** common presentations are: **diminished or absent** Moro reflex, hypotonia, lethargy, apnea.

Severe cases show **bulging fontanel, shock,** metabolic acidosis, **dropping hematocrit.** Diagnosis **confirmed by** Ultrasonography of head.

Head CT scan is indicated for intraparenchymal bleeding, particularly for fullterm infant.

Prognosis: Remember, **most infants with IVH** do **not develop hydrocephalus,** which is found in only 10-15% cases.

Grades of hydrocephalus.

Grade I: Bleeding confined to **germinal matrix** or < 10% of ventricle.

Grade II: Occupies **10-15% of ventricle.**

Grade III: > 50% of ventricle and ventricular dilation.

Grade IV: Includes grade III and **intraparenchymal bleeding,**which may not be due to extension of IVH.

75% of IVH is grade I or II. Grade I and grade II have better prognosis. Grade IV is the worst, and grade III is in between.

Treatment:

a.   Anemia: Packed RBC transfusion.

b.   Metabolic acidosis: $NaHCO_3$ (slow I.V. infusion).

c.   Seizure: Anticonvulsant.

d.   **Don't** do spinal tap in acute bleeding, but it is helpful in posthemorrhagic communicating hydrocephalus.

e.   **Hydrocephalus:** Initially **do external ventricular drain,** then **V-P shunt** (ventriculo peritoneal shunt).

77.   **Cranial injuries:**

a.   **Caput succedaneum: Diffuse, edematous** swelling over the scalp during vertex delivery. **Edema disappears spontaneously within few days.**

b.   **Cephalhematoma: Subperiosteal hemorrhage, limited to one bone only.** Swelling appears a few hours after birth because of slow precess. Underlying linear skull fracture may be present. **Most of them spontaneously resolve within 2 weeks to 3 months.** Phototherapy might required for jaundice.

c.   **Fracture of the skull:** Most common type is **linear; depressed fracture** occurs in forceps delivery and can cause neurological symptom. **Elevation of the skull is the** treatment. **Fracture of occipital bone** with separation of basal and squamous portion causes severe bleeding. It occurs in **breech delivery** with hyperextended neck.

d.   Subconjunctival, retinal hemorrhage and skin petechiae: It is **due to increased intrathoracic pressure** during passage of body in normal delivery. **No** treatment is required.

78.   Most common cause of IVH (intraventricular hemorrhage): **Asphyxia** (90% of IVH in preterm and 10% in term infant).

IVH occurs from **subependymal germinal matrix,** which in premature babies consists of **immature blood vessels** without supporting structures. This results bleeding into the ventricle. In fullterm babies, germinal matrix disappears and vascular support is increased. From germinal matrix, **neuronal and glial cells** are formed. **Most common** site of bleeding is at **the level of foramen of Monroe** (near the head of caudate nucleus).

79.   **LGA (large for gestational age) babies:**
a.   **Neonatal mortality increases** in both LGA (FT and preterm).
b.   **Birth injuries increase** significantly (fracture clavicle, cervical and brachial plexus injury, phrenic nerve paralysis, cephalhematoma, subdural hematoma).
c.   **Congenital heart disease more common than in** FT, AGA infant.
d.   ↓ **I.Q. and developmental delay more common** than in FT, AGA.

80.   **Congenital anomalies and presentations:**
a.   **Tracheoesophageal fistula: Excessive salivation,** polyhydramnios, aspiration pneumonia. Rule out VATER syndrome. Unable to pass nasogastric tube in stomach.
b.   **Choanal atresia: Respiratory distress in delivery** room. Rule out **CHARGE** syndrome. Unable to pass nasogastric tube through nares. **Diagnosis confirmed by CT scan.**
c.   **Ductal dependant lesions** (5T = Tetralogy of fallot, tricuspid atresia, truncus, transposition of great vessels, total anomalous pulmonary venous return): Cyanosis, hypotension, metabolic acidosis, murmur.
d.   **Diaphragmatic hernia:** Scaphoid abdomen, respiratory distress.
e.   **Intestinal obstruction: Bile-stained vomitus,** polyhydramnios, cystic fibrosis.
f.   Potter syndrome (renal agenesis): Oligohydramnios, pulmonary hypoplasia.
g.   Neural tube defects: ↑ alpha felo protein, polyhydramnios.
h.   Gastroschisis, omphalocele: Polyhydramnios, intestinal obstruction.
i.   Pierre-Robin syndrome: Micrognathia, cleft palate.

81.   **Hypotonia and LBW children:** Many LBW child have **hypotonia before 8 months of corrected age. It** improves spontaneously by 8 months -1 year of age. Transient hypotonia does **not** indicate poor prognosis.

VLBW (< 1500 gm) and outcomes:
a.   Mean I.Q. is 90-97, 76% do normal in school.
b.   10-20% have neurologic and developmental delay.
c.   3-6% develop C.P. (cerebral palsy).
d.   20% have a learning disorder.

82.   **Placental insufficiency syndrome:** Amniotic fluid and fetus have **meconium-stained, fetal deceleration,** and may have growth retardation. Most patients who develop this **syndrome are FT and are premature (only 20% is post term);** particularly **SGA born to a mother with toxemia, chronic hypertension and elderly primigravida.** Fetus receives **less oxygen and nutrition** due to placental insufficiency.

83. Delivery of post-term (> 42 weeks) infant: When delivery is delayed for 3 weeks, mortality also increases 3 times. **Mode and time of delivery should be decided by careful obstretic follow up** by non-stress test, biophysical profile, doppler velocimetry. In **elderly primigravida, C-section** may be indicated if pregnancy continues **2-4 weeks beyond normal,** particularly with fetal distress.

84. Most important factor in successful care of the premature infants: **Skilled, experienced nursing staff.**

85. Most important step to prevent infection in NICU: **Wash hands rigorously** from elbow down, before and after touching any patient.

86. **Drugs and their effects on premature:**
    a. $NaHCO_3$: **IVH** (intraventricular hemorrhage).
    b. Tolazoline: **Gastric hypersecretion (most common),** gastric bleeding, hypotension.
    c. Aminoglycoside: **Deafness,** renal toxicity.
    d. Phenobarbital: Drowsiness, altered state.
    e. Lasix: **Deafness,** ↓ Na, ↓ K, ↓ Cl, nephrocalcinosis, stones in biliary tract.
    f. Heparin: Bleeding, ↓ platelet, IVH.
    g. Vitamin K: Jaundice.
    h. **I.V. vitamin E: Ascites, shock.**
    i. **Indomethacin: Oliguria,** ↓ Na.
    j. Prostaglandins: **Apnea,** seizures.
    k. Morphine: **Withdrawal,** hypotension, urine retention.
    l. Pavulon: **Edema,** ↓ volume, ↓ B.P., tachycardia.
    m. Dexamethasone: **G.I. bleeding,** ↑ B.P., ↑ glucose, infection.
    n. Fentanyl: **Seizure,** withdrawal, rigid chest wall.
    o. Enteric gentamicin: **Resistant bacteria.**
    p. Chloramphenicol: **Gray syndrome,** bone marrow suppression.

87. Increased insensible water loss **(2-3 ml/kg/hour) in < 1000 gm** premature due to: **Thin skin, large surface area ,and lack of subcutaneous tissue.** Larger **premature infants (2000-2500 gm)** placed in incubator have insensible water loss of about **0.6-0.7 ml/kg/hour.**

88. Parameters to watch during fluid therapy in newborn (FT and premature): **Daily weight, (SUN) serum urea nitrogen, urine specific gravity and output,** other SMA 6.

89. Approximate fluid requirement in **FT and premature:** In premature infant, **it depends on degree of prematurity, weight loss, SUN (serum urea nitrogen), urine specific gravity.** Patient **under the warmer requires more fluid than in** incubator because of increased insensible water loss.
    FT: 80 cc/kg in day 1 and ↑ up to 100-120 cc/kg by day 2-3.
    Premature: 90-100 cc/kg in day 1 and ↑ up to 150 cc/kg by day 3-4.
    FT calorie requirement: 100 kcal/kg/day.
    Premature calorie requirement: 120 kcal/kg/day.
    Amino acid: 2.5 gm/kg/day.
    Glucose: 10 g/dl.

Intralipid: 2-3 gm/kg/day.
Na: 3-4 mEq/kg/day.
K: 1-2 mEq/kg/day.
Ca: 200-400 mg/kg/day.
Once the premature baby is stable (2-3 day of life), small nasogastric feeding should be started even with ET tube and umbilical artery catheter. **Remember, Na is required for growth.**
Approximate weight gain: 15-20 gm/day.

90. Sucking and swallowing coordination appear: At **34 weeks** gestational age, so **bottle feeding can begin after 34 weeks.** Before that ,**gavage feeding is the feeding of choice.** Continuous nasogastric (NG) or nasojejunal (NJ) feeding can be used in a patient who cannot suck, or swallow and for delayed gastric emptying. TPN should never replace oral and gavage feeding.

91. Complication of nasojejunal feeding: **Perforation.**

92. Vitamin D requirement for VLBW: Should not exceed 1500 IU/day.

93. Folic acid supplementation in preterm: It is necessary for formation of **DNA and new cells. Serum** and RBC levels are low in first few weeks and remain low for 2-3 months. Remember, folic acid supplementation does not cause increased growth or increased hemoglobin level.

    Vitamin E supplementation and deficiency in preterm:
    Deficiency: Causes hemolysis, anemia, peripheral edema, and thrombocytosis.
    It also acts as antioxidant to prevent peroxidation of PUFA (polyunsaturated fatty acids) in RBC membrane. Premature infants (< 34 weeks) are susceptible to vitamin E deficiency, so **vitamin E should be given** until 34 weeks or **until preterm doubles its birth weight. After that ,vitamin E should be discontinued and iron (prooxidant, 2 mg/kg/day) therapy should begin.**

94. Most commonly found **RDS, PDA and IVH: LBW** (highest in VVLBW).

95. ROP (retinopathy of premature) and follow up:
    Definition: This is a disease of immature, incompletely vascularized retina which was exposed to any amount of oxygen more than 21%. It is also found in patients who had hypoxic episode rather than hyperoxia.
    To avoid ROP, probably arterial oxygen tension should be kept between **50-70 mm Hg.**
    Other factors causing ROP are: ↑ CO_2, ambient light.
    Vitamin E (antioxidant) probably can reduce ROP, but it can cause sepsis, NEC, and other side effects. Vitamin E **is hyperosmolar.**

96. Increased incidence (2-20%) of kernicterus in premature infant is due to:
    a. Large dose of vitamin K given either to mother or to the baby.
    b. Meningitis in premature baby enhances kernicterus (bilirubin as high as 10 mg/dl may be harmful).

97. Ideal temperature and humidity for incubator:
    a. Humidity should be 40-60% .(It will prevent dryness, irritation; it also stabilizes body temperature and prevents heat loss in lower environmental temperature.)
    b. Incubator temperature should be kept in such a way that baby's core temperature is maintained at 36.5-37 degrees C.

98. **Definitions:**
    Premature: Live born infants delivered before 37 weeks from first day of LMP (last menstrual period).
    LBW: < 2500 gm.
    VLBW: < 1500 gm.
    VVLBW: < 750 gm (recently called immature fetus).
    IUGR: Baby is growth-retarded for his/her gestational age (< 3 percentile).
    LBW: Either premature or IUGR.
    SGA: Weight < 10 percentile.

99. VLBW infants vs. term infants: VLBW have higher incidence of rehospitalization due to prematurity, infection, psychosocial disturbances during the first year of life.

100. Most common age group for **congenital malformations: LBW** (premature and IUGR). The slower the intrauterine growth rate, the higher the malformations.

101. Most commonly found **hypoglycemia: Premature IUGR** (67%). [2nd is primi, LGA; 3rd is FT, IUGR]

102. Most commonly found **hyperglycemia: Extremely premature infant** (due to excessive intake of glucose).

103. Most commonly found **recurrent apnea: VLBW.**

104. Most commonly found NEC (necrotizing enterocolitis): LBW (highest incidence in VLBW).

105. In twin pregnancy, **outcome of twin 'B' is usually poor due to: Early** placental separation. Twin 'B' develops more respiratory distress and asphyxia.

106. Fetal transfusion syndrome in twin: Artery of donor twin gives blood to vein to recipient twin, resulting in donor twin becoming anemic and recipient twin becoming plethoric. By definition, there is difference of hemoglobin 5 gm/dl and body weight 20% between the twin.
    Donor twin: Needs P-RBC transfusion.
    Recipient twin: Needs partial exchange transfusion.

107. **Important points regarding twin:**
    a. Incidence of twin gestation is 1:80. If mother had twins previously, then the incidence is 1:20. More often in blacks.
    b. Twin mortality is higher than that of singleton.
    c. Most twins are born prematurely.

d. Maternal complications (polyhydramnios, pre-eclampsia, prolonged rupture membrane, hyperemesis gravidarum) are higher for twins than for singleton.
e. Monoamniotic twins are more asphyxiated because of entangled cord.
f. In monovular twins, weight difference usually disappears by 6 months of postnatal age.
g. Frequency of **monozygotic twins is constant throughout the world** (3.5 per 1000), but that of dizygotic varies.
h. **Twin deliveries (important):** Both have vertex presentation (do NSVD), both breech (do C-section). First twin has vertex, and second breech. First should be delivered by NSVD. Evaluate second child try vaginal delivery, if failed then do C-section.

108. **Most of the neonatal mortality occurs: Within the first several hours** and the day after birth.
a. **Highest neonatal mortality occurs in < 1000 gm (< 28 week gestation).**
b. **Lowest** neonatal mortality occurs between 3000-4000 gm.
c. Neonatal mortality **rises sharply over 4000 gm (> 42 weeks)**.
d. 40% of neonatal mortalities occur after 37 weeks and > 2500 gm.

109. **Vanishing twin syndrome:** Incidence of twin is 3-5% if ultrasonography is done around 12 weeks of gestation, but the incidence is much lower later in pregnancy, because one twin vanishes and the other persists.

110. **Prenatal diagnosis of twin:**
a. First is **uterine size bigger** than expected for gestational age.
b. Serum: ↑ alpha felo protein, ↑ hCG.
c. Diagnosis **confirmed** by: Ultrasonography.

111. **Conjoined twin (Siamese twin):** It is due to late monovular separation., It consists of two twins in one amniotic sac. Prognosis depends on site of the connection and the surgical procedure.

112. **Fetal treatment in utero under the following conditions:**

Lung immaturity	**Dexamethasone.**
Autoimmune thrombocytopenia	**Steroid, I.V. immunoglobulin,** fetal platelet transfusion.
Isoimmune thrombocytopenia	**Umbilical vein P-RBC transfusion or immunoglobulin.**
Erythroblastosis fetalis	**Umbilical vein P-RBC transfusion or intraperitoneal transfusion.**
Non-immune hydrops (anemia)	Intrauterine RBC transfusion.
Neural tube defects	**Vitamins and folate (prevention).**
Hypoxia, IUGR	**Maternal position, oxygen.**
Oligohydramnios	Amnioinfusion.

Lupus, preeclampsia	**Aspirin.**
SVT (supraventricular tachycardia)	**Digoxin,** procainamide, quinidine, propranolol.
21-Hydroxylase deficiency	Dexamethasone.
PKU	**Restrict phenylalanine.**
Fetal galactosemia	Galactose free diet.
Methyl malonic acidemia	Vitamin B_{12}.
Multiple carboxylase deficiency	Biotin.
Parvovirus	**Intrauterine RBC transfusion.**
Lyme disease	Penicillin, ceftriaxone.
Group B Streptococcus	Ampicillin.
Tuberculosis	Antituberculous drugs.
Chlamydia	Erythromycin.
Syphilis	Penicillin.
Toxoplasmosis	**Spiramycin.**
Premature labor	**Magnesium sulfate, sympathomimetic.**
Diabetes mellitus	**Insulin.**

113. **Most specific and sensitive indicator of fetal lung maturity (important): PG (phosphatidylglycerol); (also phosphatidylcholine). It does not** affect in diabetes or other high risk pregnancies.

114. **Drugs taken by their mother and their effects on the fetus:**

Dilantin and phenobarbital	**Bleeding** due to vitamin k deficiency.
Aspirin	**Bleeding** due to platelet dysfunction.
Anaesthesia with mepivacaine (if it accidentally enters the scalp)	**Bradycardia, apnea, convulsion.**
Magnesium sulfate	**Respiratory depression, hyporeflexia (first sign)**, hypotonia, meconium plug.
Oxytocin	**Hyperbilirubinemia,** hyponatremia.
Reserpine	**Nasal congestion,** drowsiness.
Excessive vitamin k	**Hyperbilirubinemia.**
Propanolol	**Hypoglycemia,** bradycardia, apnea.
Captopril	Transient renal failure, cardiovascular instability.

Narcotics, sedatives	CNS depression.
Hexamethonium bromide	Paralytic ileus.
Iodides	Neonatal goitre.
Morphine, methadone	Addiction (withdrawal symptom).
Cocaine/crack	Microcephaly, growth failure, anomalies.
Bromide	**Rash,** CNS depression.

115. **Most common organism** involved in scalp abscess due to fetal monitoring: **Staph. aureus,** gm(-) rod; **but most of them are sterile.**

116. **Confirmation of zygocity** (mono or dizygotic) in same sex by: **DNA analysis.**
    a. One boy and one girl means **"Dizygotic".**
    b. Monochorionic: Always monozygotic (two fetuses do not fuse).
    c. Dichorionic: Dizygotic (80-90%), monozygotic (10-20%) (* monozygote begins to separate in early morulation phase).

117. **Sinusoidal pattern** in fetal cardiac monitoring indicates: **Severe anemia** (due to Rh incompatibility, feto maternal transfusion). It indicates **a serious condition of the fetus and that the delivery of the fetus is urgent.**

118. L:S ratio (lecithin, to sphingomyelin) **in amniotic fluid.**
    a. Lecithin is produced by type II cells of the lung, reaching amniotic fluid through trachea.
    b. L:S ratio is **1:1 until the middle of 3rd trimester;** after that, **S remains constant and L increases.** By 35 weeks, L:S ratio become 2:1, which is considered a mature lung, i.e., the risk of hyaline membrane disease is less. Remember, even with normal (2:1) L:S ratio, hyaline membrane disease can occur in the fetus of a diabetic mother and in fetal hypothermia, asphyxia, acidosis.
    c. 20-25% of fetuses have **no** hyaline membrane disease, even with a L:S ratio lof ess than 2:1.
    d. **Contamination of specimen with meconium** reduces the reliability of the result of L:S ratio.
    e. **But the contamination of the specimen with blood** (mother or fetus) will **not** alter the significance of L:S ratio of 2:1 or more, because maternal and fetal blood L:S ratio is about 1:4. **(Please remember this point).**
    f. **In diabetic patients** the ratio should be **3:1 and above** for adequate lung maturity.

119. **Methods of assessing fetal distress:**
    a. **NST (non-stress test):**
        i. **Reactive NST** means, that with fetal movements, the heart rate **accelerates 15 beats/minute, lasting for 15 seconds.**
        ii. **Non-reactive NST:** Means **no or less** acceleration of rate and time mentioned above. It means **fetal compromise,** so do CST (contraction stress test) or BPP (biophysical profile).

b. **BPP (biophysical profile)**:
There are 5 parameters, and each has 2 points. They are:
Fetal breathing movement,
Gross body movement,
Fetal tone,
Reactive fetal heart rate,
Qualitative amniotic fluid volume.
A total score of 8 or more **is normal**, and score of 4 or less **indicates asphyxia.** It is done with the help of ultrasound.

c. **CST (contraction stress test)**: Fetal heart rate response to oxytocin stimulation. **A response rate of 3 or more late decelerations in 10 minutes** indicates fetal compromise. CST is contraindicated in prematurity, multiple gestation, incompetent cervix, placenta previa, polyhydramnios.

d. **BST (Breast stimulation test)**: It is same as CST, here oxytocin is released by breast (nipple) stimulation.

e. **Continuous fetal heart rate monitoring:** By attaching electrode to fetal presenting part or ultrasound transducer placed on maternal abdomen.

f. **Fetal scalp blood sampling:** Cervix has to be dilated, membrane should be ruptured. **A pH < 7.25 indicates fetal distress and < 7.20 indicates immediate delivery.**

120. Harlequin color change: From head to pubis, one half is red and the other is pale.

121. Mongolian spots: Most common site is **buttocks**. They have a slate blue pigmentation which is well demarcated.

122. Lanugo hair: Found in premature infant, it is soft, immature hair mostly found on scalp, face, or brow. It disappears and is replaced by vellus hair in fullterm.

123. Craniotabes: Soft areas of skull bones (near sutures) found in premature and due to intrauterine compression. It is found in parietal and occipital bones. Also associated with Wormian bones, which are found in cleidocranial dysplasia, Down syndrome, hypothyroidism, osteogenesis imperfecta, lacunar skull.

124. **Large** anterior fontanel due to: **Hypothyroidism, prematurity, vitamin D deficiency rickets,** hypophosphatasia, Trisomies (21, 18, 13), IUGR, rubella, **hydrocephalus, osteogenesis imperfecta, achondroplasia,** hypophosphatasia, syndromes (Apert, Russell-silver, Hallermann).

125. Time to pass meconium: Usually within 12 hours;
99% FT and 95% PT pass within 48 hours.

126. **Apgar score** (important points to remember):
a. Low score does **not** always signify hypoxia or acidosis: it can be low due to factors other than hypoxia/acidosis (see next).
b. It does **not** predict neonatal mortality or cerebral palsy.
c. Most cerebral palsy patients have **normal** apgar score.
d. 1 minute low apgar indicates **the need for immediate resuscitation.**
e. 5-, 10-, 15-, 20- minute scores **indicate probability of successful resuscitation.**

f.   Low apgar (0-3) score at **20 minutes indicates high morbidity and mortality.**

127.   Factors which produce **a low apgar score without** hypoxia and acidosis **(false positive low apgar).**
Immaturity, anomalies (CNS, choanal atresia), congenital (neuropathy, myopathy, pneumonia), maternal medications (magnesium sulfate, analgesics, narcotics, sedatives), delivery (precipitous, traumatic, breech causing spinal cord trauma), recovery from previous asphyxia.

128.   Factors which produce a normal **apgar score with** acidosis **(false negative normal apgar)**: High fetal catecholamine levels, maternal acidosis, found in some full term babies.

129.   Parent-infant bonding: It begins **during pregnancy and is enhanced after maternal touching and eye contact with the baby immediately after birth in the delivery room.**
Abnormal or delayed bonding due to: Prematurity, maternal and infant sickness, malformations, family stress.

130.   Lowest **neonatal mortality and maternal age: Between 20-30** (beyond this age group, there is a risk for more IUGR, intrauterine death, fetal distress).

131.   **Maternal diseases and fetal effects:**

Lupus	**Congenital heart block, ↓ WBC, ↓ Platelet** count due to maternal antibodies.
Diabetes	i. Mild (LGA, ↓ glucose due to ↑ insulin which is growth hormone for fetus). ii. Severe (IUGR due to placental vascular defect).
Hypertension	IUGR, uterine death (due to placental insufficiency and fetal hypoxia).
Endemic goitre	Hypothyroidism (due to iodine deficiency).
Graves disease	Transient hyperthyroidism (due to LATS and LATS protector antibody).
Hyperparathyroidism	**Hypocalcemia (maternal Ca inhibits fetal parathyroid gland).**
Pre-eclampsia, eclampsia	IUGR, ↓ platelet count (placental insufficiency and hypoxia).
Sickle cell disease	Preterm, IUGR (fetal hypoxia due to maternal sickling).
Rh incompatibility	Hydrops, jaundice (due to maternal antibody crossing placenta).
Myasthenia gravis	Transient myasthenia (maternal antibody block-Ach receptor in new born).

Malignant melanoma	Tumor (placenta, fetus due to metastasis).
Phenylketonuria	**Microcephaly, retardation (due to ↑ phenylalanine).**
Cyanotic heart disease	IUGR (due to ↓ fetal oxygen supply).
Cholestasis	Preterm baby (unknown).
Obesity	Macrosomia, sometimes hypoglycemia (unknown).
Myotonic dystrophy	Neonatal myotonic dystrophy (unknown).
Thrombocytopenia	i. Autoimmune: ↓ platelet count (due to nonspecific maternal antiplatelet antibody). ii. Isoimmune: ↓ platelet cout (due to baby's platelets which sensitize the mother, and form antibodies which cross placenta and produce ↓ platelet in baby. Mother's platelet count is normal).
Isoimmune neutropenia	↓ WBC (mechanism same as isoimmune thrombocytopenia).
Renal transplant	IUGR (due to uteroplacental insufficiency).

132. **Maternal medication and breast feeding:**

Antihypertensive	Usually safe for the baby. Each should be checked if given during breast feeding.
Sedatives	Sedates the baby.
Safe drugs	Weak acids, large molecules, bound to plasma and poorly absorbed from G.I. tract.

133. **Amniotic fluid volume and its abnormalities:**
Normal: 500-2000 ml.
Oligohydramnios: Less than 500 ml.
Polyhydramnios: More than 2000 ml.
Rate of increase of amniotic fluid: Less than 10 ml/day until it reaches a maximum at 34 weeks, then slowly decreases.

Polyhydramnios: Due to either decreased swallowing (anencephaly, intestinal obstruction, neuromuscular dysfunction) or increased fetal urine formation. Acute type present before 28 weeks and chronic type present in 3rd trimester.
Oligohydramnios: Due to either decreased production from lungs (hypoplastic) or decreased production from kidney (congenital anomalies, drugs), IUGR. It manifests after 20 weeks of gestational age. It is diagnosed by ultrasonography (by summation of largest pocket of fluid in each of 4 quadrants, if **sum is less than 6 cm**, it is called oligohydramnios). Oligohydramnios cause fetal deformities and lung hypoplasia (Potter syndrome).

134. Duration of labor and neonatal death:
    a. Uncomplicated labor of less than or equal to 24 hours: 0.3% death.
    b. Labor of more than 24 hours ,but less than 30 hours: 1.8% (6 times).
    c. Labor of more than 30 hours: 6.0% (20 times).

135. Organogenesis in fetus occurs: 4-12 weeks (mother should **not** take any medications until 12 weeks except required vitamin and iron).

136. Fetal growth and assessment: Remember, **serial biparietal diameter is the most important parameter for assessing fetal growth.** Another important parameter is **LMP** (last menstrual period). **Ratio of head-to-abdominal** circumference is also helpful. (Occasionally, the measurement of femoral length and total intrauterine volume is required.) Earliest assessment can be done in 12th week but it is usually done around 18-20 weeks.

     Lung maturity: The presence of phosphatidylglycerol (PG) and a L:S ratio of 2:1or more indicate lung maturity (in amniotic fluid).
     Fetal movement begins: 18-20 weeks.

137. **Fetal distress and assessment:**
    a. **Fetal tachycardia:** Heart rate **over 160 beats/min.** The reason is either **fetal** (hypoxia, anemia arrhythmia), **or maternal** (fever, hyperthyroidism, beta sympathomimetic or atropine). It is **not** found in congenital heart disease.
    b. **Fetal bradycardia:** Heart rate **less than 120 beats/min.** The reason is either **fetal** (hypoxia, heart block due to maternal lupus) or **maternal** (use of betablocker, local anaesthetic agent which crosses the placenta).
    c. **Fetal deceleration:**
        i. **Early (type I dips):** It is benign, and occurs as a result of **head compression.** It is synchronized with time and amplitude of uterine contractions.
        ii. **Late (type II dips):** It is **not** benign, and occurs as a result of **uteroplacental insufficiency.** Here deceleration **begins after** the uterine contraction has been established and **continues even when uterine contractions are over.**
        iii. **Variable: It is not** benign, and occurs as a result of **cord compression. It is** called variable because it **varies in shape, has an abrupt onset, and has no** relation to uterine contractions.
    d. **Beat-to-beat variability in heart rate:** Normal fetus should have beat-to-beat variability (in long term, it is 3-6 cycles/minute and also short term variability). **Absence** of beat-to-beat variability indicates fetal **hypoxia and compromised fetus.** Prematurity, **tachycardia and sleep** can reduce beat-to-beat variability.

138. **NEC (necrotizing enterocolitis):** Most common site is **distal ileum and proximal colon.**
     Factors causing NEC: Immature gut, hypertonic milk or medicine, early feeding, rapid feeding, infectious agents are (Clostridium difficile, C perfringens, E.coli, Staph epidermidis, rotavirus).
     Clinical presentations: Usually occur in first 14 days, but may be as late as 2 months.
     The first sign is abdominal distension with gastric residuals, guaiac (+)ve stool, perforation, shock, death.

Diagnosis: Most common diagnostic abdominal X-ray finding is pneumatosis intestinalis; portal venous gas indicates ominous sign; pneumoperitoneum means perforation.

Treatment:

a. **Nasogastric decompression** (to remove acidic gastric contents).

b. **I.V. hydration** to correct electrolytes abnormalities.

c. **Cultures** should be taken from blood, CSF, stool.

d. **Antibiotics: Anti-pseudomonas penicillin** and gentamicin.

e. Discontinue umbilical arterial line.

f. $\downarrow O_2$, $\uparrow CO_2$. Oxygen, increased ventilator rate.

g. **Surgery:**

Indications: Perforation (pneumoperitoneum or brown color paracentesis fluid), no response to medical treatment, abdominal wall erythema or palpable mass, single fixed bowel loop.

Procedure: Laparotomy, resection of necrotic bowel and external ostomy diversion.

Prognosis:

i. **10% of cases show stricture formations** (treatment is resection).

ii. **Short bowel syndrome** (due to massive resection of gut).

139. At 1 year: Preterm development is less than fullterm of same chronological age.

At 2 years: Preterm catches up in growth equal to fullterm of same age.

* Double the birth weight at 5 months.

Double the birth height at 4 years.

* First deciduous teeth to develop are the lower central incisors, then the upper central, then 3rd the upper lateral incisor.

At birth, HC > CC (head and chest circumference).

At 1 year HC= CC.

140. **Physiologic anemia:**

Full term infant: 8-12 weeks, hemoglobin 11 gm/dl.

Preterm infant: 6-8 week, hemoglobin 7-10 gm/dl.

Normal values in full term infant are 16.8 gm/dl (14-20 gm/dl), VLBW 1-2 gm/dl less than term infant.

141. **Feto maternal transfusion causing anemia:** It is more common but unrecognized unless it is severe. Even a very minute amount of fetal blood (0.1 ml) that goes to maternal circulation produces antibodies which cross the placenta and can cause severe hemolysis in the newborn.

Diagnosis confirmed by: Kleihau-Betke test (demonstrates the presence of fetal cells or hemoglobin in maternal circulation).

142. A newborn appears with severe anemia and jaundice in first **24 hours** of life. Most likely diagnosis: **Hemolytic disease.**

143. **Anemia of prematurity (at 6-8 weeks, hemoglobin 7-10 gm/dl).**

Signs and symptoms: Apnea, pallor, tachypnea, tachycardia, poor weight gain, poor feeding, lethargy.

Etiology: Repeated blood drawn for testing, reduced RBC life span, rapid growth,

transition from fetal (physiologic hypoxic state) to neonatal (normoxic state), because hypoxia stimulates erythropoietin production in utero. Oxygen availability of neonatal tissue is less than adult, because oxygen dissociation curve is shifted to the left.
Treatment: If symptomatic, then packed RBC transfusion should be given.

144.   Transfusion acquired infections are: **CMV, hepatitis B and C, HIV.**
CMV infection is almost eliminated; other two have been reduced, but not eliminated.

145.   Which antibodies are produced in Rh-hemolytic disease?
First: **19S (IgM)** gamma globulin.
Later on: **7S (IgG) which crosses the placenta** and causes hemolysis.

Rh-hemolytic disease, important points to remember:
a.   **First born child is usually not affected,** because mother did not have enough time to produce antibodies, because fetal blood goes to maternal circulation at delivery.
b.   55% of Rh(+)ve fathers are heterozygous (D/d) and can have Rh(-)ve offspring.
c.   Capacity of sensitization of mothers varies even with higher antigens exposure. Usually it is low and hemolysis occurs **only in 5% cases.**
d.   Severity of disease is increased in subsequent pregnancies. It is prevented by giving RhoGAM (anti-D gamma globulin) immediately after delivery of Rh(+)ve infant or after every abortion.
e.   When there is both ABO and Rh incompatibility, then it is better because **Rh cells are removed rapidly from the circulation by anti A or anti B** which are IgM and do not cross the placenta.
f.   **Hypoglycemia due to hyperinsulinism is secondary to hypertrophy of pancreatic islet cells.**

146.   Hypoalbuminemia in hydrops fetalis due to: **Hepatic dysfunction.**

147.   A newborn with HMD or BPD, oxygen dependent, hemoglobin should be kept: Around 14 gm/dl (to improve oxygen carrying capacity to the tissues, so oxygen requirement will be reduced).

148.   Most common antigen responsible for Rh-hemolytic disease: **D antigen (90%),**
Other are C, E.

149.   **Mother is Rh (-)ve, fetus is Rh (+)ve and** contains D antigen inherited from Rh (+)ve father. Small amount (> 1 ml) of Rh (+)ve fetal cells goes to maternal circulation during pregnancy (either by spontaneous or induced abortion, around the time of delivery) resulting in antibody formation against 'D' antigen, antibodies cross the placenta to the fetus causing hemolysis.

150.   Severity of hydrops fetalis depends on: **Severity of anemia and hypoalbuminemia.**

151.   **Rh-hemolytic disease:**

Signs and symptoms: It depends on the severity of hemolysis. Severe disease usually appears with anemia, ↑ liver and spleen, jaundice, cardiomegaly with cardiac failure and respiratory distress. **Hydrops fetalis** (generalized anasarca, pleural effusion, ascites) has poor prognosis. Jaundice may be absent at birth because placenta removes unconjugated lipid soluble bilirubin, but jaundice gets worse after birth because infant biliary system is not capable of handling huge unconjugated bilirubin **resulting in CNS toxicity and kernicterus.**

Remember, hydrops fetalis can occur due to nonimmune causes.

Peripheral smear: Polychromasia, ↑ reticulocyte and ↑ nucleated RBC.

Blood: Positive Coombs test, anemia.

152. **Definitive diagnosis** of erythroblastosis fetalis: Demonstration of blood group incompatibility and positive Coombs' test.

153. **Post natal diagnosis** of erythroblastosis fetalis:
    a. First blood grouping and cross match.
    b. If Coombs' test is positive, then do CBC with retieulocytes count and bilirubin.

154. When mother is known to be Rh(-)ve and pregnant now.
    How do you manage this pregnancy **(antenatal diagnosis)?**
    a. **Assessment of maternal IgG titre** at 12-16 weeks, 28-32 weeks and 36 weeks.
    b. **Progressively rising titre or high initial titre or titre is 1:64 and above indicates serious hemolysis.**
    c. **Indication to monitor the mother and fetus:** When mother's titre is 1:16 or higher at any time in subsequent pregnancy.
       Methods of monitoring are: Amniocentesis, ultrasound and PUBS (percutaneous umbilical blood sampling).
    d. First **ultrasonography** to look for any signs of hydrops (scalp and skin edema; pleural and pericardial effusion, ascites; hepatosplenomegaly).
    e. If any of the above signs are present, then **amniocentesis** should be done in (18-20 weeks) **to asses bilirubin concentration in amniotic fluid by spectrophotometry.**
       Three zones (zone I to III). Zone I is mild and zone II is moderate hemolysis.
       Zone III indicates severe hemolysis, but remember some fetuses with zone III do not have severe anemia, so they don't need intrauterine transfusion.
    f. If optical density 450 is in zone III or hydrops or anemia then **PUBS** should be **done to measure fetal hemoglobin level** and packed RBC can be transfused.

155. Goal for treatment of erythroblastosis fetalis:
    a. To prevent death due to anemia and hypoxia.
    b. To protect from neurotoxicity of bilirubin.
    Treatment:
    a. **In utero:**
       i. **Intrauterine transfusion through umbilical vein:**
          Indications: Hydrops, anemia (Hgb< 8 g/dl; Hct <25%).
          Procedure: Mother and baby should be sedated or baby should be paralysed, CMV negative P-RBC is used after irradiation and cross matched with mother's serum. Goal: To keep Hct 40%, it can be repeated every 2 weeks.
       ii. **Delivery of the fetus:**
          Indications: Matured lung (L:S ratio 2:1), fetal distress, problem during PUBS, >35 weeks gestational age. Baby should be delivered in any of the above

conditions.

b. **After birth:**
    i.   Immediate transfusion of o(-)ve blood.
    ii.   Phototherapy.
    iii.   "Stabilize the baby: means **to correct hypoxia, acidosis, hypothermia, hypoglycemia.**

    iv.   Exchange transfusion with whole blood if indicated. At birth Hgb < 10g/dl and bilirubin 5mg/dl or more does **not** mean immediate exchange is needed. Follow up the bilirubin every 4 hours and exchange should be done when bilirubin level reaches 20 mg/dl in fullterm stable infant.

156. Maximum rebound bilirubin after exchange transfusion: Up to 40-50% within hours because tissue bilirubin moves into the circulation.

157. Exchange transfusion: Through umbilical venous line, catheter should not be placed beyond 7 cm in fullterm when there is free flow of blood. This means bigger veins, and double volume (means 170 ml/kg, in 3 kg infant = 510 ml total volume) exchange should be done over 1 hour. Each time, 20 cc of blood in and out (except in premature and sick infant, in which case use 5-10 ml each time).

158. Late complications of Rh hemolytic disease:
a. Anemia: Iron supplement or transfusion of P-RBC.
b. Inspissated bile syndrome: Rare. Both direct and indirect bilirubin levels are elevated. Etiology is unknown. Resolves spontaneously within few weeks.
c. Portal vein thrombosis: Due to umbilical vein catheterization.

159. **Method of prevention of Rh sensitization (important):**
a. **Single dose of RhoGAM (1 ml)** within 72 hours after delivery or abortion. It reduces the risk of sensitization from 10-20% to <1% and removes 10 ml of potentially antigenic fetal cells from maternal circulation.
b. **Double doses of RhoGAM** (1st at 28-32 weeks, 2nd at birth fullterm): It is required for severe feto-maternal transfusion.

160. **'ABO' hemolytic disease:** Important points to remember:
a. Usually mother is 'O' and baby is 'A' or 'B'; if mother is 'A', then she forms anti 'B' antibodies; and if she is 'B', then she forms anti 'A' antibodies.
b. Less serious than Rh disease.
c. It occurs in 20-25% of all pregnancies. Only 10% develop hemolysis (most of them are A1 antigen).
d. Remember, **A1 antigen is stronger** and causes more hemolysis than does A2.
e. Mother has antibodies against A or B even before pregnancy. These antibodies are located in 19S (IgM) (which does not cross the placenta) and 7S (IgG) which does cross the placenta.
f. Remember, 7S **(IgG)** is the principal antibody which cause sABO hemolytic disease.
g. **Clinical presentations: Jaundice within first 24 hours** and may be anemia. Normal liver and spleen.
h. **Diagnosis:**

i. **Peripheral smear: Spherocytes. (Remember this).**
ii. Other laboratory work up: CBC with reticulocyte count and bilirubin.

i. Treatment:
    i. Phototherapy.
    ii. Exchange transfusion. (It **removes the sensitized cells and bilirubin from the circulation, corrects anemia,** if any.)

161. **Coombs' test (-)ve hemolytic diseases:**
    a. Congenital infections (CMV, toxoplasmosis, rubella, syphilis).
    b. Homozygous alpha thalassemia.
    c. RBC enzyme deficiencies (pyruvate kinase or G6PD).

162. **Single umbilical artery:** 33% of them have other congenital anomalies. **Commonly associated with trisomy 18.**

163. **Polycythemia: Definition:** Central hematocrit is 65% or higher.
Polycythemia occurs in the following situations: Infant of diabetic mother, chronic fetal hypoxia (stimulate erythropoietin production), high altitude, postmature, SGA > LGA> AGA, delayed cord clamping, twin-to-twin transfusion, trisomies (21, 18, 13), hyperthyroidism, hypothyroidism, adrenogenital syndrome, Beckwith-Wiedemann syndrome.
Clinical presentations: Tachypnea, respiratory distress, NEC, poor feeding, jaundice, seizure, cyanosis (PPHN), ↓ glucose, ↓ platelet or may be asymptomatic (15-25% cases).
All of the above clinical presentations are due to: **Viscosity.**
It is enhanced by neonatal RBC's which have reduced deformability and filterability resulting in stasis.
Treatment: Partial exchange transfusion to reduce Hct to 50%.

Formula:
Formula of exchange (ml):
$$\frac{\text{Observed-desired Hct}}{\text{Observed Hct}} \times \text{blood volume.}$$
Long term problem: Speech delay, abnormal fine-motor skills, poor school performance.

164. **Vitamin K deficiency** causing hemorrhagic disease in newborn:
Factors are: II, VII, IX, X.
All these factors decrease normally 2-3 days after birth and return to normal level by 7-10 days, so **symptoms begin 2-5 days of life appear with prolonged bleeding.** It is more common in breast-fed infant **due to lack of free vitamin K in mother and absence of bacteria responsible for vitamin k synthesis in intestine.**
Laboratory tests: ↑ PT, ↑ PTT, ↓ (II, VII, IX, X).
PIVKA (protein induced in vitamin K absence) is **a sensitive marker for vitamin K deficiency. Normal** (bleeding time, factor I, V, VIII, platelet, capillary fragility and clot retractions).
Treatment: Vitamin k_1.

165. Vitamin K deficiencies occur in following conditions:
    a. Phenobarbital and phenytoin used by pregnant mother.

b. Dicumarol and related anticoagulants.
c. Rat poison (super warfarin).

166. **Swallowed blood syndrome:** It is found in **2nd or 3rd day of life.** It is due to **swallowed maternal blood during delivery or from cracked nipple during breast feeding. Differential diagnosis from baby's blood by Apt test:** Fetal hemoglobin is resistant to alkali (remains pink), but adult blood turns into yellow-brown color.

167. **Subcutaneous ecchymoses** in premature infant is due to: **Fragile superficial blood vessels.** It disappears in 2-3 weeks.

168. **Granuloma of umbilical cord (important);**
Normal umbilical cord separates within 6-8 days after birth. **Presence of saprophytic organisms delays cord separation.**
Treatment:
a. Mild granulation tissue: Clean with alcohol several times daily.
b. Exuberant granulation tissue: Silver nitrate cauterization.

169. **Hyperthermia in the newborn is due to:**
a. Breast-fed infant due to dehydration.
b. Exposed to high environmental temperature.
c. Warm clothes in hot weather.
Clinical presentations of hyperthermia: Hot and dry skin, stupor, pallor, ↑ Na in serum, coma, convulsions.
Treatment of the above-mentioned three conditions:
a. Correct dehydration.
b. Avoid high environmental temperature.
c. Put on appropriate clothing.

170. **Cold injury of newborn:**
Signs and symptoms: Poor feeding, oliguria, bradycardia, apnea, edema, redness of extremities, ↓ glucose, ↓ pH, **massive pulmonary bleeding.**
Treatment: **Rewarming.**

171. Most common autopsy finding in neonatal cold injury: **Pulmonary hemorrhage.**

172. A newborn appears with edema and ↓ serum protein. Most likely diagnosis: **Congenital nephrosis.**

173. Most frequently used drugs causing drug withdrawal symptoms: Heroin and methadone. Heroin addiction in mother results in: **LBW (50%)** infant and half of them are **SGA.** It is due **to direct fetal growth inhibiting effect, undernutrition and infection in mother.** There is ↑ stillbirth, but **not** the congenital malformations.

Signs and symptoms: Withdrawal symptoms (irritability, tremor, **seizure,** convulsion) in first 48 hours and **symptoms exaggerate** if dose was > 6 mg/24 hour, duration > 1 year and last dose taken by mother within 24 hours. **Remember,** it reduces HMD by stimulating surfactant production and it also reduces jaundice by stimulating glucuronyl transferase.

Diagnosis: By history and physical examination, urine test (+) ve.

174. **Methadone addiction of mother: No** congenital malformation.
Signs and symptoms: 20 to 90% have withdrawal symptoms. Same as heroin, but seizures **are less** common in methadone. **Birth height and parental care is better** than in heroin addict patient.

175. **Alcohol withdrawal:**
Signs and symptoms: Rare. First 3 days infant is agitated and hyperactive, next 2 days is lethargic then becomes normal. Seizure, hypoglycemia and acidosis may occur.

176. **Cocaine addiction:** It is very popular. **Rare** withdrawal symptoms in infant. It causes **abruptio placenta,** IUGR, prematurity, small head, seizures, **developmental learning disorder.** Strong family history of child abuse, neglect, and AIDS.

177. **Phenobarbital withdrawal:** It is found in FT, AGA baby with addicted mother.
Signs and symptoms: Begins around 7 days, appears with hiccups, constant cry, irritability, mouthing movements.

178. **Treatment for all drug withdrawals:**
   a. **Phenobarbital is the preferred drug.**
   b. Paregoric.

179. **Fetal alcohol syndrome, important points to remember:**
   a. It is **directly proportional** to the amount of alcohol ingested (32% is heavy drinker, 14% is moderate drinker, 9% is abstinent).
   b. Signs and symptoms: **IUGR** (symmetric, small length, height and head circumference), facial features (short palpebral fissure, epicanthal folds, micrognathia, thin upper lip, maxillary hypoplasia).
   Heart: **VSD (most common).**
   Extremities: **Minor joints and limb abnormalities** with restriction of movements.
   Mental and motor retardation.
   c. These defects are due **to alcohol, or its breakdown products, or impairment of placental transfer of essential amino acids and zinc.** Both are important for protein synthesis.
   d. Prevention; Avoid alcohol after conception.
   e. Treatment: None.
   f. Prognosis: Poor, but depends on severity.

180. **Infants of diabetic mother** (pertinent points to remember):
   a. LGA in mild diabetes, SGA in severe uncontrolled diabetes.
   b. Polyhydramnios, high morbidity, mortality and malformation.
   c. **Pathophysiology:**
   In LGA: Maternal hyperglycemia → fetal hyperglycemia → fetal hyperinsulinemia due to beta cells hyperplasia → increased glycogen, lipid and protein synthesis → LGA infant after birth hypoglycemia due to ↑ insulin level.
   In SGA: Maternal hyperglycemia → placenta vascular changes and insufficiency → poor

nutrition → SGA infant.

Hypoglycemia due to:

↑ **insulin;** ↓ (epinephrine and glucagon), but normal (cortisol and growth hormone).

d.   **Signs and symptoms:**

LGA babies: **All organs are large except the brain.**

SGA babies: **All organs are small except the brain.**

Most common **presentation is asymptomatic hypoglycemia,**

Others are polycythemia, jaundice, ↓ calcium (after 24 hours), rarely ↓ Mg. TTNB (transient tachypnea of newborn), ↑ **RDS due to inhibitory effect of insulin on surfactant** synthesis which is stimulated by cortisol.

Cardiac: Asymmetric septal hypertrophy manifests as hypertrophic subaortic stenosis, **cardiomegaly (30%).**

Intestine: Small (L) colon syndrome.

Neurologic development and ossification center: Delayed.

e.   Treatment:

   i.   Maternal: Control diabetes well before and during pregnancy.

   ii. Infant: Normoglycemic = 5% glucose water, formula.

Hypoglycemic: I.V. glucose.

Monitor serum glucose after birth, then QIH for next 6-8 hours.

181.   Clinical features of hypothyroidism in infant: Lethargy, constipation, jaundice, poor feeding, umbilical hernia, cold extremities and mottled skin.

182.   **Hypoglycemia, important points to remember:**
   a.   **Definition:**

      Fullterm: < 35 mg/dl. (< 45 mg/dl after 3 days).

      Preterm: < 25 mg/dl (< 45 mg/dl after 3 days).

   b.   **Pathophysiology:** Four groups are at high risk for hypoglycemia.

      i.   IDM, erythroblastosis fetalis, nesidioblastosis (beta cell hyperplasia), insulinomas, Beckwith syndrome, functional beta cells hyperplasia.

      ii. IUGR (particularly premature) develops hypoglycemia due to ↓ glycogen storage, abnormal response to insulin, ↓ neoglucogenesis, ↓ cortisol, ↓ fatty acid oxidation, ↓ epinephrine, ↑ insulin.

      iii. Very immature infant develops hypoglycemia due to **increased metabolic need** and ↓ glycogen storage.

      iv. Rarely, inborn errors of metabolism (galactosemia, glycogen storage disease, fructose intolerance, MSUD, tyrosinemia, propionic and methylmalonic acidemia).

   c.   **Signs and symptoms:**

      i.   Neurologic: Lethargy, seizures, apnea, coma.

      ii. Sympathomimetic: Pallor, tachycardia, sweating.

      Remember, most common symptoms are present in SGA (IUGR) infant.

   d.   Treatment:

      i.   No seizure: I.V. glucose 200 mg/kg (2 ml/kg) 10% glucose.

      ii. Seizure: I.V. glucose 4 ml/ kg 10% glucose.

      iii. Maintenance: I.V. glucose 8 mg/kg/min, if hypoglycemia persists, then ↑ up to 12 mg/kg/min. If no improvement, then give hydrocortisone or prednisone.

      iv. Nesidioblastosis, islet cells adenoma: Surgery is indicated.

183. An asymptomatic preterm infant with uncomplicated course since birth, around 2-3 weeks of age appears with metabolic acidosis (base excess-10 to -16 mEq/l).
Most likely diagnosis: Late metabolic acidosis.
Etiology: **Increased endogenous acid formation.**
Treatment: $NaHCO_3$.
Sometimes it is due to cow's milk formula with protein and casein. In this case, give **low protein formula** with whey: casein ration 60:40.

184. Factors enhancing and appearing in neonatal infections:
   a. Maternal: Prolonged ruptured membrane (> 18 hours), fever (> 37.5 degrees C), ↑ WBC (> 18000), uterine tenderness, chorioamnionitis.
   b. Fetal: Tachycardia, distress.
   c. Others: Twins, congenital malformations (ruptured meningomyelocele, asplenia), congenital immune deficiencies; **I.M iron and galactosemia (↑ E.coli infection).**

185. **Beckwith syndrome:** Hypoglycemia, macroglossia, large-sized baby, visceromegaly (but **mild microcephaly),** omphalocele, characteristic ear lobe crease, ↑ tumors (Wilms, gonadoblastoma, hepatoblastoma), ↑ insulin secretion, chromosome 11.

186. Bacterial sepsis in newborn releases the following products:
   a. Endogenous factors:
      i.   Interleukin 1 (IL-1).
      ii. Platelet activating factor (PAF).
      iii. Tumor necrosis factor (TNF).
   b. Histamine, kinins, complement systems and other WBC products.

187. **Most** common organism causing neonatal infection: **Group B Streptococcus (mostly by type III).** Others are E.coli (K1 antigen), Staph. epidermidis, Listeria, Pseudomonas (water related infection), Serratia, candida.

188. **Neonatal bacterial sepsis:**
   a. **Pathophysiology:**
   Factors determining infection:
      i.   Immunological status of newborn, quantitative and qualitative immune deficiencies, particularly in premature, ↓ WBC (functions and mobility).
      ii. Virulence of microorganism.
      iii. Central lines.
      iv. Size of inoculum.
   b. **Signs and symptoms:** Poor feeding, lethargy, hypo or hyperthermia, abdominal distension, apnea, asphyxia (due to pneumonia).
   c. **Diagnosis:**
      i.   Confirmed by isolation of the organism in blood, CSF, urine **by culture.**
      ii. CIE. Remember, asymptomatic infant appears with transient bacteremia in group B Streptococcal infection. Positive blood culture does **not** necessarily mean definite infection: it could be contaminant.
      iii. Demonstration of organism by gram-stain.
   d. Treatment:

i. Gram negative meningitis: Cefotaxime.
ii. Pseudomonas: Ticarcillin, mezlocillin.
iii. Initial drug of choice before sensitivity: **Ampicillin and gentamicin.**
iv. Staphylococcus epidermidis: Vancomycin.
v. Staphylococcus aureus: Nafcillin.
vi. Experimental therapies: I.V. Gamma globulin, granulocyte transfusion, G-CSF (granulocyte macrophage colony stimulating factor).

189. **Neonatal conjunctivitis:**
    a. **Etiology:**
        i. Chemical (silver nitrate): first 24 hours.
        ii. Gonococcus: 2-5 days (ophthalmia neonatorum).
        iii. Chlamydia: 5-14 days (inclusion blennorrhea).
        iv. Pseudomonas (rare): 5-18 days (serious infection).
        Most common neonatal conjunctivitis: Chemical (second is chlamydia, next is gonococcus).
    b. **Appears with:** Eye discharge; remember, amount and type of discharge will never make the specific diagnosis.
    c. Diagnosis confirmed by **isolation of organism by culture.** (Gram stain for bacterial infection, gonococcal infection = gram(-)ve intracellular diplococci.)
    d. **Treatment:**
        i. Gonococcal: Ceftriaxone 25-50 mg/kg/day for 7 days (single dose may be effective), irrigation of eye with saline.
        ii. Pseudomonas and staphylococcal: Systemic antibiotics and local saline irrigation.
        iii. Chlamydia: Oral erythromycin for 14 days.
    e. **Prophylaxis (important):**
        i. If mother has untreated gonococcal infection: One dose ceftriaxone Im or I.V. (50 mg/kg, maximum 125 mg).
        ii. Silver nitrate **cannot** prevent chlamydia infection.
        iii. Mother with chlamydia infection: Oral erythromycin.
        iv. Topical antibiotic cannot prevent chlamydia pneumonia (occurs 10-20% cases) because of nasopharyngeal colonization.

190. **Bilirubin (types, formation, metabolism):**
    a. **Four types of bilirubin:**
        i. Bilirubin + albumin (delta).
        ii. Diconjugated.
        iii. Mono conjugated.
        iv. Unconjugated.
    b. **Formation of bilirubin:**
        End product of heme → biliverdin → bilirubin → bilirubin di glucuronide.
    c. In amniotic fluid: Appear at 12 weeks, disappears by 36-37 weeks. Rate of production in fetus is unknown.
    d. **Hepatic function:** UDP (uridine diphosphate) glucuronyl transferase activity first appears at 16 weeks of fetal life and helps in conjugation.
        17 to 30 weeks: 0.1% activity of adult values.
        30 to 40 weeks: 1% activity of adult values.

6 to 14 weeks after birth: Reaches adult values.

e. **Metabolism of bilirubin:**

   i. **Production:** 75% from RBC breakdown (RE system) and 25% ineffective erythropoiesis (bone marrow), tissue heme and heme protein (liver).

   ii. **Transport:** Bilirubin leaves the R.E. (reticuloendothelial) system → binds with albumin in plasma → bilirubin in liver binds with ligandin (y protein) → bilirubin glucuronide forms in liver and is excreted in intestine → either excreted in stool as stercobilinogen, or breaksdown by intestinal bacteria to unconjugated form, which is reabsorbed in enterohepatic circulation.

191. **Mechanism of neonatal jaundice (three):**

   a. ↑ bilirubin production: Normal newborn produces 8 to 10 mg/kg/day (double the amount of adult) due to ↑ RBC volume/kg, ↓ life span of RBC, larger early level bilirubin peak.

   b. ↑ Enterohepatic circulation: In intestine, conjugated bilirubin is converted to unconjugated bilirubin by beta glucuronidase.

   c. ↓ clearance of bilirubin:

      i. ↓ uptake because of ↓ ligandin in first 5 days (monkeys).

      ii. ↓ conjugation because of ↓ glucuronyl transferase activity.

      iii. ↓ excretion by liver cells in newborn.

      iv. Change of hepatic circulation; before birth, oxygenated blood supply to the liver by umbilical vein; and after birth, relative hypoxia by portal venous supply.

192. Factors modifying jaundice in newborns:

   a. **Factors ↑ jaundice:**
   Race: oriental, American Indian, Greek.
   Maternal: Diabetes, ↑ B.P., oral contraceptive.
   Drugs: Diazepam, oxytocin, epidural anesthesia.
   Infant: Premature, LBW, infection, breast-feeding, dehydration, ↓ serum zinc and mg (magnesium), ↓ vitamin E, delayed cord clamping (↑ RBC volume).

   b. **Factors ↓ jaundice:**
   Race: Black.
   Smoking.
   Drugs: Phenobarbital, phenytoin, heroin, meperidine, alcohol.

   c. **Factors have no relation to jaundice:** Parity.
   Drugs: Beta adrenergic agents.
   Low apgar score.

193. Factors affecting jaundice by different action mechanisms:

   a. Diabetes: ↑ bilirubin production.

   b. ↓ Vitamin E: Unknown, probably ↑ glucuronyl transferase enzyme activity.

   c. ↓ Zinc: Structural defects in RBC membrane and hemolysis.

   d. ↓ Magnesium: Maintains ribosome which synthesizes glucuronyl transferase enzyme, so ↓ enzyme synthesis.

194. **Physiological jaundice:** Transient hyperbilirubinemia, bilirubin >2 mg/dl, peak 2-4 days 5-6 mg/dl then reduced by day 7. Maximum bilirubin level is up to 12.9 mg/dl.
   Mechanism:

a. ↑ bilirubin load on liver cells: ↑ RBC volume, ↓ RBC survival, ↑ early labelled bilirubin, ↑ enterohepatic circulation.
b. Decreased hepatic uptake from plasma: ↓ ligandin, ↓ relative hepatic uptake deficiency.
c. Defective bilirubin conjugation: ↓ UDP glucuronyl transferase activity. ↓ UDP glucose dehydrogenase activity.
d. Defective bilirubin excretion: Excretion impaired, but not rate- limiting.
e. Diminished oxygen supply to liver after birth.

195. **Non-physiological jaundice means:**
a. Jaundice in first 24 hours.
b. Total bilirubin increases by > 5 mg/dl/day.
c. Total bilirubin (> 12.9 in fullterm, > 15 in preterm).
d. Direct bilirubin (> 1.5-2 mg/dl).
e. Duration of jaundice (> 1 week in fullterm, > 2 weeks in premature).

196. **Breast feeding jaundice:** Begins on day 4 and stays up to 10-15 days; maximum bilirubin 10-27 mg/dl.
Treatment:
Don't discontinue breast-feeding unless it reaches close to exchange level (20mg/dl), then discontinue for a few days and resume breast-feeding. **If feeding continues,** elevated level of bilirubin declines slowly from day 10 and reaches normal in 3-12 weeks. **If feeding discontinues,** then there is a prompt decline within 48 hours. Resuming breast-feeding will increase bilirubin, but not reach previous level.
Mechanism:
a. ↑ 3 alpha 20 beta pregnanediol which ↓ conjugation.
b. **↑ lipoprotein lipase and ↑ unsaturated fatty acids, (NEFA) inhibits conjugation.**
c. **Dehydration.**

197. Causes of indirect hyperbilirubinemia:
a. Breast milk.
b. Hemolytic diseases.
c. Hypothyroidism (↓ hepatic uptake and ↓ conjugation).
d. Crigler-Najjar syndrome.
e. Extravascular blood.
f. Pyloric stenosis.
(mechanism: ↑ enzyme activity, ↑ enterohepatic circulation by delayed gastric emptying time).

GROWTH AND DEVELOPMENT

1. Socialization begins at birth.

Discipline begins around 18 months. Punishment is allowed in the teaching of discipline as long as it is constructive and does not depress the child.

16-year-old wants to hang out at night. What should parents do? Show concern, but set limits.

2. Child's dependence on parents and autonomy: Children depend on parents, but there is a temporary, intermittent process of psychological separation and individuation from 1/2 year to 2 1/2 years of age. This lasts until age 3 to 4 when they develop autonomous behavior, but still need parents a lot.

3. Child's most important teachers are: Parents.

4. Teenage mother rearing a child: It is very difficult for her to plan both her own life and the child's.

5. Parents have the same policy in rearing two children: A policy might work very well for one child, but not for next. Parents feel guilty for no reason and become angry.

6. Handicapped child and his/her parents: Child who is mentally, physically, and/or emotionally handicapped or suffering from chronic diseases (e.g., BPD, PT) may receive destructive and bad behavior from parents. Doctors should recognize the problem and give support to family through social services before this happens. Doctors should learn about parents' own system of rearing a child and should respect their values as long as it is not harmful to child.

7. Preterm infant can suffer social and sensory deprivation when isolated for a prolonged period of time during hospitalization.

8. **Fatigue in adolescence due to: Iron and protein deficiency.**

9. **Increased** calorie requirement in **prepubertal and adolescent years:** For **increased growth.**

10. Water and electrolyte requirements in proportion to body surface: **Remains the same for all** ages.

11. **Development of drug metabolism in children:**
    a. First, genetic.
    b. Second, child develops the capacity to metabolize the drugs through enzyme activities.

12. Fluoride requirement in breast-fed newborn: 0.25 mg/day.

13. Side-effect of phenobarbital use: **Hyperactivity.**

14. Side-effect of dextroamphetamine: Hyperkinesis is reduced.

15. G6PD-are deficient children are more prone to have hemolysis **when exposed to:** Certain drugs. Example: Sulfadiazine and many other drugs.

16. **Important parameter to measure obesity: Skin fold thickness.** Example: Over triceps area.

17. **Development at 1m, 2m, 3m, of age:**
    1m: Begins to **smile,** follows moving objects for 90 degrees, lifts head **momentarily** to body plane or ventral suspension, holds chin up.
    2m: Smiles on **social contact, follows** moving object for 180 degree, sustains head to body plane or ventral suspension, listens to voice and coos.
    3m: **Sustains** social contact, says **'aah'** and reaches **toward the object, but misses** it, lifts head and **chest,** early **head control.**

18. **Development at 4m, 5m, 6m of age:**
    4m: Reaches for, holds, and **puts object in mouth;** has complete head control, **laughs loudly.**
    5m: **Rolls over.**
    6m: **Prefers mother,** begins **separation anxiety** from mother. Repeats vowel sounds, sits briefly with pelvic support and **rounded back.**

19. **Development at 7m, 8m, 9m:**
    7m: Transfers **object from hand to hand,** chases pellet, but can't pick it up, **babbles,** enjoys mirror, has emotional social response, **experiences separation anxiety.**
    8m: Sits **up alone with** back **straight,** for a short period pulls to standing position, recognizes strangers, **experiences separation anxiety.**
    9m: **Crawls, has less** separation anxiety, waves **bye-bye, says mama and dada, uses index** finger to move object, can stand up by holding furniture.

20. Development at 10m 11m, 12m:
    10m: Picks up **pellet with assisted pincer** movement, creeps, elevates foot on standing, begins to put object in and out of container, drops object deliberately, will not release object to let you examine it.
    11m: Takes a few sips from cup, makes a mess while eating pivots, walks holding onto furniture, **rolls ball and releases it to examiner, plays peek-a-boo, shakes head for `no', speaks one word with meaning.**
    12m: **Unassisted** pincer movement, says a few **words** beside mama and dada, plays ball, **extends the object and releases it to offered hand,** walks while holding one hand, does **postural adjustment** in dressing change.

21. Development at 15m, 18m, 2 years:
    15m: Walks alone, **says 4 to 6 words, hugs parents, builds** tower of 2 cubes.
    18m: **Runs stiffly,** says 10 words, builds tower of 3 cubes, identifies **one or more body parts.**
    2 yrs: Runs **well,** uses 50 words, builds tower of 6 cubes, puts 3 words together ("give me milk"), uses **spoon,** listens to stories, copies circle (o).

22. **Development at 3 years, 4 years, 5 years:**
    3 years: Stands **momentarily on one foot,** uses **tricycle,** copies plus (+), builds tower of 9 cubes, knows **age and sex, washes hands, unbuttons clothes, put shoes on.** Goes upstairs with alternate feet.

4 years: **Hops** on one foot, **throws ball,** uses **scissor,** draws picture of man with **2-to-4 parts** plus head. Copies cross (x), counts 4 pennies, tells a story, **uses toilet without help.**

5 years: Skips, copies square and triangle, **uses 10 syllables,** knows 4 color names, counts 10 pennies, asks for meaning of words, dresses and undresses.

23. **How to remember before test:**
    1 M: Smiles, follows object for **90 degrees.**
    2 M: Follows object **for 180 degrees.**
    3 M: Head control.
    4 M: Laughes loudly.
    5 M: Rolls over.
    6 M: Prefers mother, has separation anxiety, **has rounded back** when sit.
    7 M: Transfers object from hand to hand; babbles.
    8 M: Sits up alone; back **is straight** when sitting.
    9 M: Crawls, says bye-bye, mama dada.
    10 M: Picks up pellet with **assisted** pincer movement, creeps, doesn't release object.
    11 M: Plays peek-a-boo, releases object, knows one word with meaning.
    12 M: Says mama, dada, plus **few** other words, **uses unassisted** pincer movement, extends hand.
    15 M: Uses 4 to 6 words, 2 cubes, walks alone.
    18 M: Uses 10 words, 3 cubes, runs stiffly, knows one or more body parts.
    2 yrs: Uses 50 words, 6 cubes, runs well, copies (O) circle.
    3 yrs: Uses tricycle, 9 cubes, stands on one foot momentarily, knows age **and** sex, copies (+) plus.
    4 yrs: Hops, man's picture with 2 to 4 parts plus head, **counts** 4 pennies, goes to toilet alone, copies (x) cross.
    5 yrs: Uses 10 syllables, knows 4 color name, counts 10 pennies, copies square or triangle.
    7 yrs: Copies a diamond.

24. Ejaculation usually begins SMR 3 (sexual maturity rating), but semen is present between 3 to 4.

25. **First** puberty sign:
    Girl: Breast buds.
    Boy: Testes increase in size.

26. Motor activity and sex: Equal in both sex until 7-8 years. **Increase** faster in boy than in girl **by 9 years.**

27. **Delayed puberty in male:** Means no testicular growth by 13.5 years or by SMR 3 did not achieve within 4 year of SMR 2. Further evaluation of endocrine status is needed.

28. SMR in boy:
    Stages Features.
    1 Preadolescent type.

    2   Scanty pubic hair, pink **scrotum,** medium penis.

    3   **Curly** pubic hair, **large** scrotum and penis.

    4   **Coarse,** curly pubic hair, **dark** scrotum.

    5   Hair on medial surface of thigh of adult type.

29.   SMR in girls:

Stages Features

    1   Preadolescent type.

    2   **Sparse,** light color hair on medial **border** of labia, breasts and papilla elevated, areolar diameter increased.

    3   Dark ,curly pubic hair, breast and areola enlarged, **but** no contour separation.

    4   Coarse, curly hair, areola and papilla form secondary mound.

    5   Hair on medial side of thigh, mature **nipple** projecting.

30.   Menarche usually occurs in SMR 4. Some may begin in 3.

31.   **Delayed puberty** in females: No breast bud by 13 years, or menarche did not occur **within 5 years** of puberty changes. Needs endocrine evaluation. Outcome of adolescent in male and female **with delayed** puberty: Most are **normal.**

32.   In short stature: Most important investigation is bone age. Most important is family history.

    Short stature and outcome: Short stature boys with SMR 2-3 with height age same or more than skeletal age, he will grow later, but may not be too tall.

    Short boys with SMR **4 remain** short (because skeletal age > height age).

    Short boys with bone age **the same** as chronological age with delayed puberty: Need endocrine work up.

    SMR has better correlation for nutritional requirement than for chronological age.

33.   Normal psychologic growth of adolescent (4):

    a.   Emotional separation from family (not physical).

    b.   Develops sexual and personal character.

    c.   Sets goals and tries to achieve them.

    d.   Ego identity.

34.   Characteristics of **early** adolescence: Interested in **body changes** and secondary sexual character; has erotic thoughts, dreams and feelings, **imitates** older adolescents and adults, tries to find out his parent's economic and educational status, resulting in rejection of parental **values .**

    Characteristics of **middle** adolescence: Body image is real.There is less concern about physical changes. More freedom and responsibility. Starts to date. Peer influence is greater than parental. Few have ego identity.

    Characteristics of **late** adolescence: Starts to leave home, pursues higher education, looks for a job, **separates from peers,** ego identity may not be achieved until few years later. Adults should achieve ego identity. If the don't, then they feel inferior and have failures.

35. Young adolescents and physicians: They think doctors can do miracles and cure them immediately. If they can't, then adolescents lose faith in physicians. Doctors should be very specific about the diagnosis and treatment.

36. Chronic disease and adolescence: Obese patients in puberty feel **helpless.** Cystic fibrosis patients worry about **infertility.** Diabetic patients depends more on **doctors and parents,** so psychosocial evaluation is important.

37. Factors influencing mental maturation:
Intrinsic: Genetic.
Extrinsic: Environment.

38. Psychological development includes two factors: Cognitive means **(e.g., poor school performance)** judgement, memory, reasoning. Affective **(e.g., temper tantrum)** anger, sadness, jealousy, fear, anxiety, depression.

39. Child with **immature** speech: Early intervention is important.

40. While treating a child with difficult problem: e.g.,: **hyperkinetic child.** Physician should be aware of the family situation.

41. Most common type of child abuse:
Physical abuse (70%);
25% sexual abuse.
5% failure to thrive due to underfeeding.

42. Most common cause of failure to thrive in infancy: **Nutritional neglect** or psychological underfeeding.

43. **Munchausen syndrome by proxy:** Here children are the victims of an illness fabricated or caused by parents. Victims are < 6 years old and they may end up in the hospital.

    Example: Producing diarrhea by giving laxatives, rashes by putting caustics or rubbing on skin.
    Treatment: Report to child welfare agency and the police to protect the child.

44. **Physical abuse:**
Age group: 33% < 1 year, 33% 1-6 years, 33% over 6 years.
Premature have 3 folds higher risk.
Abuser: Mostly is related caretaker or male friend of the mother (95%).
Parents abusing their children is found in all ethnic, religious, educational, occupational and socioeconomic groups, but it is higher in the lower socioeconomic classes because of greater crisis in their lives. More than 90% of abusing parents **neither psychotic nor have criminal records,** but are lonely, angry, unhappy adults under stress. Abusive parents believe that all misbehavior by children is deliberate and severe punishment is needed to control them. Abuse occurs in family crises like loss of a job or home, marital difficulty, or birth of a sibling.

Signs and symptoms: Unexplained injury is most common presentation of physical abuse and explanation does not fit the injury. Most common site of accidental bruise is over the tibia, on the forehead, or on any bony prominence. Bruises in the lower back or on buttocks is usually due to finger marks or belt marks on the skin, choke marks on the neck, or traumatic alopecia.

Most common type of inflicted burn is hot water burn.
Most dangerous inflicted injury is subdural hematoma.
Most common cause of serious intracranial injury in first year of life is due to abuse.
Most of the subdural is not associated with fracture(skull) and bruise,but rather to the shaking or slamming of the head on the mattress.
Most common finding in abdominal injury is the rupture of liver and spleen, and duodenal trauma causing intramural hematoma and obstruction.

Diagnosis, treatment, prevention, and prognosis of child abuse.
Diagnosis: **By skeletal survey** showing recent or old fractures with calcification; if the children > 4 or 5 years and can communicate, then X-ray should be taken if needed (tenderness, limited range of motion). If X-ray is negative, but the site is tender, then X-ray should be repeated after 2 weeks to look for calcification. (Remember CPR rarely causes rib fracture in children). Medical history **does not** match with the X-ray or physical findings.

Treatment:
a. Notify to child protective services.
b. Physician should tell the parents that you are legally obligated to report any suspected injury.
c. Admit child to hospital for any medical problem.
d. Siblings should be examined within 24 hours of the report of child abuse.
e. Don't express your anger at the parents.

Prevention:
a. High-risk parents should be identified.
b. Their families need intensive support.
c. Counseling regarding discipline and nonphysical responses.
Prognosis: 80-90% families rehabilitated to provide adequate care for themselves.

45.   Most common type of sexual abuse: **Incest (sex between** family members).
Victims are 90% female; offenders are 99% male; a stepfather is 5 times more likely perpetrator than the natural father; in a day care center, a female is more often the perpetrator.

Most incest involves: Father and daughter.

Sexual abuse:
Clinical presentations: A child might disclose this relationship to her mother, a friend or even to her physician; **sexually transmitted disease is the most common presentation in prepubertal child due to sexual abuse by an adult.** Female victims prefer female physicians but it is not mandatory. Mouth, vagina, and rectum should be examined; **most**

acute genital injury occurs between the 4 and 8 o'clock positions.

Laboratory investigation:
a. Gonococcus and chlamydia culture should be obtained from mouth, rectum and vagina.
b. Serologic test for syphilis.
c. Detection of sperm (motile up to 6 hours and nonmotile up to 72 hours), acid phosphatase for 24 hours. Remember, absence of semen does not rule out intercourse.
d. Hair (pubic, scalp), fingernail scrapings, blood and sperm samples should be sent for testing.

Diagnosis: Mostly made by graphic history offered by victim, because physical examination and laboratory tests may be **normal,** even with definite sexual abuse.

Treatment: Medication to prevent pregnancy and sexually transmitted disease; mother and father of incest victim need psychotherapy and marital therapy.

Prevention: Children should tell someone for help.

Prognosis: Most incest victims can have normal adult life.

46. Most common type of failure to thrive: **Nonorganic (70%);** organic (30%).
Most common cause of nonorganic: Neglect or psychologic (50%), 20% accidental.

Failure to thrive (FTT):
Clinical manifestations:
a. Nutritional neglect: Dietary history is **not** helpful, because parents report that baby is taking enough calories.
b. Accidental neglect: Dietary history **is helpful,** because parents tell the truth and ask for help.

FTT baby appears with wasting, expressionless face, avoids eye contact. Delay in social and speech development detected after 4 months of age.

First feed the child properly for 7 days in the hospital, if no improvement then do extensive laboratory test. X-ray should be done to R/O physical abuse as well.

Treatment:
a. Notify CPA (child protective agency).
b. After hospitalization 75% are discharged home with added service for the family.
c. Written dietary instruction to parents.
d. Weekly medical follow up.

47. Most common neurodevelopmental dysfunction affecting children: **Dysfunction of selective attention span.**

48. Most serious side effect of neuroleptics (chlorpromazine, **haloperidol): Tardive dyskinesia.**
It is a choreoathetoid movement of extremities, trunk, or facial muscles. It can occur during treatment or after treatment was discontinued (withdrawal dyskinesia).
Treatment: Discontinue the medicine.

49. Language problems in children:

a. Receptive: Lack of understanding; serious problem.
b. Expressive: Lack of production of communication.

50. Etiology of mental retardation: It is complex and multifactorial.

Diagnosis of mental retardation is **confirmed by:**
a. Bayle scale of infant development.
b. Stanford-Binet intelligence scale.
c. Wechsler scales.

Treatment for mental retardation: Multidimensional and highly individualized.

51. Expression fatal illness of child to parents: Both parents should be available; physician should be polite, and honest and tell them that child has an illness from which recovery is not expected.

Management of terminal illness:
a. Physician should **not** leave decision to parents regarding child care.
b. Physician should listen to the advice of parents if it is realistic and helpful for patient.

52. Physician should tell the parents after the death of the newborn child: Mourning process for the dead infant should be complete, and steady state should be reached (around 9 months) before the woman becomes pregnant again.

IMMUNOLOGY AND ALLERGY

1. **T cell subpopulation:**
   a. Helper cells: T4 (produces antibodies IgG, IgA, some IgM in response to antigen).
   b. Suppressor cells: T8 (maintains homeostasis in immune response to tolerable level).
   c. Killer cells: Effective cells of thymus-dependent system.

2. **B cell subpopulation:** IgM, IgG, IgA, IgD and IgE.
   First **antibody appears in the body (important): IgM.**

3. **Cytokines:**
   a. **Undefined:**
      i. Chemotactic factors (eosinophil, monocyte, neutrophil).
      ii. Lymph node permeability factor.
      iii. Migration inhibition factors.
      iv. Suppressor factors.
      v. Transfer factors.
   b. **Interleukins (IL):**
      i. IL-1 (Endogenous pyrogen); promotes IL-2 synthesis.
      ii. IL-2 (T cell growth factor); T and B cell proliferation, activates killer cells.
      iii. IL-3 (B cell stimulatory factor 1); proliferation of activated B cells; promotes IgE production.
      iv. IL-5 (B cell growth factor); promotes IgA/IgM production, helps in eosinophil

growth.

v. IL-6 (B cell stimulatory factor-2).

vi. IL-7 (stimulates B cell precursor growth).

vii. Gamma interferon enhances IgM and IgG production, inhibits IL-4 effects.

4. **Assessment of T cell function:**

a. Peripheral blood lymphocyte count (normal > 1500 lymphocyte/mm3).

b. Lateral chest X-ray: Look for thymus.

c. Skin test for delayed hypersensitivity (Tuberculosis).

T4/T8 ratio (important):

a. Normal ratio is > 1.0.

b. In advanced AIDS patient, there is the loss of nearly all T4 cells, so T4/T8 ratio is reversed in terminal phase.

c. **Remember, a** reversed T4/T8 ratio is **neither** a prior diagnostic feature of AIDS **nor** an absolute sign of serious T cell deficiency.

d. Reversed ratio could be due to↑ **T8** cells (due to mild infection or error in handling specimen).

e. In AIDS patient, ratio is **not** always reversed.

5. **Assessment of B cell function:**

a. **Most commonly used markers** are the IgM molecules present on B lymphocytes surface.

b. **Most commonly used test** is quantitative measurements of serum immunoglobulin level.

c. In true immunodeficiency:

IgG <200 mg/dl and IgA and IgM are not detectable.

d. **Remember, live virus,** except φX 174, **should never be given** to a immunodeficient patient because it can cause severe disease or death.

6. B and T cells, infection and prognosis:

a. ↓ B cell: Bacterial infection, ↓ T cell = fungal (candida).

b. ↓ T and B cells: Worst prognosis.

c. ↓ T cells: Grave prognosis.

d. ↓ B cells: Better prognosis.

7. **Bruton disease or panhypogammaglobulinemia (B cell disease):**

It is mostly congenital or X linked or autosomal recessive.

Signs and symptoms: Recurrent bacterial infections (Pneumococcus, Staphylococcus, H. influenzae), pneumonia, otitis, sinusitis, meningitis, gastroenteritis, eczema, skin abscess, dermatomyositis.

Diagnosis: Absent IgA and IgM, IgG < 200 mg/dl.

Treatment: I.M. immune serum globulin (ISG).

Complications:

a. ISG: Anaphylaxis.

b. Disease: Chronic pulmonary disease (daily prophylaxis with bactrim may be helpful).

8. **Selective IgA deficiency (B Cell disease):** IgA protects the respiratory, G.I. and other

secretary areas.

Signs and symptoms: Recurrent respiratory infections and chronic diarrhea.
Associated with: SLE, rheumatoid arthritis; treatment with phenytoin.
Mode of inheritance: Autosomal recessive or dominant.
Diagnosis confirmed by: ↓ secretary IgA, but normal serum IgA.

9.   **Selective IgM deficiencies** (B cell disease): Rapid bacterial infection, atopy, ↑ spleen. It causes whipple disease, regional enteritis. Treatment: Antibiotics.

10. **DiGeorge primary T cell disease:**
Defect: It is the **result of field defect: a limited clinical disorder that has multiple causes** (previously thought a defect in 3rd and 4th pharyngeal pouch forming parathyroid and thymus gland).
Signs and symptoms: Fish mouth, hypertelorism, downward eye slanting, urinary tract anomaly, heart (interrupted aortic arch, truncus, right aortic arch); hypoparathyroidism and thymus defect do not always appear in this syndrome. **Neonate appears with hypocalcemia and tetany.**
Important point to remember: Blood transfusion given during cardiac surgery results in **serious graft-versus-host (GVHD) reaction, so blood should be irradiated.**
Treatment:
a.   **No treatment is needed,** because most patients will acquire normal immunity.
b.   Those who need therapy: Thymus transplant can be done. (Don't give thymic hormone.)
c.   Bone marrow transplant may be helpful.
d.   Calcium should be given for hypocalcemia.

11. **Nezelof syndrome:** It is a variant of DiGeorge anomaly **without parathyroid or cardiac anomaly.**

12. **Cartilage-hair hypoplasia:** Bone dysplasia (short lived dwarfism, ↓ WBC, loose skin), absence of T cell function, but limited infection (mostly by vaccinia or varicella virus). Treatment: Bone marrow transplantation may be helpful.

13. **Combined immunodeficiency disease (CID):**
Defect: Both T and B cell functions diminished.
Signs and symptoms: Wasting with or without diarrhea which is resistant to therapy, so TPN is required. Total alopecia, loose skin, candidiasis (mostly oral), pneumocystis pneumonia, encephalopathy, CBC (↓ WBC, ↓ RBC, ↑ platelet).
Treatment:
a.   **Bone marrow transplant is the preferred treatment.**
b.   Some cases respond to transplant of fetal liver alone or with thymus.
c.   Interleukin 2 may be helpful.
d.   Pneumocystic pneumonia: Pentamidine or bactrim.
e.   Varicella:
   i.   Prevention: VZIG (varicella zoster immunoglobulin).
   ii.   Treatment: Acyclovir.

14. Combined immunodeficiency disease (CID) and Letterer-Siwe syndrome (Omenn disease):
It is a variant of CID.
Enzyme: ↓ **Ectoenzyme 5 - nucleotidase is characteristic.**
Appears with pneumocystis pneumonia, skin (seborrheic dermatitis or erythematous rash).

15. **Wiskott-Aldrich syndrome: X-linked recessive, disorder is characterized by thrombocytopenia, eczema and draining ears.**
Signs and symptoms: In addition to above 3, appears with petechiae, bleeding, recurrent otitis, pneumonia, herpes conjunctivitis, ↑ **liver, spleen and lymph nodes.**
Serum: ↑ **(IgA and IgE),** ↓ **IgM,** ↓ lymphocyte, **small size platelets.**
Defect: In glycosylation of surface proteins.

Treatment:
   a. **Bone marrow transplantation is the preferred treatment.**
   b. Splenectomy to control thrombocytopenia when marrow transplant can't be done.
Reason for ↑ **infections:** Unknown. May be due to inability to form antibodies against carbohydrate antigens and poor response to other antigens, or mild dysfunction of T cells.
Death: Due to malignant reticuloendotheliosis.

16. **Ataxia-telangiectasia: It** is due to variable B and T cell deficiency, deficiency of both IgA and IgE, **autosomal recessive.**

Signs and symptoms: First neurologic sign is cerebellar ataxia. Intellectual development is normal until age 10 years, then stops. Choreoathetoid movement, mask facies. **Telangiectases are most prominent in sclera. They appear between** 1-6 years. Skin (hypo or hyperpigmentation, eczema, atopic dermatitis), recurrent sinopulmonary infection may cause bronchiectasis, growth failure. If patients survive, they don't develop secondary sex characteristics.
Diagnosis: ↓ (IgA and IgE) both in 50-70% cases, isolated ↓ IgE or IgA deficiency also occurs.
Death: Due to malignant lymphoma.

17. **Chronic mucocutaneous candidosis:**
Signs and symptoms:
   a. **Early onset:** It is severe and appears with endocrine disorders (hypoparathyroidism, hypoadrenalism), candida granuloma, candida over skin, scalp.
   b. **Late onset:** It is a milder disease and is limited to nail and oral mucosal candida infections.
   c. **Candida endocrinopathy syndrome:** Autosomal recessive, familial polyendocrinopathy and candidiasis.
   d. Biotin-dependent multiple carboxylase deficiency with candidiasis.
Diagnosis: Defects in T cell function, ↓ MIF (migration inhibitory factor), ↓ IgA (selective), ↓ Biotin.
Treatment:
   a. **I.V. Amphotericin;** but recurs after cessation of therapy.
   b. Recalcitrant cases: **Ketoconazole is the best;** variable success with clotrimazole, WBC infusion, thymosin, transfer factor.

18. **GVHD (Graft-versus host disease):** It occurs when T killer cells (immunocompetent) transfusion occurs in patient with T cell deficiency.
    a. **Acute form:** Here **blood or bone marrow** of donor and recipient differs at HLA-D locus **(rarely** occurs in tissue transplant).
    b. **Chronic form:** It is found in intrauterine blood transfusion, transplantation of bone marrow, fetal liver and thymus.

19. Adenosine deaminase (ADA) and nucleoside phosphorylase (NP) deficiency: First biochemical defect where immunodeficiency is found. ADA deficient patient has combined immunodeficiency. NP deficient patient first appears as T cell defects and then develops B cell defects.

    Signs and symptoms:
    a. ADA: Diarrhea, failure to thrive, pneumonia, candidiasis, ↑ liver and spleen, infections (bacterial, viral, fungal, protozoal).
    b. NP: Same as above; may manifest few years later.
    Diagnosis confirmed by enzyme assay in RBC.
    ADA: Squaring off the scapula and splaying of end of ribs.
    NP: Spastic tetraparesis, megaloblastic anemia, pure red cells aplasia.
    Treatment of choice: Bone marrow transplant.

20. **Complement deficiencies and diseases:**
    a. Absence of C3: Pyogenic infection (pneumococci and meningococci).
    b. ↓ C5, 6, 7, 8: Disseminated gonococci and meningococci.
    c. ↓ C9: Meningococci (meningitis).
    d. ↓ C2: Pneumococci (meningitis, pneumonia).
    e. ↓ C4: Bacteremia and meningitis.
    f. ↓ C1q: Recurrent bacterial, fungal dermatitis and meningitis.
    g. ↓ C1r: Pneumonia, meningitis.
    Remember, all of the above cause SLE, except C9.
    ↓ C7: Scleroderma, ankylosing spondylitis, rheumatoid arthritis.
    ↓ (C4, C6): Sjogren syndrome.
    ↓ (C1q, C3, C6): MPGN (Membranoproliferative glomerulonephritis).
    ↓ (C1r, C3): CGN (chronic glomerulonephritis).
    ↓ C2: H-S purpura, dermatomyositis.
    ↓ Factor D: Recurrent sinusitis, bronchitis, bronchiectasis.

    ↓ Factor H: Hemolytic uremic syndrome (H for H).
    ↓ Properdin: Meningococcal meningitis.
    ↓ CR1: SLE.
    ↓ C4 and C3→: Hereditary angioedema (important).
    Partial ↓ C1q: Severe, combined immunodeficiency disease of hypogammaglobulinemia.
    Defective opsonization of pneumococci in alternate pathway: Sickle cell disease.

    Defective complement functions: Normal newborn, anorexia nervosa.

21. Screening procedure for most of the diseases of complement system (important).

CH 50.

22. **LAD (leukocyte adhesion deficiency) (important): It** causes recurrent progressive infections of skin, subcutaneous tissue, mucous membrane and **characterized by ↓ pus formation, delayed wound healing and ↑ granulocytes count. Earliest sign is delayed separation or infection of umbilical cord.**

    Defect: Diminished or absent glycoprotein receptors or WBC surface; **normal bacterial killing, but decreased chemotaxis.**
    Diagnosis: ↑ WBC (15,000-160,000/ul) with 50-90% polymorph.
    Treatment: Antibiotics to cover (Staph.aureus, E.Coli, Pseudomonas, klebsiella, candida).
    Prenatal diagnosis: By PUBS (percutaneous umbilical blood sampling) around 20th week to demonstrate (in fetal leukocyte) **diminished or absent of glycoprotein adhesion molecules.**

23. **Phagocytic disorders (important):**
    Decreased chemotaxis of leukocytes:
    a. LAD (Leukocyte Adhesion Deficiency).
    b. Chediak-Higashi syndrome.
    c. Job syndrome (hyperimmunoglobulin E, ↑ eosinophil).
    d. Specific granule deficiency.
    Decreased bacterial killing:
    a. CGD (Chronic Granulomatous Disease).
    b. Chediak-Higashi syndrome.
    c. Specific granule deficiency.
    d. Myeloperoxidase deficiency.
    Decreased superoxide release:
    a. LAD.
    b. CGD.
    Increased superoxide release:
    a. **Neutrophil granulocyte defects (3) (WBC 2000-15000; 50-70% PMN).**
    b. Chediak-Higashi syndrome.
    c. Myeloperoxidase deficiency.
    d. Specific granule deficiency (may be normal).
    All normal activities (chemotaxis, bacterial killing, O_{2-} release).
    a. Agranulocytosis (< 1000 µl WBC).
    b. Agammaglobulinemia and related disorders.

24. **Neutrophil granule defects:**
    Two types of granules:
    a. Peroxidase positive azurophils.
    b. Peroxidase negative specific granules.
    Clinical manifestations:
    a. Hereditary MPO(myeloperoxidase deficiency): Mostly asymptomatic. May appear with candidiasis and diabetes mellitus.
    b. Congenital specific granule deficiency (SGD): Autosomal recessive; skin ulcer, bronchopneumonia or lung abscess. **Most common organism is Staphylococcus aureus** and next is candida.

c. **Chediak-Higashi syndrome (CHS):** Present in early childhood with photophobia, nystagmus, partial albinism, gingivitis, periodontitis, blond-to-dark hair, infections in skin, mucous membrane and respiratory tract with gram positive and gram negative organism.

Most common organism is S. aureus and beta hemolytic Streptococcus. Prolonged bleeding with normal platelet due to lack of ADP **which helps platelet aggregation.** Neurologic features (ataxia, motor weakness, peripheral neuropathy) develop in adulthood.

Death due to EBV or other lymphotrophic virus resulting in lymphoma like picture. **Phagocytic functions in all 3 conditions are abnormal.**

Diagnosis: By leukocyte alkaline phosphatase and peroxidase cytochemical stain.

a. MPO: Deficiency ↓ of peroxidase activity and normal alkaline phosphatase.
b. SGD: Presence of azurophilic granule peroxide and absence of alkaline phosphatase; Wright stain **showing bilobed nuclei in neutrophils.**
c. CHS: Wright stain showing **large granules** due to coalescence of specific and azurophilic granules.

Treatment of and genetic counseling for neutrophil granule defect:

a. MPO: No treatment.
b. SGD: Antibiotics, abscess drainage.
c. CHS:
    i. Ascorbic acid (it improves phagocytic function).
    ii. Antibiotics to treat active infection (prophylactic antibiotic is not effective).
    iii. **Bone marrow transplant is successful and is the preferred treatment.**
    iv. Acyclovir and prednisone provide temporary improvement.
    v. Corticosteroid, vincristine, and cyclophosphamide cannot stop the progression of the disease, but can partially arrest the infiltrative process.

Genetic counseling: Examining **neutrophil granules in fetal blood** obtained by PUBS at 20 weeks.

25. Most common inherited disorders of phagocytic function:
CGD (Chronic Granulomatous Disease).
CGD: Defect in oxidase activation of phagocytes.
X-linked recessive (55-60%) and autosomal recessive (45-55%).
Cytochrome b is **absent** in most of X-linked recessive.
Cytochrome b is **present** in most of autosomal recessive.

CGD (Chronic Granulomatous Disease):
Defects: Decreased bacterial killing, decreased superoxide release, (normal chemotaxis).
Etiology: In CGD, superoxide anion is not produced from oxygen. Bacteria is killed by hydrogen peroxide and hydroxyl radical. NADPH oxidase remains dormant unless activated by opsonized microbe and chemotactic peptide. **NAPDH then reduces oxygen** through series of reaction involving FAD (flavin adenine dinucleotide), cytochrome b.
Oxygen is reduced to superoxide anion which, after **mutation, forms H2 O$_2$ and hydroxyl radical. G6PD converts NADP to NADPH.**
Signs and symptoms: Lymphadenopathy in neck is the most common manifestation.

Chronic and recurrent pyogenic infection (pneumonia due to serratia marcescens, recurrent skin abscess and furunculosis, eczema and impetigo), granuloma causing **obstruction** of esophagus, pylorus, urethra; perianal abscess, rectal fistula, colitis causing diarrhea. Patients with chemotactic disorder appear to have rhinitis, stomatitis, conjunctivitis (mucous membrane).

Diagnosis:
a. **Screening test** is reduction of NBT (nitroblue tetrazolium) test: In CGD, **patient cannot** reduce NBT.
b. **Confirmed by** ferricytochrome reduction method to **quantify the rates of superoxide generation: Absent in CGD.**
c. Carrier detection:
   i. X-linked: 50% will **not** reduce NBT, i.e., carrier.
   ii. Autosomal: **Normal** NBT test.

Treatment of and genetic counseling for CGD:
Treatment:
a. Prophylaxis of infection: Trimethoprim sulfamethoxazole.
b. Active infection: Antibiotics, granulocyte transfusion.
c. Obstruction (gastric outlet, bladder): Prolonged antibiotics and prednisone.
d. **Preferred treatment is gamma interferon:** it reduces the number of new infections and helps fight existing infection.
e. **Serious transfusion reaction** occurs in patient with CGD who lack McLeod phenotype (lacking Kell-associated RBC antigens). **Patient should be tested for the presence of Kell antigen before transfusion.**
f. Bone marrow transplant is rarely successful.

Genetic counselling:
a. Blood from cord or placenta by fetoscopy: Diagnosis of CGD by NBT slide test. **This also detects carrier state** or from the family history.
b. Most promising method is to use probe recognizing DNA polymorphism in X-CGD gene in CVS (chorionic villi sample), but it is not yet available. (CGD gene is located on X chromosome proximal to muscular dystrophy and distal to ornithine transcarbamylase gene.)

26. **G-6-PD** (glucose 6-phosphate dehydrogenase deficiency): American blacks with RBC G6PD deficiency have normal levels of the enzymes in neutrophils. Several Caucasian patients have G-6-PD activity in neutrophil is < 5%, when it is < 1%, then NADP is **not** converted to NADPH which is required for superoxide anion formation and bacterial killing, so they present as CGD. 5% activity does not produce clinical disease.

27. **Hyperimmunoglobulin E (Job syndrome):**
Signs and symptoms: Within 2 months of age, child appears with serious infection of skin (abscess in subcutaneous tissues), pneumonia, osteomyelitis, visceral abscess, rhinitis, keratoconjunctivitis, **growth retardation.**
Most common organism is S.aureus.
Serum: ↑↑ IgE level. (Due to over-activity of T-helper cell secondary to deficiency of T-suppressor cell).

Treatment:
a. I.V. Gamma globulin prophylaxis.
b. Infection: Antibacterial, antifungal and antiviral agents should be used.
c. Drainage of abscess.

28. Most definitive abnormality found in newborn dysfunction of neutrophils (important): **Decreased leukocyte migration.**

29. **Dysfunction of neutrophils in newborn:**
Signs and symptoms: Increased incidence of sepsis, meningitis, ↓ WBC (blood and marrow), lack of WBC in lungs causing pneumonia.
Most common organism is S. aureus; C. albicans.

Defect: Decreased neutrophil migration; motile response of neutrophil depends on deformability of cell membrane and adherence to endothelial cells: these are defective in newborn. The defective movement of **lectin receptors or adhesion** sites on neutrophil and defective translocation **of C-3 receptors** from inside granules to surface membrane may be responsible for defective migration.
Treatment:
a. Recombinant human GM-CSF (stimulates neutrophil and monocyte in marrow) and G-CSF (stimulates neutrophil in marrow) and release of neutrophil from marrow; stimulates C3 receptor expression.
b. Controversial: transfusion of adult donor neutrophil in neonatal sepsis.

30. Immunologic basis of atopic diseases: **Three** forms of humoral antibody-antigen reaction, two of them occur on cell surface and the third in extracellular fluid.

a. Type I hypersensitivity reaction, mediated by IgE (immediate type or anaphylaxis). Mast cells and basophils are involved in this reaction.
b. Type II hypersensitivity (cytotoxic) interaction occurs at cell surface between antigen and antibody. IgG or IgM immunoglobulins react with antigen, stimulating the complement system. Involved cells are destroyed.
Example: Transfusion of incompatible blood.
c. Type III immunopathologic mechanism (Arthus or immune complex) involving antibody and antigen, destroying the tissue. This reaction occurs in extracellular space.
Example: Immunologic glomerulonephritis, serum sickness, arthritis.
d. Type IV, **cell**-mediated or delayed type of hypersensitivity reactions due to reaction between antigen and sensitized thymus-derived T lymphocytes.
Example: Tuberculin test, poison ivy, chemical-induced contact dermatitis, graft-versus-host disease, tissue transplant reaction.

31. Main prostaglandin produced by **mast cells: PGD2**

32. **Arachidonic acids and actions:**
a. Cyclooxygenase products:
PGD2: Constriction of (smooth muscles and bronchus), vasodilation.
TxA2: Constriction of (bronchus and microvessels), platelet aggregation.

PGE2: Dilation of (bronchus vessels, smooth muscles).
PGF2α: Bronchoconstriction, constriction of pulmonary vessels.
PGI2: Dilation of (smooth muscles and pulmonary vessels).

b. Lipoxygenase products:
Leukotrienes (LTC4, LTD4, LTE4)
Contraction (bronchus and smooth muscles), dilate microvessels, constriction of coronary and cerebral arteries.
LTB4: Chemotactic and chemokinetic for neutrophil and eosinophil.

33. Corticosteroid causing ↓ eosinophil count: Up to 6 hours following the dose.

34. Serotonin most commonly found in the body: Gastrointestinal tract. It is bronchoconstrictor.

35. RAST (radioallergosorbent test): It determines antigen-specific IgE concentration in serum. It is less sensitive than skin test.

36. Principles of treatment of allergic disorders:
a. Avoid allergens or irritants.
b. Medication (antihistamine).
c. Immunotherapy (hypo or desensitization).
d. Prophylaxis.

37. **Selective Beta2** receptors for bronchodilation: Metaproterenol, albuterol, terbutaline, isoetharine, fenoterol.
Both beta2 and beta1 receptors stimulation by: Epinephrine, isoproterenol.

38. Mechanism of action of theophylline:
It causes bronchodilatation by:
a. Relaxing bronchial smooth muscles.
b. ↑ endogenous catecholamine in circulation.
c. Stimulating contractility of fatigued diaphragm.
Remember, it has **no** inhibitory effect on cyclic AMP, because to produce this effect, the doses should be toxic.

Metabolism of theophylline: It is metabolized in liver via **cytochrome P450**-dependent, mixed function oxidase. Metabolism occurs in both first order (linear) and non-linear capacity-dependent process.

39. **Mechanism of action of cromolyn sodium:** It is **not** a bronchodilator and has no anti-inflammatory properties.
a. It prevents both antibody and non-antibody **mediated mast cell degranulation** and mediator release by blocking antigen stimulated calcium transport across the mast cell membrane.
b. **It inhibits histamine release** by regulation of phosphorylation of a mast cell protein.
c. It reduces airway hyperreactivity by unknown mechanism.
d. In inhibits bronchoconstriction caused by non-immunologic stimuli (cold air, exercise, SO_2).

Side effects:
a. Dry throat.
b. Transient bronchoconstriction due to inhalation of dry powder.

40.   Mechanism of action of nedrocromil sodium: It is different structurally from cromolyn sodium.
a. Antiallergic.
b. Anti-inflammatory.
It inhibits early and late phase reaction after antigenic challenge. Aerosols inhibit antigen, cold, fog and chemically induced bronchospasm and decrease bronchial hyperactivity.

41.   Most potent drug for treatment of allergy: **Corticosteroid.**
Anti-inflammatory effects of corticosteroid are due to:
a. Alteration in WBC number and activities.
b. Inhibition of mediator release (↓ histamine, ↓ prostaglandins).
c. Enhancement of response to agents that ↑ CAMP.
d. Increase of response to catecholamine.
Steroid therapy should be given: Alternate day therapy of prednisone or its active metabolites (prednisolone).
Complications of surface active corticosteroid (aerosols):
a. Candidiasis.
b. Dysphonia.
c. Suppress pituitary-adrenal axis (rarely).

42.   Risk of asthma to child (important):
a. One affected parent: 25%.
b. Two affected parents: 50%.
Mode of inheritance is polygenic or multifactorial.

43.   **Asthma:** It is a diffuse, obstructive lung disease with airway hyperactivity with stimuli and high degree of reversibility of obstruction. It is the most frequent admitting diagnosis in children. Both airways (small and large) are involved.

Epidemiology: 80-90% of patients appear to have asthma by 4-5 years of age, and 30% by 1 year of age. Age of onset cannot determine the prognosis, but most severely affected children usually manifest by 1 year of age, have a strong family history of asthma, and are patients with atopic dermatitis. **50% children become symptom-free by 10-20 years** of age, and only 5% develop a serious disease.

Pathophysiology: It is due to **bronchoconstriction,** mucosal hypersecretion and edema, cellular infiltration (eosinophil, basophil, neutrophil, macrophage), desquamation of epithelial and inflammatory cells. A variety of stimuli cause bronchoconstriction. Allergens bind to specific mast cells having IgE and release mediators (histamine, platelet activating factor, leukotrienes C4, D4, E4) which cause bronchoconstriction, resulting in hypoxia and hypercarbia. **Obstruction** is maximum in expiration because airway is usually smaller. **Atelectasis** causes mismatch between ventilation and perfusion. **Hypoxia and acidosis** cause pulmonary vasoconstriction, and diminished surfactant production.

Etiology: It is a combination of multiple factors (autonomic, infectious, immunologic, endocrine, psychological).

Bronchodilators: VIP (vasoactive intestinal peptide), catecholamine acting on beta adrenergic receptors.

Bronchoconstrictors: Histamine, leukotrienes (act directly on smooth muscles or through vagus nerve), adenosine.

Immunologic factors: Extrinsic asthma (allergic) mostly found in first 2 years of age (older age causes intrinsic asthma), **mostly due to ↑ IgE (but not always).**

Infection: Most due to virus (RSV, parainfluenzae; in older child, rhinovirus).

Endocrine: Increased in pregnancy, pre-menstruation, menopause, thyrotoxicosis.

Signs and symptoms: Wheezing, tachypnea, difficulty in breathing, cough; severe cases with cyanosis and respiratory failure.

Diagnosis: Remember, asthma can appear with only coughing without wheezing, because flow rates are not sufficient to produce wheezing. **Don't take chest X-ray of every asthmatic patient unless indicated. Rule out pneumonia, and foreign bodies.**

PFT (pulmonary function test): ↑ (TLC, FRC, RV); ↓ (VC, FVC, FEV1, PFR, FEF25-75).

TLC: Total Lung Capacity.

FRC: Functional Residual Capacity.

RV: Residual Volume.

VC: Vital Capacity.

FVC: Forced Vital Capacity.

FEV1: Forced Expiratory Volume.

PFR: Pulmonary Flow Rate.

FEF_{25-75}: Forced Expiratory Flow between 25-75% of vital capacity.

Treatment: Most important is bronchodilator (aerosols are preferred to epinephrine). If no response, then use aminophylline. Use steroids in severe cases.

44. Most important diagnostic evaluation in severe asthmatic (important): **ABG (arterial blood gas).**

    Early stage of asthma attack: ↓ O_2 **(1st sign)**; (↓ CO_2 ↑ pH) for hyperventilation.

    Late stage of asthma attack: ↓↓ O_2, ↑ CO_2, ↓ pH (both respiratory and metabolic) **indicate respiratory failure.**

45. **Status asthmaticus:**

    It is a severe asthma attack that is unresponsive to drugs that are usually effective.

    Treatment: Oxygen, bronchodilator (aerosols, aminophylline), corticosteroid (methylprednisolone is preferred to hydrocortisone because of its lesser effect on mineral metabolism and its lower cost), mechanical ventilation (if required), fluid therapy (do not overhydrate because of ↑ ADH secretion in asthma); no sedation.

46. Prevention of death in asthma patient: Death is rare, but it is increasing due to **unknown causes.** Death may be due to multiple factors (pollution, lack of education and/or availability of health care).

    Most important is the identification and proper care of high risk patients (ICU admission, unconsciousness from asthma, frequent hospital admissions). Psychosocial evaluation is important. Epipen (injectable epinephrine) can be provided at home to severe asthmatic patient unresponsive to aerosol therapy. But this should not delay bringing the patient to the hospital.

47. Factors influencing theophylline clearance (normal level 10-20):
    a. **Decreased clearance and increased toxicity:** Erythromycin, cimetidine, propranolol, oral contraceptives, RSV infection, cirrhosis, congestive cardiac failure, acute pulmonary edema, chronic obstructive pulmonary disease, high carbohydrate diet, prematurity, obesity, dietary methylxanthine.
    b. **Increased clearance and decreased toxicity:** Phenobarbital, dilantin, isoproterenol, terbutaline, rifampin, cigarette smoking (tobacco, marijuana), low carbohydrate, high protein.

48. **Atopic dermatitis:** It begins in infancy (first 3 months of life) and disappears by 3-5 years.
    ↑ serum IgE level found in most patients.
    Preferred treatment: Local corticosteroid.

49. **Urticaria-angioedema:** It is due to interaction of antigen with mast cell or basophil-bound IgE antibody. It is caused by histamine, leukotrienes, C3a, C5a, bradykinin.
    Urticaria: Erythematous raised skin lesions with or without itching. Usually resolves within 48 hours.
    Angioedema: Deeper layers of skin, subcutaneous tissues, mucosa, respiratory and gastrointestinal tract.

    Treatment:
    Urticaria: **Most effective is hydroxyzine (atarax). It** is the preferred drug for **cholinergic and chronic** urticaria. Next drug is diphenhydramine (benadryl). Steroid has variable effect on chronic urticaria.
    Acute attack: Use epinephrine.
    Solar urticaria: Sun screen lotion.
    Prophylaxis for cold urticaria: Cyproheptadine.
    Angioedema: Only supportive therapy (Danazol used in adults).

50. **Anaphylaxis:** It is a life-threatening ,immunologic reaction due to foreign antigen mediated by IgE.
    Histamine is the most important factor causing anaphylaxis. Other factors are ↓ factor V and VIII, ↓ (C3, C4 and kininogens), arachidonic acid metabolite, kinin, platelet activating factor.
    Signs and symptoms: First tingling sensation around mouth, difficulty in swallowing and tightness in throat and chest, urticaria, angioedema, wheezing, abdominal pain and diarrhea, cardiorespiratory arrest, and death.

    Treatment:
    Acute: Epinephrine, aminophylline, oxygen, diphenhydramine, cimetidine. (Use steroid to prevent recurrence only.)
    Prophylaxis for person at risk for anaphylaxis during contrast study:
    Prednisone and benadryl before the procedure.

51. **Serum sickness:** It is type III hypersensitivity reaction due to foreign antigen.
Signs and symptoms: Symptoms appear in 7-12 days following injection of foreign antigen. Appears with fever, malaise, generalized urticaria, purpura (sometimes) edema around face and neck, abdominal pain and diarrhea, arthritis and arthralgia in multiple **joints. A self-limited disease. Recovery in 7-10 days.**
Diagnosis: **Direct immunofluorescence study of skin lesion** showing deposit of IgM, IgA, IgE or C3.

   Treatment: Aspirin, antihistamines (steroid in severe cases).
Prevention: By desensitization. During desensitization, serum sickness can occur. Methyl prednisone cannot prevent this reaction. Some allergists give epinephrine and antihistamine before desensitization.

52. Most serious complication of serum sickness is: **Guillain-Barre syndrome and** peripheral neuritis mostly involving brachial plexus C 5-6.

53. Adverse reaction to drugs is mostly due to: **Pharmacological effects** (15% due to allergy).

54. **Drug allergy:** IgE mediated and by other mechanisms.
Penicillin allergy: Most dangerous. Anaphylaxis is not due to IgE, but, rather to **minor haptenic determinants** (penicillate, penilloate, penicillenate and its oxidation products).
Ampicillin rash: Not urticarial. Found in patient with infectious mononucleosis and hyperuricemia.
Signs and symptoms: Most common is cutaneous eruption (urticaria, eczematoid lesion), Steven Johnson syndrome, etc.
Diagnosis: Mostly by history; skin test is available for penicillin allergy.
Treatment: **Discontinuance of the drug is the best treatment** (antihistamines, epinephrine in acute cases; corticosteroid in severe cases).

55. **Insect allergy:**
Pathogenesis:
   a. **Local reaction:** Due to vasoactive or irritant material deposit in skin (not due to IgE).
   b. **Inhalant allergy** (systemic): Due to IgE mediate due to foreign insect antigen.
   c. **Honeybee venom allergy:** Due to phospholipase A.

   Signs and symptoms:
   a. Local: Mostly urticaria; others are papular, vesicular, erythematous.
   b. Systemic: Laryngeal edema, bronchospasm, ↓ B.P.
   Diagnosis by history and examination of skin lesion.

   Treatment:
   a. Local: Antihistamines.
   b. Systemic: During acute phase use epinephrine; during chronic phase, use corticosteroid, antihistamine.

56. **Ocular allergy:** It is due either to IgE mediated (conjunctivitis with ragweed hay fever) or

to cell mediate (contact dermatitis).

Treatment:
a. Contact dermatitis in eyelid: Local steroid application.
b. Allergic conjunctivitis: Eye drop (sympathomimetic drop is phenylephrine, cromolyn sodium or, in severe cases, steroid).
c. Atopic keratoconjunctivitis: Eye drop (steroid).
d. Vernal conjunctivitis: Eye drop or ointment (corticosteroid).

Vernal conjunctivitis: Most common in children. Palpebral form appears with cobblestone appearance, limbal form appears with whitish Trantas dots (at corneoscleral limbus due to eosinophil accumulation), which is characteristics of the disease.

57. **Food allergy:** It is either due to allergy, enzyme deficiency, or non-immunologic reaction to monosodium glutamate (Chinese restaurant), tyramine (cheese), nitrite (hot dog).
Cow milk allergy due to:
a. IgE (in some case) mediated.
b. Milk protein allergy (alpha lactalbumin, beta lactoglobulin and casein).

Signs and symptoms of cow milk allergy:
a. **First year of life:** Vomiting, and diarrhea with blood-streaked stool following ingestion of cow milk.
b. Older patient: Occult intestinal blood loss, pulmonary infiltrate.
c. Severe cases: Pulmonary hemosiderosis.

Diagnosis of food allergy:
a. **Elimination of food from diet** for 7 -10 days causes improvement in clinical condition.
b. Reintroduction of food (except in severe reactions) causes recurrence of symptoms within 7 days.

Treatment of food allergy: Elimination of food from diet. (Periodic attempts to reintroduce food should be tried, except in anaphylaxis because tolerance to food may develop later on.) Immunotherapy is **not** effective.

58. **JRA (Juvenile rheumatoid arthritis) (important):**
Five subtypes are:
a. **Polyarticular rheumatoid factor (RF) negative:** It is the second most common type. **90% girls. Symptoms appear any time in childhood. Multiple joints are involved.** No sacroiliitis. Rarely iridocyclitis, RF(-)ve, **ANA (antinuclear antibody) found in 25%.** No HLA. Ultimately **develops serious arthritis in only 10-15% of the cases.**
b. **Polyarticular RF positive:** Least common type. **80% girls. Multiple joints are involved.** Symptoms appear in late childhood. Rarely sacroiliitis. No eye involvement. **RF(+)ve 100%. ANA (+)ve 75%. HLADR4. Ultimate severe arthritis develops in >50% of cases.**
c. **Pauciarticular type I: Most common type. 80% girls.** Symptoms appear in **early** childhood in a **few large joints (knee, ankle, elbow).** No sacroiliitis, **most common**

is chronic iridocyclitis (30%), RF(-)ve. ANA(+)ve 90%. HLA DR5, DRW6, DRW8. Ultimately **ocular damage develops (10%), polyarthritis (20%)**.

d. **Pauciarticular type II: 90% boys.** Symptoms appear **late childhood. Affects a few** large joints (hip). **Sacroiliitis, acute iridocyclitis (10-20%). RF and ANA (-)ve. HLA B27 Ultimately spondyloarthropathy develops.**

e. **Systemic onset: 60% boys;** symptoms appear **throughout** childhood; **multiple** joints; absent (sacroiliitis and iridocyclitis); RF and ANA(-)ve; ultimately severe arthritis develops in 25% of cases.

59. **These are very important points in JRA:**
   a. HLA B27: Pauciarticular type II.
   b. Acute iridocyclitis: Pauciarticular type II.
   c. Chronic iridocyclitis: Pauciarticular type I.
   d. Spondyloarthropathy: Pauciarticular type II.
   e. Poorest prognosis: severe arthritis:
      Polyarticular RF(+)ve.
   f. Sacroiliitis: Pauciarticular type II.
   g. RF(+)ve only: Polyarticular RF(+)ve type.
   h. ANA(+)ve: Polyarticular RF(+)ve, RF(-)ve, pauciarticular type I.
   i. Reiter's disease: Pauciarticular type II (may represent).
   j. Resemble adult type: Polyarticular RF(+)ve or (-)ve.
   k. Large joints: Pauciarticular (type I and II).
   l. Mostly boys: Pauciarticular type II, systemic onset.

   Most common clinical manifestation of **JRA (systemic type).**
   Arthritis, arthralgia, high intermittent fever (100%); next rheumatoid rash, ↑ (liver, spleen, lymph nodes), ↑ WBC, delayed chronic arthritis, pleuritis, pericarditis.

60. Treatment for JRA:
   a. **Aspirin (acetylsalicylic acid) is thr preferred drug.**
   b. Tolmetin, naprosyn (nonsteroidal anti-inflammatory agent).
   c. Indication of corticosteroid use: Severe, systemic disease unresponsive to salicylate, myocarditis, pericarditis, iridocyclitis.
   d. Experimental drug is methotrexate.
   e. Physical, and occupational therapy and psychosocial support.
   f. **Iridocyclitis:** Refer to eye doctor. Topical use of steroid and dilating agent. If these fails give systemic steroid or subconjunctival injection.

61. **Non-rheumatic arthritis.**

   Diagnosis confirmed by:
   a. Septic arthritis: Isolation of organism in joint fluid.
   b. Lyme disease: Serologic. (Organism B. burgdorferi.)
   c. Osteomyelitis: Isolation of organism in blood, bone, bone scan (early), X-ray (late).
   d. Viral arthritis: Clinical, serologic or viral culture (symptomatic treatment).
   e. Genetic: Recognize the genetic syndrome/condition.
   f. Psychogenic: Clinical. (Treat with reassurance.)
   g. Childhood malignancy: Bone marrow biopsy. (Treat the malignancy.)

62. **Ankylosing spondylitis.**
    Characteristics of the disease:
    a. Involves sacroiliac joints and lumbosacral spine.
    b. Occurs mostly in males.
    c. RF and rheumatoid nodule are absent.
    d. Associated with HLAB27 and acute iridocyclitis.
    e. Aortitis causing aortic insufficiency (AI).
    f. Positive family history.
    All of the above factors differentiate it from rheumatoid arthritis.
    Treatment: **Acetylsalicylic acid (aspirin) is the preferred drug;** physical therapy.

63. **Reiter disease: HLA B27,** pauciarticular arthritis, sacroiliitis, sterile urethritis, eye abnormality, mostly in **males.** It occurs after infection **with shigella, yersinia, campylobacter, chlamydia.**
    Treatment: Salicylate or other nonsteroidal anti-inflammatory agent.
    Prognosis: Patient usually recover. Disease may recur. It rarely causes destructive arthritis.

64. **SLE (systemic lupus erythematosus):**
    Drugs causing lupus-like disease: Hydralazine, procainamide, sulfonamides, anticonvulsants. Drug-induced lupus is mild and reversible with withdrawal of drugs.
    Etiology: Unknown; it is probably due to altered immune regulation, probably genetically determined. Viruses may have some role. Mostly found in females after 8 years of age.
    Signs and symptoms: Most commonl symptoms are fever, malaise, rash, arthritis, and arthralgia. **Butterfly rash** (bluish or erythematous scaly) in malar areas over the bridge of the nose (isolated cutaneous discoid lupus is rare in children).

    Raynaud phenomenon (Triad): Vasospasm causing ischemia of the distal phalanges, then anoxic cyanosis then reactive hyperemia. It is symmetric, painful and induced by cold or emotional upset.
    Polyserositis (pericarditis, pleurisy, peritonitis): These are characteristic and cause pain in the chest and abdomen. Myocardial infarctions may occur in children and cause death.
    Heart: Endocarditis, myocarditis, pericarditis.
    Lung: Pneumonia, pulmonary bleeding, fibrosis.
    G.I.: Vasculitis causing infarction in bowel, diarrhea, vomiting.
    CNS: **Psychosis,** personality change, cerebrovascular accidents, neuritis, **convulsions.**

    Renal: Class II, and III are mild (mild hematuria and proteinuria, normal renal function). Class IV and some of III are severe forms (reduced renal function, hematuria, proteinuria, nephrotic syndrome, acute renal failure).
    Class V is mild-to-moderate type causing nephrotic syndrome.
    Remember, type IV is the most common and most severe.
    Type IV is diffuse ,proliferative nephritis.
    III is focal proliferative.
    II is mesangial lupus nephritis.
    I is no change and
    V is membranous.

65. **Diagnosis, treatment, and prognosis of lupus:**

a. **Diagnosis: It is confirmed** by demonstrating that circulating ANA (antinuclear antibody) reacts with double-stranded native DNA **(anti-DNA is specific for lupus).** Serum: ↓ C3 and C4; (+)ve Coombs' test, antiplatelet antibody. CBC: ↓ (WBC, platelet, RBC, lymphocyte).
b. Treatment:
    i. **Prednisone.**
    ii. In severe diseases, add azathioprine.
c. Prognosis: Improves with therapy. Patient needs medical and psychological support.

66. **Neonatal lupus phenomena:** It is very rare.
It occurs when the mother has an active or subclinical or other rheumatic syndrome like Sjogren syndrome. **Remember, it is associated with a maternal antibody to Ro/SSA or La/SSB. Most newborns are asymptomatic, but** have (+)ve ANA and maternal autoantibody in infants blood. **Most frequently manifested clinically with rash (trunk, extremities,** face) which usually fades over several months.

Heart: Most children with congenital heart block have mothers with antibody to Ro/SSA or La/SSB. Mother may not have clinical disease, **so for any child with congenital heart block, antibody test should be done on both baby and the mother.** Heart may be damaged permanently. Exact cause is **unknown,** but may be due to fibrosis, deposition of immunoglobulin, endocardial fibroelastosis.
Prognosis: May develop SLE as an adult age.

67. **Henoch-Schonlein purpura (anaphylactoid purpura): It is a nonthrombocytopenic purpura. Etiology: Unknown, clinical manifestations are due to vasculitis.**

Signs and symptoms: It is proceeded by URI or Streptococcal infection. Most obvious presentation is erythematous maculopapular lesion on the skin mostly over lower extremities and buttocks. It initially blanches on pressure, but this feature disappears later on.
Joints: Arthritis in bigger joints (knee, ankle).
G.I.: Colicky abdominal pain, occult blood, hematemesis; submucosal edema and hemorrhage causes narrowing and decreased gastrointestinal motility.
Renal: Hematuria, and proteinuria (which is reversible).
Diagnosis made clinically by rash, arthritis, G.I and renal manifestations.
Serum: ↑ IgA (50% cases); RF, ANA, complements are all normal.
CBC: ↑ ESR, → platelet, ↑ (eosinophil and WBC).
Treatment:
a. Nonspecific therapy.
b. Salicylate for arthritis, and fever.
c. Corticosteroid only for serious cases like intestinal bleeding, intussusception, perforation, CNS manifestations.

68. **Kawasaki disease** (mucocutaneous lymph node syndrome): Mostly occurs < 5 years of age, etiology is **unknown.** The role of a retrovirus or rickettsia has not been established.

Signs and symptoms: Fever for at least 5 days, non purulent conjunctivitis in both eyes, strawberry tongue, infected and dry fissured lip, oropharyngeal mucosal

lesion; edema, erythema and desquamation of hands and feet, polymorphic rash on the trunk, cervical lymphadenopathy.

Diagnosis: Usually made clinically.

Most important diagnostic test is echocardiogram showing coronary artery dilation or aneurysm.

Blood: ↑ ESR, ↑ C reactive protein.

Serum: RF and ANA (-)ve.

LFT: Mildly ↑ (bilirubin, SGOT, SGPT).

Treatment:

a. I.V. Gamma globulin (2g/kg): single dose over 10-12 hours. It can prevent coronary artery disease if given within first 10 days of life.

b. Salicylate: initially a high dose, then low dose maintenance therapy until coronary artery disease resolves.

c. Don't give corticosteroid.

d. Thrombolysis with streptokinase: use for active phase of coronary artery thrombosis.

e. Aortocoronary artery bypass surgery in coronary artery occlusion > 75%.

Prognosis: Recovery is complete without coronary artery disease, rarely recur. It can cause aneurysm of vessels other than coronary.

69. Polyarteritis nodosa is associated with: **Hepatitis B antigen, Streptococcal** infection, otitis media.

Polyarteritis nodosa: It causes inflammation of medium and small size arteries.

Etiology: Unknown.

Signs and symptoms: Fever, weight loss, lethargy, arthralgia and arthritis, myalgia and myositis, skin (erythematous rash, petechiae, purpura, nodular lesion, livido reticularis), peripheral neuropathy, abdominal pain, bleeding and ulceration; renal (hematuria, proteinuria, renal failure, death); CNS (stroke, seizure, encephalitis); coronary artery (myocardial infarction, heart failure); orchitis and epididymitis.

Diagnosis by clinical picture and tissue biopsy.

Serum: ↑ ESR, ↑ CRP.

Treatment:

a. Corticosteroid is the drug of choice.

b. Steroid resistent: Use cyclophosphamide.

Prognosis: Poor, death due to renal, cardiac, G.I. or CNS disease.

70. **Dermatomyositis:**

Etiology: Unknown, but cellular immune mechanism may be responsible for the disease. It occurs between 8-9 years (rarely before 2 years).

Signs and symptoms: Gradual onset, **proximal muscles myositis and weakness of** the extremities and trunk, awkward gait, Gower sign present, non-pitting edema, palatorespiratory muscles involvement causing regurgitation and respiratory difficulty.

Heart: Conduction defect and myocarditis.

* **Skin:** Heliotrope (violaceous erythema) on upper eyelid, periorbital and facial edema, butterfly rash like SLE, tight and glossy skin, extensor skin surface of joints are involved.

G.I.: Abdominal pain, melena, perforation.
Lung: Hemorrhage, interstitial disease.
Eye: Iritis, retinitis.
Soft tissue: Calcification due to calcium deposition.
Diagnosis confirmed by EMG with clinical pictures. Biopsy is helpful, but not required.
Serum: ↑ (CPK, aldolase, LDH, SGOT).

Treatment:
a. Corticosteroid is the preferred drug.
b. Management of respiratory and swallowing difficulty.
c. Physical therapy.
Prognosis: Good if treated early.
* **Late complication:** Lipodystrophy with insulin resistance and hyperandrogenism.

71. **Erythema nodosum:**
It is painful, indurated, red shiny, elevated nodule, mostly found over the shins.
Streptococcal infection (in USA) acts as a stimulus; erythema nodosum is also found in sarcoidosis, cat scratch disease, E-B virus, histoplasmosis.
Treatment: Salicylate is enough. (Steroid is not required.)
Prognosis: Good. A self-limited disease.

72. Neonatal fever, rash, and arthropathy syndrome: Rare disease, present in first week of life with maculopapular rash, high intermittent fever, meningoencephalitis, **progressive mental retardation,** chronic iridocyclitis, ↑ liver, spleen and lymph nodes, **prominent forehead.**
Etiology: Unknown.

Treatment:
a. Nonsteroidal anti inflammatory agent.
b. Physical therapy.

73. **Sjogren syndrome:** It is a rare and chronic inflammatory autoimmune disease.
Signs and symptoms:
Eyes: Photophobia, burning, blurred vision, itching.
Painless parotid (one or both sides) swelling.
Pneumonia, decreased taste sensation, angular cheilitis.
It can develop lymphoid malignancy.
Diagnosis: Clinical and biopsy (lip or glands) showing lymphocytic infiltration.
Treatment: Symptomatic (artificial tears), corticosteroid only in severe cases.

74. **Scleroderma (hard skin):**
Etiology: Unknown, mostly affects girls occurs with unpredictable slow progression or remission.

Signs and symptoms:
Morphea (focal patch) and linear scleroderma: **First signs** are patchy lesions in skin and subcutaneous tissue, pain or prickly sensation, fibrosis and scarring.

Good prognosis.

Systemic scleroderma: Always present with **Raynaud phenomenon** which may be the first clinical sign, skin (symmetric changes in extremities with induration, pigmentation, telangiectasia), small joints synovitis, aspiration from pneumonia due to esophageal dysfunction, high B.P. Also involves heart, lung, kidney, and G.I. tract.
Diagnosis is made by clinical features.
Serum: → ESR; RF and ANA is present.

Treatment: Nonspecific.
a.   Cutaneous lesion: Topical corticosteroid.
b.   Acute edematous state: Oral corticosteroid is helpful, but it does not help in any condition of scleroderma.
c.   Vigorous physical therapy.
d.   Excision of local patches does not arrest the disease.

SPORTS

1.   History of **hyperpyrexia,** lack of sweating, **convulsions,** disorientation:
Diagnosis: **Heat stroke** (due to thermoregulatory failure and dehydration). This is an **emergency situation.**
Treatment: **Reduce temperature immediately,** ensure acclimatization.

History of exhaustion, **high rectal temperature,** hypohydration, flushed skin, reduced sweating.
Diagnosis: Heat exhaustion (water depletion variety).
Treatment: Hydration.

History of exhaustion, **nausea, vomiting,** muscle cramps (due to low sodium), **normal temperature, gradual** onset:
Diagnosis: Heat exhaustion (salt depletion variety).
Treatment: Electrolyte.

History of **syncope** in upright position (rest or exercise), **high rectal temperature and pallor:**
Diagnosis: Heat syncope (due to peripheral vasodilatation and hypotension).
Treatment: Hydration.

History of **cramps** (due to low sodium), muscle spasm, **normal temperature:**
Diagnosis: Heat cramps (due to hyponatremia).
Treatment: Electrolytes.

2.   **Diabetic patient and sports:** Exercise is a very important part of treatment. Food should be given before, during (maybe), and after exercise. (Example: snacks are raisins, glucose

tablets, sugar cubes, candy).
During exercise **reduce the insulin doses** by 10-15%, even up to 50% in long run.
Injection of insulin in abdomen prevent excessive release of insulin during exercise.

3. **Diabetic patients and growth:** Well-controlled patients should have normal growth and development.

4. **Mentally retarded patients and sports:** All should engage in **noncompetitive sports.**
Individual or dual sports are better than team sports.

5. **Musculoskeletal disorder and sports:** Decision cannot be based on X-ray or history alone, but should be individualized.

Osgood-Schlatter's disease and sports:
Acute: Mild or no sports.
Chronic: Mild or moderate sports.

Rheumatic fever and sports:
Complete recovery without medicine: Moderate to severe activity.
Complete recovery with salicylate: Mild to moderate activity.
Minimal or moderate crippling: Mild to moderate activity.

Hip disorders (congenital subluxation, leg perthes, slipped capital femoral epiphysis) and sports:
Mild deformity: Moderate to severe exercise.
Moderate deformity: Mild to moderate exercise.
Severe deformity: No or mild exercise.
Swimming and non-weight-bearing activities (e.g., bicycle) are allowed.

6. **Exercise-induced asthma or asthmatic on theophylline: Either cromolyn or beta adrenergic aerosols** (salbutamol, metaproterenol, isoproterenol) should be given.
Asthmatic should do sports like any other child. No limitation of exercise.

7. **Fluid therapy and exercise:** 10-year-old child with intense exercise in hot summer day produces more than 400 cc of sweat per hour (or 350 cc/m²/hour), so 3 to 4 hours of exercise can cause **hypohydration. He should drink cold plain water** every 15 minutes or each 5 km in marathon. Commercial drinks have nothing special to contribute. **Cold water** quenches thirst and empties the stomach quickly. On the other hand, glucose water causes abdominal distension and stasis.

8. **Epilepsy and sports:** Epileptics are encouraged to engage in **non-contact sports.**
Children with generalized convulsions (well-controlled) may participate in contact sports.
There is no evidence that repeated head impacts in football worsen seizure activity.
Boxing is never recommended for any child (even non epileptic).
No gymnastic activities are allowed (e.g., rope climbing, parallel bar, ring, balance beam).
Allow swimming under supervision.
Allow skiing, bicycle as for normal children.

9.   **Spondylolisthesis and sports:**

Asymptomatic: Moderate to vigorous exercise, but no gymnastics.
Symptomatic: Back support and corrective exercise.

10.   **Spinal disease and sports:**

Mild scoliosis (30 degree): Asymptomatic; allow sports, swimming is good.
Skeletal immature child: Weight lifting should be < 10 lbs.

Bench pressing up to 50% of body weight.
Machine exercise up to 15% of body weight.
Excessive weight lifting causes hypertension and **spinal deformity.**

11.   **Eye injury in sports: Most common is due to racquet ball, not** tennis ball. Sports are
responsible for 48% of hyphema (blood in anterior chamber). Most eye injuries are beyond
the competence of pediatricians, so the general rule is **to patch the eye and refer patient
to ophthalmologist.**
Foreign body in conjunctiva: Use sterile cotton tip applicator.
Foreign body in cornea: Don't use anything because cornea is **very sensitive.**

12.   **Sports rules and problems:**

a.   **Counseling is the first step** in sports medicine.
b.   At 6 years, the child **begins to play and compare himself to others** in both skills
       and ability.
c.   At 10 years, child begins to **play contact sports.**
d.   **Every handicapped child should play sports.**
e.   For extraordinary athlete, **no special** care is needed.
f.   Sports can undermine academic performance.
g.   Boys and girls can play sports together up to prepubertal age.
h.   **Football is most injurious of sports.**
i.   In case of **stress, withdraw the adult pressure** rather than the child from sports.
j.   Parents **should not coach** their child even if they are excellent athletes.
k.   During rapid growth, **epiphyseal plate injury is** highest (like the ligament injury).
l.   **Hgb and Hct are low in 5 to 15%** of athletes, but measuring these is not needed for
       a health evaluation that determines fitness for participation in sports.
m.   Routine annual physical should be superficial because of poor cost/benefit ratio, but
       thorough health check up should be done every 3-4 years.
n.   Muscle strength peaks 1 year after PHV (peak height velocity).
o.   Boys attain PHV 2 years after girls.

13.   Most common nerve injury: Pinched cervical nerve.

High school student with spinal cord injury:
55%:   Quadriplegic.
19%:   Paraplegic.

14. In 'burning hand syndrome', site of injury: **Cervical central cord injury** (most likely will resolve spontaneously).

15. **Composition of sweat:**
    Na 40 to 80 mEq/L.
    Cl 30 to 60 mEq/L.
    K, Ca, Mg $\geq$ 5 mEq/L.

16. **Cardiac problem and sports:**

    a. Almost 85% of young athletes have **ejection type** of murmur.
    b. Patient with MVP (mitral valve prolapse) should have stress test done before engaging in sports to rule out arrythmia.
    c. Mild hypertension: No restriction of sports.
    d. Moderate hypertension: Do maximum exercise stress test to see the B.P. and EKG changes. If they are normal, then sports are allowed.
    e. Severe hypertension: No sports allowed.
    f. Patient with ectopic beat, that does not disappear after mild exercise should have maximum exercise stress test and EKG changes.
    g. Limitation of sports can cause psychological trauma, unlike the leniency of permitting participation.

17. Most common site of head injury in young athlete: **Subarachnoid bleed.**
    Post-traumatic seizure is mostly due to: Local head trauma (cortical contusion/hematoma) seizure occurs in 2.6% cases.

18. **Severity of head injury and epilepsy:**
    Epilepsy develops in 7.4% of severe injuries;
    1.6% of moderate injuries;
    0.2% of mild injuries;

19. Most common type of neck injury: **Cervical sprain.**

FLUID AND ELECTROLYTES

1. Dehydration and fluid shifting:

	ECF	ICF
Isonatremic	↓↓	↓
Hyponatremic	↓↓↓	↑
Hypernatremic	↑	↓↓

2. **Different types of dehydration (Important):**
Isonatremic dehydration:
Proportionate loss of Na and water, but patient usually receives by mouth both salt and water proportionately. Patient is symptomatic because of more ECF loss than ICF, and after replacement fluid therapy, ECF recovery is more than ICF recovery.
e.g.,: acute gastroenteritis.

Hyponatremic dehydration:
Proportionate loss of Na and water, but replacement fluid (given by caretaker or physician) contains only water or glucose water. **Loss of Na in ECF causes water to move from ECF to ICF, resulting in more ECF fluid loss, thus causing greater degree of circulatory disturbances, so patient is more symptomatic than in any other type of dehydration.** Degree of K loss is slower than Na loss, which is why osmotic gradient moves water from ECF to ICF.
e.g.,: diarrheal diseases, gastrointestinal fluid loss by drainage (NG tube, gastrostomy, ileostomy, colostomy etc). So, replacement fluid should contain Na.

Hypernatremic dehydration:
It is due to water loss (low intake or more excretion) or sodium gain (increased intake or and less excretion) or both, resulting **in high Na in ECF causing water to move into ECF from ICF, resulting in an increased ECF and decreased ICF volume. Clinical recognition of dehydration is difficult due to increase ECF volume.** Most common presentation is dehydration. **Rapid correction of fluid causes convulsion because water enters rapidly into cerebral cells causing cellular swelling and convulsion, so correction should be done over 48 hours.**

Factors which stimulate high insensible water losses:
High body temperature, high environmental temperature, low humidity, hyperventilation, premature babies with greater surface area than body weight.
In hypernatremia, kidney cannot handle high solute load. **Most important defense mechanism is 'thirst.' Patient** develops hypernatremia when **'thirst mechanism'** is disturbed which are found in unconscious patient, psychotic patient, small infants and damaged thirst center.

Hypernatremia also develops due to poor solute excretion in the following conditions:
a.   Diabetes insipidus (pituitary or renal).
b.   Immature kidney (premature infant).
c.   Renal medullary defect.
d.   Vomiting and diarrhea. (More loss of water than of Na, except in toxigenic diarrhea such as cholera, certain E. Coli infections, which act on cyclic AMP or GMP resulting in stool water containing high Na and more Na loss. But rotavirus causes malabsorptive diarrhea with low Na loss in stool.)

Clinical presentation of hypernatremia:
Symptoms:

Signs: CNS involvement is almost always appears like **lethargy, irritability,** semi-coma, hypertonicity, hyperreflexia, nuchal rigidity, muscle twitching, focal or generalized convulsion. Loss of common hemiparesis and chvostek's sign.

Skin: **Doughy, velvety-soft** or thickened skin.

Fever: It is either a cause or an effect of hypernatremia.
Blood-tinged vomitus can be found.
In **chronic hypernatremia** (one that develops over long period of time). CNS signs are **absent** except, when serum Na is very high > 175 mEq/L and osmolality > 360 Osm/Kg.
Three mechanisms of CNS involvement in hypernatremic dehydration:

Hemorrhage and thrombosis; idiogenic osmol (or osmoprotective molecule) formation, and the response to osmol formation and response to a depressed calcium concentration in ECF.
Hemorrhage and thrombosis are due to a rapid shift of fluid from entire CNS (cells, interstitial fluid and CSF) into the circulation resulting in shrinking of entire CNS from the cranium and dilation of intracranial blood vessels which causes rupture. CSF pressure falls rapidly below atmospheric pressure when hypertonic solution is infused rapidly and remains low for up to 6 hours.
Idiogenic osmols are **taurine,** aspartate, and glutamate. In hypernatremic dehydration idiogenic osmols (mainly taurine) are produced in CNS cells and **prevent efflux of water from cells resulting in further CNS cellular swelling.** It takes time to form osmols, and the same osmols remain in the cells for a long time, even after correction of osmolality and hypernatremia.

Hypernatremia and hyperglycemia: Hyperglycemia in hypernatremia is due to low insulin (transient effect). Insulin helps in active transport of glucose into the cells from serum. When insulin is low, glucose becomes extracellular obligate osmol causing increased ECF.

Hypernatremia and acidosis: It is due to cellular destruction, causing the release of hydrogen ion, resulting in acidemia.

Hypernatremia and renal function: It causes osmotic diuresis.

Hypernatremia and hemolysis: Destruction of RBC membrane by shrinking RBC.

Hypernatremia and rhabdomyolysis: Rhabdomyolysis causes renal injury in hypernatremia.

3. **THAM solution [Tris (hydroxymethyl) aminomethane]:** It is used in metabolic acidosis when, in addition to that, patient also has CO_2 retention or hypernatremia. In those two conditions, sodium bicarbonate cannot be used because it contains sodium, which will enhance hypernatremia and bicarbonate metabolize to CO_2 which will cause more respiratory acidosis rather than correct metabolic acidosis. THAM binds with H+, which is excreted in the urine.

Advantage of THAM: It lowers PCO_2 (unlike $NaHCO_3$, which increases PCO_2) and rapidly increases the pH.

Disadvantage of THAM: Apnea. It is less effective than $NaHCO_3$ in correcting metabolic acidosis.

4. **Anion Gap (Important)**
Anion gap = Na^+ - (HCO_3^- + Cl^-).

Normal anion gap is 12 mEq/L (range 8-16 mEq/L).
Increased anion gap means more than 16 mEq/L.

Measured cation =	Na^+
Unmeasured cation =	K^+, Ca^{++}, Mg^{++}
Measured anion =	HCO_3^-, Cl^-.
Unmeasured anion =	Phosphate, sulfate, protein and organic acid.

"Anion gap" refers to the difference between the combined concentration of unmeasured anion and the combined concentration of unmeasured cation; former is higher than latter.

Increased anion gap occurs under in the following conditions:
a. Renal failure (due to increased phosphate and sulfate).
b. Diabetic ketoacidosis (due to increased beta-hydroxybutyrate and acetoacetate).
c. Lactic acidosis (due to increased lactate).
d. Hyperglycemic non-ketotic coma (due to increased unidentified organic acid).
e. Disorder of various amino acids and organic acids metabolism.
f. Large amount of penicillin.
g. Salicylate poisoning (due to increased salicylate anion and organic anion due to uncoupling of oxidative phosphorylation).
h. Ethylene glycol ingestion (due to increased glycolate production).
i. Methanol ingestion (due to increased formate production).

Decreased anion gap occurs under the following conditions:
a. Nephrotic syndrome (due to decreased albumin which is anionic at pH 7.4).
b. Lithium ingestion (lithium is unmeasured cation).
c. Multiple myeloma (presence of cationic proteins).

5. **Causes of various electrolyte imbalance (Important)**
↑ **Na (hypernatremia):**

a. Diarrheal dehydration.
b. Diabetes insipidus of pituitary or renal origin.
c. Diffuse renal disease.
   e.g.: Cystinosis, dysplasia, or medullary cystic disease may be due to obligatory vasopressin-resistant hyposthenuria which stimulates nephrogenic D.I.
d. Excessive water loss in infant with diarrhea associates with high solute intake from unmodified cow's milk.

e.   Rarely due to failure of normal thirst control or poisoning with salt.

↓ Na (hyponatremia):

a.   ↑ ADH secretion (due to water retention).
b.   Acute renal failure (due to continued intake of water leads to ↑ ECF).
c.   Nephrotic syndrome in relapse (due to low plasma volume and increased interstitial fluid volume).
d.   Renal Nacl wasting.
     Ex: Low birth weight.
e.   Infant with obstructive uropathy or renal dysplasia.
f.   Spurious hyponatremia (due to hyperlipidemia or severe hyperproteinemia). It is rare in children because ↑ protein and ↑ lipid must exceed 5 gm/dl to cause ↓ Na.

↓ Na in urine:

a.   ↑ ADH secretion.
b.   Renal failure.
In both the conditions; urine contains high urea nitrogen (UN) ratio in urine/plasma (U/P).

↑ K (hyperkalemia):

a.   Excessive intake of k in chronic renal failure (CRF), particularly in dialysis patient.
b.   Smaller muscle mass in children and higher K intake in relation to body weight.
c.   Acidosis or increased catabolism due to intercurrent infection or inadequate energy intake.
d.   Primary hypoaldosteronism and hyporeninemia causes acidosis and ↑ K.
e.   Spurious ↑ K is due to hemolysis by faulty collection of blood.

↓ K (hypokalemia):

a.   Renal tubular disorders.
     e.g.,: Fanconi's syndrome
b.   RTA (renal tubular acidosis).
c.   Hyperaldosteronism and hyperreninemia.

↓ cl (hypochloremia):

a.   Associated with hyponatremia.
b.   Bicarbonate retention in metabolic alkalosis or respiratory acidosis.

↑ cl (hyperchloremia):

a.   Hypernatremia.
b.   Bicarbonate loss in metabolic acidosis, RTA (renal tubular acidosis), some forms of diarrhea.
c.   Retention of H+ (which neutralizes bicarbonate) when renal ammonia production is impaired.
Remember, retention of organic, phosphoric, or sulfuric acid does not affect cl concentration in ECF.

↓ HCO₃- (hypobicarbonatemia):

a.   Acid added to ECF (extracellular fluid).
b.   Hyperventilation causes excretion of carbonic acid.

c. Net acid input exceeds net acid excretion.
d. Bicarbonate lost in urine or gastrointestinal tract.
e. Lactic acidosis.

Remember, ↓ HCO_3 and ↓ pH = Metabolic acidosis.
↓ HCO_3 and → ↑ pH = Respiratory alkalosis.

Mixed metabolic acidosis and mild respiratory alkalosis:
Vomiting and ketosis.

Mixed metabolic acidosis and moderate-to-severe respiratory alkalosis:
Salicylate intoxication (↓↓ HCO_3).

↑ HCO_3^- (hypercarbonatemia):
Increased bicarbonate reabsorption in renal tubule.
e.g., when cl is lost or pH is low by retention of CO_2 in response to respiratory acidosis.

6. **Different diseases and related electrolytes problems (very, very important):**
   a. **Acute renal failure (ARF):**
   Serum: ↓ Na (dilutional), ↑K, ↓ pH, ↓ Ca, ↑ phosphorus, ↑ BUN, ↑ creatinine, ↑ uric acid.
   b. **Chronic renal failure (CRF):**
   Serum: **Na usually → (normal) or ↓ when Na is wasted in urine (requires** replacement therapy) or in hypertension (requires Na restriction); **K usually → (normal) but ↑ K develop** in moderate-to-severe renal insufficiency; **pH is mostly acidotic,** but sodium bicarbonate treatment is not required until serum bicarbonate level is below 20 mEq/L.
   c. **Nephrotic syndrome:**
   Serum: ↑ Cholesterol, ↑ triglyceride, ↓ albumin, ↓ Ca, C3→.
   Urine: Protein 3 to 4 +, microscopic hematuria (rarely gross hematuria), ↓ creatinine clearance due to ↓ intravascular volume causing ↓ perfusion to kidney.
   d. **Pyloric stenosis: (Hypochloremic alkalosis)**
   ↓ Na, ↓ cl, ↓ K,; ↑ HCO_3, ↑CO_2, ↑pH.
   e. **RTA (Renal tubular acidosis):**
   i. **Proximal.**
   Serum = ↓↓ K, ↓ HCO_3, ↓ Ca; ↑ Cl, ↑ osmolarity.
   Urine = ↑ K, HCO_3 (initially ↑ then →), ↑ Ca, ↓ pH.
   ii. **Distal:**
   Serum = ↓ K, ↓ HCO_3, ↓Na, ↓Ca, ↓pH; ↓Cl, → osmolarity.
   Urine = ↑ K, ↑ HCO_3, ↑ Na, ↑ Ca, ↑ pH; ↓ Cl.
   f. **Increase ADH secretion:**
   Serum = ↓ Na, ↓ Cl, ↓ BUN, → HCO_3, hypoosomolar.
   Urine = Hyperosmolar, ↑ sp.gr, ↑ ECF cause natriuresis means loss of Na in the urine.
   g. **Diabetes insipidus:**
   Serum = ↑ Na, ↑ Cl, ↑ BUN, hyperosmolar.
   Urine = Hyposmolar (50-200 mOsm/kg water) with respect to plasma, ↓ sp. gr. (1.001 to 1.005).
   h. **Congenital adrenal hyperplasia (CAH):**
   i. Salt loosing type:

Serum = ↓ Na, ↓Cl, ↑ K, ↑ Non protein nitrogen, ↑ renin, ↓ cortisol.
ii. Non salt loosing type:
Serum = → Na, → Cl, → K.

7. **Acid and base disorders (very important):**
a. **Respiratory acidosis:** ↑ CO_2 is due to pulmonary hypoventilation. That is, CO_2 production is higher than CO_2 excretion. CO_2 is the vasodilator, except in pulmonary vessels. It is compensated by metabolic alkalosis by increased absorption of bicarbonate by kidney. Remember, when CO_2 is ↑ by 10, pH goes down by 0.08.
e.g.,: pH 7.35/PCO_2 45/PO_2 80; when PCO_2 become 55 then pH will be 7.35-0.08 = 7.27.
$CO_2 + H2O \leftrightarrow H2CO_3 \leftrightarrow H^+ + HCO_3^-$.
Management: ↑ IMV rate when patient is on ventilator or improves pulmonary ventilation by any other method.

b. **Metabolic acidosis:**
It is due to the following conditions:
i. Loss of bicarbonate.
e.g.,: Diarrhea, ileostomy, ureterosigmoidostomy, acetazolamide toxicity.
ii. Increased H+ accumulation by cells.
e.g.,: Hypoxia ketosis, lactic and pyruvic acidosis, hyperglycinemia, methyl alcohol ingestion, few metabolic diseases.
iii. Kidney cannot to excrete normal acid load.
e.g.,: Renal tubular dysfunction is due to primary or secondary reason due to shock, Fanconi's syndrome; ↑ NH4 formation in liver, ↓ HCO_3 threshold in kidney.
iv. Dilutional acidosis: It is due to ↑ ECF and ↓ HCO_3 concentration.
v. Acid ingestion or administration.
Some patients with metabolic acidosis have ↑ anion gap.

Sign and symptom: Air hunger with metabolic acidosis.

Treatment:
i. First treat the underlying cause.
e.g.,: Oxygen for hypoxia, hydration for dehydration, fluid and insulin for diabetes.
ii. Maintain the circulatory, renal and pulmonary functions. If they can be maintained , sodium bicarbonate administration is not necessary in most cases.
iii. In persistent, prolonged metabolic acidosis or in cardiac arrest, sodium carbonate should be given. Never try to do rapid correction, because HCO_3- goes into cells slowly, but CO_2 produced by $NaHCO_3$- enters the cells rapidly and ultimately causes more acidosis.

Formula to correct metabolic acidosis:
$NaHCO_3$ = Body weight X Base deficit X 0.3
Infused slowly over at least a 1-hour period.

c. **Respiratory alkalosis:** ↓ CO_2 due to alveolar hyperventilation.

Sign and symptom: Light-headedness, dizziness, numbness, paresthesia, in severe cases seizure, coma.

Treatment: In hyperventilation syndrome, use rebreathing bag. Patient on mechanical ventilator reduces ventilator rate (IMV).

d. **Metabolic alkalosis:**

It is found under the following conditions:
i. Loss of H+, Cl-, K+ from stomach.
    e.g.,: pyloric stenosis, nasogastric drainage.
ii. Bronchopulmonary dysplasia as compensation for chronic respiratory acidosis.
iii. Diuretics (lasix) cause loss of K+ in urine.
iv. Loss of Cl in urine or stool; giving less Cl in feeding.
v. Cystic fibrosis.
vi. Bartter syndrome.
vii. Cushing syndrome.
viii. Hyperaldosteronism.
ix. Licorice poisoning.

Treatment:
i. To treat underlying condition and give sodium and potassium chloride, K+ should be given slowly and preferably orally.
ii. Rarely, in life threatening situation, give acid (ammonium chloride, lysine and arginine hydrochloride).

8. **Mixed acid base disturbances: (Very important)**
    Four types:
    a. **Mixed metabolic and respiratory acidosis is most common type.**
    b. Metabolic acidosis with respiratory alkalosis.
    c. Metabolic alkalosis with respiratory acidosis.
    d. Metabolic alkalosis with respiratory alkalosis.

    a. Both metabolic acidosis and respiratory acidosis **are due to hypoventilation,** which causes ↑ PCO_2 and ↓ PO_2; ↑ PCO_2 causes respiratory acidosis and ↓ PO_2 causes anaerobic metabolism resulting in an accumulation of lactic and pyruvic acid.
        e.g.,: pH 7.10, PCO_2 70 mm Hg, PO_2 45 mm Hg and base excess - 14 mEq/L.
        It can occur in dehydration from diarrhea or pneumonia with diabetic ketoacidosis.
    b. Metabolic acidosis with respiratory alkalosis is less severe occurrence, **respiratory compensation for metabolic acidosis is not very effective.**
    c. **Metabolic alkalosis with respiratory acidosis.**
        e.g.,: In BPD (bronco pulmonary dysplasia), patient has chronic respiratory acidosis with compensated metabolic alkalosis by preventing bicarbonate loss in kidney. Metabolic compensation takes a long time in respiratory acidosis; it does not occur in a few hours.
    d. Metabolic alkolosis and respiratory alkalosis is both rare.

9. **Edema and its pathophysiology:**
    Edema = Increase in interstitial fluid volume.
    Causes of edema:

a. Cardiac failure produces edema by the following mechanism:
    i. Decreased cardiac output causing congestion in atrium which fails to receive blood from the periphery and lungs resulting in both pulmonary and peripheral edema.
    ii. Decreased cardiac output reduces effective plasma volume (which is only a fraction of total plasma volume) and reduces renal blood flow, which activates secretion of both renin and angiotensin, which increases renal vascular resistance and rise in filtration fraction. This imbalance and aldosterone secretion cause sodium and water retention resulting in edema.
    iii. Decreaseds renal blood flow causes neural stimulus, which increases release of aldosterone, which causes sodium and water retention and then edema.
    iv. Slower, humeral mechanism which increases sodium and water retention and then edema.

b. **Hypoproteinemic edema:**
    It is due to loss of albumin under the following conditions.
    i. Loss of albumin in urine.
        e.g.,: nephrotic syndrome.
    ii. Loss of albumin in alimentary tract.
        e.g.,: protein losing enteropathy.
    iii. Less albumin production.
        e.g.,: malnutrition.

c. **Portal vein obstruction:** It causes increased hydrostatic pressure distal to obstruction, causing hydrostatic exudation of protein rich fluid; lymphatics cannot remove those fluids. This results in ascites.

d. **Hypervolemic edema:** It is due either to reduced or absent renal excretion.
    e.g.,: acute renal failure due to: glomerular or tubular damage; or, excessive fluid intake; or, ↑ ADH secretion; or, A-V fistula; or, hyperthyroidism ,or severe anemia.

10. **Site and mode of action of diuretics:**
    a. **Proximal tubule:** Active transport mediated by carbonic anhydrase. 90% bicarbonate is normally absorbed here. Diuretics prevent bicarbonate absorption.
        e.g.,: acetazolamide, which is carbonic anhydrase inhibitor resulting in diuresis.
    b. **Ascending limb of Loop of Henle:** Active transport of chloride normally occurs here, so sodium is absorbed along with chloride. Diuretics prevent chloride and sodium absorption.
        e.g.,: furosemide, ethacrynic acid.
        Both of them cause ↓ Na, ↓ Cl, ↓ K, ↓ Ca.
    c. **Cortical distal tubule:** Sodium is absorbed here normally; diuretics prevent sodium as well as chloride absorption. e.g.,: thiazide group of drugs.
        It also causes ↓ K.
    d. **Terminal distal tubule:** Here aldosterone normally inhibits sodium potassium exchange resulting in ↑ Na absorption; diuretics which inhibit aldosterone cause Na loss in urine. e.g.,: spironolactone.
    e. **Terminal distal tubule:** Some diuretics inhibit Na-K exchange without aldosterone.
        e.g.,: triamterene. (It also causes ↓ K.)

11. **Etiology of hyponatremia:**
    a. **Hyponatremic dehydration:** Reduction of body sodium more than of body water.

e.g.,: Diarrhea losing both sodium and water, but replaced by only water.

b. **Dilutional hyponatremia:** It is due to two reasons.

   i. **Water intoxication.** Patient drinks excessive water without enough salt intake. Patient appears with cerebral swelling and convulsions.

   ii. **Normal water intake, but salt deprivation.**
e.g.,: use of diuretics without salt replacement.
Urine contains very low sodium in dilutional hyponatremia.

c. **Increased secretion of antidiuretic hormone:**
There are two reasons:

   i. **Inappropriate secretion of ADH.** It means ↑ ADH despite normal serum osmolarity.
e.g.,: pain; anxiety; certain drugs; tumors release ADH.

   ii. **Appropriate secretion of ADH:** It means ↑ ADH when serum osmolarity is low. Here urine osmolarity is greater than plasma osmolarity, and urine sodium is greater than 20 mEq/L.
e.g.,: any hypotonic or hypoosmolar state.

d. **Infection:** Hyponatremia is due to SIADH in both acute or chronic infection. Due more to bacterial than to viral infection.
e.g.,: meningitis, tuberculosis.

e. **Edematous condition:** Any conditions can develop edema causing hyponatremia. Urine contains sodium less than 10 mEq/L.

f. **Malnutrition: It** causes asymptomatic hyponatremia, because physiologically body is adapted to low osmolarity. Correction of sodium will not improve clinical condition, or it may develop hypernatremia, so correction is not necessary.
e.g., kwashiorkor (mostly), marasmus.

g. **Pseudohyponatremia: Here** laboratory measured sodium is low, but actual sodium in the body is normal.
e.g.,: when serum glucose is high, it pulls water into the extracellular fluid resulting in low sodium measurement. When serum protein or lipid is present in higher concentration where sodium does not distribute well, then measured sodium will be low despite normal actual sodium.

12. **Fluid management in dehydration (Very important):**
5% dehydration: Present with only tachycardia.
10% dehydration: Tachycardia + sunken eyes, no tears, dry mucous membrane, loss of elasticity.
15% dehydration: Signs of 10% dehydration and shock (hypotension).
Isonatremic or isotonic dehydration: Serum sodium 135-145 mEq/L.
Hyponatremic or hypotonic dehydration: Serum sodium less than 130 mEq/L.
Hypernatremic or hypertonic dehydration: Serum sodium more than 150 mEq/L.

Principles of therapy:
Mild dehydration: Oral hydration.
Moderate dehydration: Oral hydration if there is no vomiting; otherwise; parenteral hydration.
Severe dehydration: Parenteral hydration.

Three phases of parenteral hydration:

Initial or emergency phase:

Fluid amount = 20-40 ml/kg over 1 hour.

Fluid use = 5% albumin, 0.9% Nacl, D10w, Ringer lactate.

Patient with metabolic acidosis saline administration might enhance acidosis by diluting plasma bicarbonate, but it improves acidosis when renal perfusion is increased and hydrogen ion excretion from kidney occurs.

In severe acidosis, **use solution which contains** 28 ml of 7.5% sodium bicarbonate plus 750 ml of 0.9% sodium chloride and 222 ml of 5% dextrose water, so total solution is 1 L. This solution contains Na 140 mEq/L, Cl 115 mEq/L and HCO_3 25 mEq/L.

But pyloric stenosis with dehydration results in hypochloremic metabolic alkalosis. Fluid therapy should be 0.9 Nacl. **Remember, never give K in emergency phase.**

In severe dehydration with poor circulation, use of bicarbonate percussors like lactate [Ringer lactate] or acetate may cause problems like acidosis because they cannot convert to bicarbonate.

Purpose: to increase plasma volume and maintain the circulation.

Indication for using emergency phase:

a.   In isonatremic and hyponatremic dehydration, when degree of dehydration is 10% and above.

b.   In hypernatremic dehydration with shock, i.e., dehydration is 15% and above; here 5% albumin is preferred.

Calculation of Fluid in isonatremic dehydration (5%, 10%, 15%): (wt = 10 kg).

In 5% dehydration (present with only tachycardia) =

(Na = 135, K = 4.0, BUN = 20)

Deficit = 50 ml/kg = 50 X 10 = 500 ml.

Maintenance = 100 ml/kg = 100 X 10 = 1000 ml om 24 hours.

(Ist 10 kg = 100 ml/kg, 10-20 kg = 50 ml/kg, more than 20 kg = 20 ml/kg).

Total = 500 + 1000 = 1500 ml over 24 hours.

Half (750 ml) over first 8 hours = Repletion phase.

Next half (750 ml) over next 16 hours = Recovery phase.

Fluid: D5 water + Nacl (55 mEq/L) + $NaHCO_3$ (20 mEq/L); add K acetate (20 mEq/L) after urine output or ringer lactate. Use of $NaHCO_3$ is controversial.

10% dehydration:

Appears with sunken eyes, dry mucous membrane, no tears, has normal B.P.

Na = 135, K = 4.0,   BUN = 30.

Deficit = 100 ml/kg = 100 x 10 = 1000 ml.

Maintenance = 100 x 10 = 1000 ml.

Total = 1000 + 1000 = 2000 ml.

Emergency phase = 20ml/kg over 1 hour = 200 ml.

Repletion phase = next 7 hours = half of remaining fluid (total 900 ml) that means 128 ml/hour.

Recovery phase = next 16 hours = other half (900 ml) should be given = 56 ml/hour.

Fluid in emergency phase = 5% albumin, 0.9% Nacl, D10w, ringer lactate.

Fluid in repletion and recovery phase = same as 5% dehydration.

15% dehydration (same as 10% dehydration + hypotension).

Na = 135, K = 4.0, BUN = 60-90.

Deficit = 150 ml/kg = 150 X 10 = 1500 ml.

Maintenance = 100 X 10 = 1000 ml.

Total = 1500 + 1000 = 2500 ml.

Emergency phase: first give 20 ml/kg over 1/2 hour. If no improvement, give another 20 ml/kg over next 1/2 hour.

Repletion phase = next 7 hours = half of remaining fluid (total 1050 ml) = 150 ml/hour.

Recovery phase = next 16 hours = other half (1050 ml) = 66 ml/hour.

Fluid = same as 10% dehydration.

Calculation of fluid in hyponatremic dehydration (5%, 10%, 15%) (wt 10 kg).
Calculation same as isonatremic dehydration of the same degree **except the calculation of Na deficit.**

e.g.,:   Na = 120, K = 4.0.

Sodium deficit:

Body weight X (desired Na -actual Na) X 0.6 = 10 X (135-120) X 0.6 mEq = 90 mEq.

Maintenance sodium:

3 to 4 mEq/kg/day = 30-40 mEq/day.

Total sodium requirement = 120-130 mEq/day.

Total correction time = 24 hours.

Fluid in this case = Na 120-130 mEq/day, D5 water; add K acetate (20 mEq/L) after urine output.

Indication for rapid correction of sodium:

Hyponatremic seizure which usually occurs when Na is less than 120 mEq/l.

e.g.,:   Water intoxication.

Tx: 3% solution of Nacl at a rate 1 ml/min to maximum 12 ml/kg of the body weight.

Remember: do not use hypotonic solution.

Calculation of fluid in hypernatremic dehydration (usually 10%; 15%) = (wt = 10 kg).

Appears with doughy skin, irritability.

Always calculate at least 10% dehydration, because recognition of clinical dehydration is difficult due to good ECF volume despite severe intracellular dehydration.

10% dehydration:

Na = 170 mEq/L, BUN = 25 mg/dl.

Deficit = 100 ml/kg = 100 x 10 = 1000 ml.

Maintenance for 48 hours = 1000 + 1000 = 2000 ml.

Total = 1000 + 2000 = 3000 ml over 48 hours.

Fluid should be corrected **equally over 48 hours** = 62.5 ml/hour.

Exception from other types of dehydration in that emergency phase is not required because of good ECF volume which maintains circulation.

Fluid = D5 water + NaCl (30 mEq/L) + add K acetate (maximum 40 mEq/L) after urine output. (Some authorities suggest 2 to 3% of glucose instead of 5% glucose.)

15% dehydration and shock = (Na = 170 mEq/L, BUN = 50 mg/dl).

Deficit = 150 ml/kg = 150 X 10 = 1500 ml.

Maintenance for 48 hours = 1000 + 1000 = 2000 ml.

Total = 1500 + 2000 = 3500 ml.

Emergency phase = 5% albumin 20 ml/kg = 200 ml over 1 hour.
(Albumin is used because of shock.)
Remaining fluid = 3500 -200 = 3300 ml over 48 hours, i.e., 69 ml/hour).
Fluid = same as 10% dehydration.
Remember, serum Na level should not drop more than 10 mEq every 24 hours.
Rapid correction causes convulsions because water enters rapidly into cerebral cells
causing cellular swelling and convulsion.

13. **A few important points to remember in hypernatremic dehydration:**
    a. Clinical hypotension is **not** seen because of good ECF volume, despite dehydration of 15% and above, **unlike** iso-and hyponatremic dehydration.
    b. Because of hyperosmolarity, patient appears with cerebral damage with hemorrhage and thrombosis or subdural effusion.
    c. Seizure is common in this dehydration. Usually found when serum Na was corrected too rapidly during rehydration. Remember, serum Na should not drop more than 10 mEq/L in 24 hours.
    d. Seizure is treated with I.V. administration of 3-5 ml/kg of 3% Nacl solution or by hypertonic mannitol.
    e. Diagnosis of cerebral damage due to hypernatremias by high protein level in CSF.
    f. Prevention of seizure is very important, so undertake rehydration therapy carefully.

14. **Salt poisoning (Important):**
    Definition: Excessive amount of salt intake within short period of time.

    History: A 8-month-old child has had H/O diarrhea for 2 days. Its mother mistakenly gave baby homemade formula with too much salt. Baby shows vomiting, irritability, and stiffening of the body.

    On examination: Patient is tachypneic, but comatose. Hypertonicity, and/or hyperreflexia is present. Skin is dry and warm, but there is good turgor. Eyes and fontanelles are not sunken.

    Laboratory values: Na 180 mEq/L, K= 4.0 mEq/L, HCO_3 = 10 mEq/L, BUN = 35 mg/dl.

    Fluid = Na+ 25 mEq; K+ 40 mEq (after urine output), cl- 25 mEq, acetate or lactate 40 mEq. Glucose is not required because it is associated with hyperglycemia, but 2% solution can be used.

    Treatment: First start I.V. with the above solution. In the mean time prepare for **2 or 3 repeated peritoneal dialysis** treatments. If Na is more than 200, use commercial dialysis fluid (45 ml/kg) with 4.25% glucose for 1 hour. When Na level goes down, use dialysis fluid with 1.5% glucose.
    Exchange transfusion is **not** the substitute treatment.
    Seizure = Use phenobarbital.
    Heart failure = Use digoxin.

    Goal of treatment: **Rapid removal of sodium from the body,** unlike hypernatremic dehydration. Along with sodium, glucose is also high. Rapid removal of Na would cause shift of waters from ECF into the cells, but ↑ glucose will prevent that. Slow metabolism of glucose will hydrate the cells and prevent damage.

15. **Breast feeding and diarrhea:** Patient with mild dehydration and no vomiting is usually treated with oral rehydrating solution for 1 to 2 hours, before resuming the breast feeding. **Patient usually recovers while breast feeding.**

16. **Bronchial asthma and fluid-electrolytes:**
Fluid: It should be restricted due to ↑ ADH secretion in status asthmaticus. Endogenous and exogenous steroids, and endogenous production of water as hydrogen containing energy substrate is oxidized. Hyperventilation, however, increases water requirement due to increase metabolism.

Excess fluid in asthma causes pulmonary edema due to the following three factors.
a. Negative pleural pressure.
b. Increased capillary pressure due to fluid overload.
c. Decreased oncotic pressure.
So, small concentrated urine in asthma patient should not be considered dehydration.

↑ **ADH secretion due to:** Mild dehydration, stress, epinephrine (beta adrenergic drug), decreased stimulation of atrial volume receptor due to decreased left atrial filling from decreased pulmonary blood flow.

Electrolytes: Only maintenance electrolytes are necessary, because steroid causes sodium retention by preventing sodium loss in kidney.

17. **Cystic fibrosis and salt:** Cystic fibrosis patient loses a lot of salt in the sweat.
Tx: ↑ Fluid containing salt, chicken soup, beef broth. Both have high sodium.

18. **Other diseases that may produce ↑ Nacl in the sweat:** Ectodermal dysplasia; nephrogenic diabetes insipiency; untreated adrenal insufficiency; hypothyroidism and malnutrition.
But the level of Nacl in sweat in these diseases are never as high as in cystic fibrosis.

19. **Sports and fluid (Very important): Pure, plain, cold water.** Cold water reduces gastric emptying time, so stomach empties out quickly. Glucose water increases gastric emptying time, so stomach remains distended. Full stomach causes injury during sports.

20. **Fluid and surgery: (Important)**

Preoperative: Patient should have adequate hydration before surgery. Vital signs should be normal and acidosis should be corrected. Adequate amount of carbohydrate, glucose, and electrolytes should be given either orally or parenterally. Oral feeding should be stopped at least 3 hours before surgery.

Intraoperative: When pleural or abdominal cavity is open, there is increased water loss. This should be corrected with volume expander, glucose, and saline as needed. Blood transfusion is usually avoided until there is significant blood loss. No K should be given because K level is high due to tissue trauma and hypoxia. Stress hyperglycemia can occur; glucose infusion should be adjusted. Patient should have good urine output, normal O_2 saturation in pulse oximeter, normal ABG if required.

Postoperative: Fluid intake should be restricted for 24 hours (less than 85 ml/Kcal metabolized) due to ↑ ADH secretion which is appropriate to fluid restriction and volume contraction. Maintenance Na intake should be low due to low calorie requirement during and after surgery. **Most common complication of fluid therapy during and after surgery** is overhydration.

21. **Most common cause of infantile diarrhea: Rotaviruses.**
It is a RNA virus. Infection occurs in dry seasons in tropical areas and in winter months in temperate zones. It is transmitted by hand to skin to mouth and is prevented by meticulous hand washing.
Second most common organism in the infant is enterotoxigenic E. coli which may be the most common cause in older children.

Salmonellae: Most common type in U.S.A. is S. typhimurium. It invades **distal small bowel and colon.** Diarrhea is mostly due to osmotic malabsorption, increased motility, and partly by toxins.
Diagnosis confirmed by culture.

Shigella: Most common type is S. flexneri and S. sonnei. Initially they invade the small intestine, and later the large intestine. Diarrhea is mostly due to toxins and partly to osmotic malabsorption. Shigella toxin can cause convulsions.

E. coli: It has pathogenic and nonpathogenic strain. Some strain can cause invasive and malabsorptive diarrhea. It can mimic mild salmonella or shigella infection. Enterotoxigenic strain release toxin.

Yersinia enterocolitica, Campylobacter fetus: Both are invasive organisms that characteristically cause abdominal pain and mild diarrhea.

22. **Enterotoxin and mechanism of action:**

Enterotoxin causes diarrhea in infant by two major organisms: Vibrio cholerae and enterotoxigenic E. coli. Staph. aureus also produces toxin. The toxin rapidly and irreversibly adheres to GM1 monosialogangliosides in the cell wall of the intestine resulting in formation of adenylate cyclase which stimulates cyclic AMP (3', 5' monophosphate). This causes active chloride secretion and passive secretion of sodium and potassium, ultimately causing water and electrolyte loss.

23. **Most common parasitic intestinal infection in AIDS patient:** Crytosporidial infection.

24. **Most common tumor causing diarrhea in infant: Ganglioneuromas.**
It produces diarrhea by producing VIP (vasoactive intestinal peptide). VIP is also produced in pheochromocytoma and bronchogenic carcinoma.

25. **Congenital chloride diarrhea (Gamble-Darrow syndrome):** Autosomal recessive. It is due to impaired chloride absorption, probably by affecting chloride bicarbonate exchange mechanism. It appears with life-long watery stools with chloride concentration around 150 mEq/L. Early mortality is high.

26. **Mechanism of noninfectious secondary diarrheas:** It is due to maldigestive, osmotic, and secretary process. Secretary process is due to prostaglandin stimulation of adenyl or guanyl cyclase.
Ex: Monosaccharide and disaccharide deficiency (lactase), toddler diarrhea, diarrhea are due to unbound bile acids and fatty acids.

27. **Adrenal hypofunction in HIV patient:** In HIV, patient's **most common adrenal opportunistic infection is due** to **cytomegalovirus** (51%). The next most common is Mycobacterium avium intracellulare (12%), then Cryptococcus species (7%). Addison disease is the result.

28. **Periodic paralysis and K imbalance:**
Familial recurrent paralysis are two types:
    a. **Early onset:** It starts early in life, appears with paralysis while patient is at rest after exercise. **High K level** in the serum stimulates the attack.
    b. **Late onset:** It starts late in childhood, and is stimulated by high carbohydrate intake. **Serum K level is low.**
    Treatment: Give K.

29. **Exercise and ↑ ADH:** ↑ ADH is due to water loss and emotional stress.

30. **Athletic pseudonephritis:** After excessive exercise, the presence of RBC, RBC casts, sugar in the urine is called athletic pseudonephritis.
Treatment: Rest. After one week, urine becomes normal.

31. **Running and hemoglobinuria:** Running on hard surface causes breakdown of RBC in the soles of the feet.
Treatment: Wearing cushions on the soles of the feet.

32. **Exercise in land and water:**
Land exercise: PO_2 and PCO_2 is usually within normal limit.
Swimming and diving: ↓ PO_2 and ↑ PCO_2 commonly occurs due to breath-holding and hypoventilation. ↑ **PCO_2 is stronger respiratory stimulus than** ↓ **PO_2.** In breath-holding PO_2 falls more rapidly than PCO_2 rises.

In normal individual, breath-holding causes no problem, because there is normal physiologic response. **But hyperventilation before swimming and diving should not be done because it causes ↓↓ PCO_2 resulting lack of respiratory stimulation which can cause drowning.**

33. Few important points about patients with liver failure:
    a. ↑ ADH is due to ↓ effective plasma volume.
    b. Hyperventilation commonly occurs which causes respiratory alkalosis and

compensatory renal metabolic acidosis resulting in low bicarbonate in ECF.

c. Encephalopathy is aggravated by shift of NH_3 to the brain due to alkalemia.

d. Prolonged diuretic use causes ↓ K which causes metabolic alkalosis due to replacement of K by hydrogen in cells, so ↓ hydrogen in ECF.

34. A 12-month-old child was brought to the emergency room with history of sudden onset of limp. This required resuscitation followed by a shaking movement of the body, but no seizure. Sepsis work-up was negative.

Serum Na^+ = 140 →, K^+ = 8.5 ↑, HCO_3^- = 13.0 ↓.
BUN: 10.0 →, Cr = 0.4 mg/dl →,
Renin = 0.2 ng/ml/hr ↓, aldosterone = 3.5 ng/dl ↓.
Key finding = ↑ K, ↓ HCO_3, BUN →, Cr →, ↓ renin, ↓ aldosterone.
Diagnosis: Hyporeninemic hypoaldosteronism.

Treatment:
a. **For ↑ K:** Discontinue K in fluid, $NaHCO_3$ infusion, calcium gluconate, sodium polystyrene sulfonate.
Mechanism of action: $NaHCO_3$ = Alkali moves K back into the cells. Calcium Gluconate = Blocks the action of K in the heart.
Sodium polystyrene sulfonate = Releases Na^+ for K^+ (1 mEq for 1 mEq) while passing through intestinal tract.
b. **Specific:** Fludrocortisone.

35. A child with chronic renal failure was treated with vitamin D_3 and $CaCO_3$ tablet to prevent renal osteodystrophy. What is the most likely complication?
Diagnosis: Hypercalcemia.
Signs and symptoms: Anorexia, dizziness.
Treatment: Discontinue the medication for a few days.

36. A child appears with history of sore throat, and fever then develops vomiting and diarrhea with dark brown stool, guaiac negative.

Physical examination: Pale, puffy eyelid, diffuse abdominal tenderness.
Laboratory: ↑ BUN 90, ↓ Na 129.
Hct is normal.
Platelet count is 250000 (normal).

Diagnosis: Abnormal renal function is due to acute post Streptococcal glomerulonephritis.
Differential diagnosis: Hemolytic uremic syndrome:
Presentation can mimic above presentation but there is ↓ **Hct and ↓ platelet count for hemolysis.**

37. **Few important points regarding therapy for dehydration (Important):**
a. **Oral redehydration therapy is always preferred, except** in preterm infant, patient with circulatory failure, and patient with persistent vomiting.
b. Oral redehydrating solution should contain glucose and electrolytes. Amino acids are

better absorbed than protein. Medium chain triglyceride are better absorbed than long chain. Remember, **unmodified skim milk causes hypernatremia due to high solute load, so it should not be used.**

c. Milk, milk products, and food products should not be used for 24-36 hours because it increases the stool volume by osmosis. Gradual resumption of those food products is necessary so that all the needed calories can be provided within 3 to 5 days. **For the first 24 to 36 hours, use oral rehydrating solution to reduce stool volume, but not to rest the intestine.**

d. Diarrhea should be alleviated within a few days. If not, look for serious problem.

e. If patient is on breast feeding, try to continue it. Remember, breast feeding may soften or loosen stool, but not make it watery.

f. Parenteral hydration has been discussed previously.

NUTRITION

1. Fluoride-vitamin given together: It is better to give both together because it is convenient, economical, and equally effective (i.e., no difference from their being given separately).

2. Best way to give fluoride: Empty stomach (100% biovailability), between meals, at bedtime. It not only helps in active mineralization of bone and teeth, but also prevents caries.

3. Best indicator for dietary fluoride intake: Fluoride concentration in drinking water. For infants major source of fluoride is formula mixed with fluoride.

4. Effect of foods on teeth: Among all sugars, sucrose causes most dental caries because cariogenic Streptococcal mutants breaks down sucrose into glucose and fructose, which are polymerized respectively to dextran and levans, these sticky polymers keep bacteria on teeth surface resulting in plaque. Lactic acid, produced from by-product of fructose-levan, dissolves enamel and forms cavities. Starch and sugar together stays in mouth longer than does sugar alone, and cause more damage.
Fats have best results of preventing teeth from having caries by coating teeth, thus reducing sugar retention. Proteins also protect teeth by increasing urea level in saliva, resulting in increase of buffering activity of saliva. Daily cleaning, proper fluoride intake, moderate amount of sugar (no need to eliminate completely) and dental check up by 3 years of age are all recommended to keep teeth in good shape.

5. Vitamin supplement for gum, oral mucosa, and tongue: Proper balanced diet is good enough. There is no need for vitamin supplements.

6. Prenatal fluoride supplementation to mother for prevention of caries in offspring: It has no effect and is not recommended.

7. TPN effects on liver and G.I. tract: TPN (total parenteral nutrition) causes increased bilirubin, alkaline phosphatase and transaminases after 2 weeks. Risk of cholestaisis is

maximum during early phase and in preterm infant.

8. Vitamins in TPN for preterm: Should contain all components of vitamin B, and increased amounts of vitamin D and vitamin K.

9. Neonatal sepsis presents with: Lethargy, hypo-or hyperthermia, hyperbilirubinemia, hyperglycemia, hypertriglyceridemia - last two are due to intolerance of glucose and lipid.

10. Breast milk/colostrum and severe preterm infant: Neither is needed to enhance caloric intake. Breast milk contains secretary IgA, lactoferrin, leukocytes and other substances that inhibit bacterial growth and antigen penetration.

11. Athlete and weight control: Athlete should neither gain more than 1 to 2 lbs/wk, nor lose more than 2 to 3 lbs/wk.
    Athletes should gain muscle mass and lose fat. If they gain more weight, it is due to fat. If they lose more than they should, they lose muscle mass.

12. Food recommended before competition: No food at least for $2_{1/2}$ hours before competition, adequate calories from carbohydrates, take plenty of liquid, and familiar food. Avoid excess sugar (which causes diarrhea), fats, well-marbled meats and rich desserts because they are not easily digestible. Excess proteins and fats causes difficulty in respiration.

13. Iron deficiency in athlete who does strenuous exercise is due to decreased iron absorption. Loss of iron through sweat, urine, stool due to hemolysis.

14. Protein and calorie intake and strenuous exercise: Additional 25 to 45 gm of protein and 600 to 1,200 kcal (i.e., beyond regular daily requirement) per day. (Does not need large amount of protein).

15. In athlete, caloric distribution should be:
    55 to 75% carbohydrates
    25 to 30% fat
    15 to 20% protein.

16. Metabolism at rest and exercise: During rest and less intense exercise for few minutes, body gets energy by aerobic metabolism any exercise more than that results in anaerobic metabolism.

17. Exercise and water: Athlete should drink plain, cold water (up to 100 to 250 ml every 15 minutes). Water maintains body temperature, and transports nutrients and waste products. Water is important for body's biochemical reaction. Best way to monitor dehydration in athlete is body-weight loss (not thirst). If loss is more than 3% of body weight during exercise session, then the advice is to stop exercise and take adequate fluid.

18. Nutrition and athlete: most important is well-balanced diet. There is no need for extra nutrients, but, athlete does need extra water and calories to compensate for water and energy loss.

19. Fat and cholesterol: Should not be restricted during first 2 years of life.

20. Full term infant and formula: In first 6 months infant does not need vitamin and mineral supplements if being given adequate iron-containing formula. In second 6 months it does not need vitamin and mineral supplement if being given iron-containing formula and adequate solid foods. After 4 months, give iron containing formula. Infant who is given ready-to-use formula needs fluoride supplementation, but for concentrated or powdered formula, fluoride is not needed unless community water contains less than 0.3 ppm of fluoride.

21. Full term infant on breast milk: Need supplementation of vitamin D (400 IU/d), fluoride shortly after birth and vitamin B_{12} if mother is strictly vegetarian, and iron supplementation after 6 months in healthy infant. Does not need supplementation of vitamin A, B_{12}, E.

22. Water requirement in infant: Infant on breast or formula does not need water supplementation except in hot weather. Infant on solid food does need water because of high renal solute load.

23. Preterm infant on TPN: In obstructive jaundice, discontinue copper and manganese from TPN. In renal problem, discontinue selenium and chromium from TPN. Cysteine, an essential amino acid for newborns, lowers pH of TPN. This allows more Ca and P in TPN. Ca and P are still not enough for their needs, but enough to prevent metabolic bone diseases.

24. Preterm infants: Should get extra vitamin D (at least 500 IU/day), vitamin E (0.7 IU per 100 kcal), folic acid (50 mcg/day). No need to give vitamin C. Like fullterms, they should get equal amount of vitamins A, K, B_1, B_2, B_6, B_{12}, niacin, pantothenic acid and biotin. Iron (2 to 3 mg/kg/d) supplementation is definite when weight around 2 kg, but if it is given earlier, then vitamin E should be given simultaneously.

25. Newborns on TPN: Usually develop essential fatty acids deficiency in a week's time. MCT oil does not have essential fatty acid, but intralipid does.

26. Toxic effects of trace element:
Chromium: Non-toxic in human.
Cobalt: Myocardial degeneration, polycythemia.
Copper: Wilson disease, liver damage.
Manganese: Neurologic damage.
Molybdenum: Gout-like syndrome, antagonist of copper.
Selenium: Garlic odor, loss of hair-fingernail.
Zinc: ↓HDL, ↑copper deficiency, kidney and CNS damage.
Aluminum : Toxic to renal-insufficient patient due to accumulation of aluminum resulting in osteomalacia and encephalopathy.

27. Deficiency of trace element:
Chromium: Glucose utilization defect.
Cobalt: Not known in humans.
Copper: Sideroblastic anemia, ↓WBC, ↓growth, ↓pigmentation, osteoporosis, glucose

intolerance.

Manganese: Large joints, short broad limbs, spine defect, ataxia, decrease glucose tolerance, abnormal lipid metabolism.

Molybdenum: Neurologic manifestation.

Selenium: Cardiomyopathy.

Zinc: Skin lesion, diarrhea, ↓growth , ↓sexual maturation, ↓wound healing, ↓cell mediated immunity.

28. Only reliable indicator for deficiency of chromium and zinc: Beneficial effect after supplementation of the respective trace elements.

29. Vitamin E is useful to prevent: Retinopathy of prematurity, hemolytic anemia in preterm infant, severe neuropathy in biliary atresia, and muscle weakness in cystic fibrosis.

30. Breast fed infant having diarrhea for several days is due to: Vitamin K deficiency, needs Vitamin K 1 mg I.M. every 5 to 7 days as long as diarrhea persists.

31. Vitamin C in large doses causes: Nephrolithiasis, decreased B_{12} absorption; scurvy in fetus of mother who ingested Vitamin C throughout pregnancy.

32. Feeding recommended in different clinical conditions causing failure to thrive: Cardiac patients with failure need salt restriction; carnitine may be useful in some cardiac conditions. Respiratory patients to lower CO_2 production, dietary fat should be increased 60% of the total calories.
Renal patients restrict protein or amino acid less than 1 g/kg/day.

Hepatocellular disease (e.g., Viral hepatitis): In mild cases, restrict protein to less than 2 g/kg/d; fat and carbohydrate as tolerated by the patient. In severe cases (e.g., Reye syndrome), restrict protein to less than 1 g/kg/d and more carbohydrate (60-70%) of total calories, usually do not tolerate fat.

Obstructive jaundice - same as hepatocellular disease, in addition fat soluble vitamins and MCT (medium chain triglyceride).

33. Toddler diarrhea (or sloppy stool syndrome, irritable colon syndrome or chronic nonspecific infantile diarrhea): Onset is between 6 months and 1 year of age, appears with persistent lose stool, but normal weight gain and normal intestinal morphology. Two categories of patients: those who improve with dietary changes and those who do not.

Dietary history may include some or all of the following: Greater caloric intake than required; intake of large amount of juice or hypertonic liquid; watery stools more in the afternoon and evening; normal stools between loose stools; weight percentile is higher than height percentile.

Patient who does not improve with dietary changes usually has a strong similar family history in parents and siblings. Follow up examination is needed to document weight gain. Gradual recovery over 3 to 4 years is usual.

34. The Feingold hypothesis: There is a probable correlation between the diet containing synthetic colors, flavors, natural food containing salicylates (e.g., apple, orange, grape, plum, tomatoes, cucumbers) and behavioral disturbances like hyperactivity, attention deficit disorder, and minimal brain dysfunction. It is controversial, but hyperactive children may benefit from additive-free diet.

35. IgE-mediated hypersensitivity and prognosis: Children less than 3 years of age will become asymptomatic (44%) in 1 to 7 years, but those more than 3 years of age will remain symptomatic. Infants with milk allergy will tolerate milk (70% to 80%) by 4 years.

36. Diagnosis of food allergy: History will suggest to do the following tests. Skin testing with 1:20 weight-volume glycerinated extract. After skin prick, wheal formation equal to or greater than 3 mm in diameter is a positive result.

    Children older than 3 years - prick test as mentioned above. If negative, then there is no food allergy; if positive, then conduct double blind food challenge if clinical symptoms (diarrhea, vomiting, rash) appear, for that indicates a true food allergy; but if no clinical symptoms that means positive skin test and no food allergy. False negative is rare (<5%).

    Children younger than 3 years - conduct double blind food challenge. If positive, conduct skin prick test to determine immediate type of immunologic response. If open food challenge is negative then double blind food challenge is not necessary. RAST (radioallergosorbent test) - it determines antigen-specific IgE in the serum. It offers no advantage over skin test except in skin with atopic dermatitis. Food challenge test should be done to confirm the diagnosis.

37. Definition in different food-related conditions: Food hypersensitivity or allergy - immunologic reaction from food or its additive due to IgE (immediate allergy within 2 hours) or IgG, IgM, lymphocytes (delayed allergy from 2 to 48 hours).

    Food anaphylaxis: severe reaction due to IgE and release of chemical mediators.
    Food anaphylactoid reaction: anaphylaxis like reaction due to chemical mediators (non IgE).
    Food idiosyncrasy - allergy like symptoms-signs but non immune mechanism.
    Food toxicity - toxic effect due to toxin released from food or bacteria.
    Adverse food reaction: abnormal symptoms and signs due to food and food additive.
    Food pharmacologic reaction - clinical symptoms and signs due to pharmacologic effect from food and food additives.
    Food metabolic effect: clinical symptoms and signs due to the substance produced after metabolism of food.

38. Stop the breast feeding when mother is taking following medicines: (Effects on breast fed newborn are noted.)

    a. Chloramphenicol: Theoretical risk of idiosyncratic bone marrow suppression, so stop the breast feeding.
    b. Metronidazole: Vitro mutagen, so avoid breast feeding.
    c. Fluroquinolones: Not evaluated yet, but stop breast feeding because of theoretical risk

of cartilage development of weight bearing joints. norfloxacin, ofloxacin. (e.g., ciprofloxacin, norfloxacin, ofloxacin).

39. Breast feeding is allowed when mother is taking following medications: Isoniazid (may be hepatotoxic to newborn), tetracycline (may cause dental staining in newborn, but it is poorly absorbed), trimethoprim-sulfamethoxazole and dapsone (some experts do not recommend breast feeding), erythromycin, amoxicillin, acyclovior, aztreonam, cefadroxil, cefotaxime, cefazolin, cefoxitin, cefprozil, ceftriaxone, ceftazidime, clindamycin, chloroquine, quinine, kanamycin, moxalactam, ticarcillin, pyrimethamine, rifampin, streptomycin, sulbactam, nalidixic acid, nitrofurantoin.

40. Vitamins, their deficiencies and excesses:
Vitamin A:
Deficiency: Night blindness, photophobia, blindness, dry skin, defective enamel of teeth, epiphyseal bony defect and growth retardation.
Excess: Increased intracranial pressure, dry skin, painful swelling of long bones and hepatosplenomegaly. Large amount of retinoid used for acne may cause severe malformations in the fetus.

Vitamin B_1 (Thiamine):
Deficiency: Beriberi which includes edema, cardiac failure, polyneuritis, constipation; Wernicke-encephalopathy which includes ataxia and confusion.
Excess: None

Vitamin B_2 (Riboflavin):
Deficiency: Ariboflavinosis; photophobia, burning of eyes, corneal vascularization, growth retardation.
Excess: None.

Vitamin B_6 (Pyridoxine):
Deficiency: Convulsion, hypochromic anemia, oxaluria, rarely peripheral neuritis in patients receiving INH.
Excess: Sensory neuropathy.

Vitamin B_{12} (Cobalamine):
Deficiency: Juvenile pernicious anemia due to defective absorption of vitamin B_{12}. It is also due to gastrectomy, inflammatory small bowel disease, celiac disease; homocystinuria and methylmalonic aciduria.
Excess: None.

Niacin:
Deficiency: Pellagra; deficiency syndrome of multiple B-vitamin.
Excess: Vasodilation by nicotinic acid only, itching, flushing and hepatotoxcicty.
Folacin:
Deficiency: Megaloblastic anemia due to malabsorption.
Excess: None.
Biotin:
Deficiency: Dermatitis, seborrhea.

Excess: None.

Vitamin C (Ascorbic acid):
Deficiency: Scurvy, delayed wound healing.
Excess: Oxaluria.

Vitamin D:
Deficiency: Rickets, osteomalacia, growth retardation and infantile tetany.
Excess: Soft tissues calcification; polyuria, nocturia, diarrhea, loss of weight.

Vitamin E:
Deficiency: Hemolysis in preterm infants, defective neural integrity.
Excess: Unknown.

Vitamin K:
Deficiency: Bleeding disorder; bone metabolic defect.
Excess: Hyperbilirubinemia in preterm infants.

41.   Nutritional requirements:
Water: Infants water content is 70-75% of the body weight.
Adults water content is 60-65% of the body weight.
Infants daily consumption of fluid is 10-15% of the body weight.
Adults daily consumption of fluid is 2-4% of the body weight.
Fullterms water requirement is 70-150 ml/kg/day.
Preterms water requirement is 85-170 ml/kg/day.
Preterms fecal water loss 3-10% of intake, evaporative loss from skin and lungs 40-50% of intake, excretory loss from kidney 40-50% or more.
Water deficiency: Dehydration, thirst, oliguria, anuria, death.
Water excess: Stomach discomfort, water intoxication, convulsion, cardiac failure and edema.

Calories:
Distribution of calories in milk, formula and diet should be: Protein (9-15%), carbohydrate (45-55%) and fat (35-45%).

Basic caloric requirement in infants 55 kcal/kg/day but it decreases to 25-30 kcal/kg/day when patients become mature. When patients have fever, basal metabolism increases by 10% for each degree rise of temperature in centigrade.

Proteins:
Proteins are metabolized to amino acids and oligopeptides. Amino acids are important for growth and repair in different body cells and tissues.
Deficiency: Fatigue, hypoproteinemic edema, malnutrition (kwashiorkor, marasmus), negative nitrogen balance.
Excess: Probably not harmful but certain anomalies in amino acids and protein metabolism

Carbohydrates:

It constitutes no more than 1% of the total body weight, stored as glycogen in the liver and muscles but supplies maximum body energy. Infants liver size is 10% of adult size and muscle mass is 2%, so the glycogen content is 3.5% of the adult's amount.

Deficiency: Ketosis, weight loss.

Excess: Weight gain, inborn errors of sugar metabolism.

Fats:

It forms cellular membrane and supplies second highest amount of energy source next to carbohydrates. Fat soluble vitamins are A, D, E, K. Triglycerides constitutes 98% of the fat and remaining 2% by fatty acids, cholesterol, phospholipids, mono and diglycerides. Liver synthesize transport proteins (VDLD, LDH, HDL). Short and medium chain triglycerides usually digested by pancreatic lipase and bile salts, then it is converted to free fatty acids by cellular mucosal lipase, after that fatty acids pass through intestinal veins to portal vein to liver without esterification to triglycerides or formation of chylomicron. Patients with absorptive intestinal problem need short and medium chain triglycerides.

Deficiency: Underweight, craving for fat.

Excess: Overweight, abdominal symptoms in hyperlipidemia.

Essential fatty Acid:

Linoleic acid and linolenic acid are essential fatty acids because it is not synthesized in our body. Linoleic acid should constitute 1-2% of total dietary calories.

Deficiency: Increased serum level of trienoic acid in comparison to tetranoid acid; dry thick skin.

Excess: Membrane destruction, increase peroxidation.

42.   Vitamins and bacteria:
Vitamin k, biotin and pantothenic acid are synthesized by bacteria.

43.   Maternal concern and child's eating habits:
When the mother develops fear or guilt for child's eating habits then these emotional factors might cause lot of nutritional problems to the child, e.g., mother's concern for child underweight may lead to obesity and vice versa.

44.   Important points in infants feeding:
   a. Mother should be happy and relaxed. Maternal tension cause feeding problems to the baby.
   b. Every infant has its own feeding pattern which should not be compared to other infants.
   c. After the first month of life, 90% of the infant develops 'self-regulation' means feeding amount and interval.
   d. Infant can lose weight up to first 5-7 days of life, but after that they should gain weight.
   e. Weight gains is the most important parameter for appropriate feeding.
   f. Crying does not always necessarily mean hunger.
   g. Compulsive parents do better with specific instructions.
   h. Any maternal questions should be answered properly.

45.   Important points in breast feeding:
   a. Human milk is the best milk.
   b. Less commonly causes intestinal absorptive problems, colic, eczema.

c. Breast milk contains lactoferrin which inhibits the growth of E. Coli bacteria.

d. Lipase can kill Giardia lamblia and Entamoeba histolytica.

e. Infants do not need iron supplementation but they do need fluoride and vitamin D.

f. Infants of mothers with high anti poliomyelitis titres may be protected from attenuated polio virus vaccine but it does not affect active immunization efficacy.

g. There are psychological advantages for both the mother and the baby but mothers should not feel bad if she is unable or unwilling to nurse the child.

46. Contraindications to breast feeding:
HIV, CMV, active T.B., herpetic lesions in the breast, DIC, sepsis, nephritis, profuse bleeding, breast abscess, eclampsia, typhoid fever, malaria, neurosis, psychosis, malnutrition, substance abuse. Erythroblastosis fetalis, herpetic lesions (oral or genitalia), mastitis, retracted and inverted nipple are not a contraindication.

47. Fluoride and vitamin given simultaneously: It is better to give both together because it is convenient, economical and equally effective (i.e., no difference than when given separately).

48. Best way to give fluoride: On an empty stomach (100% bioavailability), between meals, or at bedtime. It helps in active mineralization of bones and teeth as well as prevents caries.

49. Best indicator for dietary fluoride intake: fluoride concentration in drinking water. For infants the major source of fluoride is formula mixed with fluoride.

50. Nutrition (Table - deficiencies):

DEFICIENCY	DISEASES
Zinc	Acrodermatitis enteropathica
Copper	Menkes syndrome
Vitamin D	Rickets
Chloride	Chloride loosing diarrhea
Vitamin B	Pernicious anemia
Fat	Abetalipoproteinemia
Carbohydrate	Disaccharidase deficiency (lactase, sucraseisomaltase, glucose-galactose malabsorption)
Protein	Enterokinase deficiency, defect in amino acid transport (e.g., cystinuria, methionine absorption defect, blue diaper syndrome, Hartnup disease)
Pancreatic lipase	Fat malabsorption
Pancreatic trypsinogen	Protein malabsorption

STATISTICS

1. Null hypothesis: When we compare two groups in a study and notice some differences between them, the null hypothesis may suggest that the observed differences are due just to random variations in the data. If you accept null hypothesis, you think that observed differences are due to such random variations, but if you reject the null hypothesis, you think that observed differences are not due to random variations. Null hypothesis may be true or false.

   Type I (alpha) error means null hypothesis is true, but rejected.
   Type II (beta) error means null hypothesis false, but accepted.
   No error means either null hypothesis is true and accepted or is false and rejected.

2. The P value: P value <0.01 means the result is statistically significant because the probability of random variation alone is very small.

3. Incidence of the exposed and non exposed groups:

Disease (e.g.,: Cancer)		Present	Absent
Exposure	Present	A(80)	B(20)
(e.g., smoking)	Absent	C(30)	D(70)

   Incidence rate of exposed group = A/A+B = 80/80+20 = 80%
   Incidence rate of non-exposed group = C/C+D = 30/30+70 = 30%
   Incidence rate = Only new disease cases over a period of time divided by population at risk, so, incidence means new cases.
   Prevalence rate = Total number of disease cases at a given time divided by total population, so, prevalence means all cases.

4. Sensitivity and specificity: (test of VDRL for syphylis):

	Disease present	Disease absent
Positive Screening	A (90)	B (20)
Negative Screening	C (10)	D (80)

   Sensitivity = A/A+C = 90/100 = 90%
   Specificity = D/B+D = 80/100 = 80%

   Sensitivity = Persons with the disease and positive screening test divided by Number of persons tested with disease (*100)
   i.e., sensitivity of a test means it gives a positive finding when the person has the disease.

   Specificity = Persons without the disease and negative screening test is divided by Number of persons tested without diseases (*100)
   i.e., specificity of a test means it gives a negative finding when the person does not have the

disease.

In syphilis, RPR and VDRL have high sensitivity, so the test can give high false positive and few false negative results, but FTA-ABS has high specificity which gives correct diagnosis.

A = True positive,	D = True negative
B = False positive,	C = False negative

5. Cases Control Studies:

	Liver failure	Normal liver
Alcoholic	(A) 70	(B) 20
Non-alcoholic	(C) 30	(D) 80

Cases = A/A+C = 70/100 = 70%
Controls = B/B+D = 20/100 = 20%

6. Relative risk = Incidence rate among exposed group divided by Incidence rate among non exposed group
Attributal risk = Incidence rate among exposed group minus Incidence rate among nonexposed group [e.g.,. Incidence of the rate of cancer in the smoking group minus the incidence rate in the non-smoking group.]

Absolute risk =Incidence.

7. Mean = Sum of the numbers associated with the observations divided by the number of observations.
Median = Middle number.
Mode = Most frequently occurring number.

8. Probability of a disease condition:

Probability = Total number of times disease occurs divided by Total number of times disease can occur. [e.g., Total premature birth = 60; total RDS = 20. Probability = 20/60 = 33%]

9. Chi-square test:

This test most commonly used for differences between proportions, i.e., comparing effects of two different medications used in two different groups.

ABBREVIATED TERMS

AI	aortic incompetence
ALL	acute lymphocytic leukemia
A-P	anteroposterior
ARDS	adult respiratory distress syndrome
AS	aortic stenosis
ASD	atrial septal defect
AV	arteriovenous
B/L	bilateral
BPD	bronchopulmonary dysplasia
CMV	cytomegalovirus
ESR	erythrocytes sedimentation rate
G/C	gonococcus
GE	gastroesophageal
H/O	history of
IV	intravenous
IVP	intravenous pyelography
JRA	juvenile rheumatoid arthritis
KTW	Klippel-Trenaunay-Weber syndrome
(L)	left
LGA	large for gestational age
MI	mitral incompetence
MPS	mucopolysaccharidosis
MS	mitral stenosis
MVP	mitral valve prolapse
PCP	pneumocystis carinii pneumonia
PDA	patent ductus arteriosus
PIE	pulmonary interstitial emphysema
PIP	positive inspiratory pressure
PPD	purified protein derivative
PS	pulmonic stenosis
(R)	right
R/O	ruled out
SCFE	slipped capital femoral epiphysis
SGA	small for gestational age
TA	tricuspid atresia
TAPVR	total anomalous pulmonary venous return
TB	tuberculosis
TOF	tetralogy of Fallot
TORCH	toxoplasmosis, rubella, cytomegalovirus, herpes
TTNB	transient tachypnea of the newborn
UPJ	ureteropelvic junction obstruction
VSD	ventricular septal defect

DIAGRAMS

In this section we have provided diagrams of both the radiological pictures and of the clinical presentations of different diseases as well as brief descriptions. We were unable to provide diagrams for some diseases, but descriptions were given. Description numbers correspond to diagram numbers. (e.g.,: item no. 1 is the description of diagram no. 1). All the diagrams were placed at the end. (Diagram stands as 'D'.)

Diagram no.   Description

1. Voiding cystourethrogram (VCU) demonstrats severe reflux in (R) side: dilated ureter, pelvis and calyces.

2. VCU demonstrats (L) ectopic kidney: (L)-sided kidney is down to bony pelvis. UTI is a common complication of ectopic kidney.

3. Legg-Perthes disease (avascular necrosis of femoral head): Hip X-ray appeares as flattened (R) femoral head.

4. SCFE (slipped capital femoral epiphysis): usually found in obese children, who complain of pain in knee. Hip x-ray appears as (a) separation of epiphysis from metaphysis and (b) widening of epiphyseal line. (B/L) SCFE is found in renal osteodystrophy.

5. Scoliosis (Clinical or x-ray): lateral bending of vertebral column, which may be associated with MVP (mitral valve prolapse).

6. Thrombocytopenia absent radius (TAR) syndrome:thrombocytopenia, absent radius, renal anomaly. Picture shows an absence of radius (x-ray or clinical presentation).

7. Choanal atresia: absence of opening of posterior nares, patient shows signs of cyanosis which crying usually improves. CT scan will confirm diagnosis.

8. Rickets: Swelling of wrists, bowing of legs, rachitic rosaries of chest wall. In younger children, craniotabes and delayed closure of fontanelle are found. X-ray shows widening, flaring, cupping, and fraying of metaphysis of longbones.

9. Wilms' tumor: painless abdominal mass with H/O gross hematuria. IVP shows distortion of renal pelvis and calyces of that side.

10. Neuroblastoma: distended abdomen; calcifications are noted in X-ray. Adrenal tumor displaces kidney, but VCU or IVP would not show abnormal pelvis and calyces unlike Wilms' tumor.

11. Thalassemia major: enlargement of skull and facial bones due to compensatory bone marrow hyperplasias. Skull x-ray shows hair-on-end appearance due to widening of diploic

spaces and atrophy of skull bones.

12. Intussusception: abdominal colicky pain, bloody stool and palpable sausage-shaped abdominal mass. Barium enema is helpful in confirming diagnosis.

Treatment: If it is not reduced by enema, then surgery is needed. Barium enema shows filling defects or cupping where barium cannot go further.

13. Pyloric stenosis (target sign in sonogram): visible peristalsis of abdomen. Abdominal x-ray shows dilated stomach. Abdominal sonogram shows narrow pylorus (confirmatory).

14. NEC (necrotizing enterocolitis): characteristic abdominal x-ray shows intramural air (pneumatosis intestinalis); dilated loops of intestine; bubbly appearance; in advanced stage of disease, air is noted in portal system and free air is noted under diaphragm.

15. Hirschsprung disease: multiple dilated loops of bowel, but no air fluid level is found in abdominal x-ray. Barium enema shows narrow aganglionic segment with proximal dilatation.

16. Meconium ileus: multiple dilated loops of small bowel; no air fluid level, but bubbly appearance due to intestinal air present in sticky meconium; found in cystic fibrosis.

17. Duodenal obstruction (atresia): Abdominal x-ray shows "double-bubble" sign, one bubble due to stomach air above stomach fluid level; other bubble due to duodenal air above duodenal fluid or contents. It is found commonly in Down Syndrome. There is gasless abdomen distal to bubbles. Annular pancreas can mimic duodenal obstruction.

18. Intestinal malrotation: Due to Ladd bands crossing and compressing duodenum, mimicing duodenal obstruction in x-ray picture. Emergency barium enema study shows undescended cecum. Ladd bands, arising from cecum, obstruct duodenum and end in abdominal wall. Upper G.I. series shows abnormal jejunal position and ligament of Treitz in (R) upper quadrant.

19. Jejunal atresia: "Triple bubble" sign (one bubble for stomach, one for duodenum, and one for jejunum). Bilious vomiting is present.

20. Foreign body (coin) in esophagus:

X-ray anteroposterior (AP) view reveals full coin shadow.
X-ray lateral view reveals edge of coin.
Patient shows signs of dysphagia, e.g., does not want to eat or drink.

21. Foreign body (coin) in trachea:

X-ray anteroposterior view reveals edge of coin.
X-ray lateral view reveals full coin shadow.
Patient shows signs of (a) inspiratory stridor as foreign body obstructs upper airway and (b) wheezing in lower airway obstruction.

22. Gastroesophageal (G.E) reflux: barium study shows reflux of barium from stomach to esophagus resulting in regurgitation, aspiration, and failure to thrive.

23. Hiatal hernia: barium study shows longitudinal gastric folds above diaphgram.

24. Severe esophagitis: barium study shows ragged mucosa which is complication of GE reflux. Infant cries due to pain.

25. Esophageal varices: barium study shows varices in lower part of esophagus. Esophageal bleeding could be complication of ruptured varices.

26. Perforated esophagus: gastrograffin study shows leak from esophagus to mediastinum.

27. Tracheoesophageal (TE) fistula and esophageal atresia: x-ray of neck and upper chest shows coiled NG/OG (nasogadtric/orogastric) tube due to blind upper end of esophagus. Associated vertebral fusion and cardiomegaly due to VSD would suggest VATER syndrome (in VACTER anomaly, 'C' stands for cardiac). (V for vertebral defect, A for anal atresia, TE for tracheoesophageal fistula, R for radial bone hypoplasia and renal defects.)

28. Ulcerative colitis: Barium enema study shows spiculation (ulceration) and loss of haustration in later stages of disease. Biopsy to confirm diagnosis.

29. Crohn disease (Regional enteritis): cobblestone patterns (or irregular mucosas) and thickened bowel with segmented lesions are found in barium studies.

30. Pancreatic pseudocyst: sonogram or CT scan shows large cyst (hollow) over pancreas. Small cyst usually resolvs spontaneously, but large cyst requires drainage.

31. Congenital diaphragmatic hernia: x-ray of chest and abdomen shows presence of intestine (fluid and air-filled loops) inside chest. Most common site is in (L) chest cavity, and heart is shifted to (R) side. (Important for exam.)

32. Retropharyngeal abscess: lateral x-ray neck shows retropharyngeal soft tissue swelling that is more than half of width of adjacent single vertebra, air is present in that area, and abnormal cervical vertebral lordosis is noted. (Important for exam.)

33. Choanal stenosis: narrowing of posterior nares, unable to pass catheter through affected side. CT scan to confirm diagnosis.

34. Acute sinusitis: x-ray shows opacification of maxillary and ethmoidal sinuses. Sinus mucosal thickness more than 4 mm indicates presence of bacteria.

35. Hypertrophic adenoid: lateral neck x-ray shows obliteration of nasopharyngeal air column due to adenoidal hypertrophy.

36. Agenesis or hypoplastic lung: chest x-ray shows small lung volume in that side with mediastinal shift to same side. Lung scan to confirm the diagnosis.

37. Vascular ring: barium study of esophagus shows compression on esophagus by vascular ring. Echocardiogram or MRI to confirm diagnosis.

38. Pulmonary atelectasis (small): chest x-ray shows white uniform density in that area. It is commonly found in (R) upper lobe, but can occur anywhere in lungs. Postextubation atelectasis is common. (Important for examination.)

39. Pulmonary atelectasis (massive): chest x-ray shows complete collapse of one lung with mediastinal shift to that side; compensatory overdistension of other lung is common. (Important for examination.)

40. Congenital lobar emphysema: chest x-ray shows radiolucent (dark) lobe (mostly [L] upper) which pushes mediastinum to other side. Lung volume is decreased on opposite side, increased on same side. (Important for examination.)

41. Pneumatoceles (cyst) or bullous emphysema: chest x-ray shows large cyst with air fluid level or small cyst (dark areas represent air and white areas represent fluid). It is due to ruptured alveoli. It may resolve spontaneously. (Important for examination.)

42. Staphylococcal pneunomonia: chest x-ray shows initial bronchopneumonia, then involvement of whole lobe (mostly [R] side), pleural effusion, empyema, pyopneumothorax, and pneumatocele. Pneumonia with pneumatocele is therefore probably due to Staphylococcal infection. (Important for examination.)

43. Pneumococcal pneumonia: chest x-ray shows positive infiltrate before clinical rales, lobar involvement is common in older children; pleural effusion may be present. X-ray findings may remain positive for up to 3 to 4 weeks after treatment. (Important for examination.)

44. Viral pneumonia: diffuse infiltrates starting from perihilar regions, hyperinflation on both sides. In RSV pneumonia (first 2 years of age), clinical improvement occurs first, followed by radiological clearing. Nonspecific x-ray pictures. Measles causes giant cell pneumonia in nonimmunized or immunocompromised children.

45. Aspiration pneumonia: alveolar (sometimes reticular) infiltrates are noted in both lungs. History is very suggestive. 90% are symptomatic within one hour of aspiration, and nearly all of them within two hours.

46. Hydrocarbon pneumonia: first few hours after aspiration of hydrocarbon chest x-ray is normal, then rapidly develops basilar infiltrates. History of aspiration is suggestive. Patient usually recovers completely by one week after initial sickness.

47. Pneumocystis carinii pneumonia (PCP) (important): bilateral granular infiltrates extend from hilar regions to periphery with hyerexpanded lungs; common in immunodeficient patients. Treatments of choice are trimethorprim and sulfamethoxazole. Pentamidine is also effective, but it can cause azotemia. In AIDS patients with PCP pneumonia, prednisone may be useful.

48. Pulmonary hemorrhage: butterfly white densities in perihilar region. It could be found in patient on mechanical ventilator, post-surfactant therapy. Chest x-ray may be non-specific, ranging from patchy densities to massive densities (white), depending on the amount of bleeding.

49. Respiratory distress syndrome (RDS): fine reticulogranular patterns with air bronchogram. It is found in preterm newborns, and borderline term infants of diabetic mothers, because insulin suppresses surfactant production. Group B Streptococcus infection cannot be distinguished from RDS.

50. Pulmonary interstitial emphysema (PIE): air accumulates in interstitial tissues after leaking from alveoli. Chest x-ray shows signs of multiple areas of black pockets or dots (air) within white lung tissues. It can lead to pneumothorax and pneumomediastinum. It is caused by high PIP (positive inspiratory pressure) and high MAP (mean airway pressure).

51. Pneumothorax: chest x-ray has shown edge of collapsed lung (white) and dark areas (air) of pneumothorax between lungs and chest wall, or between lungs and diaphragm.

52. Pneumodiastinum:

    anteroposterior view of chest x-ray shows dark (hyperlucent) areas due to air in each side of heart border. Air between sternum and heart shadow has been noted in lateral film. In penumopericardium, heart is surrounded by air, including bottom, and patient is usually very symptomatic (tachycardia), which is unusual in penumomediastinum.

53. Chylothorax: mostly due to rupture of thoracic duct during operations. Chest x-ray appears as white dense shadows over pleuras. Definitive diagnosis is made by examining of pleural fluid which has triglycerides in chylous fluid. In pseudochylous milky fluid, there is increased cholesterol.

54. Pulmonary hemosiderosis: chest x-ray may vary from minimal infiltrates to massive involvements. It is due to alveolar hemorrhages causing hemosiderin deposits in lungs.

    Four types:
    a. Idiopathic form
    b. Heiner syndrome-cows milk hypersensitivity.
    c. Goodpasture syndrome-glomerulonephritis.
    d. With myocarditis.

55. Emphysema with Alpha-1 antitrypsin deficiency: overinflated (B/L) lungs show depressed diaphragm.

56. Pulmonary edema: diffuse perihilar white densities mimic butterfly distributions (important). It could be due to fluid overload, PDA, or ARDS (adult respiratory distress syndrome).

57. Meconium aspiration: patchy infiltrates (white areas are collapsed alveoli or consolidations, and dark areas are trapped air), flat diaphragm, increased A-P diameter (lateral film and clinical examination), and coarse streaking of lungs.

58. BPD (bronchopulmonary dysplasia): chest x-ray of BPD appears as complete opacification (white) with air bronchogram or multiple bubbly small lucent areas (air trapped in interstitial tissues) surrounded by white irregular dense areas (fibrotic lung tissues), hyperinflation, flattened diaphragm.

59. Cystic fibrosis: X-ray sinuses shows opacity (white) due to secretions occupying sinuses. Chest x-ray shows increased streaky densities with overdistension mostly in upper lobes. Pathologic findings are initial bronchiolitis (smaller airways) and later on bronchitis (larger airways).

60. Hemothorax: blood is noted in pleural cavities. Chest x-ray has shown white dense shadows in pleura over lungs. It is called hemopneumothorax if air is present.

61. Fracture clavicle (important): broken clavicular bone is due to traumatic delivery.

62. Epiglottitis (important): lateral x-ray of neck shows signs of swollen epiglottis.

63. Dextrocardia with situs inversus: heart is one (R) side, liver is on (L) side, and stomach is on (R) side. R/O Kartagener's syndrome

64. Subcutaneous calcifications: calcium infiltrations (IV).

65. (R) femoral head is outside acetabulum: hip dislocation.

66. X-ray appeared as hyperexpanded (R) lung with mediastinal shift to (L) side (important): foreign body (peanut) aspiration in (R) bronchus causing obstruction resulting air trapping in expiration.

67. Pneumoperitoneum: air is noted between diaphragm and liver. R/O perforation of intestine.

68. Fracture parietal bone (x-ray): linear dark line (not corrugated) over parietal bone. Corrugated lines indicate normal blood vessels. It can lead to leptomeningeal cyst.

69. Hirschsprung's disease: abdominal distension and constipation. X-ray shows dilated intestines.
Barium - proximal dilation with narrow distal segment.
Diagnosis is confirmed by biopsy of narrow segment, which is aganglionic.

70. Lacunar skull (important): X-ray of the skull shows honeycomb appearance, associated with spina bifida, occipital meningomyelocele. It is due to defective membranous bone formation with unknown etiology. Intracranial pressure may be normal, increased, or decreased.

71. Wormian bones: skull x-ray shows small bones between skull bones within skull sutures. R/O hypothyroidism, cleidocranial dystosis, lacunar skull, osteogenes imperfecta or Down syndrome.

72. Depressed skull fracture (newborn): H/O traumatic delivery, skull x-ray shows depressed localized area in parietal bone.

73. Serofibrinous pleurisy and effusion: chest x-ray shows homogenous densities (white) over lung fields, with pleural effusions obliterating costophrenic and cardiophrenic angles. Shift of fluids are noted during clinical examinations.

74. Leptomeningeal cyst: meninges protrude through fracture line.

    Physical exam: Cystic masses over scalp that increase in size when patient cries or coughs. X-ray: Large defects (dark area) in parietal bone.

75. IVH (intraventricular hemorrhage): head sonogram shows blood (white) within ventricle, with or without ventricular dilatation. Sonogram is diagnosis of choice in newborn.

76. Cephalhematoma (Important): CT scan of head shows collection of blood (white) between skull bone and periosteum, but normal intracranial structures.

77. Dandy Walker malformation: CT scan of head shows dilated fourth ventricle due to developmental failure of roof of fourth ventricle. Child shows signs of occipital prominence. Occipital skull transillumination is positive.

78. Arnold-Chiari malformation: herniation of cerebellar tonsils through foramen magnum into cervical canal. Sonogram of head shows elongated 4th ventricle and downward displacement of cerebellum.

79. Aqueductal stenosis: CT scan of head shows dilated both lateral ventricles and 3rd ventricle, but non-dilated 4th ventricle.

80. Pituitary tumor: skull x-ray shows enlarged sella turcica with erosion, which may be associated with calcification.

81. Brain abscess: CT scan with contrast of head shows ring of abscess.

82. Posterior fossa infratenterial tumor: MRI of head shows high signal tumor in cerebellum. Cerebellar astrocytoma is most common posterior fossa tumor in children.

83. Supratentorial tumor: CT scan of head shows calcified mass. Craniopharyngioma is the most common supratentorial (pituitary) tumor.

84. Choroid plexus papilloma: CT scan of head shows echogenic (white) choroid plexus with dilated lateral ventricles.

85. Absent septum pellucidum: CT scan of head shows absent septum cavum pellucidum and dilated lateral ventricles.

86. Agenesis of corpus callosum: CT scan shows dilated 3rd ventricle (middle) and bat-wing appearance of lateral ventricle communicating with 4th ventricle.

87. Spiral long bones fracture (important): it is not necessarily evidence of child abuse.

88. Posterior fossa tumor: visual defects, headache, vomiting, ataxic gait. R/O cerebellar astrocytoma, medulloblastoma, brain-stem glioma or ependymoma in order of descending frequency of occurrence.

89. Vascular ring: barium swallow shows indentation of esophagus due to pressure effects from vascular ring. Inspiratory stridor is usual presentation.

90. Appendicitis:
X-ray abdomen-Calcified appendicolith.
Sonogram- Enlarged, edematous appendix.

91. Mycoplasma pneumonia: Steven-Johnson syndrome may be associated. In early stage, x-ray shows interstitial infiltrate and later segmental distributions. Pleural effusions in 20% of cases. First there is clinical improvement, then radiologic clearing as in RSV.

92. Klebsiella pneumonia (important): lobar infiltrates with bulging fissure are suggestive of this.

93. TTNB (transient tachypnea of newborn): fluid lines in fissures, hyperaerated lungs, flat diaphragm, highly visible pulmonary vascular marking, and (rarely) small pleural effusion.

94. Pulmonary embolism causing infarction: normal chest x-ray. Diagnosis is confirmed either by pulmonary angiogram (invasive procedure), or by pulmonary perfusion that appears as perfusion defects in both lungs.

95. Diaphragmatic paralysis (R) side: elevation of (R) side of diaphragm due to (R) phrenic nerve paralysis.

96. Medullary nephrocalcinosis: x-ray shows scattered calcification over kidney area (at T_{12} level up to L_3 vertebrae and over 11th and 12th ribs). Sonogram shows medullary calcification before x-ray. Excretion of excessive calcium shows white shadows over kidney areas. (e.g.,: Idiopathic, William syndrome).

97. IVP (intravenous pyelography) study has shown obstruction of (R) ureter by stone: prolonged excretion of dye in side of obstruction (kidney shows white shadows for dye in obstructed side).

98. Chondrodysplasia punctata: stippled calcification are found in growth plates. In Conradi-Hunermann type, there are characteristic asymmetric lower limbs.

99. Campomelic dysplasia: most important findings are slender long bones bent at midpoint resulting in skin dimple over soft tissues. Severe respiratory distress is due to narrow thorax and upper airways.

100. Osteogenesis imperfecta (important): broken bones are due to osteoporosis, blue sclera, conductive deafness. Type II is lethal, type IV is least problematic, types I and II are in between.

101. Achondrogenesis I: extremely soft skull bones, very short extremities, small barrel shaped chest, short and square femurs, large head compared to body, and short neck. X-ray shows no ossifications in vertebrae and very poor in skull.

102. Achondrogenesis II: normal head compared to body, short neck, and very short extremities. X-ray: skull is poorly ossified but better than type I.

103. Epidural hematoma: CT scan of head shows hyperdense biconcave image (white shadow).

104. Subdural hematoma:
    a. Acute: CT scan of head shows hyperdense (white) shadow, which is difficult to distinguish from surrounding bones. MRI is more helpful.
    b. Chronic: CT scan of head shows hypodense shadow, which is easy to diagnose.

105. Skull x-ray of sarcoidosis: sarcoid granulation tissues deposit inside skull bones, causing destruction of both inner and outer layer of bones. It appears as multiple, small and large dark areas (radiolucent) in skull bones.

106. Parietal foramen (important): X-ray of skull shows interparietal foramen (dark shadow) over posterosuperior angle of parietal bones. It is normal.

107. Marfan syndrome (important): long thin person shows signs of much larger lower segment (pubis to heel) than upper segment (head to pubis), ectopic lens, long thin fingers (arachnodactyly), aortic insufficiency. Most common morbidity in children is MVP (mitral valve prolapse), which causes arrhythmias, endocarditis, emboli, and cardiac failure.

108. Granuloma annulare: non scaly, annular lesion, raised papular border with atrophic depressed center. (Fungal infection is scaly).

109. Picture of retina shows pigmented spots: H/O gradual loss of vision. Retinitis pigmentosa is diagnosis.

110. Milk bottle caries: most of upper and lower teeth are damaged except lower central teeth which are protected by tongue.

111. Retinoblastoma: opacity has noted through pupil, poor vision, cat's eye appearance in dark.

112. Chorioretinitis: retinal atrophy and pigmentation.
    R/O TORCH infection.

113. Retinopathy of prematurity (ROP): fibrosis and ridge formation in temporal part of retina. It is found in premature infants.

114. SLE (important): butterfly rashes over bridge of nose.

115. Pulmonary arteriovenous fistula: localized enhancement of pulmonary vascularity. Large fistulas may appear in X-ray, but small fistulas can be diagnosed by fluoroscopy (abnormal

vascular pulsation) or MRI. Pulmonary angiogram will demonstrate extent and distribution of fistulas. R/O Rendu-Osler-Weber syndrome.

116. Posterior urethral valve (important): dilation of posterior urethra has been shown in VCU study.

117. Duplication of ureter: double ureter is in (R) side as IVP shows.

118. (R) Ureteropelvic junction obstruction (important): dilated renal pelvis and distended calyces as IVP shows. This is most common of UPJ obstruction in children, and most common etiology is congenital stenosis.

119. Retinal hemorrhage: R/O child abuse.

120. Unilateral intracranial calcification and cerebral atrophy: R/O Sturge-Weber syndrome. (Periventricular calcification is found in CMV, and diffuse calcification is noted in toxoplasmosis).

121. DiGeorge syndrome: absence of thymus is noted in chest X-ray, and there is defect in parathyroid gland, due to field defect which causes embryologic abnormalities in 3rd and 4th pharyngeal pouch.

122. Zinc deficiency (acrodermatitis enteropathica): psoriasiform or eczematous or vesicobulous lesions are distributed symmetrically in checks, lips, hands, feet, and perineum.

123. Staphylococcal impetigo: bullous noncrusted lesions are noted over skin.

124. Streptococcal impetigo: nonbullous crusted lesions are noted over skin.

125. Papular urticaria: R/O insect bite.

126. Urticaria pigmentosa: most common form of mastocytosis. Skin lesions are urticarial or bullous fade and recur in same parts of body until they are fixed and hyper pigmented.

127. Pityriasis rosea: it is a benign condition that may be preceded by URI symptoms and joints pain. First lesion is herald patch which is solitary, round, or oval lesion located over trunk. It is followed by oval-shaped maculopapular rashes which are distributed over skin lines.

128. IgA dermatosis: Central crust is surrounded by Rosette-like blisters; due to deposition of IgA and occasionally C3 at dermoepidermal junction. Initial treatment of choice is oral sulfapyridine or dapsone. If there is no response, use either corticosteroid or combination of all drugs.

129. Incontinentia pigment (Bloch-Sulzberger disease): hyperpigmented (if dark) lesions (either linear or whorled) are noted over body.

130. Osteosarcoma: bony erosions and soft tissues calcification are found in X-ray of long bones. Initial presentation is pain at site of tumor which is missed until x-ray is taken.

131. Lung metastasis in osteosarcoma: chest x-ray has shown multiple areas of white nodular densities in lungs. These are lesions of primary osteosarcoma of long bone.

132. Fanconi syndrome (constitutional aplastic pancytopenia): this syndrome shows signs of absent (or rudimentary) thumb, pancytopenia, increased fetal hemoglobin (Hb F 5-15%), and high percentage (10-70%) of chromatid breaks in chromosomal studies.

133. Maroteaux-Lamy syndrome (MPS VI = mucopolysaccharidoses VI): mimics Hurler disease, but there is no mental retardation. Patient shows signs of coarse face, large head, short neck, short trunk, umbilical hernia, claw hands, and other joint deformities.

134. Methylamalonic acidemia: Patients show signs of triangular face and large forehead. Laboratory findings are hyperammonemia, hyperglycinemia, ketosis, pancytopenia, and excessive quantities of methylmalonic acid in body fluids.

135. Rheumatic fever: acute migratory polyarthritis, fever, rashes, subcantaneus nodules and, later on, carditis, which leads to valvular damage.

136. Midline scalp defect: Trisomy 13.

137. Localized alopecia (loss of hair) of head of newborn: due to positional.

138. Trichotillomania: broken hairs are due to hair pull.

139. Alopecia totalis: total absence of hair in scalp due to maldevelopment of hair follicles.

140. Fungal infection in scalp: localized erythema, scaling.

141. Adhesions of labial minoras in newborn: adhesions are resolved by local application of estrogen cream. Sometimes gentle manipulations are required to separate adhesions.

142. Urticaria: erythematous rashes with whales, itchiness.

143. (L) facial palsy in newborn: patient is unable to close (L) eyes due to pressure on facial nerve, causing edema.

144. ITP (idiopathic thrombocytopenic purpura): superficial bruises with petechiae are noted.

145. Picture has shown microcephaly: R/O congenital TORCH infections.

146. Arthrogryposis multiplex congenita: flexion contractures of joints with muscle wasting. It could be due to inutero position because of oligohydramnios, primary muscular hypoplasia, or (most commonly) due to unknown etiology.

147. Meningomyelocele: most commonly found over lumbosacral regions, with or without ruptured membrane. It needs surgical repair. After surgery, hydrocephalus usually develops. It is commonly associated with Arnold-Chiari malformation. Sonogram should be done before surgery in order to confirm that diagnosis.

148. Spina bifida: skin dimple or lipoma or tuft of hairs present over spina bifida. X-ray shows bifid spine.

149. Caput: Swelling and elongation over the parietal and occipital regions.

150. Encephalocele: Swelling over the occipital region.

151. Breech presentation: both feet are touching the face.

152. Cornelia deLange syndrome: bushy eyebrows, downward turn of upper lip.

153. Neuroblastoma (important): abdominal distension, sweating. IVP shows downward displacement of kidney in tumor side because it is an adrenal tumor.

154. Klumpke's paralysis (newborn): loss of finger grip and claw hand.

155. Brachial plexus injury (newborn): arm is adducted, inwardly rotated and extended, but normal finger grip is noted in Erb's paralysis. Loss of Moro reflex in affected side.

156. Back of both thighs appeared as asymmetric skin folds: R/O congenital dislocation of one hip joint. Palpable click in physical examinations.

157. Potter's syndrome: flat face, low set ears, antimongoloid slant in both eyes, renal agenesis; deformed extremities due to pressure effects from oligohydramnios.

158. Cerebral dystrophy: facial asymmetry, antimongoloid slants, both eyes bulging and pseudostrabismus.

159. Bruise over periorbital regions: R/O child abuse.

160. Widely spaced 1st (great) and 2nd toes: R/O Down syndrome.

161. Hyperthyroidism in newborn: exopthalmos, tachycardia, restlessness.

162. Parotitis: painful swelling in front and below ear over parotid regions.

163. Thrombocytopenic purpura: purpuric rashes over body caused by platelet destructions due to maternal antiplatelet antibodies which cross placenta.

164. Polyarthritis: swollen bigger joints (e.g.,: knee, ankle).

165. Newborn with (B/L) skin redness over knee areas: R/O drug withdrawal (e.g.,: from methadone, heroin). It may be due to rubbing of knees against bed while in prone position.

166. Diastasis recti: midline abdominal bulging due to weakness in rectus abdominis muscles.

167. Holoprosencephaly (midline facial defect): hypotelorism (smaller than normal distance between eyes), midline cleft lip and palate, one nasal orifice, frontal lobar defect in brain.

168. Gynecomastia (prepubertal boys): prepubertal boys - it is due either to obesity or to increased breast tissues. No further investigation is needed.

169. Breast enlargement:
Newborn   Due to maternal estrogen.
Young child   Small breast enlargement may be normal if genitalia are normal for age.
Large breast   R/O prolactinoma.

170. Neonatal acne: acne is present over face and body.

171. Mastitis: enlarged breast with redness and tenderness. Staphylococcal infection is common.

172. Small newborn with thin hairs: normal premature child.

173. Post-mature newborn: long nails, dry peeling skin, loss of subcutaneous fats.

174. Cushing syndrome: moon face with obesity in upper part of body (over abdomen).

175. Child abuse, different signs of: when adult put child in hot water tub, child showed signs of hot water burn over buttocks and feet (sparing back of leg and thigh), because child folded legs to protect himself. Small tiny areas of burn may be from cigarettes. Human bites leave teeth marks on body parts.

176. Picture shows spastic child: extended stiff lower extremities, hypertonia, increased tendon reflexes; lower limbs diplegia is most common. It is due to cerebral palsy.

177. Brushefield spots in iris: Down syndrome.

178. Reiter syndrome: includes sterile urethritis, arthritis, ocular inflammation, pustules, erythematous cheeks with exfoliating rashes.

179. Swelling over parietal bone in newborns: R/O cephalhematoma.

180. Thanatophoric dysplasia (important): very large head, very short upper and lower extremities, depressed nasal bridge, frontal bossing, bulging eyes, very narrow chest (pear-shaped), sometimes clover-leaf skull. X-ray of lumber vertebrae - inverted U-shaped and flat. Shortening of long bones in X-ray and bowing of femurs. Small foramen magnum. (Narrow pear-shaped chest, large head, short extremities).

181. Achondroplasia (important): large head, short proximal limbs (rhizomelic), depressed nasal bridge, frontal bossing, small maxillae, large protruding mandible, short stature, trident fingers (thumb, 2nd and 3rd digits, 4th and 5th digits), dental malocclusions. Hypotonia resolves by 2 to 3 years of age. Normal development if there is no hydrocephalus. Normal chest. (Normal chest, large head, short proximal limbs.)

182. Hypochondroplasia (important): normal head, nasal bridge, maxilla and mandible. Stocky and muscular build. Hands and feets are short and broad (not trident), straight legs, normal chest. (All normal with short stocky built.)

183. Neurofibromatosis: cafe-au-lait spots are noted on skin.

184. Pierre-Robin syndrome: micrognathia, pseudomacroglossia, and cleft palate.

185. Treacher-Collins syndrome: small deformed ears with downward slanting of both eyes.

186. Hurler syndrome (autosomal recessive): coarse face, corneal clouding, gibbus, stiff joints, hernias, growth retardation. X-ray shows dolichocephalic thick skull, boot-or J-shaped sella turcica, ovoid vertebral bodies in lower thoracic and upper lumber regions.

187. Trisomy 18 (Important): rockerbottom feet, hyperextended lower extremities, microcephaly with occipital prominence, clenched fingers, and flexed upper extremities.

188. Precocious puberty in male child: pubic hairs, axillary hairs, and enlarged penis. R/O adrenal cortical tumor.

189. Precocious puberty in female child: pubic hairs, enlarged breasts, and clitoris. R/O ovarian tumor.

190. Osteopetrosis (marble bones): large head, fractured bones, deafness, blindness, hydrocephalus.

191. Erythema multiforme (important): bullous lesions, crust formations with plaques all over body, mostly on face, scalp, and trunk.

192. Talipes equinovarus: heel raised, inward foot deformity, bony deformities.

193. Urinary bladder extrophy (newborn): anterior abdominal wall defects. Visible red/pink bladder mucosas. (Short penis due to epispadius.) X-ray of pelvic bones shows widely separated symphisis pubis.

194. Gastroschisis: visible matted intestines outside abdominal wall, not covered with mucous membranes. Abdominal wall is well-formed.

195. Omphalocele: midline mass covered with mucous membrane. Defective development of anterior abdominal wall.

196. Pseudohypogonadism (obesity): normal genitalia which appear small due to obesity. Normal breast enlargement.

197. Hydrocephalus: very large head, positive transillumination. Head sono-dilated ventricles.

198. Asymmetrical SGA: normal head, but small body for gestational age.

199. Symmetrical SGA: both head and body are small for gestational age.

200. Hallerman-Streiff- Francois syndrome: Bird-like face; small eyes, big sharp nose; antimongoloid slants in both palpebral fissures.

201. Acrocephaly: round head due to early fusions of coronal suture. (e.g., Apert syndrome).

202. Scaphocephaly (dolichocephaly): long narrow (anteroposteriorly) head due to closure of sagittal suture.

203. Craniopharyngioma: a 6-year-old child with pubic hairs and short stature.

204. Infectious mononucleosis: fever, generalized lymph nodes enlargement, exudative tonsillitis, petechiae on palate, macular rashes with or without ampicillin therapy.

205. Measles: Koplik's spots are found on buccal mucosa initially, then maculopapular rashes all over face and behind ears; rashes progressively become more confluent; fever, conjunctivitis and coryza.

206. German measles (Rubella): pink macular rashes, generalized enlargement of lymph nodes mostly in suboccipital region and mild fever.

207. Mumps: unilateral or bilateral enlargement of parotid glands which are painful, tender, fever, earache, and trismus.

208. Periorbital cellulitis: cellulitis around eye with fever mostly due to Hemophilus influenza.

209. Precocious puberty:
      Girls Hypertrophied clitoris, pubic hair. R/O adrenal tumor or (ovarian) gonadal tumor.
      Boys Short stature, pubic hairs, enlarged penis. R/O pituitary tumor. Exogenous steroid can cause precocious secondary sexual characters. In female, normal breasts with enlarged genitalia cannot be physiological.

210. Congenital adrenal hyperplasia:
      Female Enlarged clitoris (looks like male infant with hypospadias and undescended testes).
      Male Normal genitalia at birth.

211. Hypothyroidism:
      Newborn Prolonged jaundice, umbilical hernia, and constipation.
      Children Coarse face, hoarse voice, and dry skin.

212. Conjunctivitis: eye discharge, redness in conjunctiva. Children with unilateral purulent discharge always R/O GC infection and sexual abuse. It could be due to virus, chlamydia, or bacterial infections.

213. Squint/strabismus: asymmetric corneal reflex. Patient needs further evaluation by ophthalmologist.

214. Nail-patella syndrome: absent or hypoplastic nails and absent patellae.

215. Ectodermal dysplasia: absent or hypoplastic teeth, bald head, absent eyebrows, inadequate sweat glands and poor temperature control. Diagnosis is confirmed by biopsy of palm or

216. Menkes kinky-hair syndrome: twisted hairs are sparsely distributed on scalp and eyebrows.

217. Progeria: alopecia, growth retardation, loss of subcutaneous fat. Patient appears old.

218. (KTW) Klippel-Trenaunay-Weber syndrome: asymmetric limbs due to hypertrophy of one limb with cutaneous hemangiomas due to arterio-venous fistulas; may be associated with lymphangiomas and protein-losing enteropathy.

219. Down syndrome: upward slanting of both eyes, protruding tongue, epicanthic folds, Brushfield's's spots. Atlantoaxial cervical joints fusion and absence of 12th rib may be appear in X-ray finding. So X-ray of cervical vertebrae is important before participation in sports is allowed. VSD is most common cardiac defect.

220. Russell-Silver syndrome: triangular face, craniofacial dysostosis, asymmetric limbs (not due to A-V fistula-like KTW syndrome), intrauterine growth retardation.

221. Lesch -Nyhan syndrome: self-mutilation (biting of self) not due to impaired sensation or increased uric acid level but rather due to compulsive behavior. Choreiform or athetoid movements, mental retardation, increased reflexes.

222. Mucopolysaccharidoses: Hurler (type 1), Hunter (II). Large protruding tongue, short stature, hepatosplenomegaly, skeletal defects. Hurler syndrome patients usually have cloudy corneas.

223. Cockayne syndrome: dorsal kyphosis (backward vertebral enlargement), short stature, retinal pigments, loss of subcutaneous fats.

224. Metatarsus varus (feet): inward curving of metatarsal bones.

225. Bow leg: outward curve of tibias; considered normal in first two years of life.

226. Knock-knee (genu valgum): both knees are closer together than normal due to femoral condyles' unequal growth.

227. Amniotic band: limb is cut off due to amniotic band.

228. Monilial dermatitis in diaper area: satellite beefy red lesions over diaper area, including groin.

229. Duchenne muscular dystrophy: hypertrophied calf muscles in both legs.

230. Neurofibromatosis: cafe-au-lait spots, shagreen patches with multiple pigmented lesions.

231. Leukemia: neonatal-subcutaneous deposits of leukemic cells. ALL is most common in children. ALL patients show signs of fever, bruises, pallor, recurrent infections. Blast cells are found in blood as well as in bone marrow.

232. Multiple pigmented nevi: may be found in neurofibromatosis.

233. Keloid: increased scar formations after trauma, burn and incision.

234. Erythema nodosum: multiple tender, raised, erythematous nodules are present over pretibial regions. Etiology may be unknown or due to infection streptococcus, mycoplasma, T.B. Sarcoidosis or drug sensitivity and presentation of inflammatory bowel diseases.

235. Diaper dermatitis in newborns: erythematous lesions over diaper areas except in groin which does not come in contact with diaper.

236. Torticollis: head is tilted due to pain in sternocleidomastoid muscle.

237. Isolated cleft lip/cleft palate: not associated with any syndrome.

238. Kawasaki disease: fever, cracked lips, enlarged lymph nodes, erythematous rashes, thrombocytosis and later on peeling of skin of hands and feet.

239. Alopecia areata: localized hair loss in scalp, total hair loss is very rare. Smooth, bald head.

240. Chocolate brown discoloration of teeth: it is due to tetracycline mistakenly given to younger children.

241. Eczema: excoriated itchy plaques of skin over antecubital fossas, behind knees and over face.

242. Seborrhoeic dermatitis: Scaly, greasy, erythematous plaques over scalp.

243. Pyloric stenosis: picture of abdomen shows visible peristalsis in infant around 2 to 6 weeks of age.

244. Herpes zoster: extremely painful vesicles distributed along dermatomes. It does not cross midline.

245. Herpes Simplex: painful blisters and ulcers are distributed outside and or inside mouth and on lips.

246. Chicken pox (varicella): rashes appears in crops and then progress from macules to papules, papules to vesicles, vesicles to crusts.

247. Erysipelas: spreading cellulitis which has well-defined margin caused by Streptococcus.

248. Hyperthyroidism:
     Newborn: irritability, tachycardia, poor weight gain.
     Children: goitre, proptosis, tremor; there may be rapid growth.

249. Cushing syndrome: Moon face, hirsutism, acne, truncal obesity, and short stature.

250. Congenital cataract (one eye or both eyes): (L) opaque (white) lens, R/O congenital rubella, galactosemia.

251. Congenital glaucoma: corneal clouding and enlarged eyeball.

252. Toxic epidermal necrolysis or scalded skin syndrome: painful red color skin with positive Nikolsky's sign, which is separation of epidermis from dermis due to edema. It is due to Staphylococcus phage types 71 or 22.

253. Meningitis: opisthotonos (arching of back), high-pitched cry, bulging fontanelle, neck stiffness, lethargy and convulsion.

254. Forearm with positive PPD: indurated erthyematous, swollen skin. Chest X-ray should be done to R/O active TB.

255. Meningococcemia: shock, purpuric rashes with bluish discoloration in a very sick child.

256. Turner syndrome (female only): webbed neck, short stature, delayed secondary sexual characters, no mental retardation, bicuspid aortic valve and aortic coarctation.

257. Noonan syndrome (male only): known as Male Turner Syndrome, normal chromosomes, mental retardation, pulmonary stenosis. Male child has Webbed neck and short stature.

258. Sturge-Weber syndrome: facial hemangiomas (port wine stains) are found along distribution of trigeminal nerve; seizures, mental retardation. Meningeal hemangioma may be an associated features in this syndrome.

259. Waardenburg syndrome: white forelock, congenital sensorineural deafness, may be associated with skin vitiligo and heterochromic iris.

260. Scabies: very itchy, excoriated, papular rashes are found mostly between fingers but may be noted on any other parts of body.

261. Psoriasis: silvery, scaly, erythematous plaques are usually noted in elbows, scalp, knees and back.

262. Hemangioma (cavernous): usually noted in skin and mucous membrane which shows swelling with bluish discolorations.

263. Histiocytosis: patients show signs of seborrheic skin rashes or skin deposits of histiocyte, enlarged liver and spleen; skull x-ray shows lytic bone lesions due to eosinophilic granuloma.

264. Osteogenesis imperfecta: H/O repeated fractures of bones, deformed body parts, and short stature.

265. Cystic hygroma: most commonly is found in neck appeared as ill-defined cystic mass, R/O Turner syndrome. Transillumination test is positive.

266. Picture showing poor head control: it is a floppy baby. R/O Down syndrome, hypothyroidism, cerebral palsy, and neuromuscular disorder. Shows signs of floppy child.

Good head control usually noted around 3 months of age.

267. Picture showing "Setting-sun" eye sign: due to hydrocephalus with increased intracranial pressure. V-P shunt is treatment. Staph. epidermidis is most common organism causing infection.

268. Coloboma of iris: cleft in one iris. R/O Wilms' tumor.

269. Congenital ptosis: drooping of one eyelid or both eyelids. Bilateral ptosis could be due to myasthenia gravis.

270. Microopthalmos (small eye): R/O congenital rubella and other TORCH infections.

271. Subconjunctival hemorrhage: blood under conjunctiva; usually resolves spontaneously within a few weeks.

272. Prune-belly syndrome: lax abdominal muscles due to dilated urinary apparatus; horseshoe kidney, double ureters, dysplastic kidney, pelvic kidney. Posterior urethral valve is noted in male infant with this syndrome.

273. Hypospadias: abnormal urethral opening with chordee (ventral curvature). Circumcision is contraindicated in hypospadias.

274. Inguinal hernia/hydrocele: surgery is needed to repair inguinal hernia to avoid strangulation,yet hydrocele can resolve spontaneously in younger children.

275. Nephrotic syndrome: periorbital edema, pain in abdomen, proteinuria, hypovolemia.

276. Angioneurotic edema: urticaria along with marked edemas are noted around eyes and mouth.

277. Steven-Johnson syndrome: bullous lesions over skin, mucous membrane of mouth, conjunctiva. Erythema multiforme appeared as target lesions.

278. Dermoid cyst: benign, nontender swelling mostly noted in midline or external angular regions of orbit.

279. Oral thrush: ulcerated, painful, erythematous white plaques. It may be normal in newborns, but usually found in patients with immune deficiencies.

280. Syndactyle/polydactyle: "Syndactyle" means two fingers are fused together; "polydactyle" means more than five fingers in hands or feet.

281. Hemorrhagic knee in hemophiliac: swelling of one knee joint with bluish discoloration of overlying skin due to trauma.

282. JRA (juvenile rheumatoid arthritis): recurrent painful swelling of bigger joints.

283. DeLange syndrome: hirsutism, short stature, failure to thrive, bushy eyebrows, down-turned mouth, small chin and nose.

284. Lowe syndrome: joint hypermobility, hypotonia, mental retardation, cataract, blindness and renal tubular defects.

285. Crown syndrome: ocular proptosis (protruding eye ball) due to shallow orbits, hypertelorism, craniosynostosis of coronal, lambdoid and sagittal sutures.

286. Tuberous Sclerosis: hypopigmented skin, adenoma sebaceum (on cheek), periungual fibromas, cafe-au-lait spots, shagreen patches, tubers (granulomas) inside brain appeared as irregular calcification. Earliest clinical sign is white leaf macule, but most commonly recognized one is adenoma sebaceum.

287. Picture appeared as dry skin: due to dehydration which causes loss of skin elasticity.

288. Impetigo (maculo-vesiculo-pustular lesion): multiple crusted lesions with oozing due to Streptococcal infections (Gr A betahemolytic), secondary Staphylococcal infections may occur.

289. Child abuse: picture appeared as calcification over posterior aspects of ribs, which are common places of child abuse.

290. (L) ventricular enlargement with rib notching appeared in chest x-ray: R/O aortic coarctation.

291. Oral thrush in newborns: white patches inside mouth. These patches cannot be removed by rubbing, indicating candida infection. Milk white deposits could be removed easily.

292. Crohn disease: multiple perineal fistulas.

293. Phimosis: unable to separate prepuce from glans penis.

294. Nephrotic syndrome: generalized edema with H/O proteinuria.

295. Midline swelling in neck: R/O thyroglossal cyst.

296. Picture of protruding tongue:
    Normal eye   Hypothyroidism.
    Outward-upward eye slanting   Down syndrome.
    Large baby with visceromegaly   Beckwith-Wiedemann syndrome.

297. (B/L) lymphedemas of feet: R/O Turner syndrome.

298. Undescended vs. retractile testis: scrotum is not formed in an undescended testes, but is well formed in retractile testes. Retractile testes is due to excessive cremasteric reflex. Further evaluation (sonogram) is needed for an undescended testis.

299. Cri-du-chat syndrome: cat-like cry, deletion of short arm of chromosome, appears with microcephaly, micrognathia, antimongoloid slant, hypertelorism and prominent ears.

300. Hypoplasia of unilateral depressor anguli oris muscle: when baby cries, hypoplastic side of mouth does not move, but normal side moves downward and outward. Normal eye lids closure. Normal facial appearance when baby is not crying.

301. McCune -Albright syndrome (polyostotic fibrous dysplasia): premature breasts development, margin of cafe-au-lait spots are irregular (regular margins in neurofibromatosis), precocious puberty, and fibrous dysplasia of bones, resulting in their thickening.

302. Prader-Willi syndrome: obese child, short height, and mental retardation.

303. Williams Syndrome: growth retardation, elfin face, heart murmur due to supravalvular aortic stenosis, and hypercalcemia.

304. Ectodermal dysplasia: bald head, absence of eye brows, and peg-shaped teeth.

305. Scarlet fever: white or red strawberry tongue.

306. Myasthenia gravis: (B/L) ptosis of eyelids.

307. Rectal prolapse: R/O cystic fibrosis.

308. Umbilical polyp: smooth rounded red mass over umbilical area; due to failure of obliteration of vitelline duct.

309. Ehlers-Danlos syndrome: hyperextensible bruised skin, blue sclera.

310. Picture of molluscum contagiosum: can appear in any part of body, spread from one part to another; self-limited disease, caused by DNA virus.

311. Dactylitis: swollen, painful fingers. It could be due to JRA, sickle cell disease.

312. Picture shows proptosis of one eyeball: R/O retroorbital mass, which could be due to metastasis from abdominal neuroblastoma.

313. Tearing of one eye: nasolacrimal duct obstruction which improves with massages locally in that area.

314. Pyogenic arthritis: swollen, hot, tender single joint; fever and increased ESR.

315. Genital warts: R/O sexual abuse in children.

316. Grape-like structures protruding through vagina in newborn: vaginal adenocarcinoma, a highly malignant tumor.

317. Child shows signs of facial nerve and VI cranial nerve paralysis: R/O brain-stem tumor (glioma) which shows signs of facial palsy and diplopia. Mobius syndrome shows signs of congenital facial palsy and abduction weakness, usually on both sides, but asymmetric.

318. Pectus excavatum: narrowing of thoracic cavity in midline.

319. Pigeon chest: prominent sternum and ribs.

320. Absence of 12th rib: R/O Down syndrome.

321. Narrow thorax and short extremities: asphyxiating thoracic dystrophy.

322. Campomelia or bent limbs: osteogenesis imperfecta, campomelic dysplasia, hypophosphatasias, and skeletal dysplasias.

323. Heliotropic (violaceous) erythema: dermatomyositis. Sometimes appears as butterfly rashes like SLE.

324. Oxycephaly: head bulges upward.

325. Female child with (B/L) inguinal swelling: R/O testicular feminization syndrome. Result of chromosome study is 46 xy (male). Sonogram should be done to look for gonadal tissues.

326. Rubinstein-Taybe syndrome: broad thumb.

327. Multiple lentigenes (LEOPARD) syndrome: large pigmented (dark) freckles (lentigenes) over skin. Autosomal dominant, pulmonic stenosis, cryptorchidism, hypogonadism, obstructive cardiomyopathy, growth retardation and sensoneural deafness.

328. Balanoposthitis: swollen, red prepuce with H/O difficulty in urination.

329. Seckel's dwarfism: short stature, microcephaly with prominent nose.

330. Angioneurotic edema: (B/L) puffy eyes with respiratory difficulties.

331. Hemifacial hypertrophy or hypertrophy of one leg: R/O Wilms' tumor.

332. Sternomastoid muscle localized swelling: traumatic delivery - hematoma.
Non-traumatic delivery - tumor.

333. Fundus appeared as optic disc edema, tortuous blood vessels: due to increased intracranial pressure.

334. Sprengel's deformity: one scapula is higher than other due to failure of descent of scapula from neck.

335. Claw hand deformities: R/O Cornelia de Lange syndrome or Klumpke paralysis.

336. Infant of diabetic mother: LGA, plethoric, plump face, hairs are distributed over ears. In LGA babies, all organs are large except brain.

337. Newborn with skin petechiae- due to thrombocytopenia: in autoimmune thrombocytopenia both mother's and baby's platelets are low in count.
Isoimmune thrombocytopenia, mother's platelets are normal, but baby's platelets are low in count.
R/O infection patient needs antibiotics. It could be due to virus infections or TORCH infections.

338. Henoch-Schonlein purpura: Purpuric rashes distributed over lower extremities; arthralgia, arthritis, microscopic hematuria.

339. Bilateral lateral rectus paralysis: R/O intracranial tumor.

340. Sex maturity rating (SMR) of breast, genitalia of female and genitalia of male:

    SMR 1   Preadolescent
    SMR 2   Early adolescent
    SMR 3, 4   Middle adolescent
    SMR 5   Late adolescent.

341. Trisomy 13 (see diagram 167): midline facial defects with cleft lip and palate, central apnea.

342. Purulent vaginal discharge in children (no diagram): R/O sexual abuse and gonococcal infection.

343. Werdnig-Hoffmann disease (see diagram 266): hypotonic floppy baby with tongue fasciculations. Respiratory failure is usual cause of death.

344. Cyanotic newborn (no diagram): R/O cyanotic congenital heart disease or other conditions, which lead to cyanosis-like sepsis or persistent pulmonary hypertension.

345. Cavernous sinus thrombosis (no diagram): drowsiness, fever,purulent nasal discharges, signs of increased intracranial pressure, swelling over eyeball area.

346. Anal fissures (no diagram): H/O painful defecations with fresh blood-streaked stools.

347. Umbilical granuloma (no diagram): granulation tissues, over umbilical area, appears pink..

348. Behcet syndrome (See diagram 29): barium studies mimic Crohn disease. Underlying pathology of multi-system vasculitis would cause oral-genital ulcers and uveitis by which this syndrome can be differentiated from Crohn disease.

349. Streptococcal pneumonia (no diagram): x-ray of chest shows diffuse bronchopneumonia with or without pleural effusions. After 8 to 10 weeks, x-ray pictures become normal.

350. Hemophilus influenza pneumonia (no diagram): lobar infiltrates, but no special features

(unlikely to be given in examination).

351. Pseudomonas pneumonia (no diagram): serious necrotizing bronchopneumonia, but no special X-ray features. It is common in immunodeficient patients, malignancies, preterm babies on ventilators. Ceftazidime with aminoglycosides is treatment of choice.

352. Pulmonary alveolar proteinosis (no diagram): butterfly white densities in perihilar regions, or (B/L) lower lobe densities or nodular densities. Diagnosis is confirmed by biopsy. Repeated pulmonary lavage is treatment of choice.

353. Hamman-Rich syndrome (idiopathic diffuse interstitial fibrosis of lung) (no diagram): granular, reticular or nodular lung densities (white).

354. Adult respiratory distress syndrome (ARDS) (see diagram 56): chest x-ray shows pulmonary edema. It can occur in any age group. Pulmonary damage (non-cardiac causes) in ARDS is due to shock, infections, DIC, drug overdoses, toxic inhalations, traumas, aspirations.

355. Fetal aspiration syndrome or aspiration pneumonia (see diagram 45): Aspirated lung fields has shown coarsely granular patterns (patchy white) with irregular lung aeration; due to aspiration of amniotic fluids which contain epithelial cells, vernix caseosa, and (sometimes) meconium.

356. Wilson-Mikity syndrome (see diagram 58): chest x-ray picture same as BPD.

357. Hydrothorax (see diagram 60): due to either cardiac or renal diseases. Chest x-ray appears as white dense shadows over pleuras.

358. Empyema (lung) (see diagram 73): chest x-ray picture mimics serofebrinous pleurisy. No shift of fluid noted during clinical examinations.

359. Short sternum (no diagram): R/O Trisomy 18.

360. Hunter syndrome (x-linked recessive): no corneal clouding and no gibbus. Coarse face, stiff joints, hernias, growth retardation as in Hurler syndrome.

361. Scleroderma (no picture): shiny edematous or atrophic skin.

362. Raynaud phenomenon (no picture): characteristic triad - distal fingers first shows signs of blanching due to vasospasm, then cyanosis due to hypoxia, finally redness due to hyperemia. It is found in SLE and scleroderma.

363. Facial dilated capillaries with H/O ataxia (No picture): R/O ataxia-telangiectasia.

364. Horner syndrome: ptosis, pupillary constrictions, enopthalmos, absence of sweating on that side.

365. Rheumatoid arthritis (no picture): swollen smaller joints. (e.g., fingers).

366. Collodion body (newborns) (no picture): whole body is covered with thick layers of collodion.

367. Biliary atresia (no picture): cholestatic jaundice (greenish color skin), distended abdomen. Clinical signs and symptoms appeared after 6 weeks of age. Clay-colored stool may be present.

368. Jaundice in first 24 hours (no picture): R/O hemolytic jaundice.

369. Breast-milk jaundice (no picture): H/O breast-feeding, but R/O other causes of jaundice.

370. Physiologic jaundice (no picture): Mild jaundice usually appears in 3rd day of life. R/O other causes of jaundice.

371. Newborn with only facial redness - (No picture): R/O cord around neck or facial presentation.

372. Peri-umbilical redness (no picture); R/O umbilical infection.

373. Mongolian spot newborn (no picture): Bluish discoloration of skin mostly over lumbosacral regions. It is normal.

374. Imperforate anus (no picture):
Female: meconium usually passes through vagina due to rectovagina fistula.
Male: mecpmoim usually passes through urethra due to rectourethral fistula.

375. Cerebral edema (no picture): CT scan of head shows inability to distinguish between cerebral cortex and medulla, narrow slit-like ventricles.

376. Trichobezoar (no picture): H/O swallowing hairs which ultimately forms a hair mass, shaped like stomach, which obstruct the pylorus. Barium study shows filing defect within the stomach.

377. Gastroenteritis (no picture): Abdominal X-ray shows multiple dilated loops of bowel with air-fluid level.

378. Small intestinal obstruction (no picture): Abdominal X-ray shows multiple air-fluid level in small intestine.

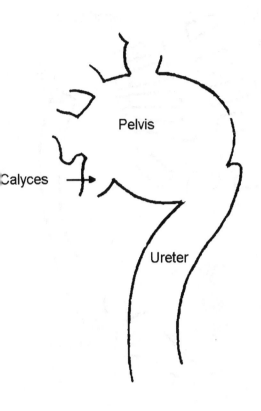

D.1- VCU Showing reflux (R) Side

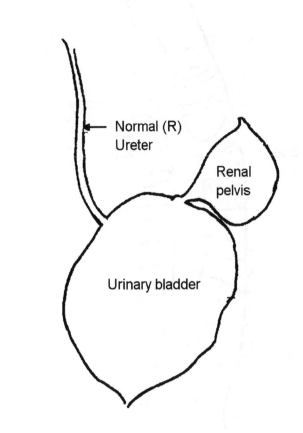

D.2- VCU Showing ectopic kidney (L)

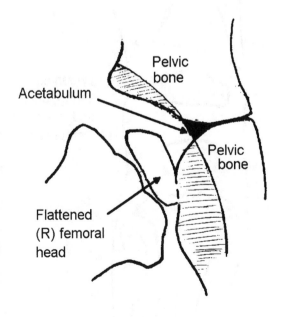

D.3- Legg Perthes disease (X-ray)

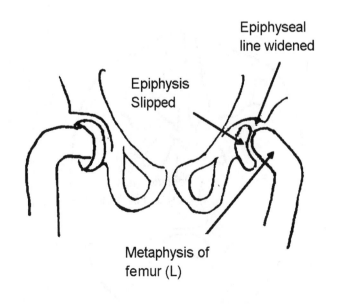

D.4- Slipped capital femoral epiphysis (X-ray)

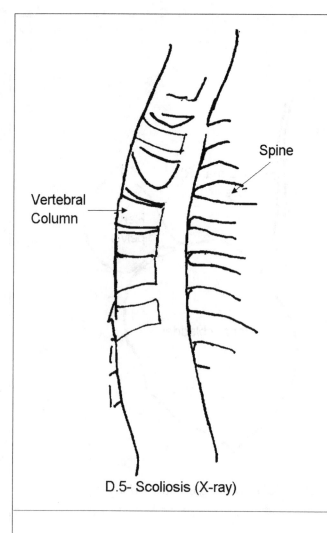

Vertebral
Column

Spine

D.5- Scoliosis (X-ray)

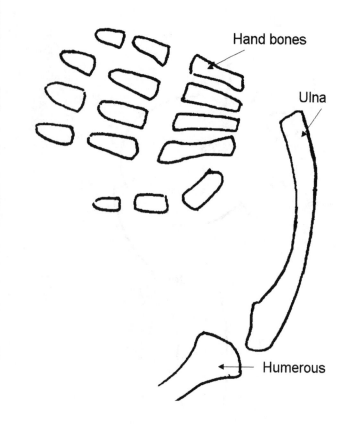

Hand bones

Ulna

Humerous

D.6- TAR syndrome (absent radius in X-ray)

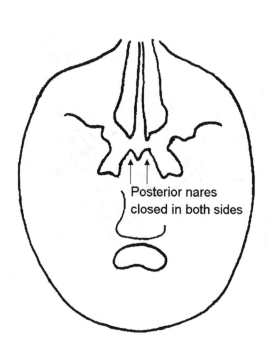

Posterior nares
closed in both sides

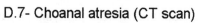

D.7- Choanal atresia (CT scan)

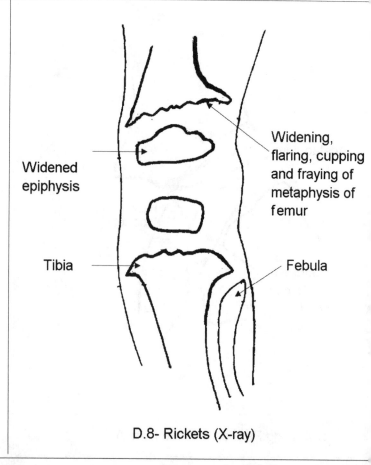

Widened
epiphysis

Widening,
flaring, cupping
and fraying of
metaphysis of
femur

Tibia

Febula

D.8- Rickets (X-ray)

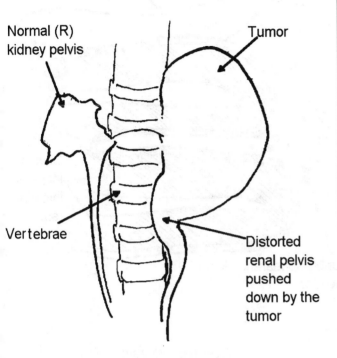

Normal (R) kidney pelvis

Tumor

Vertebrae

Distorted renal pelvis pushed down by the tumor

D.9- Wilms' tumor (L) kidney (IVP)

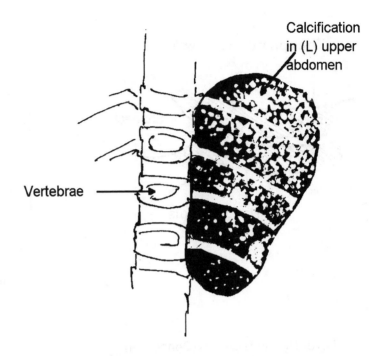

Calcification in (L) upper abdomen

Vertebrae

D.10- Neuroblastoma (L) adrenal (X-ray)

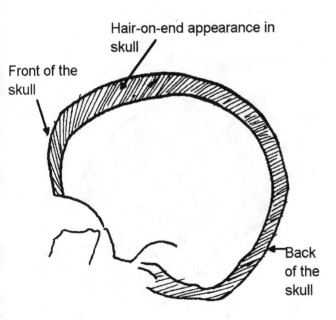

Hair-on-end appearance in skull

Front of the skull

Back of the skull

D.11- Thalassemia major (skull X-ray)

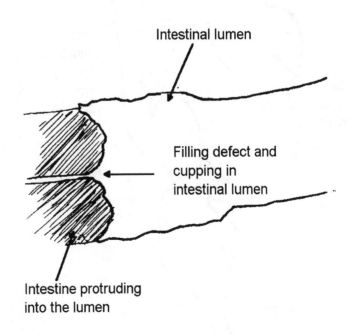

Intestinal lumen

Filling defect and cupping in intestinal lumen

Intestine protruding into the lumen

D.12- Intussuception (barium enema)

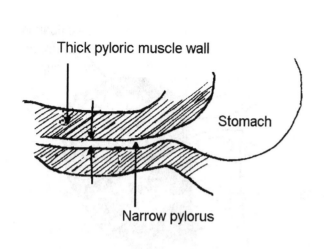

Thick pyloric muscle wall

Stomach

Narrow pylorus

D.13- Pyloric Stenosis (Sonogram)

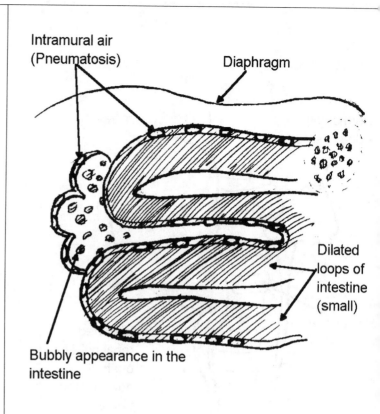

Intramural air (Pneumatosis)

Diaphragm

Dilated loops of intestine (small)

Bubbly appearance in the intestine

D.14- NEC (X-ray)

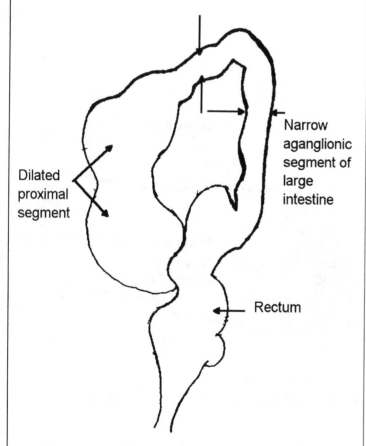

Dilated proximal segment

Narrow aganglionic segment of large intestine

Rectum

D.15- Hirschsprung disease (barium enema)

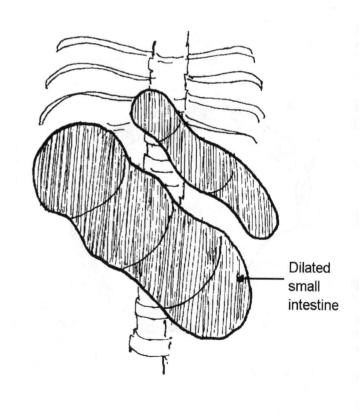

Dilated small intestine

D.16- Meconium ileus (X-ray)

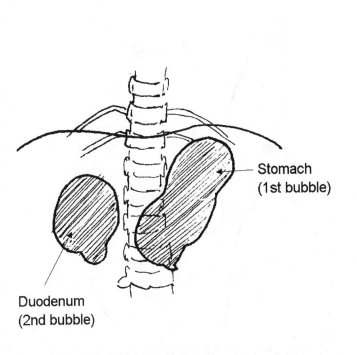

Stomach
(1st bubble)

Duodenum
(2nd bubble)

D-17: Duodenal atresia (X-ray)

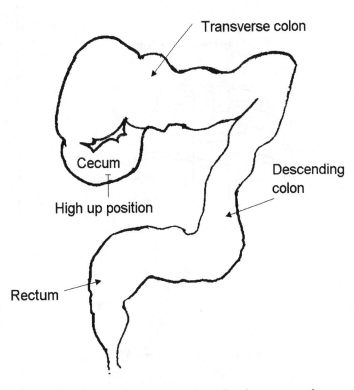

Transverse colon

Cecum

High up position

Descending
colon

Rectum

D-18: Intestinal malrotation (barium enema)

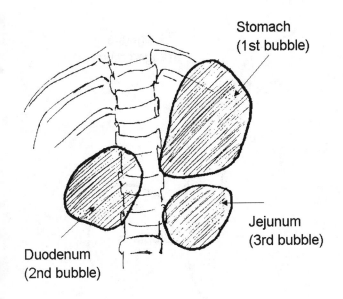

Stomach
(1st bubble)

Jejunum
(3rd bubble)

Duodenum
(2nd bubble)

D-19: Jejunal atresia (X-ray)

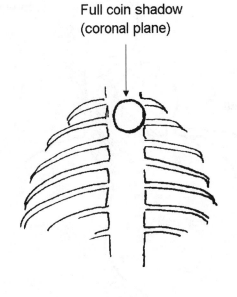

Full coin shadow
(coronal plane)

D-20: Esophageal foreign body (X-ray - AP View)

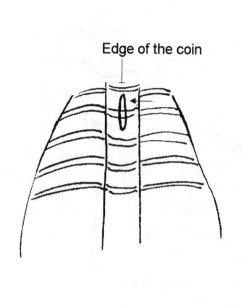

Edge of the coin

D-21: Tracheal foreign body(X-ray-AP View)

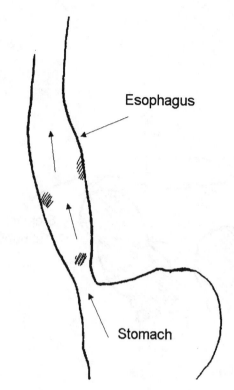

Esophagus

Stomach

D-22: Gastroesophageal reflux (barium study)

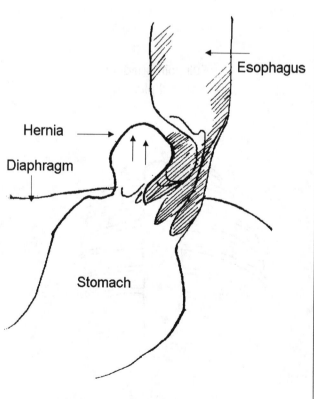

Esophagus

Hernia

Diaphragm

Stomach

D-23: Hiatal hernia (barium study)

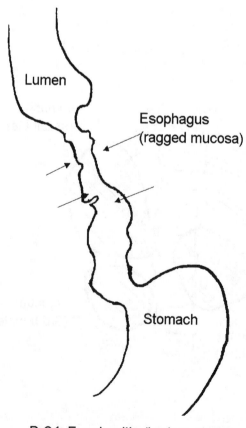

Lumen

Esophagus
(ragged mucosa)

Stomach

D-24: Esophagitis (barium study)

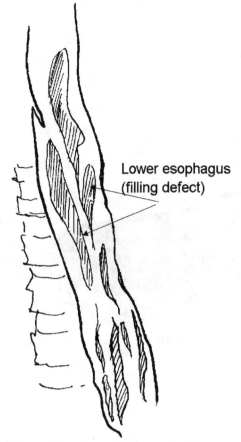

Lower esophagus
(filling defect)

D-25: Esophageal varices (barium study)

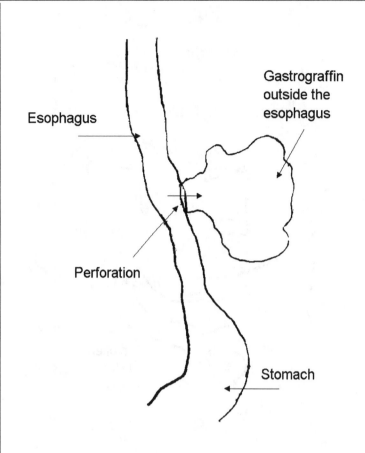

Gastrograffin
outside the
esophagus

Esophagus

Perforation

Stomach

D-26: Perforated esophagus (barium study)

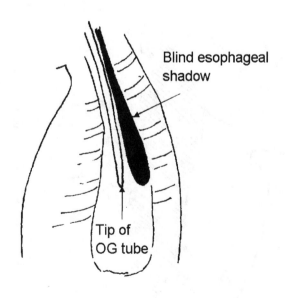

Blind esophageal
shadow

Tip of
OG tube

D-27: TE fistula & esophageal atresia
(X-ray neck & chest)

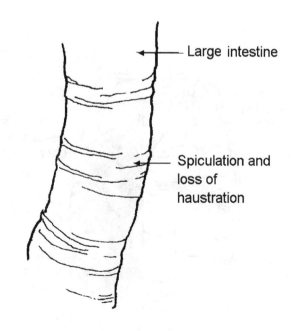

Large intestine

Spiculation and
loss of
haustration

D-28: Ulcerative colitis (barium enema)

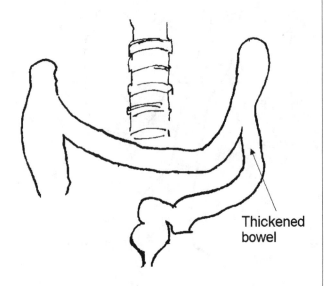

Thickened
bowel

D-29: Crohn disease (barium study)

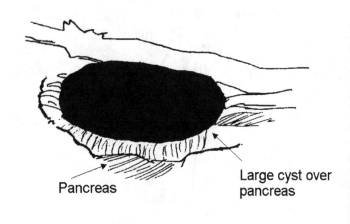

Pancreas

Large cyst over
pancreas

D-30: Pancreatic pseudocyst (Sonogram)

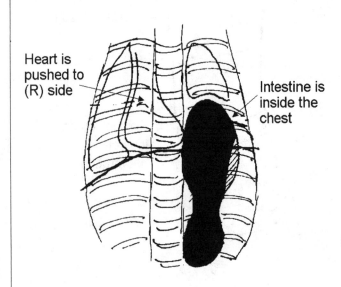

Heart is
pushed to
(R) side

Intestine is
inside the
chest

D-31: Congenital diaphragmatic hernia (X-ray)

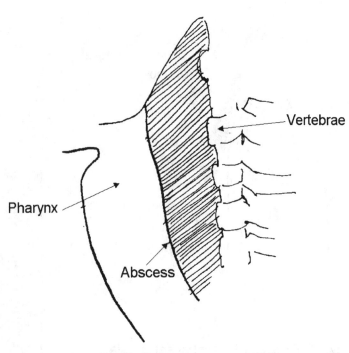

Vertebrae

Pharynx

Abscess

D-32: Retropharyngeal abscess (lateral X-ray neck)

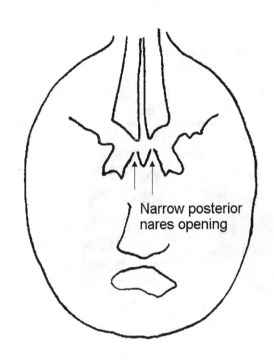

Narrow posterior
nares opening

D-33: Choanal Stenosis (CT Scan)

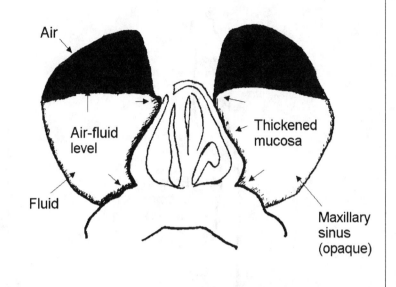

Air

Air-fluid
level

Fluid

Thickened
mucosa

Maxillary
sinus
(opaque)

D-34: Acute Sinusitis (X-ray)

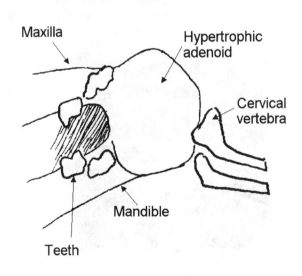

Maxilla

Hypertrophic
adenoid

Cervical
vertebra

Mandible

Teeth

D-35: Hypertrophic adenoid (lateral X-ray neck)·

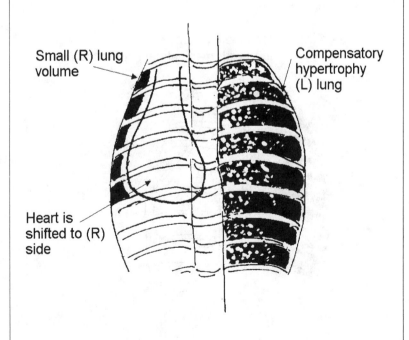

Small (R) lung
volume

Compensatory
hypertrophy
(L) lung

Heart is
shifted to (R)
side

D-36: Hypoplastic (R) lung (X-ray)

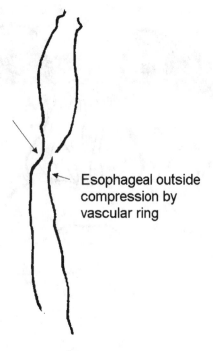

Esophageal outside
compression by
vascular ring

D-37: Vascular ring (barium study)

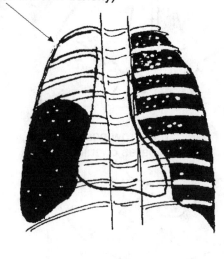

(R) upper lobe atelactasis
(white uniform density)

D-38: Pulmonary atelactasis (X-ray)

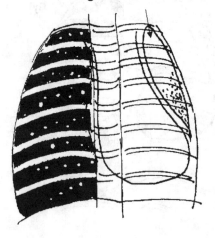

Complete collapse of (L)
lung with mediastinal shift to the (L)

D-39: Massive pulmonary atelactasis (X-ray)

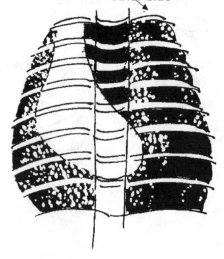

(L) upper lobe emphysema
pushing mediastinum to the
other side

D-40: Congenital lobar emphysema (X-ray)

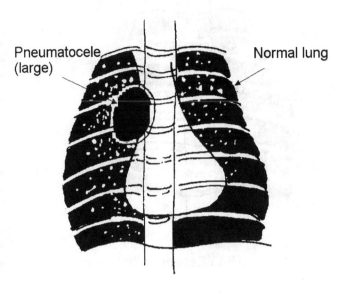

Pneumatocele
(large)

Normal lung

D-41: Pneumatocele (X-ray)

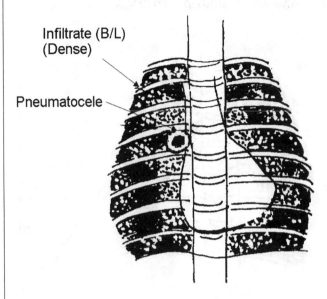

Infiltrate (B/L)
(Dense)

Pneumatocele

D-42: Staphylococcal pneumonia (X-ray)

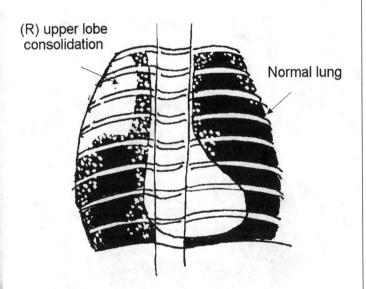

(R) upper lobe
consolidation

Normal lung

D-43: Pneumococcal pneumonia (X-ray)

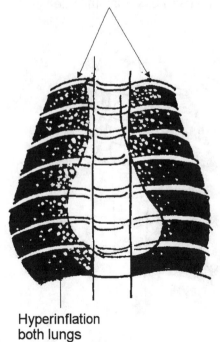

Diffuse (B/L) infiltrate (nondense)

Hyperinflation
both lungs

D-44: Viral pneumonia (X-ray)

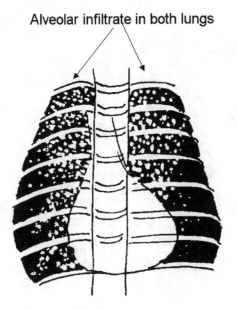

Alveolar infiltrate in both lungs

D-45: Aspiration pneumonia (X-ray)

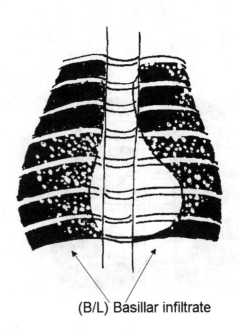

(B/L) Basillar infiltrate

D-46: Hydrocarbon pneumonia (X-ray)

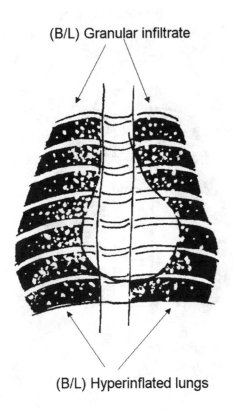

(B/L) Granular infiltrate

(B/L) Hyperinflated lungs

D-47: Pneumocystis carinii pneumonia (X-ray)

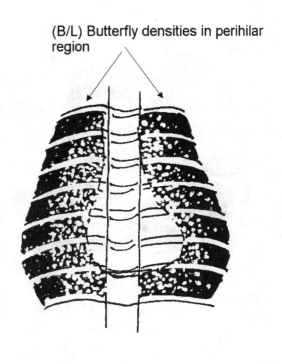

(B/L) Butterfly densities in perihilar region

D-48: Pulmonary hemorrhage (X-ray)

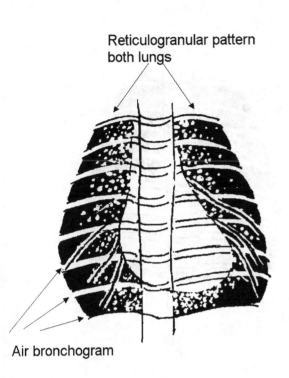

Reticulogranular pattern
both lungs

Air bronchogram

D-49: Respiratory distress syndrome (X-ray)

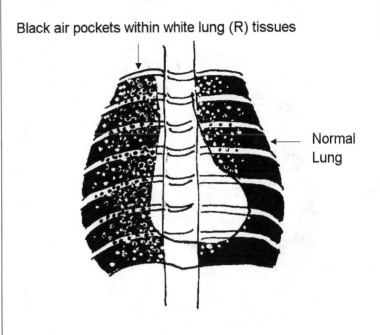

Black air pockets within white lung (R) tissues

Normal
Lung

D-50: Pulmonary interstitial emphysema (R) (X-ray)

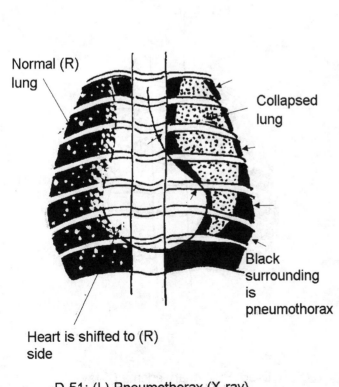

Normal (R)
lung

Collapsed
lung

Black
surrounding
is
pneumothorax

Heart is shifted to (R)
side

D-51: (L) Pneumothorax (X-ray)

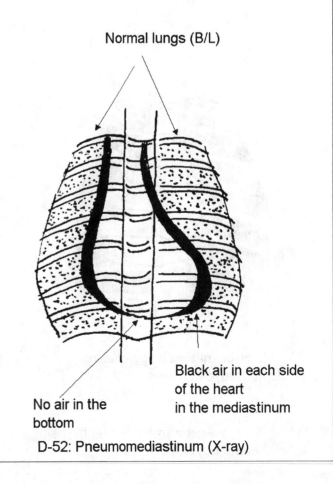

Normal lungs (B/L)

No air in the
bottom

Black air in each side
of the heart
in the mediastinum

D-52: Pneumomediastinum (X-ray)

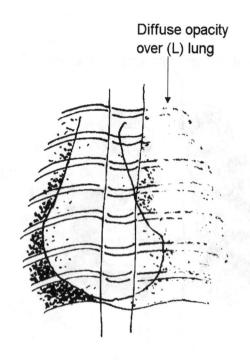

Diffuse opacity
over (L) lung

D-53: Chylothorax (L) (X-ray)

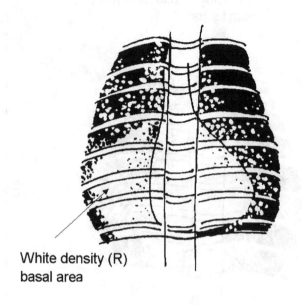

White density (R)
basal area

D-54: Pulmonary hemosiderosis (X-ray)

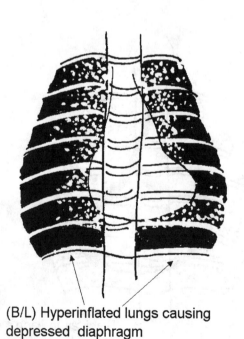

(B/L) Hyperinflated lungs causing
depressed diaphragm

D-55: Emphysema with Alpha-1-antitrypsin
         deficiency (X-ray)

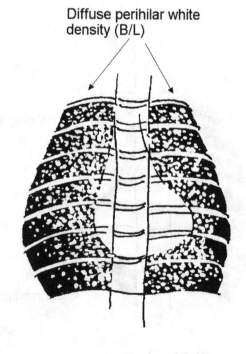

Diffuse perihilar white
density (B/L)

D-56: Pulmonary edema (X-ray)

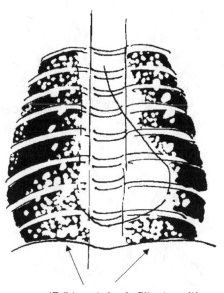

(B/L) patchy infiltrate with
flat diaphragm

D-57: Meconium aspiration (X-ray)

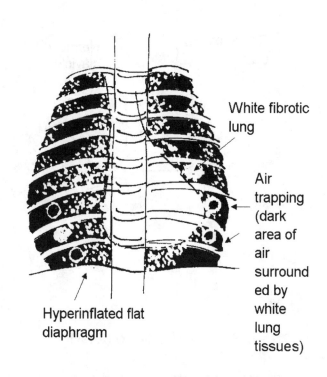

White fibrotic
lung

Air
trapping
(dark
area of
air
surround
ed by
white
lung
tissues)

Hyperinflated flat
diaphragm

D-58: Bronchopulmonary dysplasia (X-ray)

Streaky density & overdistension (B/L)
upper lobe

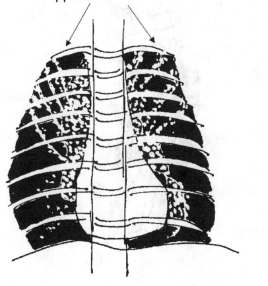

D-59: Cystic fibrosis (X-ray)

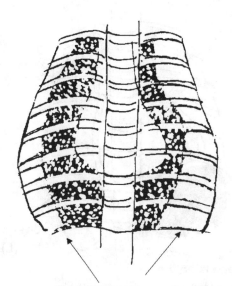

(B/L) White dense shadow in the
pleura

D-60: Hemothorax (X-ray)

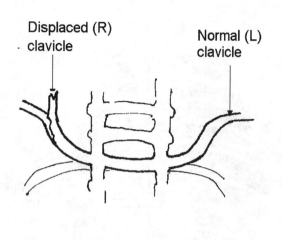

Displaced (R) clavicle

Normal (L) clavicle

D-61: Fracture clavicle (R) (X-ray)

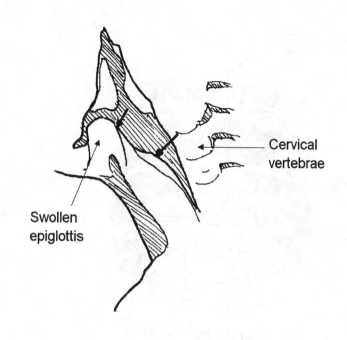

Swollen epiglottis

Cervical vertebrae

D-62: Epiglottitis (lateral X-ray neck)

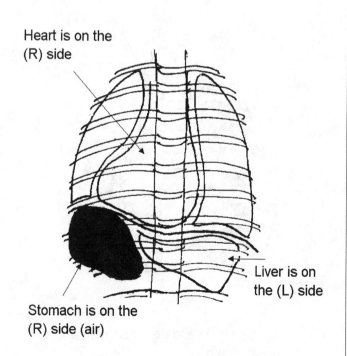

Heart is on the (R) side

Liver is on the (L) side

Stomach is on the (R) side (air)

D-63: Dextrocardia (X-ray) with situs inversus

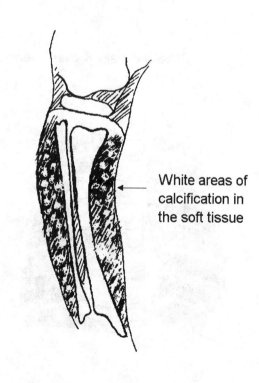

White areas of calcification in the soft tissue

D-64: Subcutaneous calcification (X-ray)

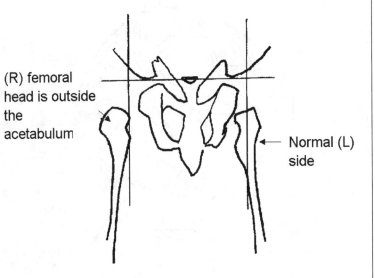

(R) femoral head is outside the acetabulum

Normal (L) side

D-65: Dislocated (R) hip (X-ray)

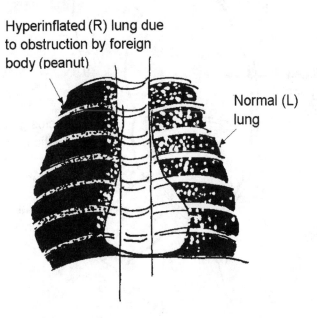

Hyperinflated (R) lung due to obstruction by foreign body (peanut)

Normal (L) lung

D-66: Foreign body in (R) bronchus (X-ray) (End expiration film)

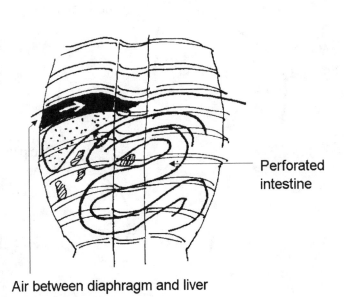

Perforated intestine

Air between diaphragm and liver

D-67: Pneumoperitoneum (X-ray)

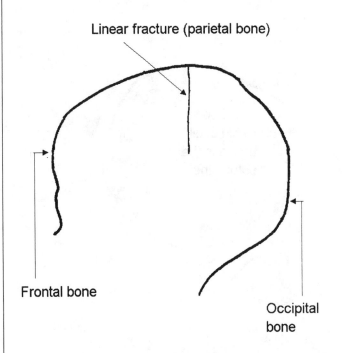

Linear fracture (parietal bone)

Frontal bone

Occipital bone

D-68: Parietal bone fracture (X-ray)

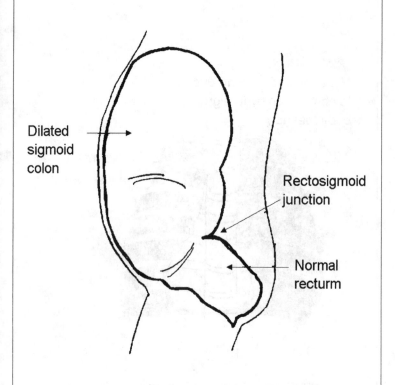

Dilated
sigmoid
colon

Rectosigmoid
junction

Normal
recturm

D-69: Hirschsprung disease (barium enema)

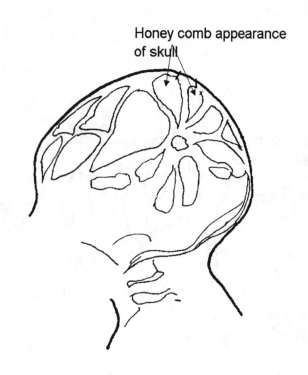

Honey comb appearance
of skull

D-70: Lacunar skull (X-ray-lateral)

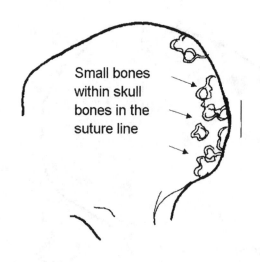

Small bones
within skull
bones in the
suture line

D-71: Wormian bones (Skull X-ray-lateral)

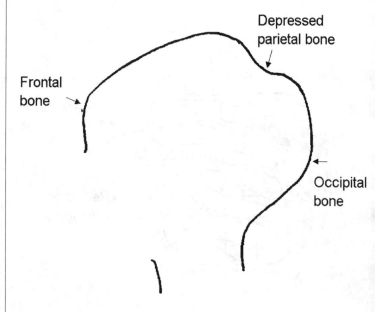

Depressed
parietal bone

Frontal
bone

Occipital
bone

D-72: Depressed skull fracture (X-ray skull-lateral)

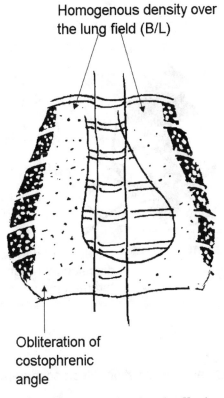
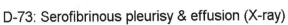

Homogenous density over the lung field (B/L)

Obliteration of costophrenic angle

D-73: Serofibrinous pleurisy & effusion (X-ray)

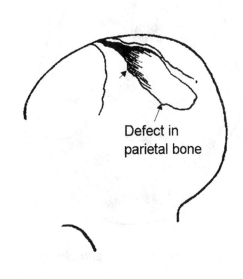

Defect in parietal bone

D-74: Leptomeningeal cyst (skull X-ray lateral)

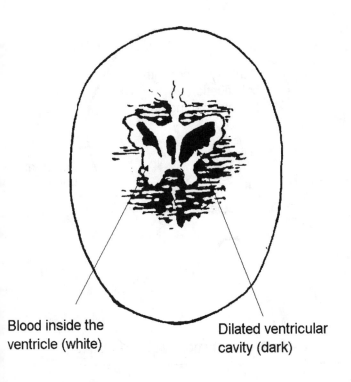

Blood inside the ventricle (white)

Dilated ventricular cavity (dark)

D-75: Intraventricular hemorrhage (Sonogram)

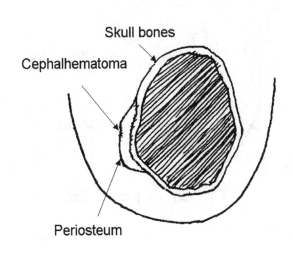

Skull bones

Cephalhematoma

Periosteum

D-76: Cephalhematoma (CT Scan head)

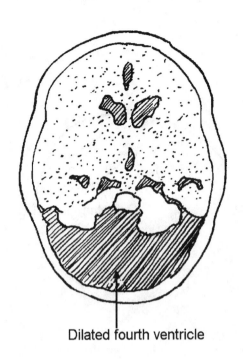

Dilated fourth ventricle

D- 77: Dandy Walker malformation (Head CT Scan)

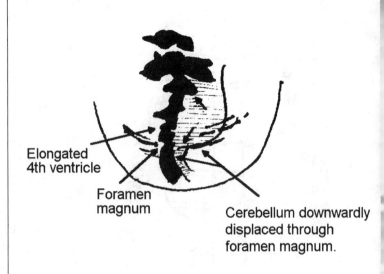

Elongated
4th ventricle

Foramen
magnum

Cerebellum downwardly
displaced through
foramen magnum.

D-78: Arnold Chiari malformation (Head sonogram)

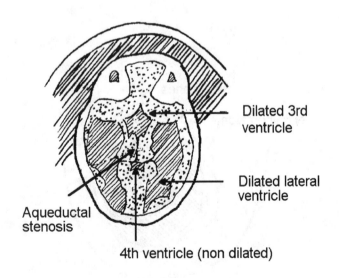

Dilated 3rd
ventricle

Dilated lateral
ventricle

Aqueductal
stenosis

4th ventricle (non dilated)

D-79: Aqueductal stenosis (Head CT Scan)

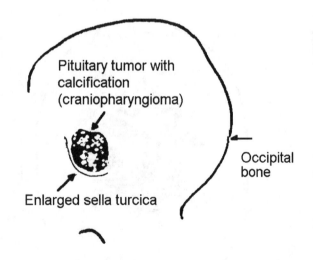

Pituitary tumor with
calcification
(craniopharyngioma)

Occipital
bone

Enlarged sella turcica

D-80: Pituitary tumor (skull x-ray lateral)

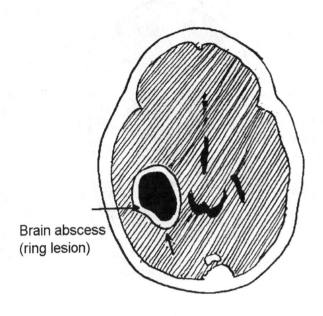

Brain abscess
(ring lesion)

D-81: Brain abscess (Head CT scan)

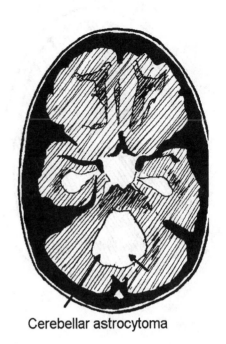

Cerebellar astrocytoma

D-82: Posterior fossa tumor (Head MRI)

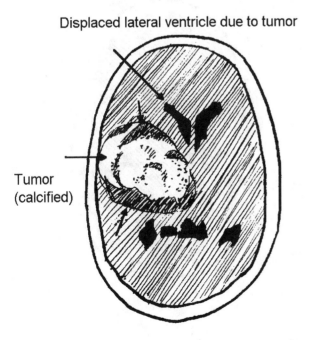

Displaced lateral ventricle due to tumor

Tumor
(calcified)

D-83: Supratentorial tumor (Head CT scan)

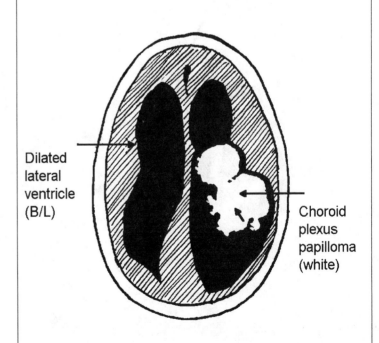

Dilated
lateral
ventricle
(B/L)

Choroid
plexus
papilloma
(white)

D-84: Choroid plexus papilloma (Head CT scan)

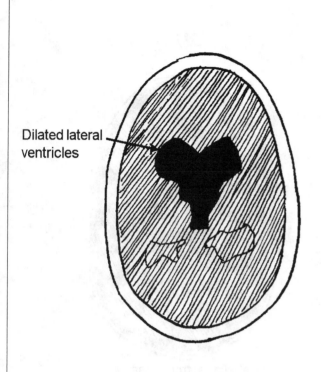

Dilated lateral
ventricles

D-85: Absent septum pellucidum (Head CT scan)

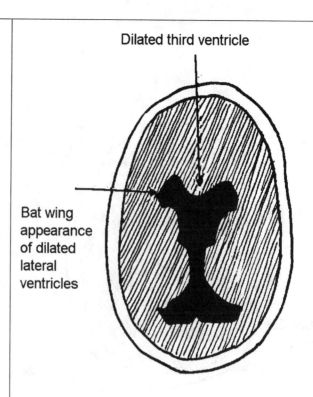

Dilated third ventricle

Bat wing
appearance
of dilated
lateral
ventricles

D-86: Agenesis of corpus callosum (Head CT scan)

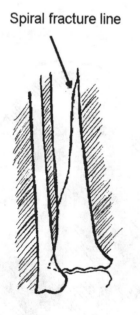

Spiral fracture line

D-87: Spiral tibial fracture (X-ray)

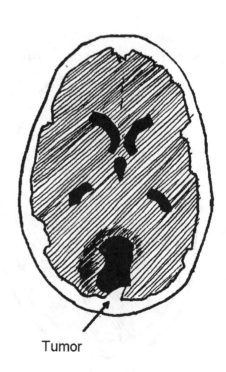

Tumor

D-88: Posterior fossa tumor (Head CT Scan)

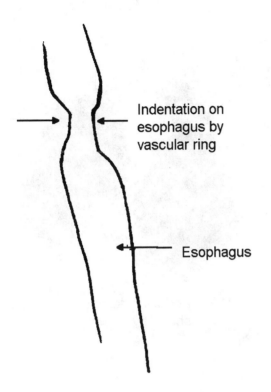

Indentation on esophagus by vascular ring

Esophagus

D-89: Vascular ring (barium study)

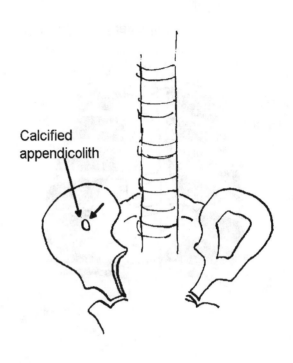

Calcified appendicolith

D-90: Appendicitis (abdominal X-ray)

(L) upper lobe infiltrate (later stage)

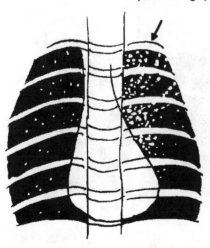

D-91: Mycoplasma pneumonia (X-ray)

(R) upper lobe pneumonia

Buldging fissure

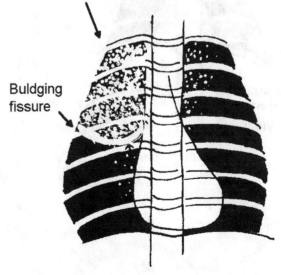

D-92: Klebsiella pneumonia (X-ray)

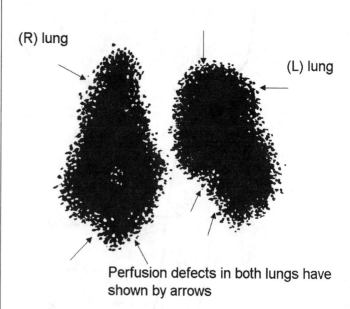

Hyperaerated both lungs

Fluid in the fissure

Flat diaphragm

D-93: TTNB (Transient tachypnea of the new born) (X-ray)

(R) lung

(L) lung

Perfusion defects in both lungs have shown by arrows

D-94: Pulmonary embolism (lung perfusion scan)

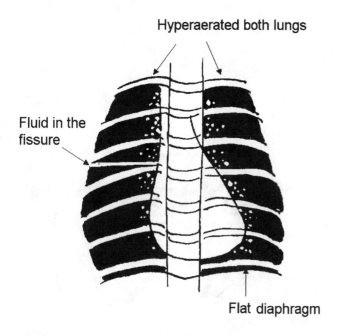

Elevation of (R) diaphragm

Stomach gas shadow

Normal (L) diaphragm

D-95: (R) diaphragmatic paralysis (X-ray)

(B/L) Scattered calcification over the kidney areas

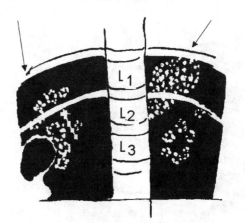

L₁

L₂

L₃

D-96: Medullary nephrocalcinosis (X-ray)

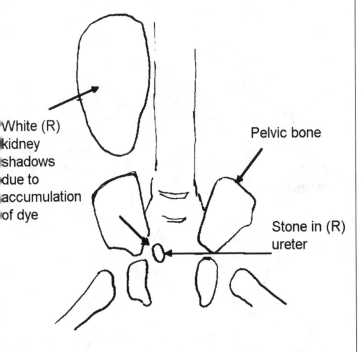

White (R)
kidney
shadows
due to
accumulation
of dye

Pelvic bone

Stone in (R)
ureter

D-97: Obstruction in (R) ureter (IVP study)

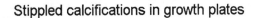

Stippled calcifications in growth plates

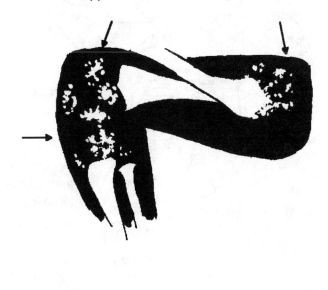

D-98: Chondrodysplasia punctata (X–ray)

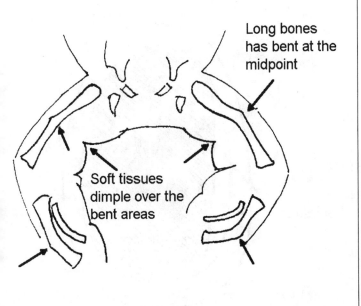

Long bones
has bent at the
midpoint

Soft tissues
dimple over the
bent areas

D-99: Campomelic dysplasia (X-ray)

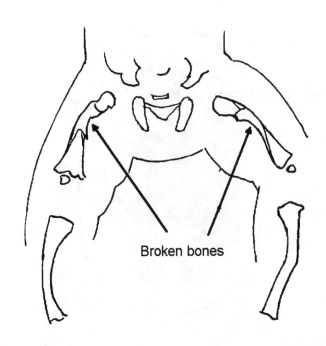

Broken bones

D-100: Osteogenesis imperfecta (X-ray)

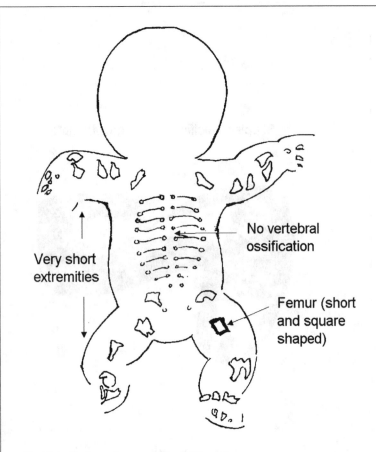

Very short
extremities

No vertebral
ossification

Femur (short
and square
shaped)

D-101: Achondrogenesis I (X-ray)

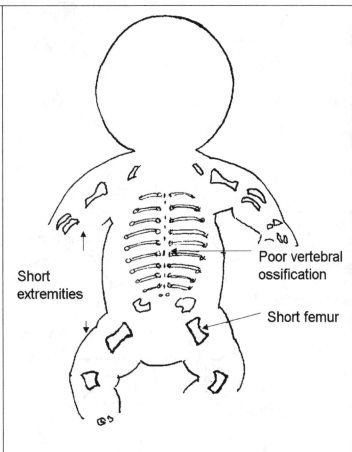

Short
extremities

Poor vertebral
ossification

Short femur

D-102: Achondrogenesis II (X-ray)

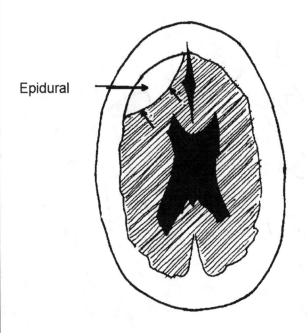

Epidural

D-103: Epidural hematoma (CT Scan)

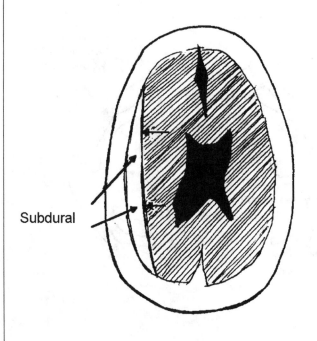

Subdural

D-104: Subdural hematoma (CT Scan)

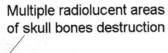

Multiple radiolucent areas
of skull bones destruction

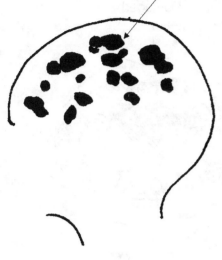

D-105: Sarcoidosis (skull X-ray)

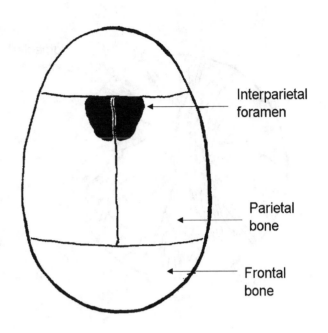

Interparietal
foramen

Parietal
bone

Frontal
bone

D-106: Parietal foramen (X-ray)

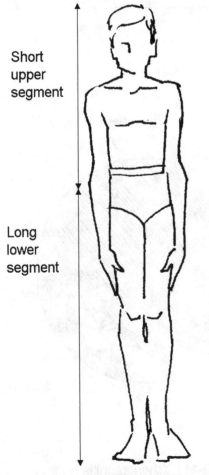

Short
upper
segment

Long
lower
segment

D-107: Marfan syndrome

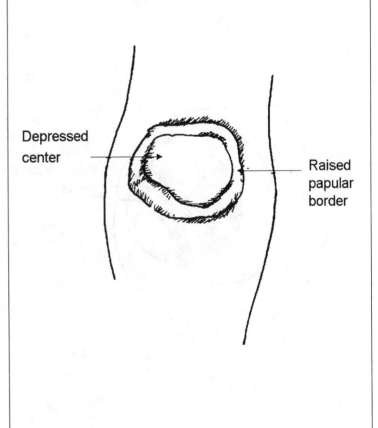

Depressed
center

Raised
papular
border

D-108: Granuloma annulare

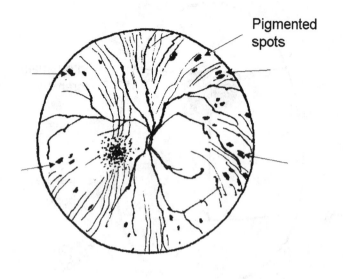

Pigmented spots

D-109: Retinitis pigmentosa (Retinal diagram)

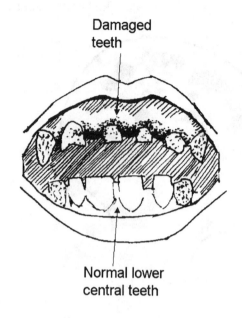

Damaged teeth

Normal lower central teeth

D-110: Milk bottle caries

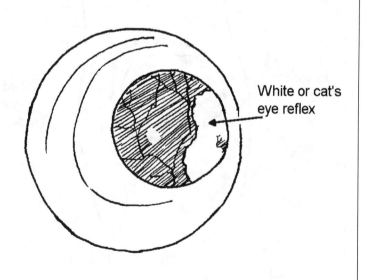

White or cat's eye reflex

D-111: Retinoblastoma (retina)

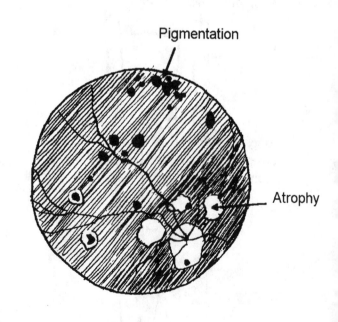

Pigmentation

Atrophy

D-112: Chorioretinitis (retina)

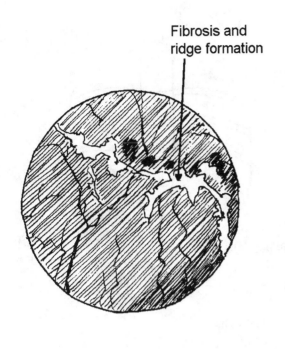

Fibrosis and
ridge formation

D-113: Retinopathy of prematurity

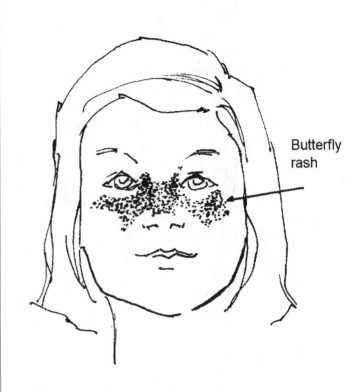

Butterfly
rash

D-114: Systemic lupus erythematosus

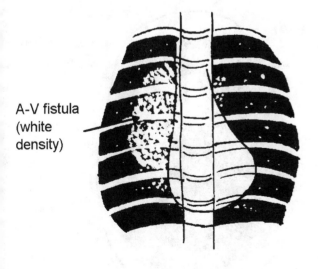

A-V fistula
(white
density)

D-115: Pulmonary A-V fistula (X-ray)

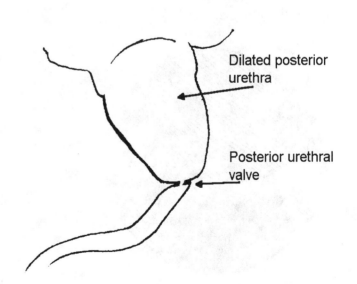

Dilated posterior
urethra

Posterior urethral
valve

D-116: Posterior urethral valve (VCU study)

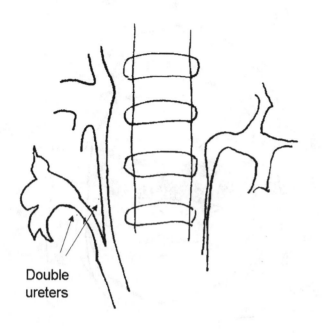

Double
ureters

D-117: Double ureters (R) side (IVP Study)

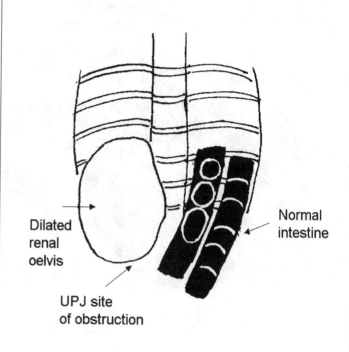

Dilated
renal
oelvis

Normal
intestine

UPJ site
of obstruction

D-118: (R) Ureteropelvic junction obstruction (IVP study)

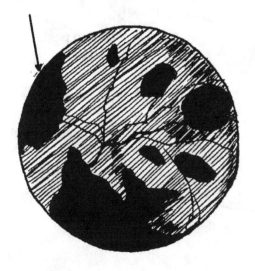

Hemorrhage

D-119: Retinal hemorrhage (retina)

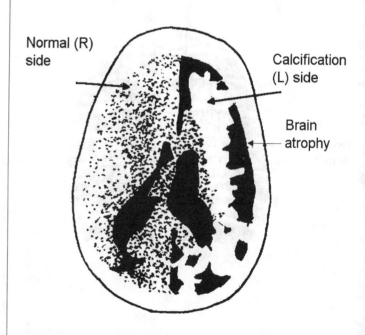

Normal (R)
side

Calcification
(L) side

Brain
atrophy

D-120: Sturge-Weber syndrome (CT scan head)

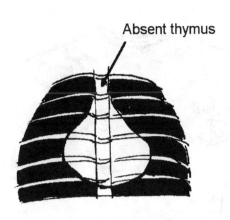

Absent thymus

D-121: DiGeorge syndrome (X-ray)

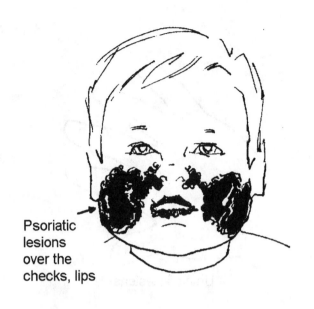

Psoriatic lesions over the checks, lips

D-122: Zinc deficiency

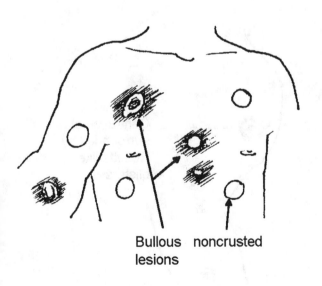

Bullous noncrusted lesions

D-123: Staphylococcal impetigo

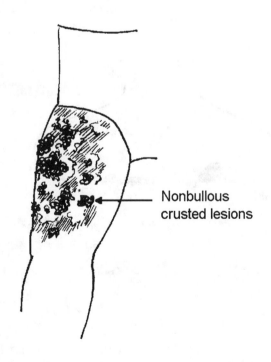

Nonbullous crusted lesions

D-124: Streptococcal impetigo

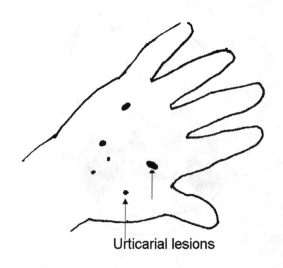

Urticarial lesions

D-125: Papular urticaria

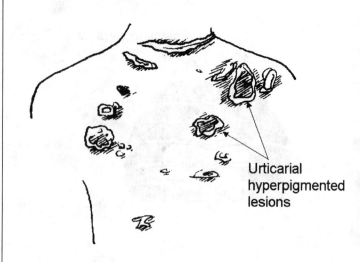

Urticarial hyperpigmented lesions

D-126: Urticaria pigmentosa

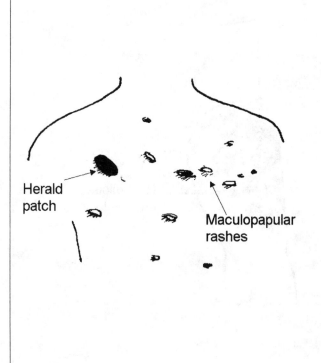

Herald patch

Maculopapular rashes

D-127: Pityriasis rosea (Christmas tree pattern)

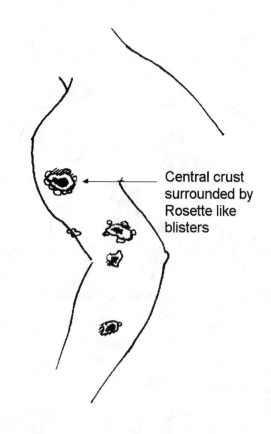

Central crust surrounded by Rosette like blisters

D-128: IgA dermatosis

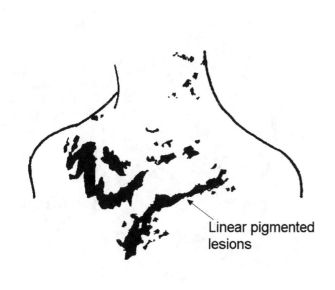

D-129: Incontinentia pigmenti

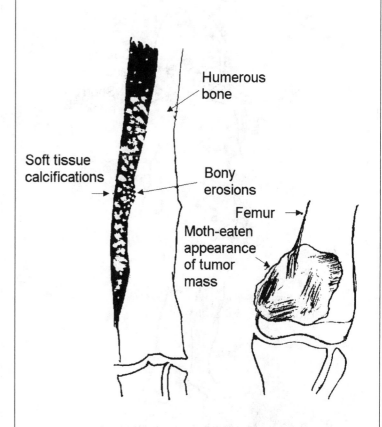

D-130: Osteosarcoma (X-ray humerous & femur)

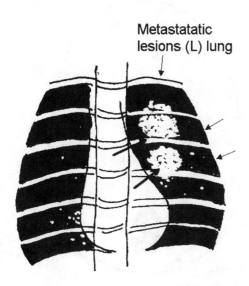

D-131: Lung metastasis of osteosarcoma

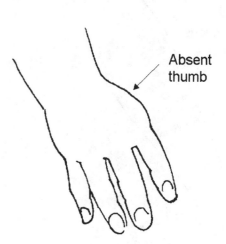

D-132: Fanconi syndrome

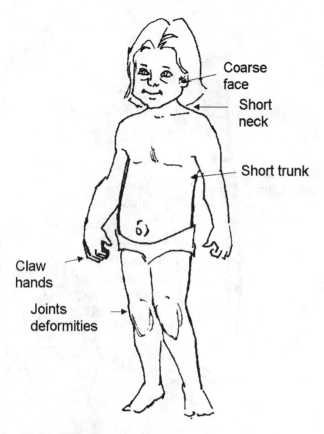

Coarse face

Short neck

Short trunk

Claw hands

Joints deformities

D-133: Maroteaux-Lamy syndrome

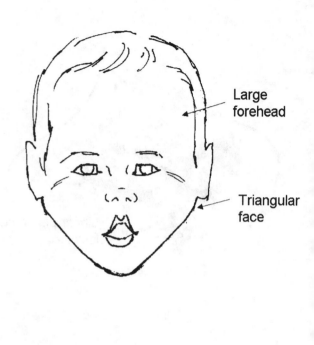

Large forehead

Triangular face

D-134: Methylmalonic acidemia

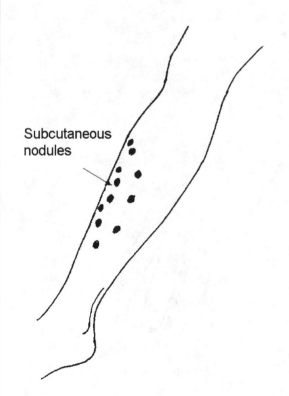

Subcutaneous nodules

D-135: Subcutaneous nodules in rheumatic fever

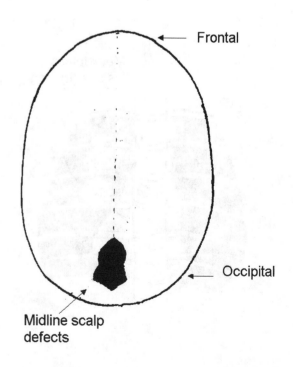

Frontal

Occipital

Midline scalp defects

D-136: Midline scalp defects (Trisomy 13)

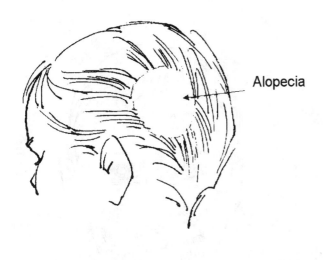

Alopecia

D-137: Localized alopecia of newborn

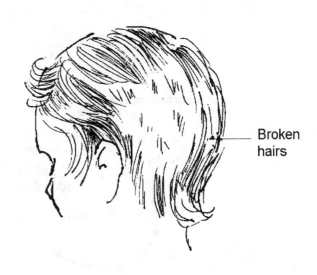

Broken hairs

D-138: Trichotillomania

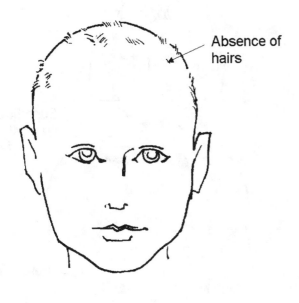

Absence of hairs

D-139: Alopecia totalis

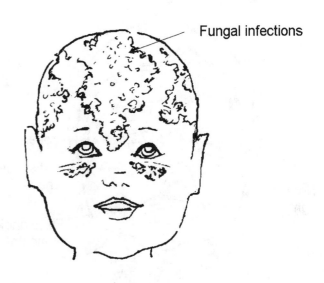

Fungal infections

D-140: Fungal scalp infections

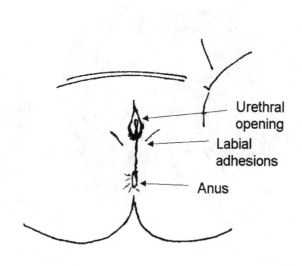

Urethral
opening

Labial
adhesions

Anus

D-141: Labial adhesions

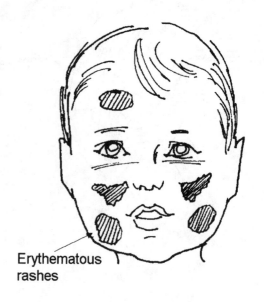

Erythematous
rashes

D-142: Urticaria

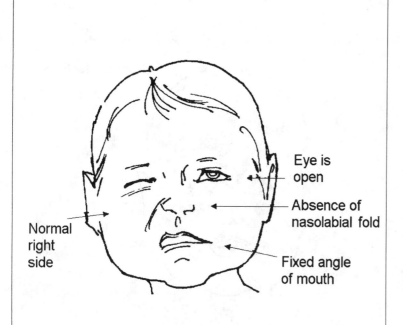

Eye is
open

Absence of
nasolabial fold

Normal
right
side

Fixed angle
of mouth

D-143: Left facial palsy

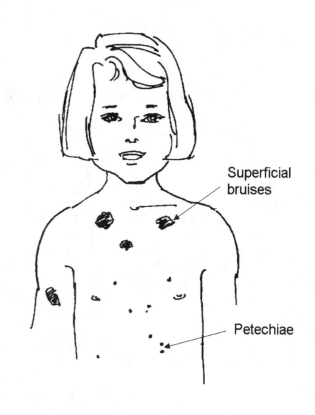

Superficial
bruises

Petechiae

D-144: Idiopathic thrombocytopenic purpura(ITP)

Small head

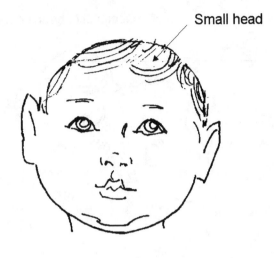

D-145: Microcephaly

Flexion contractures of joints

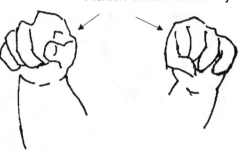

D-146: Arthrogryposis

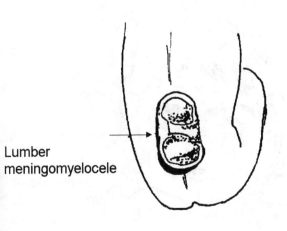

Lumber
meningomyelocele

D-147: Meningomyelocele

Spina bifida
underneath
the skin
dimple

Lower
back
region

D-148: Spina bifida

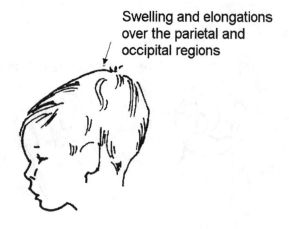

Swelling and elongations
over the parietal and
occipital regions

D-149: Caput

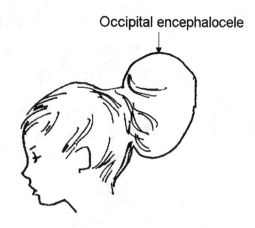

Occipital encephalocele

D-150: Encephalocele

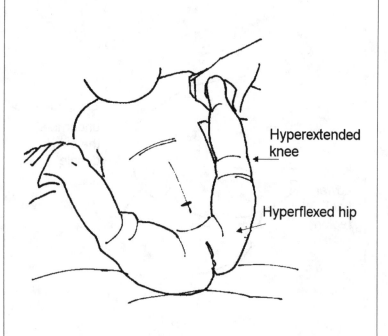

Hyperextended
knee

Hyperflexed hip

D-151: Breech presentation

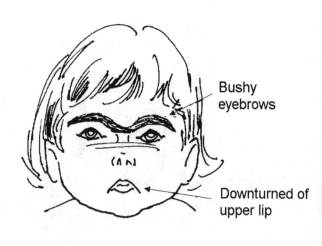

Bushy
eyebrows

Downturned of
upper lip

D-152: Cornelia deLange syndrome

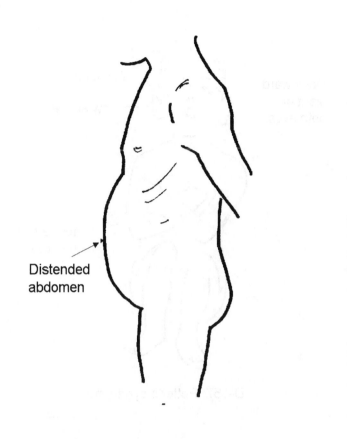

Distended
abdomen

D-153: Abdominal distension

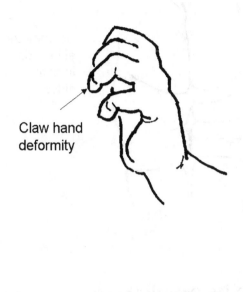

Claw hand
deformity

D-154: Klumpke paralysis

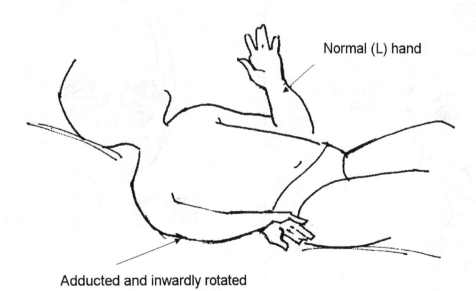

Normal (L) hand

Adducted and inwardly rotated

D-155: Brachial plexus palsy (R) side

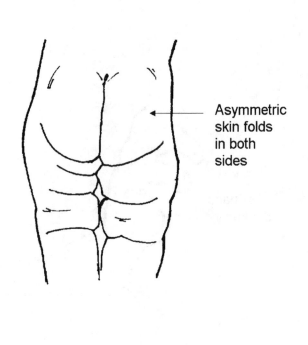

Asymmetric
skin folds
in both
sides

D-156: Dislocated hip joint

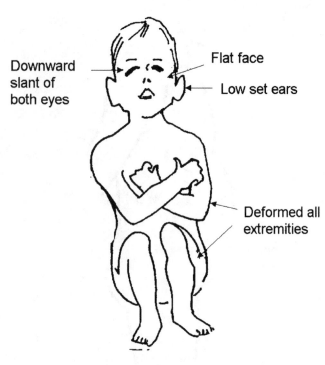

Downward
slant of
both eyes

Flat face

Low set ears

Deformed all
extremities

D-157: Potter's syndrome

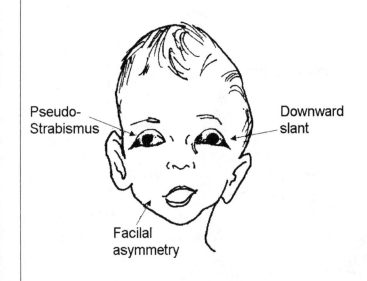

Pseudo-
Strabismus

Downward
slant

Facilal
asymmetry

D-158: Cerebral dystrophy

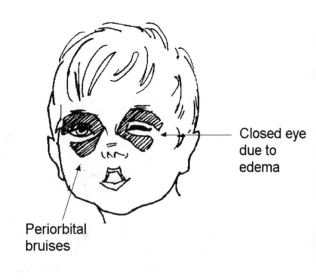

Closed eye
due to
edema

Periorbital
bruises

D-159: Periorbital bruises (Child abuse)

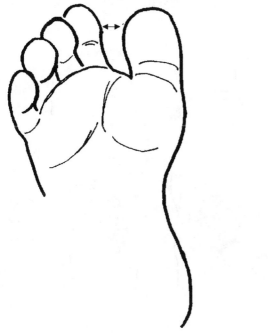

Wider space between 1st & 2nd toes

D-160: Down syndrome

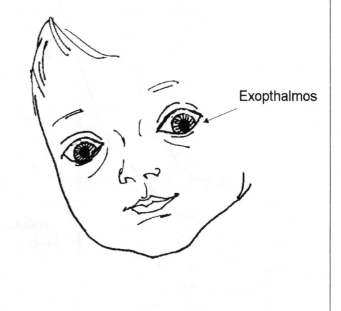

Exopthalmos

D-161: Hyperthyroidism

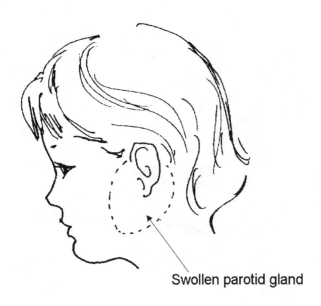

Swollen parotid gland

D-162: Parotitis

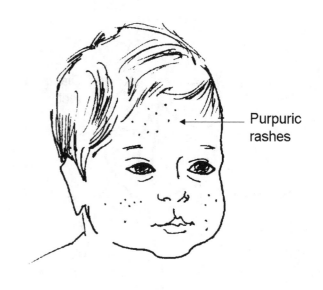

Purpuric rashes

D-163: Thrombocytopenic purpura

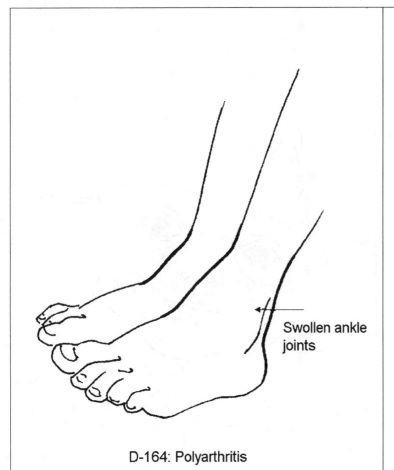

Swollen ankle joints

D-164: Polyarthritis

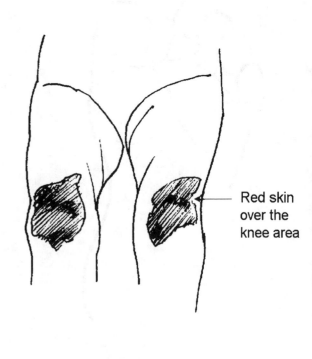

Red skin over the knee area

D-165: (B/L) Skin redness over the knee

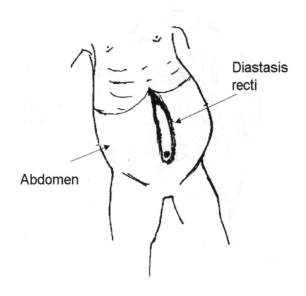

Diastasis recti

Abdomen

D-166: Diastasis

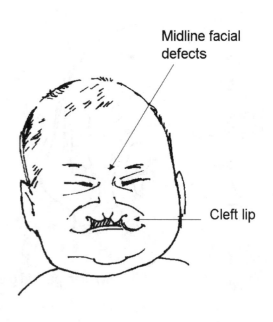

Midline facial defects

Cleft lip

D-167: Holoprosencephaly

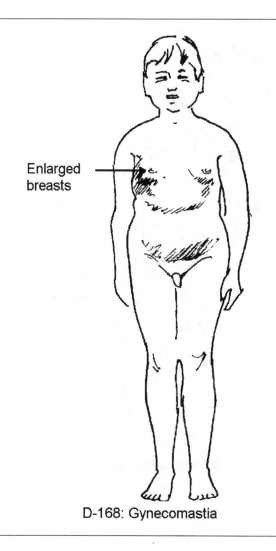

Enlarged breasts

D-168: Gynecomastia

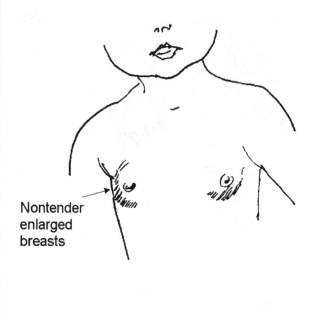

Nontender enlarged breasts

D-169: Breast enlargement (B/L)

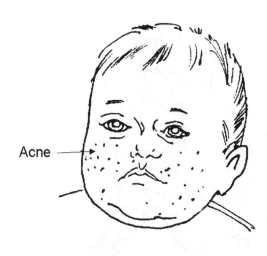

Acne

D-170: Neonatal acne

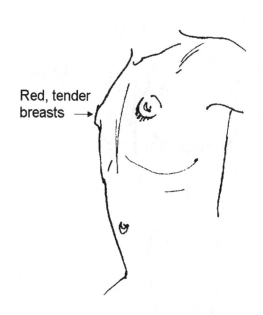

Red, tender breasts

D-171: Mastitis

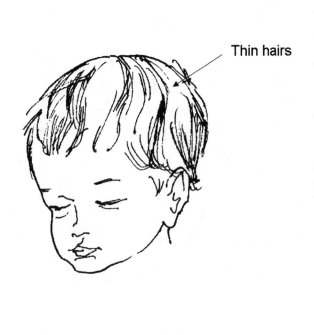

Thin hairs

D-172: Normal premature

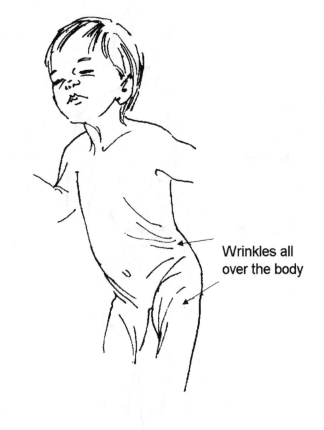

Wrinkles all over the body

D-173: Postmature newborn

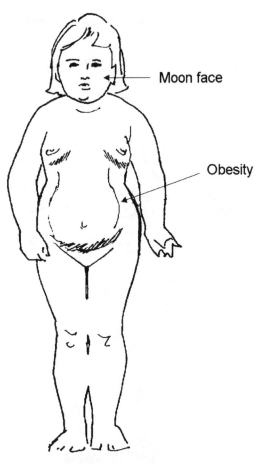

Moon face

Obesity

D-174: Cushing syndrome

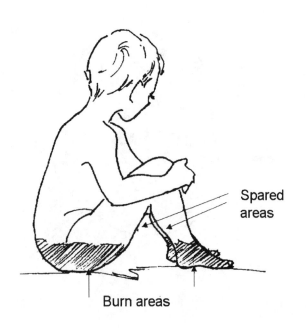

Spared areas

Burn areas

D-175: Hot water burn (Child abuse)

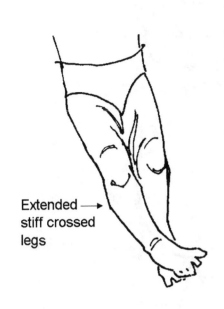

Extended → stiff crossed legs

D-176: Spastic child (cerebral diplegia)

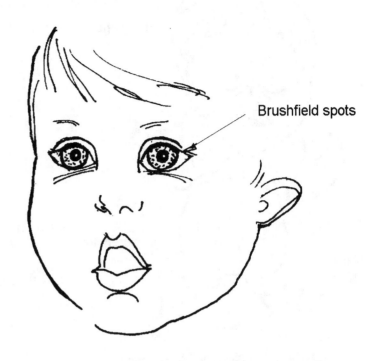

Brushfield spots

D-177: Brushfield spots in iris (Down syndrome)

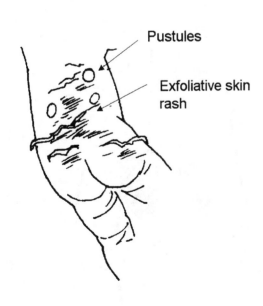

Pustules

Exfoliative skin rash

D-178: Reiter syndrome

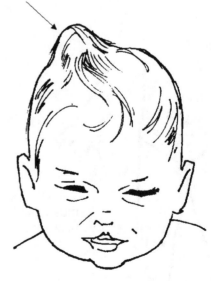

(R) parietal cephalhematoma

D-179: Cephalhematoma

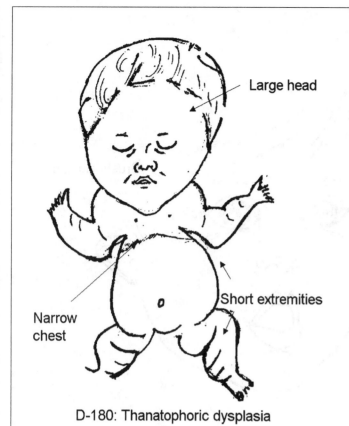

Large head

Narrow chest

Short extremities

D-180: Thanatophoric dysplasia

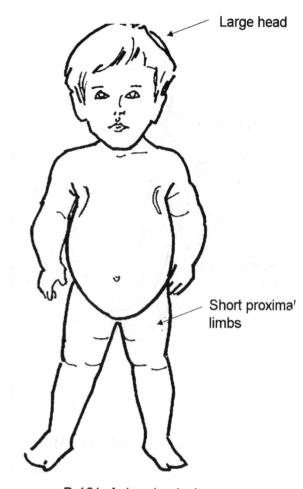

Large head

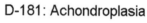

Short proxima' limbs

D-181: Achondroplasia

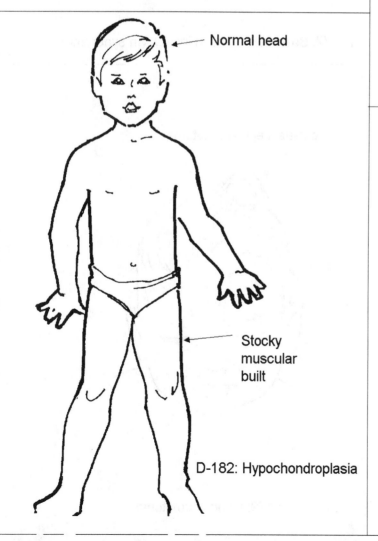

Normal head

Stocky muscular built

D-182: Hypochondroplasia

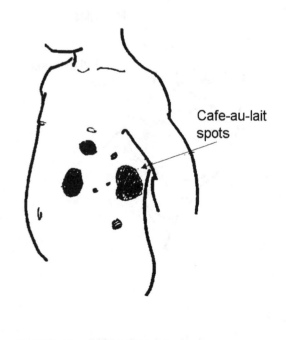

Cafe-au-lait spots

D-183: Neurofibromatosis

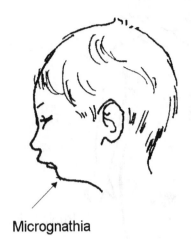

Micrognathia

D-184: Pierre-Robin syndrome

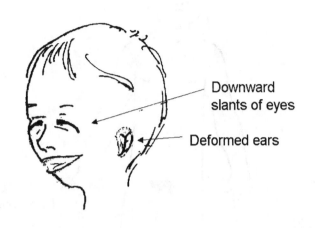

Downward slants of eyes

Deformed ears

D-185: Treacher Collins syndrome

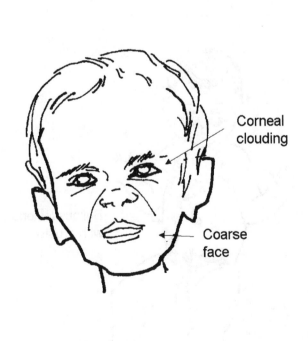

Corneal clouding

Coarse face

D-186: Hurler syndrome

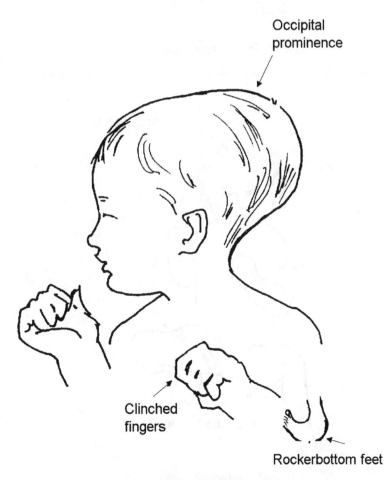

Occipital prominence

Clinched fingers

Rockerbottom feet

D-187: Trisomy 18

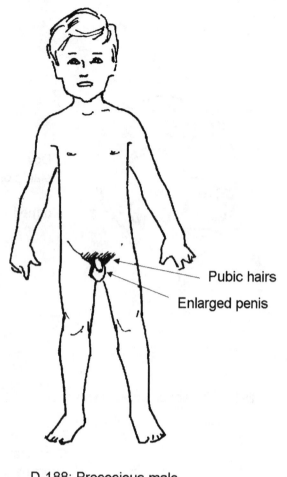

Pubic hairs

Enlarged penis

D-188: Precocious male

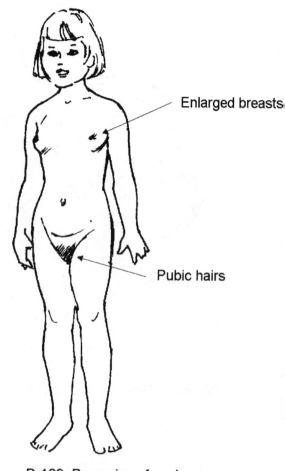

Enlarged breasts

Pubic hairs

D-189: Precocious female

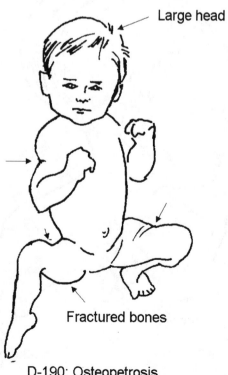

Large head

Fractured bones

D-190: Osteopetrosis

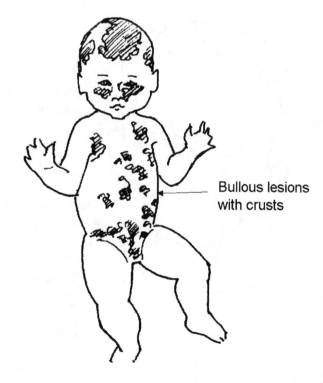

Bullous lesions
with crusts

D-191: Erythema multiforme

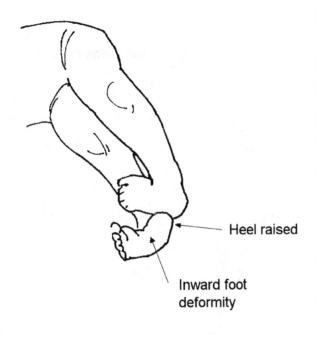

Heel raised

Inward foot
deformity

D-192: Talipes equinovarus

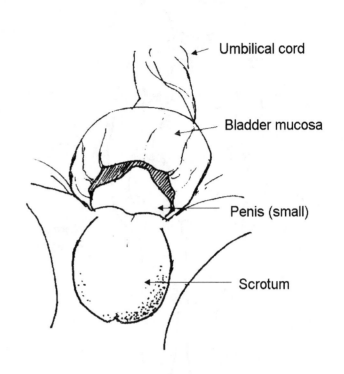

Umbilical cord

Bladder mucosa

Penis (small)

Scrotum

D-193: Urinary bladder extrophy

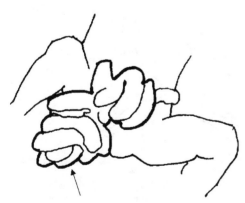

Matted intestines
(not covered with mucosa)

D-194: Gastroschisis

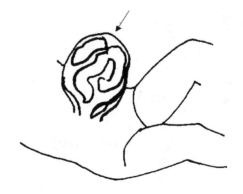

Midline mass covered with mucosa

D-195: Omphalocele

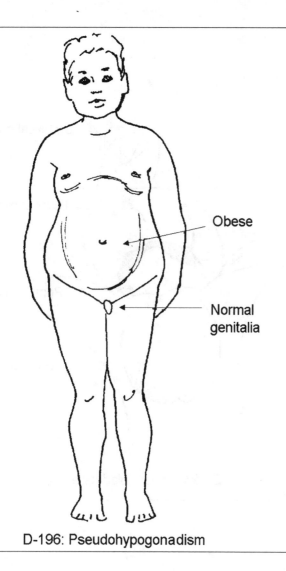

Obese

Normal
genitalia

D-196: Pseudohypogonadism

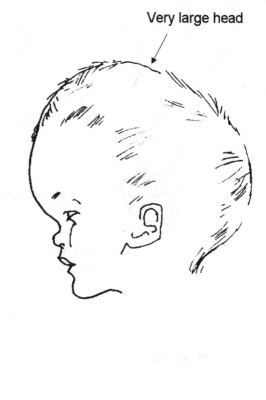

Very large head

D-197: Hydrocephalus

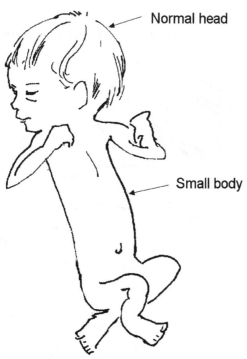

Normal head

Small body

D-198: Asymmetric SGA

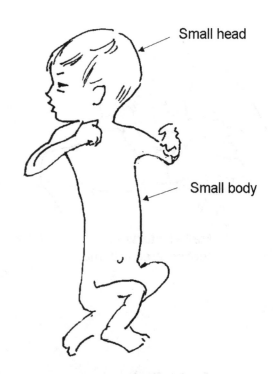

Small head

Small body

D-199: Symmetric SGA

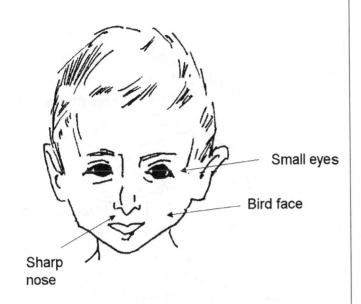

Small eyes

Bird face

Sharp
nose

D-200: Hallerman-Streiff-Francois syndrome

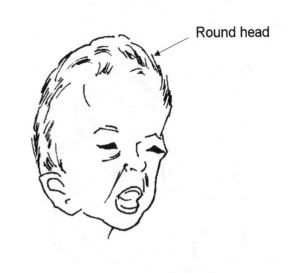

Round head

D-201: Acrocephaly

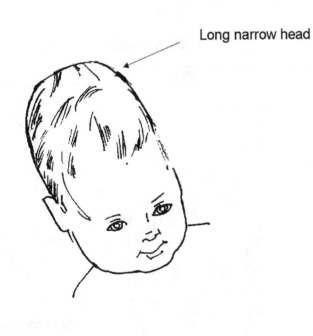

Long narrow head

D-202: Scaphocephaly

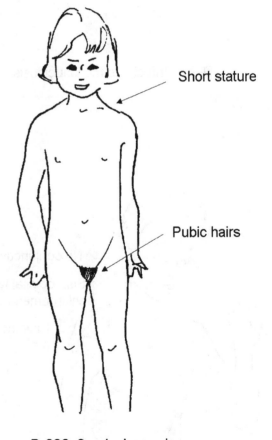

Short stature

Pubic hairs

D-203: Craniopharyngioma

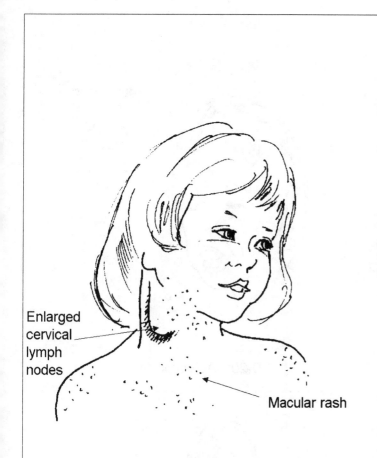

Enlarged cervical lymph nodes

Macular rash

D-204: Infectious mononucleosis

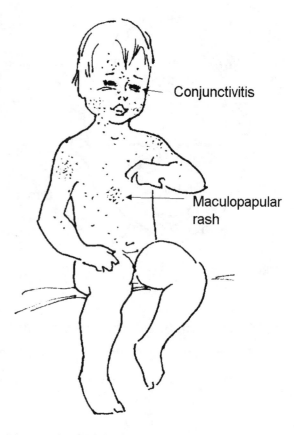

Conjunctivitis

Maculopapular rash

D-205: Measles

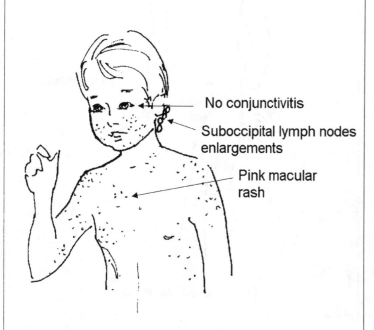

No conjunctivitis

Suboccipital lymph nodes enlargements

Pink macular rash

D-206: German measles (Rubella)

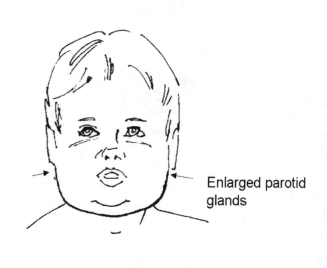

Enlarged parotid glands

D-207: Mumps

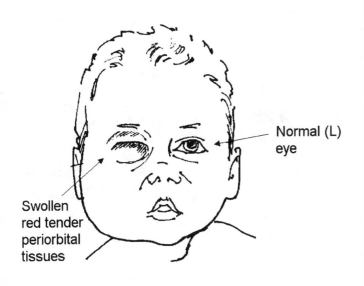

Normal (L) eye

Swollen red tender periorbital tissues

D-208: Periorbital cellulitis (R)

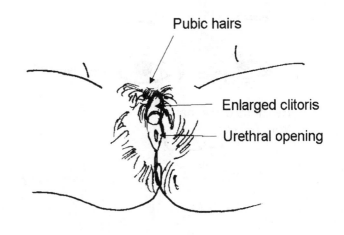

Pubic hairs

Enlarged clitoris

Urethral opening

D-209: Precocious puberty (Girl)

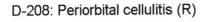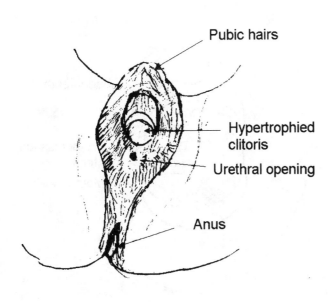

Pubic hairs

Hypertrophied clitoris

Urethral opening

Anus

D-210: Congenital adrenal hyperplasia

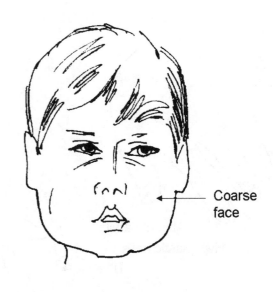

Coarse face

D-211: Hypothyroidism

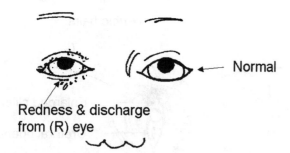

Normal

Redness & discharge
from (R) eye

D-212: Conjunctivitis (R) eye

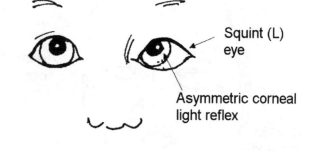

Squint (L)
eye

Asymmetric corneal
light reflex

D-213: Squint (L) eye

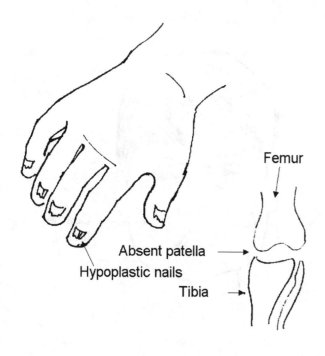

Femur

Absent patella

Hypoplastic nails

Tibia

D-214: Nail-patella syndrome

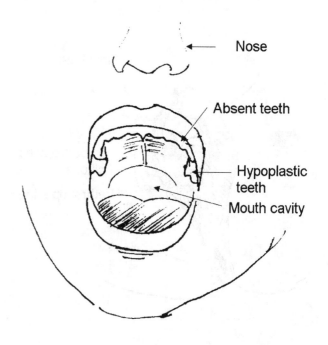

Nose

Absent teeth

Hypoplastic
teeth

Mouth cavity

D-215: Ectodermal dysplasia

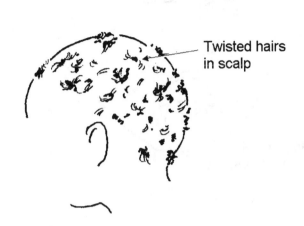

Twisted hairs
in scalp

D-216: Menkes kinky hair syndrome

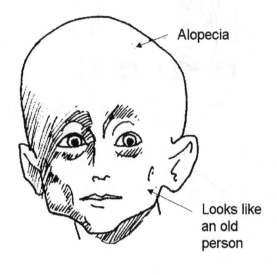

Alopecia

Looks like
an old
person

D-217: Progeria

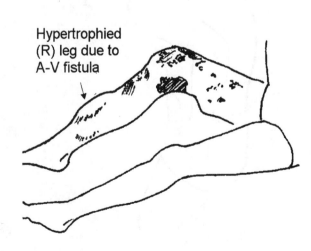

Hypertrophied
(R) leg due to
A-V fistula

D-218: Klippel-Trenaunay-Weber syndrome

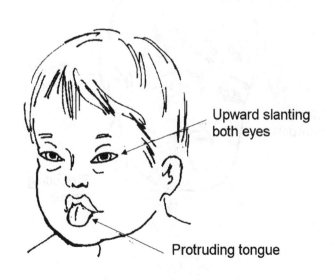

Upward slanting
both eyes

Protruding tongue

D-219: Down syndrome

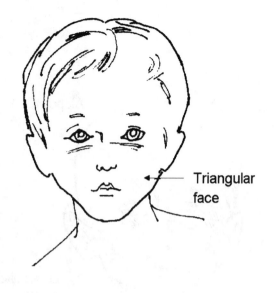

Triangular face

D-220: Russell-Silver syndrome

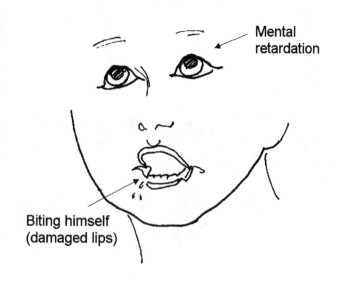

Mental retardation

Biting himself (damaged lips)

D-221: Lesch-Nyhan syndrome

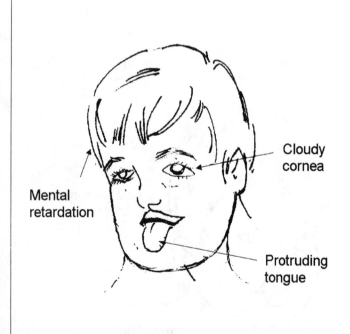

Cloudy cornea

Mental retardation

Protruding tongue

D-222: Mucopolysaccharidoses

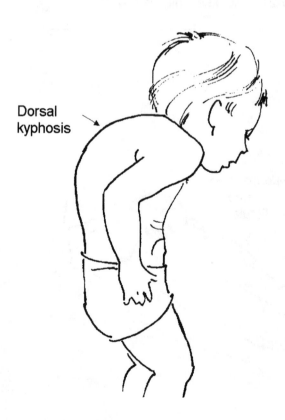

Dorsal kyphosis

D-223: Cockayne syndrome

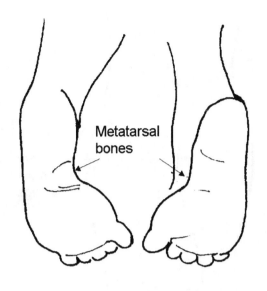

Metatarsal
bones

D-224: Metatarsus varus

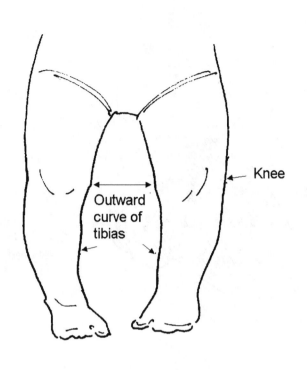

Knee

Outward
curve of
tibias

D-225: Bow legs

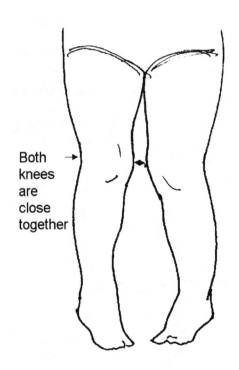

Both
knees
are
close
together

D-226: Knock knee

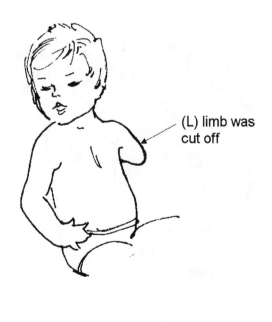

(L) limb was
cut off

D-227: Amniotic band

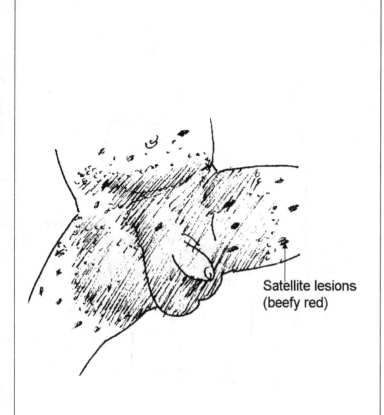

D-228: Monilial diaper dermatitis

Satellite lesions
(beefy red)

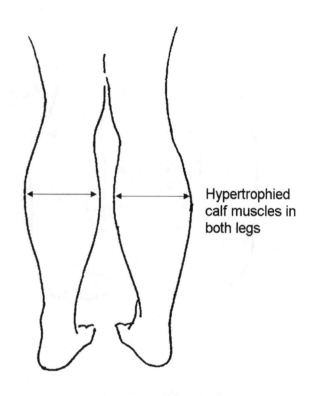

Hypertrophied
calf muscles in
both legs

D-229: Duschenne muscular dystrophy

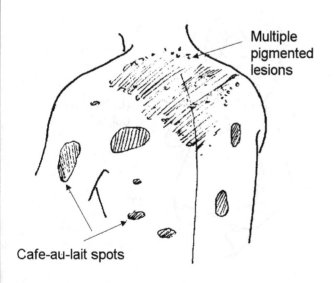

Multiple
pigmented
lesions

Cafe-au-lait spots

D-230: Neurofibromatosis

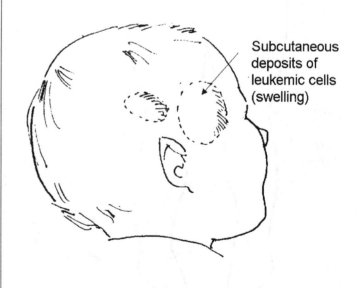

Subcutaneous
deposits of
leukemic cells
(swelling)

D-231: Leukemia

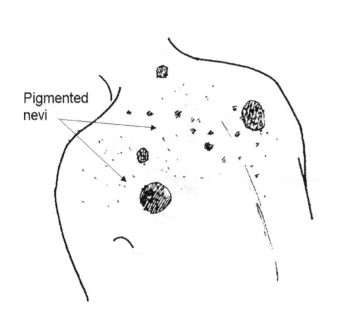

Pigmented
nevi

D-232: Multiple pigmented nevi

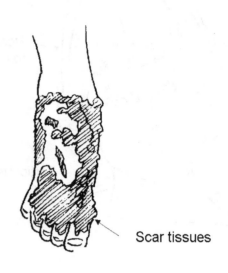

Scar tissues

D-233: Keloid

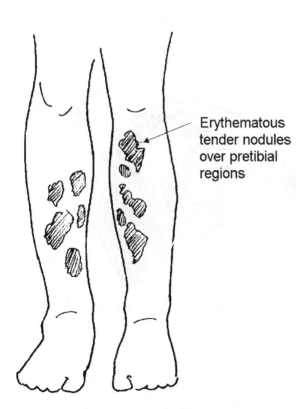

Erythematous
tender nodules
over pretibial
regions

D-234: Erythema nodosum

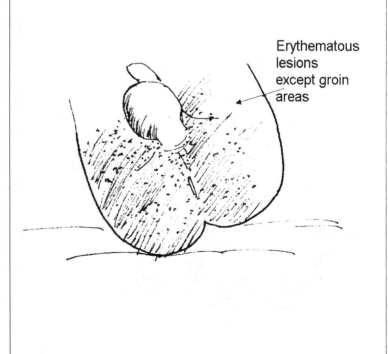

Erythematous
lesions
except groin
areas

D-235: Diaper dermatitis

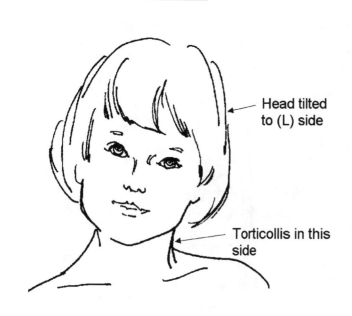

Head tilted
to (L) side

Torticollis in this
side

D-236: Torticollis (L) side

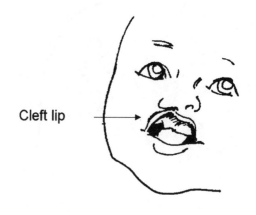

Cleft lip

D-237: Isolated cleft lip

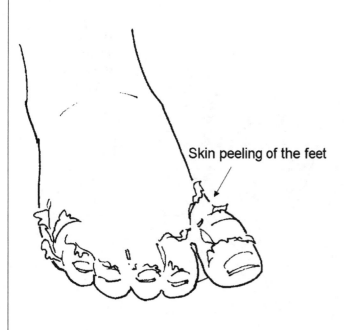

Skin peeling of the feet

D-238: Kawasaki disease

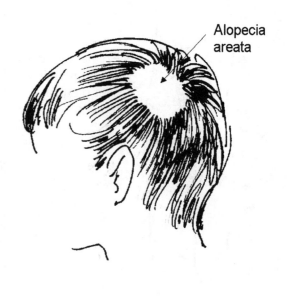

Alopecia
areata

D-239: Alopecia areata

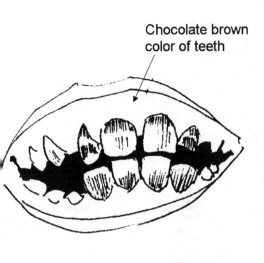

Chocolate brown
color of teeth

D-240: Chocolate brown teeth

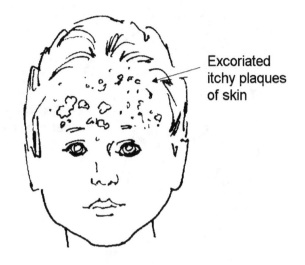

Excoriated
itchy plaques
of skin

D-241: Eczema

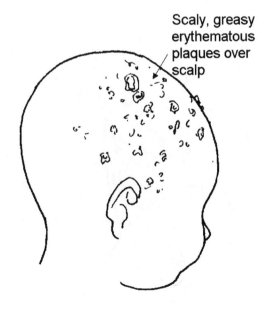

Scaly, greasy
erythematous
plaques over
scalp

D-242: Seborrhoeic dermatitis

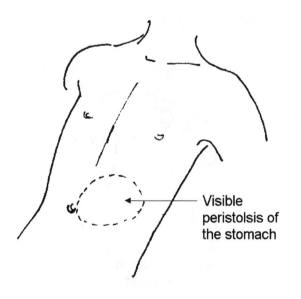

Visible
peristolsis of
the stomach

D-243: Pyloric stenosis

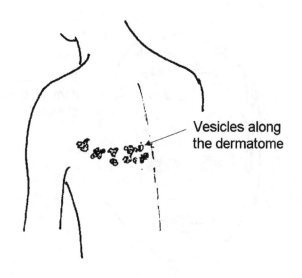

Vesicles along the dermatome

D-244: Herpes zoster

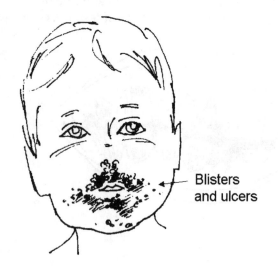

Blisters and ulcers

D-245: Herpes simplex

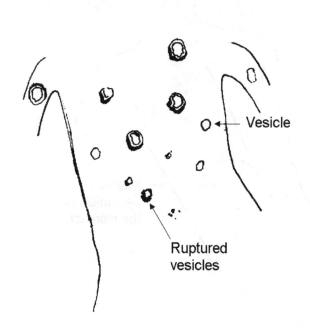

Vesicle

Ruptured vesicles

D-246: Chicken pox

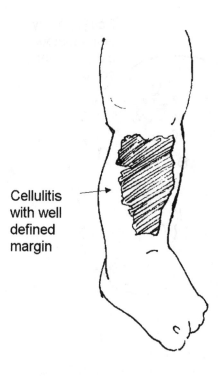

Cellulitis with well defined margin

D-247: Erysipelas

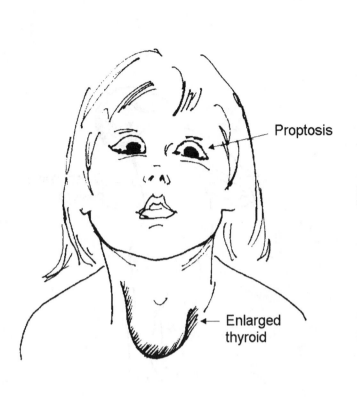

D-248: Hyperthyroidism

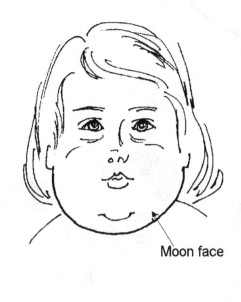

D-249: Cushing syndrome

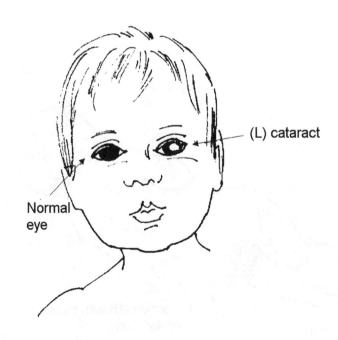

D-250: Congenital cataract

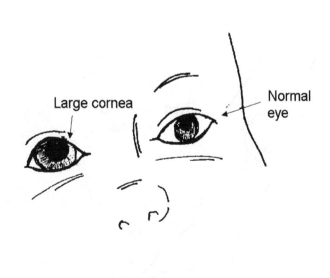

D-251: Congenital glaucoma (R) eye

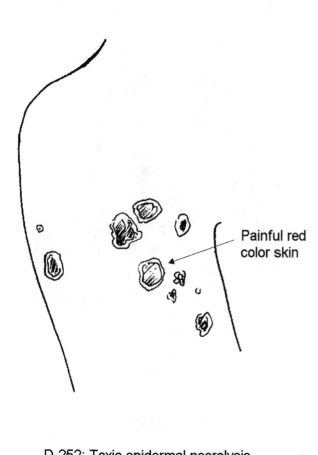

Painful red
color skin

D-252: Toxic epidermal necrolysis

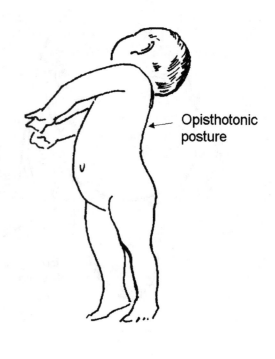

Opisthotonic
posture

D-253: Meningitis

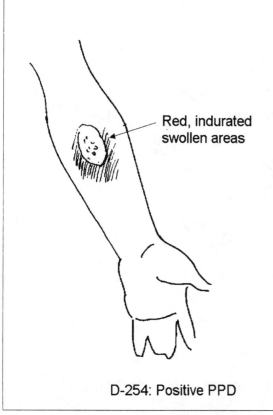

Red, indurated
swollen areas

D-254: Positive PPD

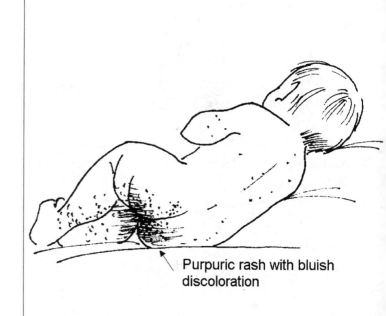

Purpuric rash with bluish
discoloration

D-255: Meningococcemia

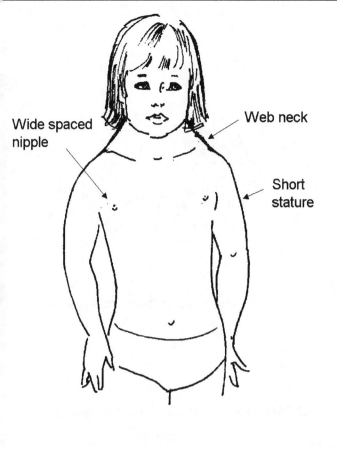

Wide spaced nipple

Web neck

Short stature

D-256: Turner syndrome (45 XO)

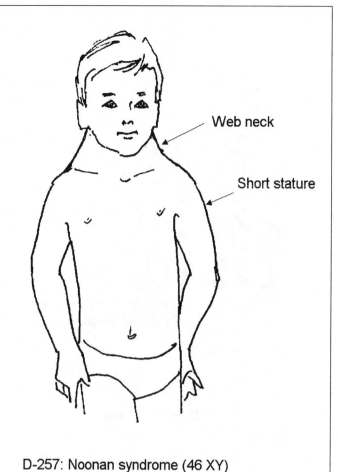

Web neck

Short stature

D-257: Noonan syndrome (46 XY)

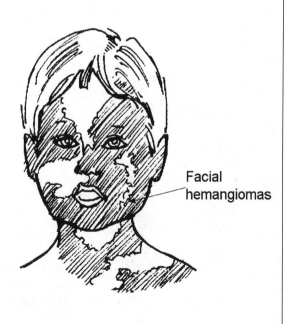

Facial hemangiomas

D-258: Sturge-Weber syndrome

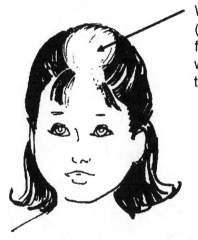

White forelock (white forehead, white hairs in the middle)

D-259: Waardenburg syndrome

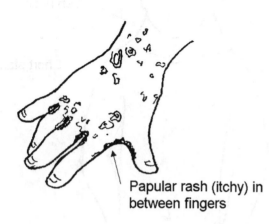

Papular rash (itchy) in
between fingers

D-260: Scabies

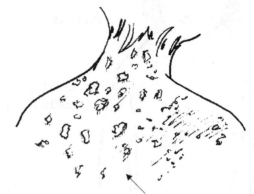

Silvery, scaly erythematous plaques

D-261: Psoriasis (back of neck & chest)

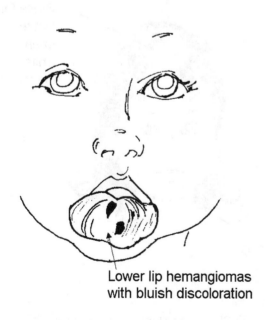

Lower lip hemangiomas
with bluish discoloration

D-262: Cavernous hemangiomas (lip)

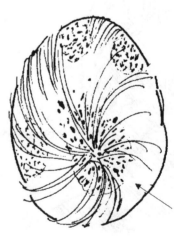

Seborrheic
skin rash
over the scalp

D-263: Histiocytosis (scalp)

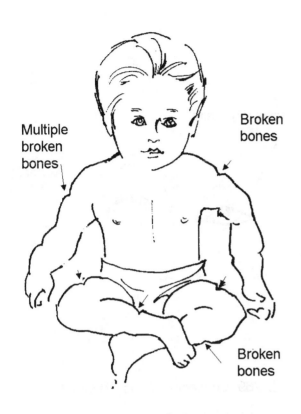

Multiple broken bones

Broken bones

Broken bones

D-264: Osteogenesis imperfecta

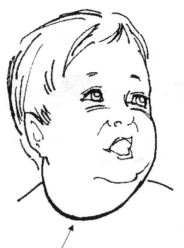

Swollen cystic mass over the neck

D-265: Cystic hygroma

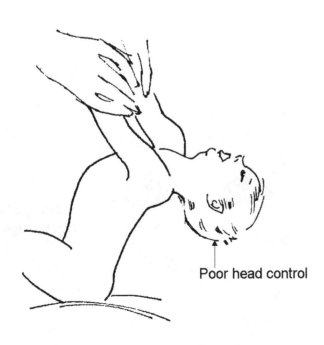

Poor head control

D-266: Floopy baby (6 months old)

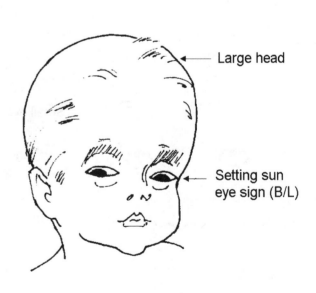

Large head

Setting sun eye sign (B/L)

D-267: Hydrocephalus

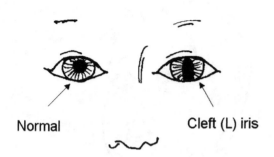

Normal   Cleft (L) iris

D-268: Coloboma of (L) iris

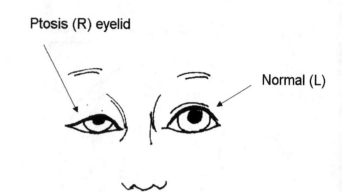

Ptosis (R) eyelid

Normal (L)

D-269: Congenital ptosis (R) eyelid

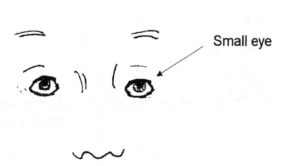

Small eye

D-270: Microopthalmias (B/L)

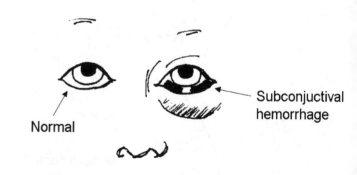

Normal

Subconjuctival hemorrhage

D-271: Subconjunctival hemmorrhage

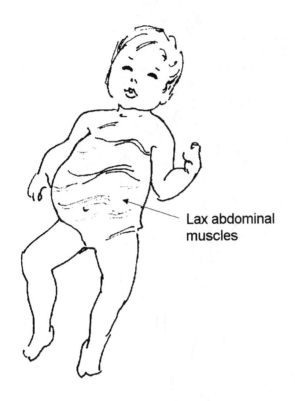

D-272: Prune belly syndrome

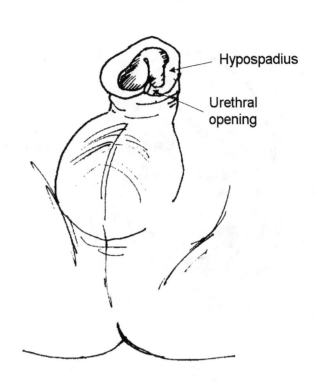

D-273: Hypospadius (First degree - mild)

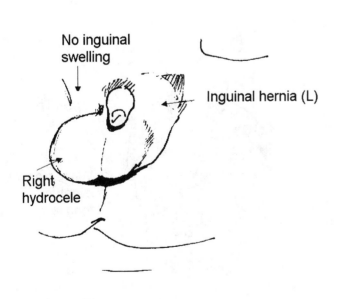

D-274: Inguinal hernia (L) side

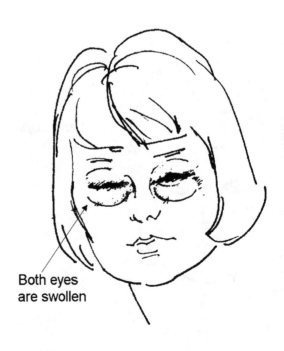

D-275: Nephrotic syndrome

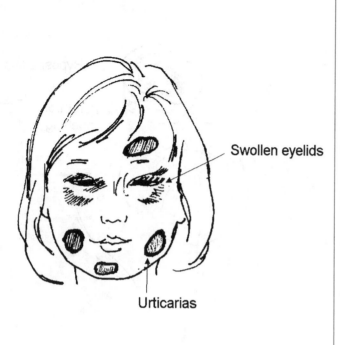

Swollen eyelids

Urticarias

D-276: Angioneurotic edema

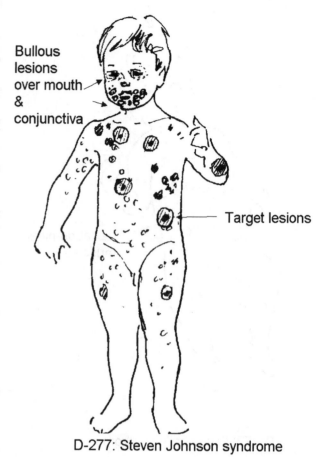

Bullous lesions over mouth & conjunctiva

Target lesions

D-277: Steven Johnson syndrome

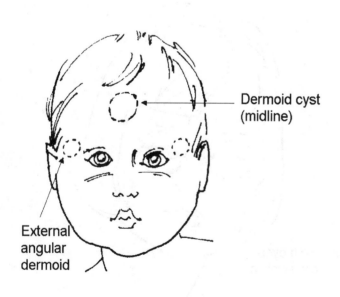

Dermoid cyst (midline)

External angular dermoid

D-278: Dermoid cysts

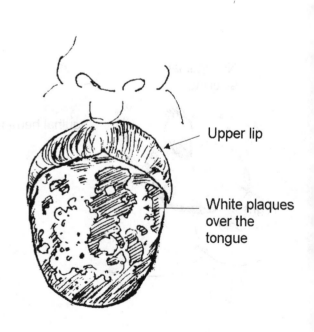

Upper lip

White plaques over the tongue

D-279: Oral thrush

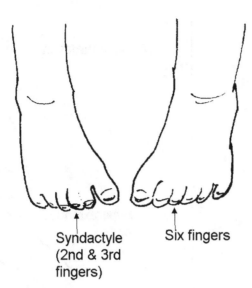

Syndactyle
(2nd & 3rd
fingers)

Six fingers

D-280: Polydactyle/syndactyle

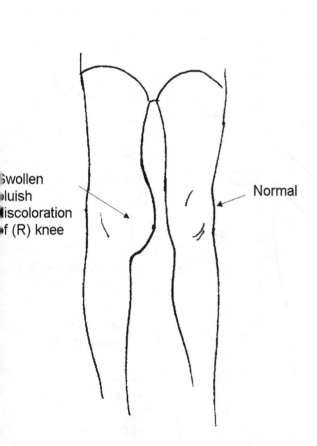

Swollen
bluish
discoloration
of (R) knee

Normal

D-281: Hemorrhagic knee (hemophilliac)

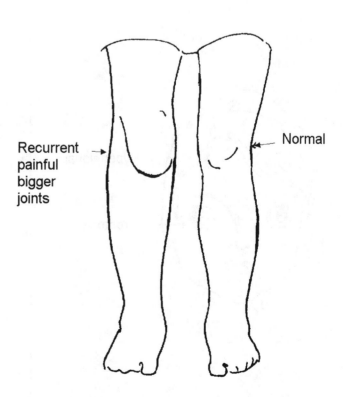

Recurrent
painful
bigger
joints

Normal

D-282: Juvenile rheumatoid arthritis (JRA)

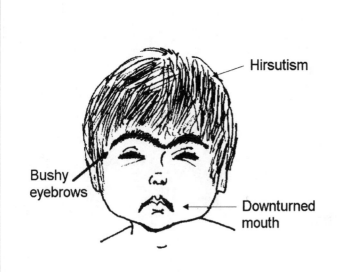

Hirsutism

Bushy
eyebrows

Downturned
mouth

D-283: DeLange syndrome

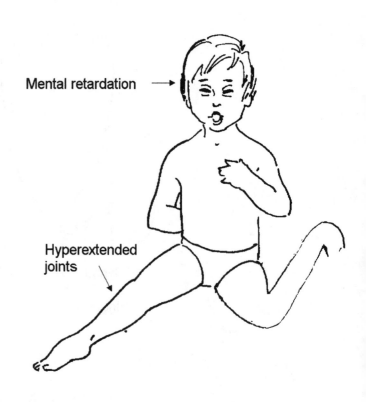

Mental retardation

Hyperextended
joints

D-284: Lowe syndrome

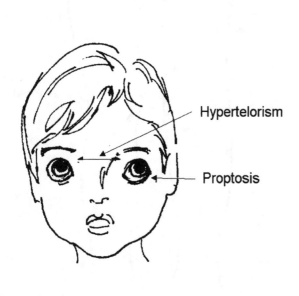

Hypertelorism

Proptosis

D-285: Crouzon syndrome

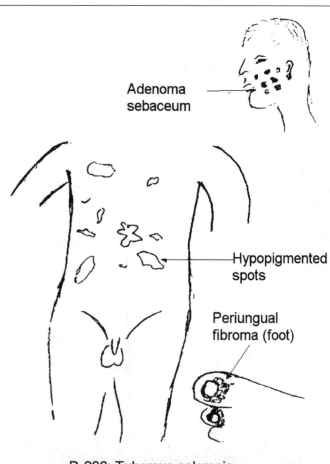

Adenoma
sebaceum

Hypopigmented
spots

Periungual
fibroma (foot)

D-286: Tuberous sclerosis

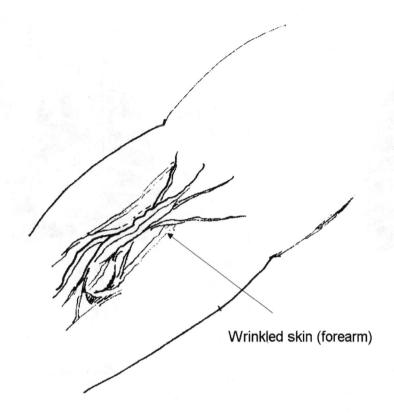

Wrinkled skin (forearm)

D-287: Dry skin (dehydration)

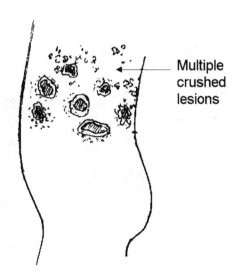

Multiple
crushed
lesions

D-288: Impetigo

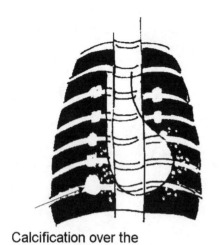

Calcification over the
posterior aspect of ribs

D-289: Child abuse

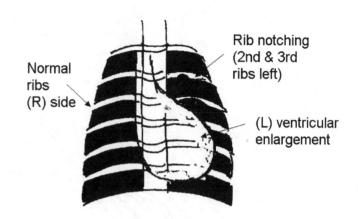

Normal
ribs
(R) side

Rib notching
(2nd & 3rd
ribs left)

(L) ventricular
enlargement

D-290: Aortic coarctation

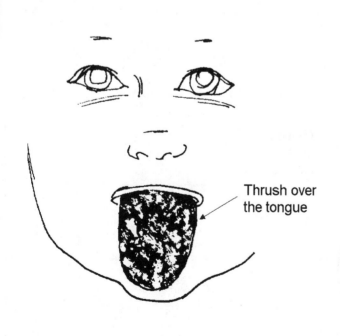

Thrush over
the tongue

D-291: Oral thrush

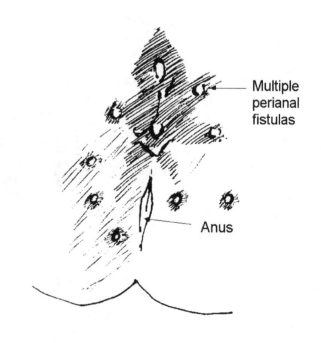

Multiple
perianal
fistulas

Anus

D-292: Crohn disease

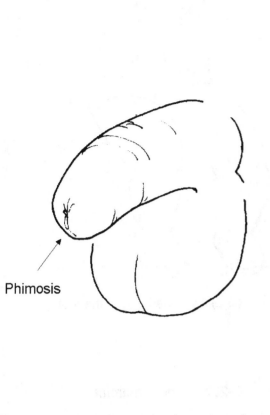

Phimosis

D-293: Phimosis

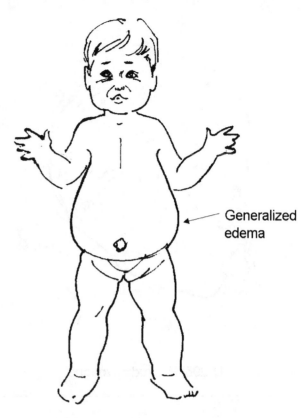

Generalized edema

D-294: Nephrotic syndrome

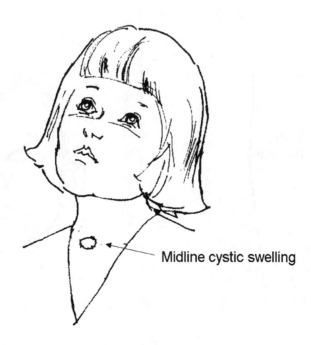

Midline cystic swelling

D-295: Thyroglossal cyst

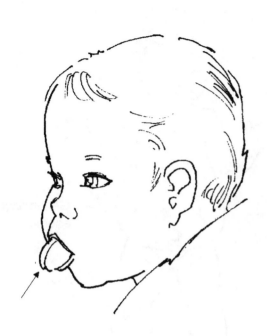

D-296: Protruding tongue

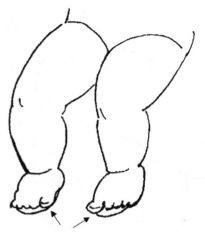

(B/L) Lymphedema of the feet

D-297: Turner syndrome

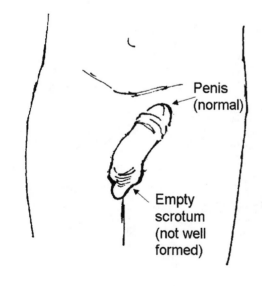

Penis
(normal)

Empty
scrotum
(not well
formed)

D-298: Undescended testes

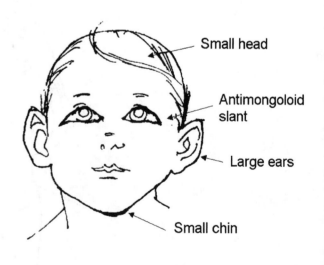

Small head

Antimongoloid
slant

Large ears

Small chin

D-299: Cri-du-chat syndrome

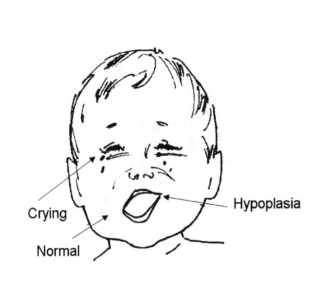

Crying

Normal

Hypoplasia

D-300: Hypoplasia of depressor angulioris muscle
(L) side

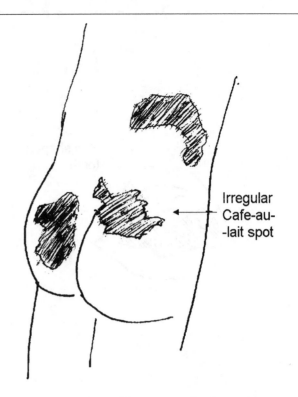

Irregular
Cafe-au-
-lait spot

D-301: McCune-Albright syndrome

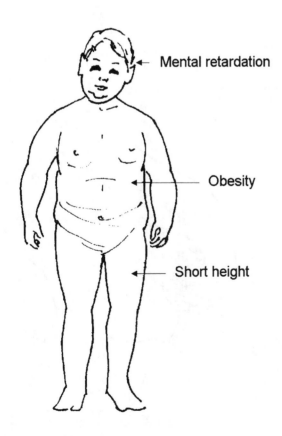

Mental retardation

Obesity

Short height

D-302: Prader-Willi syndrome

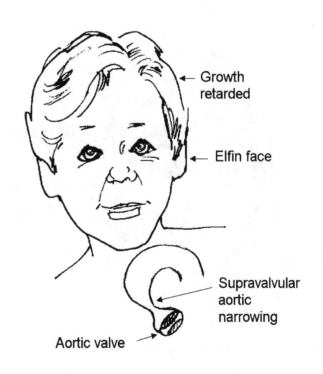

Growth
retarded

Elfin face

Supravalvular
aortic
narrowing

Aortic valve

D-303: William syndrome

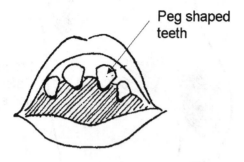

Peg shaped teeth

D-304: Ectodermal dysplasia

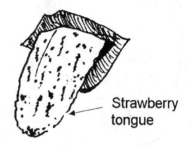

Strawberry tongue

D-305: Scarlet fever

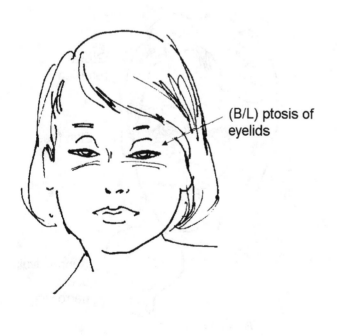

(B/L) ptosis of eyelids

D-306: Myasthenia gravis

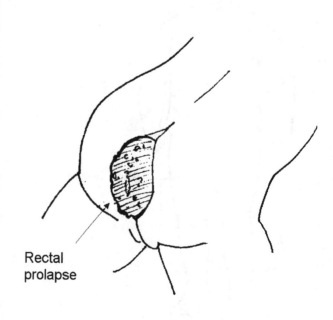

Rectal prolapse

D-307: Cystic fibrosis

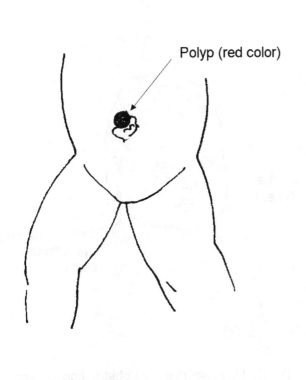

Polyp (red color)

D-308: Umbilical polyp

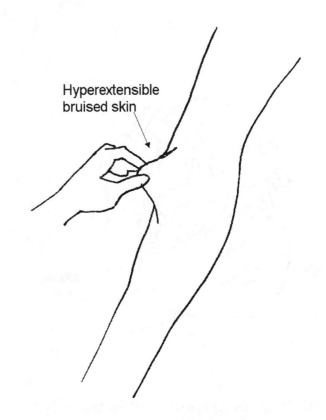

Hyperextensible bruised skin

D-309: Ehlers-Danlos syndrome

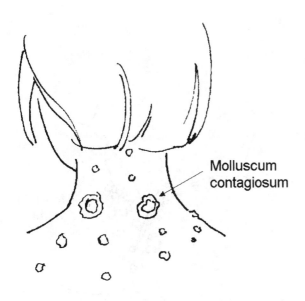

Molluscum contagiosum

D-310: Molluscum contagiosum

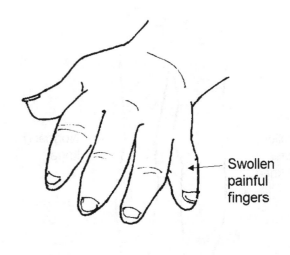

Swollen painful fingers

D-311: Dactylitis

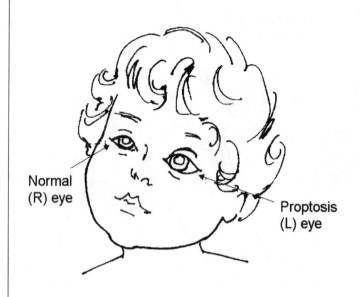

Normal
(R) eye

Proptosis
(L) eye

D-312: Proptosis (L) eye (Retroorbital mass)

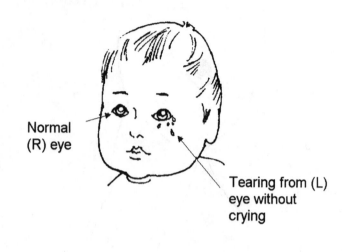

Normal
(R) eye

Tearing from (L)
eye without
crying

D-313: Nasolacrimal duct obstruction (L) side

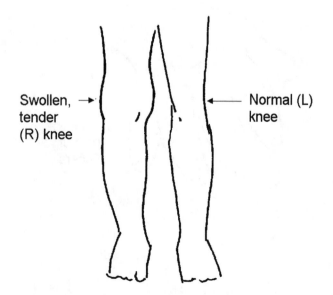

Swollen,
tender
(R) knee

Normal (L)
knee

D-314: Pyogenic arthritis (R) knee joint

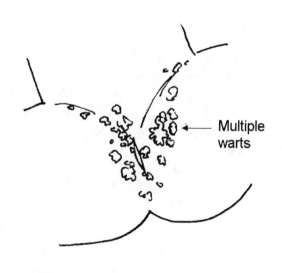

Multiple
warts

D-315: Genital warts (R/O sexual abuse)

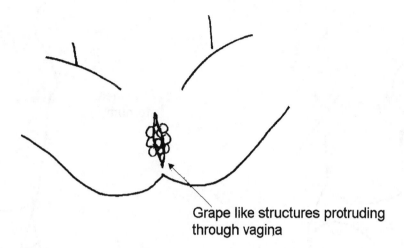

Grape like structures protruding through vagina

D-316: Vaginal adenocarcinoma (newborn)

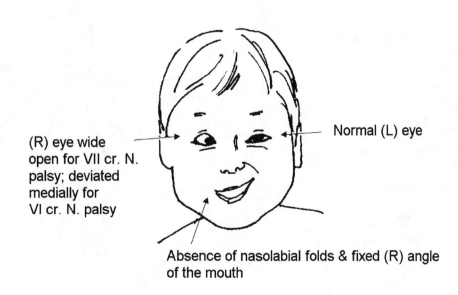

(R) eye wide open for VII cr. N. palsy; deviated medially for VI cr. N. palsy

Normal (L) eye

Absence of nasolabial folds & fixed (R) angle of the mouth

D-317: (R) Facial and VI cranial nerve paralysis

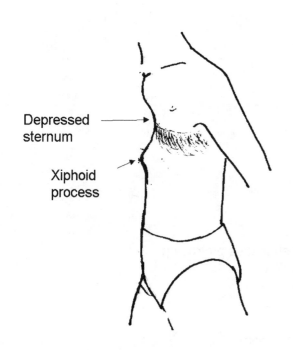

Depressed
sternum

Xiphoid
process

D-318: Pectus excavatum

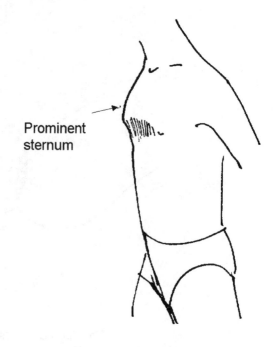

Prominent
sternum

D-319: Pigeon chest

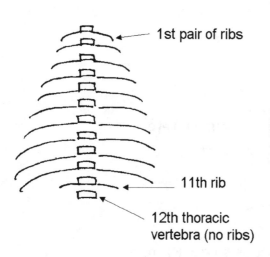

1st pair of ribs

11th rib

12th thoracic
vertebra (no ribs)

D-320: Absent 12th ribs (B/L) (X-ray)

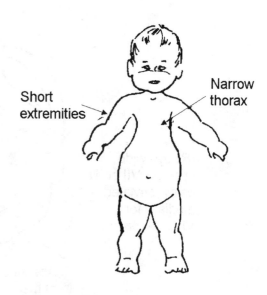

Short
extremities

Narrow
thorax

D-321: Asphyxiating thoracic dystrophy

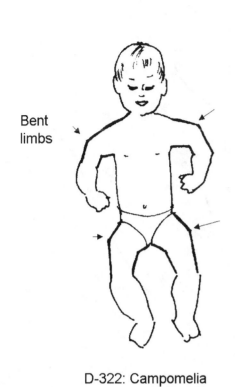

Bent limbs

D-322: Campomelia

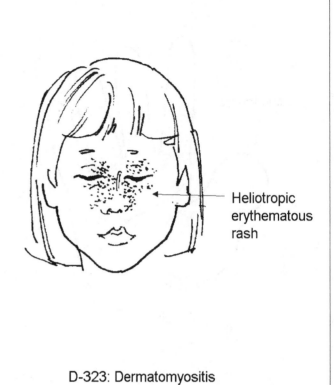

Heliotropic erythematous rash

D-323: Dermatomyositis

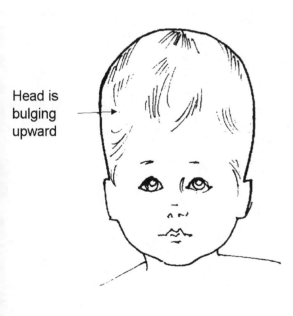

Head is bulging upward

D-324: Oxycephaly

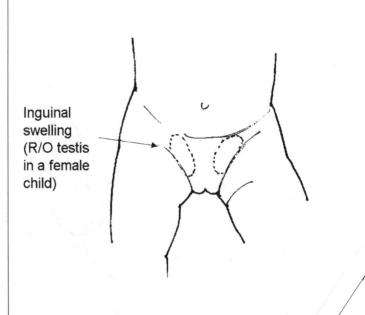

Inguinal swelling (R/O testis in a female child)

D-325: Testicular feminization synd

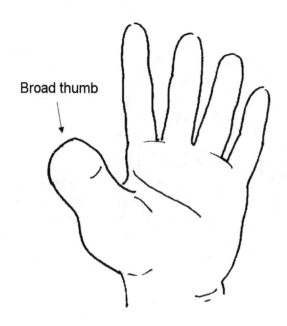

Broad thumb

D-326: Rubinstein Taybe syndrome

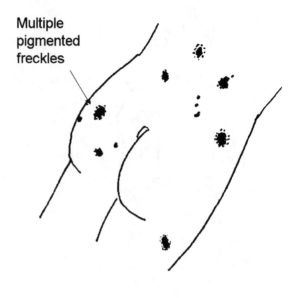

Multiple pigmented freckles

D-327: LEOPARD syndrome

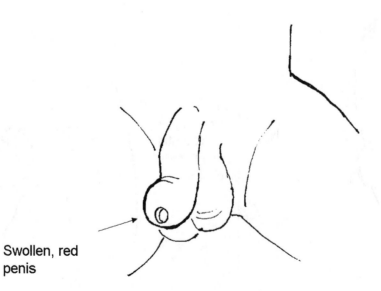

Swollen, red penis

D-328: Balanoposthitis

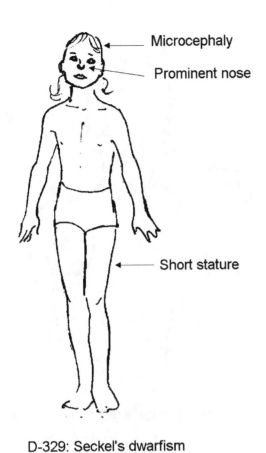

Microcephaly

Prominent nose

Short stature

D-329: Seckel's dwarfism

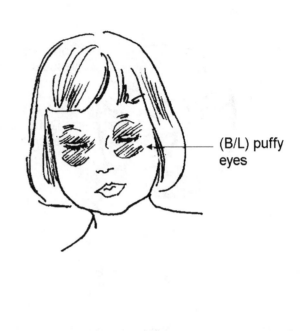

(B/L) puffy eyes

D-330: Angioneurotic edema

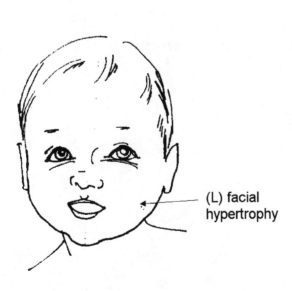

(L) facial hypertrophy

D-331: Hemifacial hypertrophy

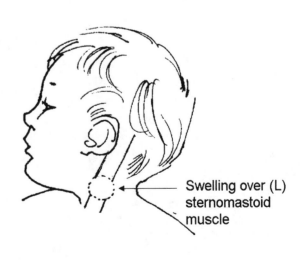

Swelling over (L) sternomastoid muscle

D-332: Sternomastoid (L) muscle hematoma/tumor

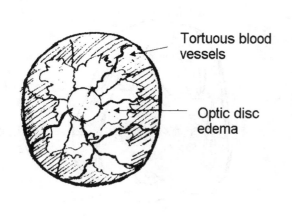

Tortuous blood
vessels

Optic disc
edema

D-333: Optic disc edema

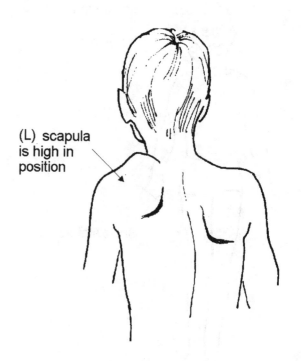

(L) scapula
is high in
position

D-334: Sprengel's deformity

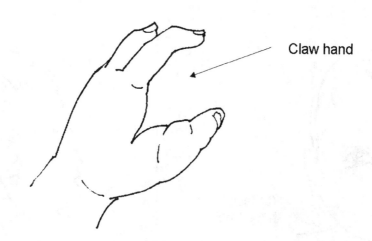

Claw hand

D-335: Claw hand deformity

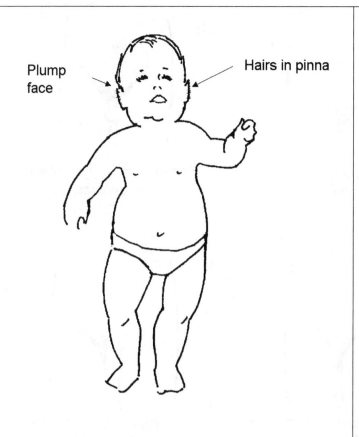

Plump face

Hairs in pinna

D-336: LGA newborn

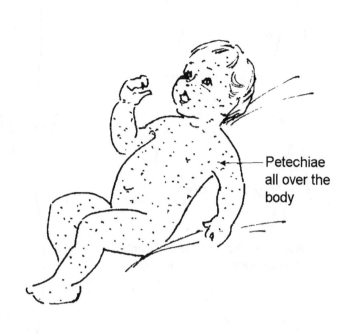

Petechiae all over the body

D-337: Skin petechiae (thrombocytopenia)

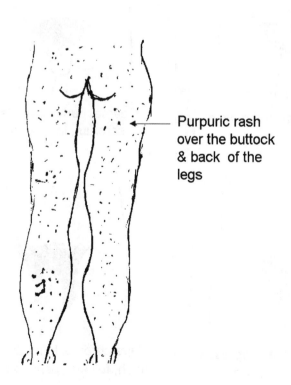

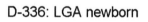

Purpuric rash over the buttock & back of the legs

D-338: Henoch-Schonlein purpura

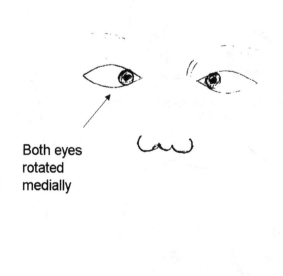

Both eyes rotated medially

D-339: (B/L) Lateral rectus paralysis

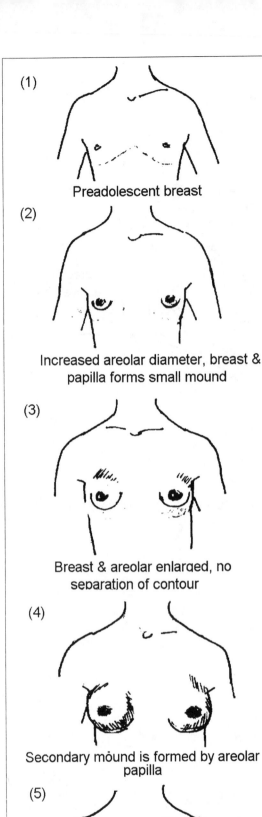

(1) Preadolescent breast

(2) Increased areolar diameter, breast & papilla forms small mound

(3) Breast & areolar enlarged, no separation of contour

(4) Secondary mound is formed by areolar papilla

(5) Prominent nipple

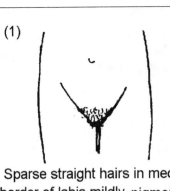

(1) Sparse straight hairs in medial border of labia mildly pigmented

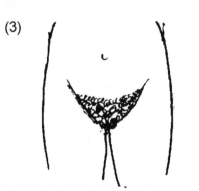

(2) Begining to curl with increasing amount & darkness

(3) Abundant, coarse and curly hairs

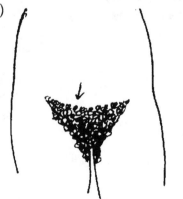

(4) Triangular shape and spread to medial side of thighs

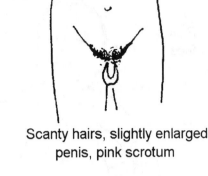

(1) Scanty hairs, slightly enlarged penis, pink scrotum

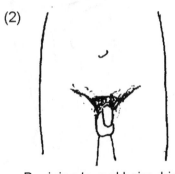

(2) Begining to curl hairs, bigger penis & scrotum

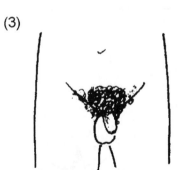

(3) Coarse, curly hairs; dark scrotum, large penis

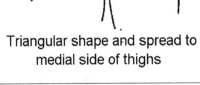

(4) Hairs spreads to medial side of thigh, full size penis & scrotum

D-340: Sex maturity rating (SMR) of female & male

INDEX